BLUEPRINTS
OBSTETRICS &
GYNECOLOGY

Fifth Edition

BLUEPRINTS
OBSTETRICS & GYNECOLOGY

Fifth Edition

Tamara Callahan, MD, MPP
Assistant Professor
Department of Obstetrics and Gynecology
Vanderbilt University Medical Center
Nashville, Tennessee

Aaron B. Caughey, MD, MPP, MPH, PhD
Associate Professor
Fellowship Program Director
Division of Maternal-Fetal Medicine
Department of Obstetrics, Gynecology, and Reproductive Sciences
University of California, San Francisco
San Francisco, California

Wolters Kluwer | Lippincott Williams & Wilkins
Health

Philadelphia · Baltimore · New York · London
Buenos Aires · Hong Kong · Sydney · Tokyo

Acquisitions Editor: Charley Mitchell
Sr. Managing Editor: Stacey Sebring
Editorial Assistant: Catherine Noonan
Marketing Manager: Jennifer Kuklinski
Production Editor: Kevin Johnson
Art Director: Doug Smock
Compositor: Maryland Composition/ASI

Library of Congress Cataloging-in-Publication Data

Blueprints obstetrics and gynecology / Tamara L. Callahan, Aaron B. Caughey. — 5th ed.
    p. ; cm. — (Blueprints)
  Rev. ed. of: Blueprints obstetrics & gynecology / Tamara L. Callahan, Aaron B. Caughey. 4th ed. c2007.
  Includes bibliographical references and index.
  ISBN 978-0-7817-8249-4
  1. Gynecology—Outlines, syllabi, etc. 2. Obstetrics—Outlines, syllabi, etc. 3. Gynecology—Examinations, questions, etc. 4. Obstetrics—Examinations, questions, etc. I. Callahan, Tamara L. II. Caughey, Aaron B. III. Callahan, Tamara L. Blueprints obstetrics & gynecology. IV. Series.
  [DNLM: 1. Pregnancy Complications—Examination Questions. 2. Genital Diseases, Female—Examination Questions. WQ 18.2 B6585 2009]
  RG112.C35 2009
  618.0076—dc22

        2008024493

DISCLAIMER

Contents

Contributors

Contributors to the 5th Edition
Marisa R. Adelman, MD
Stephanie Beall, MD
Lynne A. Black
Daniel H. Biller, MD
Nicole S. Carroll, MD
Michael E. Cole, MD
Nari Heshmati, MD
Celeste O. Hemingway, MD
Beth Colvin Huff, MSN, NP
Lucy Koroma, MSN, WHNP
Christopher M. Sizemore, DO
Merielle M. Stephens, MD
Susan H. Tran, MD
Sarah E. Little, MD
Jin Chang, DO
Brian L. Shaffer, MD
Yvonne W. Cheng, MD, MPH

Contributors to Previous Editions
Annette Chen, MD
Bruce B. Feinberg, MD
Linda J. Heffner, MD, PhD
Sara Newmann, MD, MPH
Susan H. Tran, MD
Jing Wang, MD

Preface

In 1997, the first five books in the Blueprints series were published as board review for medical students, interns, and residents who wanted high-yield, accurate clinical content for USMLE Steps 2 and 3. Twelve years later, we are proud to report that the original books and the entire Blueprints brand of review materials have far exceeded our expectations.

The feedback we've received from our readers has been tremendously helpful and pivotal in deciding what direction the fifth edition of the core books would take. To ensure that the fifth edition of the series continues to provide the content and approach that made the original Blueprints a success; we have expanded the text to include the most up-to-date topics and evidence-based research and therapies. Information is provided on the latest changes in the management of cervical dysplasia, preeclampsia, cervical insufficiency, and preterm labor. The newest and future techniques in contraception and sterilization and hormone replacement therapies are covered, as are contemporary treatment options for uterine fibroids and invasive breast cancer.

The succinct and telegraphic use of tables and figures was highly acclaimed by our readers, so we have redoubled our efforts to expand their usefulness by adding a significant amount of updated and improved artwork including a new section of color plates. In each case, we have tried to include only the most helpful and clear tables and figures to maximize the reader's ability to understand and remember the material. Our readers also asked for an enhanced art program, so a tri-color system is being used in this edition to increase the usefulness of the figures and tables.

We have likewise changed our bibliography to include updated evidence-based articles as well as references to classic articles and textbooks in both obstetrics and gynecology. These references are now provided at the end of the book and are further expanded in the on-line references. It was also suggested that the review questions should reflect the current format of the boards. We are particularly proud to include new and revised board-format questions in this edition with full explanations of both correct and incorrect options provided in the answers.

What we've also learned from our readers is that Blueprints is more than just board review for USMLE Steps 2 and 3. Students use the books during their clerkship rotations, subinternships, and as a quick refresher while rotating on various services in early residency. Residents studying for USMLE Step 3 often use the books for reviewing areas that were not their specialty. Students in physician assistant, nurse practitioner, and osteopath programs use Blueprints either as a companion or in lieu of review materials written specifically for their areas.

When we first wrote the book, we had just completed medical school and started residency training. Thus, we hope this new edition brings both that original viewpoint as well as our clinical experience garnered over the past 12 years. However you choose to use Blueprints, we hope that you find the books in the series informative and useful.

Tamara L. Callahan, MD, MPP, and Aaron B. Caughey, MD, MPP, MPH, PhD

Acknowledgments

I would like to express my sincere and deep appreciation to my coauthor, Dr. Caughey, and to the OB/Gyn residents at Harvard and Vanderbilt who gave liberally of their time and expertise to make this book something of which we can all be proud. Without the extraordinary talent and commitment of these physicians, this project would not have been possible. This accomplishment is also credited in no small part to Michael, Mom, Dad, Jai, Tonya, Brian, Carol, Oneeka, and E—the incredible core of family and friends who lovingly and selflessly shepherded me through the most joyous and darkest times in my life. And to my angels, Connor and Jaela, being your mother has been an indescribable honor and an immeasurable joy—a blessing that I try to earn each and every day. I would also like to acknowledge my mentors, Dr. William F. Crowley, Jr., Dr. Janet Hall, Dr. Linda J. Heffner, Dr. Nancy Chescheir, Dr. Robert Barbieri, and Dr. Nancy E. Oriol, whose strength, insight, leadership, and drive are exemplary of what it means to be an active contributor to academic medicine and women's health. Lastly, I'd like to thank the many medical students and residents who have shared their input and enthusiasm with us along this exciting journey. Their support has been paramount to the success of this project and to our quest to make this book the very best it can be. It has truly been a privilege to be a small part of their never-ending learning experience.

Tamara L. Callahan, MD, MPP

I would like to acknowledge and extend my thanks to everyone involved in the fifth edition of our book, most importantly my coauthor, Dr. Callahan, as well as all of those who contributed to the first four editions including Drs. Newmann, Tran, Chen, Feinberg, Wang, and Heffner, and the staff at both Blackwell and LWW. I would also like to thank my colleagues and mentors for the supportive environment in which I work including the residents and faculty in the department of Obstetrics and Gynecology at UCSF, Drs. Washington, Norton, Kuppermann, Ames-Castro, Repke, Blatman, and Norwitz as well as the students, staff, and faculty at UC Berkeley's Health Services and Policy Analysis program and the Department of Economics. I would also like to acknowledge the suggestions and critiques from medical students around the country and particularly at Harvard and UCSF who keep pushing us to produce better editions of this work. Finally, to my family, Bill, Carol, Ethan, Becca, Owen, Samara, Stan, Adeline, Big & Mugsy, Nicole, Aidan, Ashby, our little Beignet, and of course, Susan, whose continued patience and support during all of my projects keeps me on task and productive.

Aaron B. Caughey, MD, MPP, MPH, PhD

Abbreviations

3β-HSD	3β-hydroxysteroid dehydrogenase	CKC	cold-knife conization (biopsy)
5-FU	5-fluorouracil	CMV	cytomegalovirus
17α-OHP	17α-hydroxyprogesterone	CNS	central nervous system
ABG	arterial blood gas	CPD	cephalopelvic disproportion
ACTH	adrenocorticotropic hormone	CPK	creatine phosphokinase
AD	autosomal dominant	CRS	congenital rubella syndrome
ADH	antidiuretic hormone	CSF	cerebrospinal fluid
AED	antiepileptic drug	CT	computed tomography (CAT scan)
AFE	amniotic fluid embolus	CVA	cerebrovascular accident
AFI	amniotic fluid index	CVAT	costovertebral angle tenderness
AFLP	acute fatty liver of pregnancy	CVD	collagen vascular disorders
AFP	α-fetoprotein	CVS	chorionic villus sampling
AGUS	atypical glandular cells of undetermined significance	CXR	chest x-ray
		DA	developmental age
AIDS	acquired immunodeficiency syndrome	D&C	dilation and curettage
ALT	alanine transaminase	D&E	dilation and evacuation
AMA	advanced maternal age	DCIS	ductal carcinoma in situ
APA	antiphospholipid antibody	DES	diethylstilbestrol
AR	autosomal recessive	DEXA	dual-energy x-ray absorptiometry
ARDS	adult respiratory distress syndrome	DHEA	dehydroepiandrosterone
AROM	artificial rupture of membranes	DHEAS	dehydroepiandrosterone sulfate
ART	assisted reproductive technology	DHT	dihydrotestosterone
ASC	atypical squamous cells	DIC	disseminated intravascular coagulation
ASC-H	atypical squamous cells cannot exclude high-grade squamous intraepithelial lesion	DMPA	depot medroxyprogesterone acetate (Depo-Provera)
		DTRs	deep tendon reflexes
ASC-US	atypical squamous cells of undetermined significance	DUB	dysfunctional uterine bleeding
		DVT	deep venous thrombosis
AST	aspartate transaminase	ECG	electrocardiogram
AV	arteriovenous	EDC	estimated date of confinement
AZT	zidovudine	EDD	estimated date of delivery
β-hCG	beta human chorionic gonadotropin	EFW	estimated fetal weight
BID	twice a day	EIF	echogenic intracardiac focus
BP	blood pressure	ELISA	enzyme-linked immunosorbent assay
BPP	biophysical profile	EMB	endometrial biopsy
BUN	blood urea nitrogen	EMG	electromyography
BV	bacterial vaginosis	ERT	estrogen replacement therapy
CAH	congenital adrenal hyperplasia	ESR	erythrocyte sedimentation rate
CBC	complete blood count	FAS	fetal alcohol syndrome
CCCT	clomiphene citrate challenge test	FH	fetal heart
CF	cystic fibrosis	FHR	fetal heart rate
CHF	congestive heart failure	FIGO	International Federation of Gynecology and Obstetrics
CIN	cervical intraepithelial neoplasia		

FIRS	fetal immune response syndrome	IUI	intrauterine insemination
FISH	fluorescent in situ hybridization	IUP	intrauterine pregnancy
FNA	fine-needle aspiration	IUPC	intrauterine pressure catheter
FSE	fetal scalp electrode	IUT	intrauterine transfusion
FSH	follicle-stimulating hormone	IVC	inferior vena cava
FTAABS	fluorescent treponemal antibody absorption	IVF	in vitro fertilization
		IVP	intravenous pyelogram
FTP	failure to progress	JVP	jugular venous pressure
G	gravidity	KB	Kleihauer-Betke test
GA	gestational age	KOH	potassium hydroxide
GBS	group B streptococcus	KUB	kidneys/ureter/bladder (x-ray)
GDM	gestational diabetes mellitus	LBW	low birth weight
GFR	glomerular filtration rate	LCHAD	long-chain hydroxyacyl-CoA dehydrogenase
GH	gestational hypertension		
GI	gastrointestinal	LCIS	lobular carcinoma in situ
GIFT	gamete intrafallopian transfer	LDH	lactate dehydrogenase
GLT	glucose loading test	LDL	low-density lipoprotein
GnRH	gonadotropin-releasing hormone	LEEP	loop electrosurgical excision procedure
GSI	genuine stress incontinence	LFT	liver function test
GTD	gestational trophoblastic disease	LGA	large for gestational age
GTT	glucose tolerance test	LGV	lymphogranuloma venereum
GU	genitourinary	LIQ	lower inner quadrant
HAART	highly active antiretroviral therapy	LH	luteinizing hormone
Hb	hemoglobin	Lletz	large loop excision of the transformation zone
HbH	hemoglobin H disease		
hCG	human chorionic gonadotropin	LMP	last menstrual period
hCS	human chorionic somatomammotropin	LOQ	lower outer quadrant
		LOT	left occiput transverse
Hct	hematocrit	LSIL	low-grade squamous intraepithelial lesion
HDL	high-density lipoprotein		
HELLP	hemolysis, elevated liver enzymes, low platelets	LTL	laparoscopic tubal ligation
		Lytes	electrolytes
HIV	human immunodeficiency virus	MAO	monoamine oxidase
HLA	human leukocyte antigen	MESA	microsurgical epididymal sperm aspiration
hMG	human menopausal gonadotropin		
HPI	history of present illness	MHATP	microhemagglutination assay for antibodies to T. pallidum
HPL	human placental lactogen		
HPV	human papillomavirus	MI	myocardial infarction
HR	heart rate	MIF	müllerian inhibiting factor
HRT	hormone replacement therapy	MLK	myosin light-chain kinase
HSG	hysterosalpingogram	MRI	magnetic resonance imaging
HSIL	high-grade squamous intraepithelial lesion	MRKH	Mayer-Rokitansky-Kuster-Hauser (syndrome)
HSV	herpes simplex virus	MSAFP	maternal serum α-fetoprotein
I&D	incision and drainage	MTHFR	methyl tetrahydrofolate reductase
ICSI	intracytoplasmic sperm injection	NPO	nil per os (nothing by mouth)
ID/CC	identification and chief complaint	NPV	negative predictive value
Ig	immunoglobulin	NRFT	nonreassuring fetal testing
IM	intramuscular	NSAID	nonsteroidal anti-inflammatory drug
INH	isoniazid	NST	nonstress test
INR	International Normalized Ratio	NSVD	normal spontaneous vaginal delivery
ITP	idiopathic thrombocytopenia purpura	NT	nuchal translucency
IUD	intrauterine device	NTD	neural tube defect
IUFD	intrauterine fetal demise or death	OA	occiput anterior
IUGR	intrauterine growth restricted	OCP	oral contraceptive pill

OCT	oxytocin challenge test	SNRIs	serotonin-norepinephrine reuptake inhibitor
OI	ovulation induction	SPT	septic pelvic thrombophlebitis
OP	occiput posterior	SROM	spontaneous rupture of membranes
OT	occiput transverse	SSRIs	selective serotonin reuptake inhibitors
OTC	over-the-counter	STD	sexually transmitted disease
P	parity	STI	sexually transmitted infection
PBS	peripheral blood smear	SUI	stress urinary incontinence
PCOD	polycystic ovarian disease	SVT	superficial vein thrombophlebitis
PCOS	polycystic ovarian syndrome	SVT	supraventricular tachycardia
PCR	polymerase chain reaction	TAB	therapeutic abortion
PDA	patent ductus arteriosus	TAC	transabdominal cerclage
PE	physical exam	TAHBSO	total abdominal hysterectomy and bilateral salpingo-oophorectomy
PE	pulmonary embolus		
PET	preeclampsia/toxemia	TBG	thyroid binding globulin
PFTs	pulmonary function tests	TENS	transcutaneous electrical nerve stimulation
PID	pelvic inflammatory disease		
PIH	pregnancy-induced hypertension	TFTs	thyroid function tests
PMDD	premenstrual dysphoric disorder	TIBC	total iron-binding capacity
PMN	polymorphonuclear leukocyte	TLC	total lung capacity
PMOF	premature ovarian failure	TNM	tumor/node/metastasis
PMS	premenstrual syndrome	TOA	tubo-ovarian abscess
PO	per os (by mouth)	TOLAC	trial of labor after cesarean
POCs	products of conception	TOV	transposition of the vessels
POP	progesterone-only contraceptive pills	tPA	tissue plasminogen activator
Pop-Q	pelvic organ prolapse quantification system	TPAL	term, preterm, aborted, living
		TRH	thyrotropin-releasing hormone
PPCM	peripartum cardiomyopathy	TSE	testicular sperm extraction
PPD	purified protein derivative	TSH	thyroid-stimulating hormone
PPROM	preterm premature rupture of membranes	TSI	thyroid-stimulating immunoglobulins
		TSS	toxic shock syndrome
PPS	postpartum sterilization	TSST	toxic shock syndrome toxin
PPV	positive predictive value	TTTS	twin-to-twin transfusion syndrome
PROM	premature rupture of membranes	UA	urinalysis
PSTT	placental site trophoblastic tumor	UAE	uterine artery embolization
PT	prothrombin time	UG	urogenital
PTL	preterm labor	UIQ	upper inner quadrant
PTT	partial thromboplastin time	UOQ	upper outer quadrant
PTU	propylthiouracil	UPI	uteroplacental insufficiency
PUBS	percutaneous umbilical blood sampling	US	ultrasound
PUS	pelvic ultrasound	UTI	urinary tract infection
QD	each day	V/Q	ventilation/perfusion ratio
QID	four times a day	VAIN	vaginal intraepithelial neoplasia
RBC	red blood cell	VBAC	vaginal birth after cesarean
RDS	respiratory distress syndrome	VD	volume of distribution
ROM	rupture of membranes	VDRL	Venereal Disease Research Laboratory
ROT	right occiput transverse	VIN	vulvar intraepithelial neoplasia
RPR	rapid plasma reagin	VLDL	very low density lipoprotein
RR	respiratory rate	VS	vital signs
SAB	spontaneous abortion	VSD	ventricular septal defect
SCC	squamous cell carcinoma	VZIG	varicella zoster immune globulin
SERM	selective estrogen receptor modulators	VZV	varicella zoster virus
		WBC	white blood cell
SGA	small for gestational age	XAFP	expanded maternal serum alpha feto-protein (test)
SHBG	sex hormone binding globulin		
SIDS	sudden infant death syndrome		
SLE	systemic lupus erythematosus	XR	x-ray

Part 1

Obstetrics

Pregnancy and Prenatal Care

PREGNANCY

Pregnancy is the state of having products of conception implanted normally or abnormally in the uterus or occasionally elsewhere. Pregnancy is terminated by spontaneous or elective abortion or delivery. A myriad of physiologic changes occur in a pregnant woman, which affect every organ system.

DIAGNOSIS

In a patient who has regular menstrual cycles and is sexually active, a period delayed by more than a few days to a week is suggestive of pregnancy. Even at this early stage, patients may exhibit signs and symptoms of pregnancy. On physical examination, a variety of findings indicate pregnancy (Table 1-1).

Many over-the-counter (OTC) urine pregnancy tests have a high sensitivity and will be positive around the time of the missed menstrual cycle. These urine tests and the hospital laboratory serum assays test for the beta subunit of human chorionic gonadotropin (β-hCG). This hormone produced by the placenta will rise to a peak of 100,000 mIU/mL by 10 weeks of gestation, decrease throughout the second trimester, and then level off at approximately 20,000 to 30,000 mIU/mL in the third trimester.

A viable pregnancy can be confirmed by ultrasound, which may show the gestational sac as early as 5 weeks on a transvaginal ultrasound, or at a β-hCG of 1,500 to 2,000 mIU/mL, and the fetal heart as soon as 6 weeks, or a β-hCG of 5,000 to 6,000 mIU/mL.

TERMS AND DEFINITIONS

From the time of fertilization until the pregnancy is 8 weeks along (10 weeks gestational age [GA]), the conceptus is called an **embryo**. After 8 weeks until the time of birth, it is designated a **fetus**. The term **infant** is used for the period between delivery and 1 year of age. Pregnancy is divided into trimesters. The **first trimester** lasts until 12 weeks but is also defined as up to 14 weeks GA, the **second trimester** from 12 to 14 until 24 to 28 weeks GA, and the **third trimester** from 24 to 28 weeks until delivery. An infant delivered prior to 24 weeks is considered to be **previable**, from 24 to 37 weeks is considered **preterm**, and from 37 to 42 weeks is considered **term**. A pregnancy carried beyond 42 weeks is considered **postterm**.

Gravidity (G) refers to the number of times a woman has been pregnant, and **parity** (P) refers to the number of pregnancies that led to a birth at or beyond 20 weeks GA or of an infant weighing more than 500 g. For example, a woman who has given birth to one set of twins would be a G1 P1, as a multiple gestation is considered as just one pregnancy. A more specific designation of pregnancy outcomes divides parity into **term** and **preterm** deliveries and also adds the number of **abortuses** and number of **living** children. This is known as the TPAL designation. Abortuses include all pregnancy losses prior to 20 weeks, both therapeutic and spontaneous, as well as ectopic pregnancies. For example, a woman who has given birth to one set of preterm twins, one term infant, and with two miscarriages would be a G4 P1-1-2-3.

■ TABLE 1-1 Signs and Symptoms of Pregnancy

Signs
Bluish discoloration of vagina and cervix (Chadwick sign)
Softening and cyanosis of the cervix at or after 4 weeks (Goodell sign)
Softening of the uterus after 6 weeks (Ladin sign)
Breast swelling and tenderness
Development of the linea nigra from umbilicus to pubis
Telangiectasias
Palmar erythema
Symptoms
Amenorrhea
Nausea and vomiting
Breast pain
Quickening—fetal movement

The prefixes nulli-, primi-, and multi- are used with respect to gravidity and parity to refer to having 0, 1, or more than 1, respectively. For example, a woman who has been pregnant twice, one ectopic pregnancy and one full term birth, would be multigravidous and primiparous. Unfortunately, this terminology often gets misused with individuals referring to women with a first pregnancy as primiparous, rather than nulliparous. Obstetricians also utilize the term "grand multip," which refers to a woman whose parity is greater than or equal to 5.

DATING OF PREGNANCY

The GA of a fetus is the age in weeks and days measured from the last menstrual period (LMP). **Developmental age** (DA) or conceptional age or embryonic age is the number of weeks and days since fertilization. Because fertilization usually occurs about 14 days after the first day of the prior menstrual period, the GA is usually 2 weeks more than the DA.

Classically, **Nägele's rule** for calculating the **estimated date of confinement** (EDC), or estimated date of delivery (EDD), is to subtract 3 months from the LMP and add 7 days. Thus, a pregnancy with an LMP of 8/05/08 would have an EDC of 5/12/09. Exact

dating uses an EDC calculated as 280 days after a certain LMP. If the date of ovulation is known, as in assisted reproductive technology (ART), the EDC can be calculated by adding 266 days. Pregnancy dating can be confirmed and should be consistent with the examination of the uterine size at the first prenatal appointment.

With an uncertain LMP, ultrasound is often used to determine the EDC. Ultrasound has a level of uncertainty that increases during the pregnancy but it is rarely off by more than 7% to 8% at any GA. A safe rule of thumb is that the ultrasound should not differ from LMP dating by more than 1 week in the first trimester, 2 weeks in the second trimester, and 3 weeks in the third trimester. The dating done with crown-rump length in the first half of the first trimester is probably even more accurate, to within 3 to 5 days.

Other measures used to estimate gestational age include pregnancy landmarks such as auscultation of the fetal heart (FH) at 20 weeks by nonelectronic fetoscopy or at 10 weeks by Doppler ultrasound, as well as maternal awareness of fetal movement or "quickening," which occurs between 16 and 20 weeks.

Because ultrasound dating of pregnancy only decreases in accuracy as the pregnancy progresses, determining and confirming pregnancy dating at the first interaction between a pregnant women and the healthcare system is imperative. A woman who presents to the emergency department may not return for prenatal care, so dating confirmation should occur at that visit. Pregnancy dating is particularly important because a number of decisions regarding care are based on accurate dating. One such decision is whether to resuscitate a newborn at the threshold of viability, which may be at 23 or 24 weeks of gestation depending on the institution. Another is the induction of labor at 41 weeks of gestation. Since 5% to 15% of women may be oligo-ovulatory, they ovulate beyond the usual 14th day of the cycle. Thus, their LMP dating may overdiagnose a prolonged (≥41 weeks' gestation) or postterm pregnancy (≥42 weeks' gestation). Thus, early verification or correction of dating can correct such misdating.

PHYSIOLOGY OF PREGNANCY

Cardiovascular

During pregnancy, **cardiac output** increases by 30% to 50%. Most increases occur during the first trimester, with the maximum being reached between 20 and 24 weeks' gestation and maintained until delivery. The increase in cardiac output is first due to an increase in stroke volume then is maintained by an increase in heart rate as stroke volume decreases to near prepregnancy levels by the end of the third trimester. **Systemic vascular resistance** decreases during pregnancy, resulting in a fall in arterial blood pressure. This decrease is most likely due to the elevated progesterone leading to smooth muscle relaxation. There is a decrease in systolic blood pressure of 5 to 10 mm Hg and in diastolic blood pressure of 10 to 15 mm Hg that nadirs at week 24. Between 24 weeks' gestation and term, blood pressure slowly returns to prepregnancy levels but should never exceed them.

Pulmonary

There is an increase of 30% to 40% in tidal volume (V_T) during pregnancy (Fig. 1-1) despite the fact that the total lung capacity is decreased by 5% due to the elevation of the diaphragm. This increase in V_T decreases the expiratory reserve volume by about 20%. The increase in V_T with a constant respiratory rate leads to an increase in minute ventilation of 30% to 40%, which in turn leads to an increase in alveolar (PAo_2) and arterial (Pao_2) Po_2 levels and a decrease in $PAco_2$ and $Paco_2$ levels.

$Paco_2$ decreases to approximately 30 mm Hg by 20 weeks' gestation from 40 mm Hg prepregnancy. This change leads to an increased CO_2 gradient between mother and fetus and is likely caused by elevated progesterone levels that either increase the respiratory system's responsiveness to CO_2 or act as a primary stimulant. This gradient facilitates oxygen delivery to the fetus and carbon dioxide removal from the fetus. Dyspnea of pregnancy occurs in 60% to 70% of patients. This is possibly secondary to decreased $Paco_2$ levels, increased V_T, or decreased total lung capacity (TLC).

Gastrointestinal

Nausea and vomiting occur in more than 70% of pregnancies. This has been termed "**morning sickness**" even though it can occur anytime throughout the day. These symptoms have been attributed to the elevation in estrogen, progesterone, and hCG. It may also be due to hypoglycemia and can be treated with frequent snacking. The nausea and vomiting typically resolve by 14 to 16 weeks' gestation. **Hyperemesis gravidarum** refers to a severe form of morning sickness in which women lose greater than 5% of their prepregnancy weight and go into ketosis.

During pregnancy, the stomach has prolonged gastric emptying times, and the gastroesophageal sphincter has decreased tone. Together, these changes lead to reflux and possibly combine with decreased esophageal tone to cause ptyalism, or spitting, during pregnancy. The large bowel also has decreased motility, which leads to increased water absorption and constipation.

Renal

The kidneys increase in size and the ureters dilate during pregnancy, which may lead to increased rates of pyelonephritis. The glomerular filtration rate (GFR) increases by 50% early in pregnancy and is maintained until delivery. As a result of increased

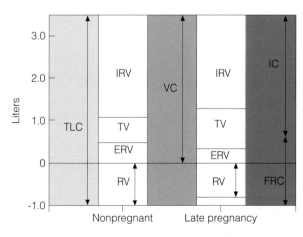

TLC–total lung capacity
VC–vital capacity
IC–inspiratory capacity
FRC–functional residual capacity
IRV–inspiratory reserve volume
TV–tidal volume
ERV–expiratory reserve
RV–residual volume

Figure 1-1 • Lung volumes in nonpregnant and pregnant women.

GFR, blood urea nitrogen and creatinine decrease by about 25%. An increase in the renin-angiotensin system leads to increased levels of aldosterone, which results in increased sodium resorption. However, plasma levels of sodium do not increase because of the simultaneous increase in GFR.

Hematology

Although the plasma volume increases by 50% in pregnancy, the red blood cell volume increases by only 20% to 30%, which leads to a decrease in the hematocrit, or dilutional anemia. The white blood cell (WBC) count increases during pregnancy to a mean of 10.5 million/mL with a range of 6 to 16 million. During labor, stress may cause the WBC count to rise to over 20 million/mL. There is a slight decrease in the concentration of platelets, probably secondary to increased plasma volume and an increase in peripheral destruction. Although 7% to 8% of patients' platelets may be between 100 and 150 million/mL, a drop in the platelet count below 100 million/mL or over a short time period is not normal and should be investigated promptly.

Pregnancy is considered to be a hypercoagulable state, and the number of thromboembolic events increases. There are elevations in the levels of fibrinogen and factors VII–X. However, the actual clotting and bleeding times do not change. The increased rate of thromboembolic events in pregnancy may also be secondary to the other elements of Virchow triad, an increase in venous stasis and vessel endothelial damage.

Endocrine

Pregnancy is a hyperestrogenic state. The increased estrogen is produced primarily by the placenta, with the ovaries contributing to a lesser degree. Unlike estrogen production in the ovaries, where estrogen precursors are produced in ovarian theca cells and transferred to the ovarian granulosa cells, estrogen in the placenta is derived from circulating plasma-borne precursors produced by the maternal adrenal glands. Fetal well-being has been correlated with maternal serum estrogen levels with low estrogen levels being associated with conditions such as fetal death and anencephaly.

The hormone hCG is composed of two dissimilar alpha and beta subunits. The alpha subunit of hCG is identical to the alpha subunits of luteinizing hormone (LH), follicle-stimulating hormone (FSH), and thyroid-stimulating hormone (TSH), whereas the beta subunits differ. Levels of hCG double approximately every 48 hours during early pregnancy, reaching a peak at approximately 10 to 12 weeks, and thereafter declining to reach a steady state after week 15.

The placenta produces hCG, which acts to maintain the corpus luteum in early pregnancy. The corpus luteum produces progesterone, which maintains the endometrium. Eventually the placenta takes over progesterone production and the corpus luteum degrades into the corpus albicans. Progesterone levels increase over the course of pregnancy. Progesterone causes relaxation of smooth muscle, which has multiple effects on the gastrointestinal, cardiovascular, and genitourinary systems. **Human placental lactogen (hPL)** is produced in the placenta and is important for ensuring a constant nutrient supply to the fetus. hPL, also known as human chorionic somatomammotropin (hCS), causes lipolysis with a concomitant increase in circulating free fatty acids. hPL also acts as an insulin antagonist, along with various other placental hormones, thereby having a diabetogenic effect. This leads to increased levels of insulin and protein synthesis. Levels of **prolactin** are markedly increased during pregnancy. These levels decrease after delivery but later increase in response to suckling.

There are two major changes in thyroid hormones during pregnancy. First, estrogen stimulates thyroid binding globulin (TBG) leading to an elevation in total T3 and T4 but free T3 and T4 remain relatively constant. Second, hCG has a weak stimulating effect on the thyroid, likely as its alpha subgroup is similar to TSH. This leads to a slight increase in T3 and T4 and a slight decrease in TSH early in pregnancy. Overall, however, pregnancy is considered a euthyroid state.

Musculoskeletal and Dermatologic

The obvious change in the center of gravity during pregnancy can lead to a shift in posture and lower back strain. Numerous changes in the skin occur during pregnancy, including spider angiomata and palmar erythema secondary to increased estrogen levels and hyperpigmentation of the nipples, umbilicus, abdominal midline (the **linea nigra**), perineum, and face (**melasma** or **chloasma**) secondary to increased levels of melanocyte-stimulating hormone and the steroid hormones.

Nutrition

Nutritional requirements increase during pregnancy and breastfeeding. The average woman requires 2,000 to 2,500 kcal/day. The caloric requirement is increased by 300 kcal/day during pregnancy and by 500 kcal/day when breastfeeding. Most patients should gain between 20 and 30 pounds during pregnancy. Overweight women are advised to gain less, between 15 and 25 pounds; underweight women are advised to gain more, 28 to 40 pounds.

In addition to the increased caloric requirements, there are increased nutritional requirements for protein, iron, folate, calcium, and other vitamins and minerals. The protein requirement increases from 60 g/day to 70 or 75 g/day. Recommended calcium intake is 1.5 g/day. Many patients develop iron deficiency anemia because of the increased demand on hematopoiesis both by the mother and the fetus. Folate requirements increase from 0.4 to 0.8 mg/day and are important in preventing neural tube defects.

All patients are advised to take prenatal vitamins during pregnancy. These are designed to compensate for the increased nutritional demands of pregnancy. Furthermore, any patient whose hematocrit falls during pregnancy is advised to increase iron intake with oral supplementation (Table 1-2).

■ **TABLE 1-2** Recommended Daily Dietary Allowances for Nonpregnant, Pregnant, and Lactating Women

	Nonpregnant Women by Age					Pregnant Women	Lactating Women
	11 to 14	15 to 18	19 to 22	23 to 50	51+		
Energy (kcal)	2,400	2,100	2,100	2,000	1,800	+300	+500
Protein (g)	44	48	46	46	46	+30	+20
Fat-soluble vitamins	800	800	800	800	800	1,000	1,200
Vitamin A activity (RE) (IU)	4,000	4,000	4,000	4,000	4,000	5,000	6,000
Vitamin D (IU)	400	400	400	—	—	400	400
Vitamin E activity (IU)	12	12	12	12	12	15	15
Water-soluble vitamins							
Ascorbic acid (mg)	45	45	45	45	45	60	80
Folacin (μg)	400	400	400	400	400	800	600
Niacin (mg)	16	14	14	13	12	+2	+4
Riboflavin (mg)	1.3	1.4	1.4	1.2	1.1	+0.3	+0.5
Thiamin (mg)	1.2	1.1	1.1	1	1	+0.3	+0.3
Vitamin B_6 (mg)	1.6	2	2	2	2	2.5	2.5
Vitamin B_{12} (μg)	3	3	3	3	3	4	4
Minerals							
Calcium (mg)	1,200	1,200	800	800	800	1,200	1,200
Iodine (μg)	115	115	100	100	80	125	150
Iron (mg)	18	18	18	18	10	+18	18
Magnesium (mg)	300	300	300	300	300	450	450
Phosphorus (mg)	1,200	1,200	800	800	800	1,200	1,200
Zinc (mg)	15	15	15	15	15	20	25

From Gabbe SG, Niebyl JR, Simpsen JL. *Obstetrics: Normal and Problem Pregnancies*, 4th ed. New York: Churchill Livingstone, 2002:196. IU, International Unit.

PRENATAL CARE

Prenatal visits are designed to screen for various complications of pregnancy and to educate the patient. They include a series of outpatient office visits that involve routine physical examinations and various screening tests that occur at different points in the prenatal care. Important issues of prenatal care include initial patient evaluation, routine patient evaluation, nutrition, disease states during the pregnancy, and preparing for the delivery.

INITIAL VISIT

This is often the longest of the prenatal visits because it involves obtaining a complete history and performing a physical as well as a battery of initial laboratory tests. It should occur early in the first trimester, between 6 and 10 weeks, although occasionally patients will not present for their initial prenatal visit until later in their pregnancy.

History

The patient's history includes the present pregnancy, the last menstrual period, and symptoms during the pregnancy. After this, an obstetric history of prior pregnancies including date, outcome (e.g., SAB [spontaneous abortion], TAB [therapeutic abortion], ectopic pregnancy, term delivery), mode of delivery, length of time in labor and second stage, birth weight, and any complications. Finally, a complete medical, surgical, family, and social history should be obtained.

Physical Examination

A complete physical examination is performed, paying particular attention to the patient's prior medical and surgical history. The pelvic examination includes a Pap smear, unless one has been done in the past 6 months, and cultures for gonorrhea and chlamydia. On bimanual examination, the size of the uterus should be consistent with the gestational age from the LMP. If a woman is unsure of her LMP or size and dates are not consistent, one should obtain an ultrasound for dating. Accurate dating is crucial for all subsequent obstetrical evaluations and interventions.

Diagnostic Evaluation

The panel of tests in the first trimester includes a complete blood count, primarily for hematocrit, blood type, antibody screen, rapid plasma reagin (RPR) or VDRL screening for syphilis, rubella antibody screen, hepatitis B surface antigen, urinalysis, and urine culture. If a patient has no history of chickenpox, a titer for varicella zoster virus (VZV) antibodies is sent. A purified protein derivative (PPD) is usually placed during the first or second trimester. A urine pregnancy test should be sent if the patient is not entirely certain she is pregnant. If there has been any bleeding or cramping, a β-hCG level should be obtained. While there is some debate over the use of routine toxoplasma titers, they are often ordered as well. All patients are counseled about human immunodeficiency virus (HIV) and testing should be offered routinely (Table 1-3). In addition, first trimester screening tests for aneuploidy with nuchal translucency (NT) by ultrasound and serum markers are increasingly being obtained in most women via referral to a prenatal diagnosis unit. In addition to this battery of tests, there are a variety of other screens offered to high-risk patients (Table 1-4).

ROUTINE PRENATAL VISITS

Blood pressure, weight, urine dipstick, measurement of the uterus, and auscultation of the fetal heart are performed and assessed on each follow-up prenatal care visit. Maternal blood pressure decreases during the first and second trimester and slowly returns to baseline during the third trimester; elevation may be a sign of preeclampsia. Maternal weight is followed serially throughout the pregnancy as a proxy for adequate nutrition. Also, large weight gains toward the end of pregnancy can be a sign of fluid retention and preeclampsia. Measurement of the uterine fundal height in centimeters corresponds roughly to the weeks of gestation. If the fundal height is progressively decreasing or is 3 cm less than gestational age, an ultrasound is done to more accurately assess fetal growth. After 10 to 14 weeks, Doppler ultrasound is used to auscultate the fetal heart rate. Urine is routinely dipped for protein, glucose, blood, and leukocyte esterase. Protein may be indicative of preeclampsia, glucose of diabetes, and leukocyte esterase of urinary tract infection (UTI). Pregnant women are at an increased risk for complicated UTIs such as pyelonephritis given increased urinary stasis

■ TABLE 1-3 Routine Tests in Prenatal Care

Initial Visit and First Trimester	Second Trimester	Third Trimester
Hematocrit	MSAFP/triple or quad screen	Hematocrit
Blood type and screen	Obstetric ultrasound	RPR/VDRL
RPR/VDRL	Amniocentesis for women interested in prenatal diagnosis	GLT
Rubella antibody screen		Group B strep culture
Hepatitis B surface antigen		
Gonorrhea culture		
Chlamydia culture		
PPD		
Pap smear		
Urinalysis and culture		
VZV titer in patients with no history of exposure		
HIV offered		
Early screening for aneuploidy (nuchal translucency plus serum markers)		

■ TABLE 1-4 Initial Screens in Specific High-Risk Groups

High-Risk Group	Specific Test
African American, Southeast Asian, MCV <70	Sickle-cell prep for African Americans; Hgb electrophoresis
Family history of genetic disorder (e.g., hemophilia, sickle-cell disease, fragile X syndrome), maternal age 35 or older at time of EDC	Prenatal genetics referral
Prior gestational diabetes, family history of diabetes, Hispanic, Native American, Southeast Asian	Early glucose loading test
Pregestational diabetes, unsure dates, recurrent miscarriages	Dating sonogram at first visit
Hypertension, renal disease, pregestational diabetic, prior preeclampsia, renal transplant, SLE	BUN, Cr, uric acid and 24 hour urine collection for protein and creatinine clearance (to establish a baseline)
Pregestational diabetes, prior cardiac disease, hypertension	Electrocardiogram (ECG)
Pregestational diabetes	Hgb A1C, ophthalmology for eye exam
Graves disease	Thyroid-stimulating immunoglobulins (can cause fetal disease)
All thyroid disease	TSH, possibly free T4
PPD+	Chest x-ray after 16 weeks' gestation
Systemic lupus erythematosus (SLE)	AntiRho, antiLa antibodies (can cause fetal complete heart block)

from mechanical compression of the ureters and progesterone-mediated smooth muscle relaxation.

At each visit, the patient is asked about symptoms that indicate complications of pregnancy. These symptoms include vaginal bleeding, vaginal discharge or leaking of fluid, and urinary symptoms. In addition, after 20 weeks, patients are asked about contractions and fetal movement. Vaginal bleeding is a sign of possible miscarriage or ectopic pregnancy in the first trimester, and of placental abruption or previa as the pregnancy advances. Vaginal discharge may be a sign of infection or cervical change, whereas leaking fluid can indicate ruptured fetal membranes. While irregular (Braxton Hicks) contractions are common throughout the third trimester, regular contractions more frequent than five or six per hour may be a sign of preterm labor and should be assessed. Changes in or absence of fetal movement should be evaluated by auscultation of the fetal heart in the previable fetus and with further testing such as a nonstress test or biophysical profile in the viable fetus.

First-Trimester Visits

During the first trimester patients—particularly nulliparous women—need to be familiarized with pregnancy. The symptoms of pregnancy and what will occur at each prenatal visit should be reviewed. At the second prenatal visit, all of the initial labs should be reviewed with the patient. Patients with poor weight gain or decreased caloric intake secondary to nausea and vomiting may be referred to a nutritionist. Patients treated for infections noted at the initial prenatal visit should be cultured for test of cure. Additionally, early screening for aneuploidy, with an ultrasound for nuchal translucency (NT) and correlation with serum levels of PAPP-A and free β-hCG, is offered between 11 and 13 weeks of gestation to all women.

Second-Trimester Visits

During the second trimester, much of the screening for genetic and congenital abnormalities is done. This allows a patient to obtain an elective termination if there are abnormalities. Screening for **maternal serum alpha fetoprotein** (MSAFP) is usually performed between 15 and 18 weeks. An elevation in MSAFP is correlated with an increased risk of neural tube defects and a decrease is seen in some aneuploidies including Down syndrome. The sensitivity of aneuploidy screening is augmented using β-hCG and estriol along with

MSAFP called the **triple screen**. The addition of inhibin A to this screening test further enhances the ability to detect abnormalities and is known as the **Quad screen**. Between 18 and 20 weeks' gestation, most patients are offered a screening ultrasound. This provides the opportunity to screen for common fetal abnormalities. Also noted are the amniotic fluid volume, placental location, and gestational age.

The fetal heart is usually first heard during the second trimester and the first fetal movement, or "quickening," is felt in the second trimester, usually between 16 and 20 weeks' gestational age. Most patients have resolution of their nausea and vomiting by the second trimester, although some continue with these symptoms throughout their pregnancy. Because the risk of spontaneous abortions decreases after 12 weeks of gestation, childbirth classes and tours of the labor floor are usually offered in the second and third trimesters.

Third-Trimester Visits

During the third trimester, the fetus is viable. Patients will begin to have occasional Braxton Hicks contractions and, if these contractions become regular, the cervix is examined to rule out preterm labor. Prenatal visits increase to every 2 to 3 weeks from 28 to 36 weeks and then to every week after 36 weeks. In addition, patients who are Rh negative should receive RhoGAM at 28 weeks. Beyond 32 to 34 weeks Leopold maneuvers (see Fig. 3-1) are performed to determine fetal presentation. Either as a routine or if there is any question, an office ultrasound may be used at 35 to 36 weeks to confirm fetal presentation. In the setting of breech presentation, women are offered external cephalic version of the fetus at 37 to 38 weeks of gestation.

Beyond 37 weeks, which is considered term, the cervix is usually examined at each visit. Because a vigorous examination of the cervix known as "sweeping" or "stripping" the membranes has been demonstrated to decrease the probability of progressing postterm or requiring an induction of labor, this is commonly offered at all term pregnancy prenatal visits.

Third-Trimester Labs

At 27 to 29 weeks, the third-trimester labs are ordered. These consist of the hematocrit, RPR/VDRL, and **glucose loading test** (GLT). At this time, the hematocrit is getting close to its nadir. Patients with a hematocrit below 32% to 33% (hemoglobin less than

11 mg/dL) are usually started on iron supplementation. Because this will cause further constipation, stool softeners are given in conjunction. The GLT is a screening test for gestational diabetes. It consists of giving a 50-g oral glucose loading dose and checking serum glucose 1 hour later. If this value is greater than or equal to 140 mg/dL, a **glucose tolerance test** (GTT) is administered, though some institutions utilize a lower threshold of 130 mg/dL or 135 mg/dL.

The GTT is the diagnostic test for gestational diabetes. It consists of a fasting serum glucose measurement and then administration of a 100-g oral glucose loading dose. The serum glucose is then measured at 1, 2, and 3 hours after the oral dose is given. This test is indicative of gestational diabetes if there is an elevation in two or more of the following threshold values: the fasting glucose, 95 mg/dL; 1 hour, 180 mg/dL; 2 hour, 155 mg/dL; or 3 hour, 140 mg/dL.

In high-risk populations, vaginal cultures for gonorrhea and chlamydia are repeated late in the third trimester. These infections are transmitted vertically during birth and should be treated if cultures or DNA tests return positive. At 36 weeks, screening for group B streptococcus is also performed. Patients who have a positive culture should be treated with intravenous penicillin when they present in labor to prevent potential neonatal group B streptococcus infection.

ROUTINE PROBLEMS OF PREGNANCY

BACK PAIN

Low back pain in pregnancy is quite common, particularly in the third trimester when the patient's center of gravity has shifted and there is increased strain on the lower back. Mild exercise—particularly stretching—may release endorphins and reduce the amount of back pain. Gentle massage, heating pads, and Tylenol can be used for mild pain. For patients with severe back pain, muscle relaxants or occasionally narcotics can be used.

CONSTIPATION

The decreased bowel motility secondary to elevated progesterone levels leads to increased transit time in the large bowel. In turn, there is greater absorption of water from the gastrointestinal tract. This can result in constipation. Increased PO fluids, particularly water, should be recommended. In addition, stool softeners

or bulking agents may help. Laxatives can be used, but are usually avoided in the third trimester because of the theoretical risk of preterm labor.

CONTRACTIONS

Occasional irregular contractions that do not lead to cervical change are considered Braxton Hicks contractions and will occur several times per day up to several times per hour. Patients should be warned about these and assured that they are normal. Dehydration may cause increased contractions, and patients should be advised to drink many (10 to 14) glasses of water per day. Regular contractions, as often as every 10 minutes, should be considered a sign of preterm labor and should be assessed by cervical examination. If a patient has had several days of contractions and no documented cervical change, this is reassuring to both the obstetrician and the patient that delivery is not imminent.

DEHYDRATION

Because of the expanded intravascular space and increased third spacing of fluid, patients have a difficult time maintaining their intravascular volume status. Dietary recommendations should include increased fluids. As mentioned above, dehydration may lead to uterine contractions, possibly secondary to cross-reaction of vasopressin with oxytocin receptors.

EDEMA

Compression of the inferior vena cava (IVC) and pelvic veins by the uterus can lead to increased hydrostatic pressure in the lower extremities and eventually to edema in the feet and ankles. Elevation of the lower extremities above the heart can ease this. Also, patients should be advised to sleep on their sides to decrease compression. Severe edema of the face and hands may be indicative of preeclampsia and merits further evaluation.

GASTROESOPHAGEAL REFLUX DISEASE

Relaxation of the lower esophageal sphincter and increased transit time in the stomach can lead to reflux and nausea. Patients with reflux should be started on antacids, advised to eat multiple small meals per day, and avoid lying down within an hour of eating. For patients with continued symptoms, H_2 blockers or proton pump inhibitors can be given.

HEMORRHOIDS

Patients will have increased venous stasis and IVC compression, leading to congestion in the venous system. Congestion of the pelvic vessels combined with increased abdominal pressure with bowel movements secondary to constipation can lead to hemorrhoids. Hemorrhoids are treated symptomatically with topical anesthetics and steroids for pain and swelling. Prevention of constipation with increased fluids, increased fiber in the diet, and stool softeners may prevent or decrease the exacerbation of hemorrhoids.

PICA

Rarely, a patient will have cravings for inedible items such as dirt or clay. As long as these substances are nontoxic, the patient is advised to maintain adequate nutrition and encouraged to stop ingesting the inedible items. However, if patients have been consuming toxic substances, immediate cessation along with a toxicology consult is advised.

ROUND LIGAMENT PAIN

Usually late in the second trimester or early in the third trimester, there may be some pain in the adnexa or lower abdomen. This pain is likely secondary to the rapid expansion of the uterus and stretching of the ligamentous attachments, such as the round ligaments. This is often self-limited but may be relieved with warm compresses or acetaminophen.

URINARY FREQUENCY

Increased intravascular volumes and elevated glomerular filtration rate (GFR) can lead to increased urine production during pregnancy. However, the most likely cause of urinary frequency during pregnancy is increasing compression of the bladder by the growing uterus. A urinary tract infection may also be present with isolated urinary frequency but is often accompanied by dysuria. A urinalysis and culture should therefore be ordered to rule out infection. If no infection is present, patients can be assured that the increased voiding is normal. Patients should be advised to keep up PO hydration despite urinary frequency.

VARICOSE VEINS

The lower extremities or the vulva may develop varicosities during pregnancy. The relaxation of the venous smooth muscle and increased intravascular pressure probably both contribute to the pathogenesis. Elevation of the lower extremities or the use of pressure stockings may help reduce existing varicosities and prevent more from developing. If the problem does not resolve by 6 months' postpartum, patients may be referred for surgical therapy.

PRENATAL ASSESSMENT OF THE FETUS

Throughout pregnancy, the fetus is screened and diagnosed by a variety of modalities. Parents can be screened for common diseases such as cystic fibrosis, Tay-Sachs, sickle-cell disease, and thalassemia. If both parents are carriers of recessive genetic diseases, the fetus can then be diagnosed. Fetal karyotype and genetic screens can be obtained via amniocentesis or chorionic villus sampling (CVS). The fetus can be imaged and many of the congenital anomalies diagnosed via second trimester ultrasound. First and second trimester genetic screening and prenatal diagnosis is discussed further in Chapter 3. Other fetal testing includes fetal blood sampling, fetal lung maturity testing, and assessment of fetal well-being.

ULTRASOUND

Ultrasound can be used to date a pregnancy with an unknown or uncertain LMP and is most accurate in the first trimester. To detect fetal malformations, most patients undergo a routine screening ultrasound at 18 to 20 weeks. Routinely, an attempt is made to identify placental location, amniotic fluid volume, gestational age, and any obvious malformations. Of note, most patients will think of this ultrasound as the time to find out the fetal sex. While determination of fetal sex is medically indicated in some settings (e.g., history of fragile X syndrome or other X-linked disorders) it is not necessarily a part of the routine Level I obstetric ultrasound. This point of clarification is useful to discuss with patients to establish proper expectations for the ultrasound.

In high-risk patients, careful attention is paid to commonly associated anomalies such as cardiac anomalies in pregestational diabetics. Fetal echocardiography and, rarely, MRI are used to augment assessment of the fetal heart and brain, respectively.

In the third trimester, ultrasound can be used to monitor high-risk pregnancies by obtaining **biophysical profiles** (BPP), fetal growth, and fetal Doppler studies. The BPP looks at five categories and gives a score of either 0 or 2 for each: amniotic fluid volume, fetal tone, fetal activity, fetal breathing movements, and the **nonstress test** (NST), which is a test of the fetal heart rate. A BPP of 8 to 10 or better is reassuring. Ultrasound with Doppler flow studies can also be used to assess the blood flow in the umbilical cord. A decrease, absence, or reversal of diastolic flow in the umbilical artery is progressively more worrisome for placental insufficiency and resultant fetal compromise.

ANTENATAL TESTING OF FETAL WELL-BEING

Formal antenatal testing includes the NST, the oxytocin challenge test (OCT), and the BPP. The NST is considered formally reactive (a reassuring sign) if there are two accelerations of the fetal heart rate in 20 minutes that are at least 15 beats above the baseline heart rate and last for at least 15 seconds. An OCT or contraction stress test (CST) is obtained by getting at least three contractions in 10 minutes and analyzing the fetal heart rate (FHR) tracing during that time. The reactivity criteria are the same as for the NST. In addition, late decelerations with at least half of the contractions constitute a positive test and are worrisome. Commonly, most antenatal testing units use the NST beginning at 32 to 34 weeks of gestation in high-risk pregnancies and at 40 to 41 weeks for undelivered patients. If the NST is nonreactive, the fetus is assessed via ultrasound. If the fetal heart tracing has any worrisome decelerations or the BPP is not reassuring, an OCT is usually performed or, in more severe cases, consideration is given to delivery.

FETAL BLOOD SAMPLING

Percutaneous umbilical blood sampling (PUBS) is performed by placing a needle transabdominally into the uterus and phlebotomizing the umbilical cord. This procedure may be used when the fetal hematocrit needs to be obtained, particularly in the setting of Rh isoimmunization, other causes of fetal anemia, and hydrops. PUBS is also used for fetal transfusion, karyotype analysis, and assessment of fetal platelet count in alloimmune thrombocytopenia.

FETAL LUNG MATURITY

To test for fetal lung maturity, an amniotic fluid sample obtained through amniocentesis is analyzed. Classically, the lecithin to sphingomyelin (L/S) ratio has been used as a predictor of fetal lung maturity. Type II pneumocytes secrete a surfactant that uses phospholipids in its synthesis. Commonly, lecithin increases as the lungs mature, whereas sphingomyelin decreases beyond about 32 weeks. The L/S ratio should therefore increase as the pregnancy progresses. Repetitive studies have shown that an L/S ratio of greater than 2 is associated with only rare cases of **respiratory distress syndrome** (RDS). Examples of other fetal lung maturity tests include measuring the levels of phosphatidylglycerol (PG), saturated phosphatidyl choline (SPC), the presence of lamellar body count, and surfactant to albumin ratio (S/A).

KEY POINTS

- A urine pregnancy test will often be positive at the time of the missed menstrual cycle.
- Physiologic changes during pregnancy, mediated by the placental hormones, affect every organ system.
- Cardiovascular changes include a decrease in systemic vascular resistance and blood pressure and an increase in cardiac output.
- The initial prenatal visit is used to screen for many of the problems that can occur in pregnancy and to verify dating of the pregnancy.
- Much of the screening for genetic and congenital abnormalities is performed in the second trimester.
- Blood pressure, weight gain, fundal height, fetal heart rate, and symptoms including contractions, vaginal bleeding or discharge, and perceived fetal movement are assessed at each prenatal visit.
- Many of the routine problems of pregnancy are related to hormonal effects of the placenta.
- It is important to discuss the side effects of pregnancy in order to best prepare the patient.
- While pregnancy is often the cause of many somatic complaints, other causes should still be ruled out as in the nonpregnant patient.
- Common screening tests for fetal abnormalities include MSAFP and the triple screen.
- The fetus may be diagnosed with abnormalities using amniocentesis, CVS, and ultrasound.
- Fetal status can be assessed antepartum with ultrasound, NST, BPP, and OCT.

Early Pregnancy Complications

ECTOPIC PREGNANCY

An **ectopic pregnancy** is one that implants outside the uterine cavity. Implantation occurs in the fallopian tube in up to 99% of the cases (Fig. 2-1). Implantation may also occur on the ovary, the cervix, the outside of the fallopian tube, the abdominal wall, or the bowel. The incidence of ectopic pregnancies has been increasing over the past 10 years, and now occurs in more than 1:100 pregnancies. This is thought to be secondary to the increase in assisted fertility, sexually transmitted infections (STIs), and pelvic inflammatory disease (PID). Patients who present with vaginal bleeding and/or abdominal pain should always be evaluated for ectopic pregnancy because a ruptured ectopic pregnancy is a true emergency. It can result in rapid hemorrhage, leading to shock and eventually death.

RISK FACTORS

Several risk factors predispose patients to extrauterine implantation (Table 2-1). Many affect the fallopian tubes, causing either tubal scarring or decreased peristalsis of the tube. One of the strongest risk factors is prior ectopic pregnancy. Since the advent of assisted reproductive technologies (ART), it has been noted that there is an increased risk of ectopic pregnancies in such pregnancies. Use of an intrauterine device (IUD) for birth control leads to an increased rate of ectopic pregnancy in those women who become pregnant because the IUD has prevented normal intrauterine implantation.

DIAGNOSIS

The diagnosis of ectopic pregnancy is made by history, physical examination, laboratory tests, and ultrasound. On history, patients often complain of unilateral pelvic or lower abdominal pain and vaginal bleeding. Physical examination may reveal an adnexal mass that is often tender, a uterus that is small for gestational age, and bleeding from the cervix. Patients with ruptured ectopic pregnancies may be hypotensive, unresponsive, or show signs of peritoneal irritation secondary to hemoperitoneum.

On laboratory studies, the classic finding is a beta human chorionic gonadotropin (β-hCG) level that is low for gestational age and does not increase at the expected rate. In patients with a normal **intrauterine pregnancy** (IUP), the trophoblastic tissue secretes β-hCG in a predictable manner that should lead to doubling (or at least an increase of 2/3 or more) approximately every 48 hours. An ectopic pregnancy has a poorly implanted placenta with less blood supply than in the endometrium; thus the level of β-hCG does not double every 48 hours. The hematocrit may be low or may drop in patients with ruptured ectopic pregnancies.

Ultrasound may reveal an adnexal mass or an extrauterine pregnancy (Fig. 2-2). A gestational sac with a yolk sac seen in the uterus on ultrasound indicates an intrauterine pregnancy. However, there is always a small risk of **heterotopic pregnancy**, a multiple gestation with at least one IUP and at least one ectopic pregnancy. This is of particular concern in the setting of IVF pregnancies when more than one embryo was utilized. At early gestations, neither

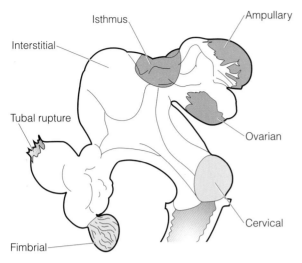

Figure 2-1 • Sites of ectopic pregnancies.

■ **TABLE 2-1** Risk Factors for Ectopic Pregnancy
History of STIs or PID
Prior ectopic pregnancy
Previous tubal surgery
Prior pelvic or abdominal surgery resulting in adhesions
Endometriosis
Current use of exogenous hormones including progesterone or estrogen
In vitro fertilization and other assisted reproduction
DES-exposed patients with congenital abnormalities
Congenital abnormalities of the fallopian tubes
Use of an IUD for birth control

an IUP nor an adnexal mass can be seen on ultrasound.

Patients who cannot be definitively diagnosed with an ectopic versus an IUP are labeled rule-out ectopic. If such patients are stable on exam, they may be followed with serial β-hCG levels every 48 hours. β-hCG levels that do not double (or increase by at least 2/3) every 48 hours are suspicious for ectopic pregnancy. As a guideline, an IUP should be seen on transvaginal ultrasonography with a β-hCG between 1,500 and 2,000 mIU/mL. A fetal heartbeat should be seen with β-hCG >5,000 mIU/mL.

TREATMENT

If a patient presents with a ruptured ectopic pregnancy and is unstable, the first priority is to stabilize with intravenous fluids, blood products, and pressors if necessary. The patient should then be taken to the operating room where exploratory laparotomy can be

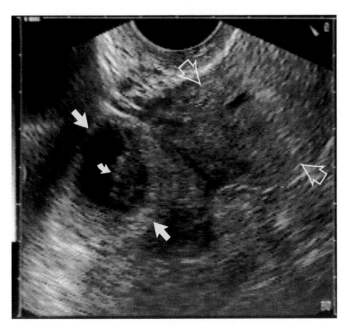

Figure 2-2 • Endovaginal view of a right adnexal ectopic pregnancy with a gestational sac (*large arrows*) and fetal pole (*small arrow*). The uterus is seen to the right of the image, with a small amount of endometrial fluid (*hollow arrows*).

performed to stop the bleeding and remove the ectopic pregnancy. If the patient is stable with a likely ruptured ectopic pregnancy, the procedure of choice at many institutions is an exploratory laparoscopy that can be performed to evacuate the hemoperitoneum, coagulate any ongoing bleeding, and resect the ectopic pregnancy. Resection can be either through a salpingostomy, where the ectopic pregnancy is removed leaving the fallopian tube in place or a salpingectomy where the entire ectopic pregnancy is removed. In the rare case of a cornual (or interstitial) ectopic pregnancy, a cornual resection can be performed.

Patients who present with an unruptured ectopic pregnancy can be treated either surgically as above or medically. **Methotrexate** therapy for treatment of the ectopic pregnancy is used at most institutions for uncomplicated, nonthreatening, ectopic pregnancies. It is appropriate to use methotrexate for patients who have small ectopic pregnancies (as a general rule, less than 4 cm and without a fetal heartbeat) and for those patients who will be reliable with follow-up.

Care of such women involves assessment of baseline transaminases and creatinine, IM methotrexate, and serially following the β-hCG levels. Commonly, the β-hCG level will rise the first few days after methotrexate therapy, but should fall by 10% to 15% between days 4 and 7 of the treatment. If such a fall is not achieved, the patient requires a second dosage of methotrexate. Additionally, these women should be monitored for signs and symptoms of rupture—increased abdominal pain, bleeding, or signs of shock—and advised to come to the emergency room immediately with such symptoms.

SPONTANEOUS ABORTION

A **spontaneous abortion**, or miscarriage, is a pregnancy that ends before 20 weeks' gestation. SABs are estimated to occur in 15% to 25% of all pregnancies. This number may be even higher because losses that occur at 4 to 6 weeks' gestational age are often confused with late menses. The type of SAB is defined by whether any or all of the **products of conception** (POC) have passed and whether or not the cervix is dilated. Definitions are as follows:

- **Abortus**—fetus lost before 20 weeks' gestation, less than 500 g, or less than 25 cm.
- **Complete abortion**—complete expulsion of all POC before 20 weeks' gestation (Fig. 2-3).

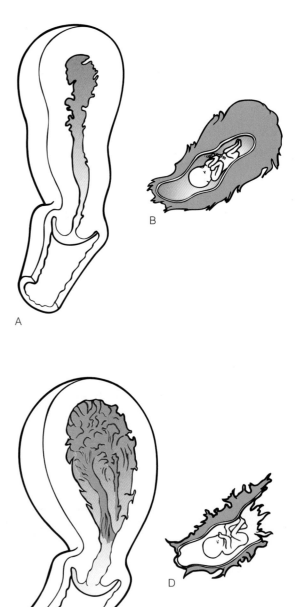

Figure 2-3 • (A) Complete abortion. **(B)** Product of complete abortion. **(C)** Incomplete abortion. **(D)** Product of incomplete abortion.

- **Incomplete abortion**—partial expulsion of some but not all POC before 20 weeks' gestation.
- **Inevitable abortion**—no expulsion of products, but vaginal bleeding and dilation of the cervix such that a viable pregnancy is unlikely.
- **Threatened abortion**—any vaginal bleeding before 20 weeks, without dilation of the cervix or expul-

sion of any POC (i.e., a normal pregnancy with bleeding)

- **Missed abortion**—death of the embryo or fetus before 20 weeks with complete retention of all POC.

FIRST-TRIMESTER ABORTIONS

It is estimated that 60% to 80% of all SABs in the first trimester are associated with abnormal chromosomes. This percentage may be higher because many abortions likely occur even before implantation. Other factors associated with SABs include infections, maternal anatomic defects, immunologic factors, and endocrine factors. A large number of first-trimester abortions have no obvious cause.

DIAGNOSIS

Most patients present with bleeding from the vagina (Table 2-2). Other findings include cramping, abdominal pain, and decreased symptoms of pregnancy. The physical examination should include vital signs to rule out shock and febrile illness. A pelvic examination can be performed to look for sources of bleeding other than uterine and for changes in the cervix suggestive of an inevitable abortion. The laboratory tests ordered include a quantitative level of β-hCG, complete blood count, blood type, and antibody screen. An ultrasound can assess fetal viability and placentation. As ectopic pregnancies can also present with vaginal bleeding, this must also be considered in the differential diagnosis.

TREATMENT

The treatment plan is based on specific diagnosis and on the decisions made by the patient and her caregivers. Initially, all pregnant and bleeding patients

■ **TABLE 2-2** Differential Diagnosis of First-Trimester Bleeding
Spontaneous abortion
Postcoital bleeding
Ectopic pregnancy
Vaginal or cervical lesions or lacerations
Extrusion of molar pregnancy
Nonpregnancy causes of bleeding

need to be stabilized if hypotensive. A complete abortion can be followed for recurrent bleeding and signs of infection such as elevated temperature. Any tissue that the patient may have passed at home and at the hospital should be sent to pathology, both to assess that POC have passed and for chromosome analysis if applicable.

An incomplete abortion can be allowed to finish on its own if the patient prefers expectant management, but can also be taken to completion with either a dilation and curettage (D&C) or administration of prostaglandins (e.g., misoprostol) to induce cervical dilatation and uterine contractions. Inevitable abortions and missed abortions are similarly managed.

A patient with a threatened abortion should be followed for continued bleeding and placed on pelvic rest with nothing per vagina. Often, the bleeding will resolve. However, these patients are at increased risk for preterm labor (PTL) and preterm premature rupture of membranes (PPROM). Finally, all Rh-negative pregnant women who experience vaginal bleeding during pregnancy should receive RhoGAM.

SECOND-TRIMESTER ABORTIONS

Second-trimester abortions (12 to 20 weeks' gestational age) have multiple etiologies. Infection, maternal uterine or cervical anatomic defects, maternal systemic disease, exposure to fetotoxic agents, and trauma are all associated with late abortions. Abnormal chromosomes are not a frequent cause of late abortions. Late second-trimester abortions and periviable deliveries are also seen with PTL and incompetent cervix. As in first-trimester abortions, the treatment plan is based on the specific clinical scenario.

Incomplete and missed abortions can be allowed to finish on their own but are often taken to completion with a D&E (dilation and evacuation). The distinction between a D&C and D&E depends on gestational age at the time of procedure (i.e., first or second trimester). The fetus is larger in the second trimester making the procedure more difficult. Between 16 and 24 weeks, either a D&E may be performed or labor may be induced with high doses of oxytocin or prostaglandins. The advantage of a D&E is that the procedure is self-limited and performed faster than an induction of labor. However, aggressive dilation is necessary prior to the procedure with laminaria (small rods of seaweed that are placed in the cervix the day prior to the procedure and expand as they absorb water, thereby dilating the cervix) and there is a significant risk of uterine perforation and cervical lacerations. An induction of labor can take longer, but allows completion of the abortion without the inherent risks of instrumentation. With either method, great care should be taken to ensure the complete evacuation of all POC.

In the second trimester, the diagnoses of PTL and incompetent cervix need to be ruled out. Particularly in the setting of inevitable abortions or threatened abortions, the etiology is likely to be related to the inability of the uterus to maintain the pregnancy. PTL begins with contractions leading to cervical change, whereas an incompetent cervix is characterized by painless dilation of the cervix. In the case of an incompetent cervix, an emergent cerclage may be offered. PTL can potentially be managed with tocolysis.

INCOMPETENT CERVIX

Patients with an **incompetent cervix** or cervical insufficiency present with painless dilation and effacement of the cervix, often in the second trimester of pregnancy. As the cervix dilates, the fetal membranes are exposed to vaginal flora and risk of increased trauma. Thus, infection, vaginal discharge, and rupture of the membranes are common findings in the setting of incompetent cervix. Patients may also present with short-term cramping or contracting, leading to advancing cervical dilation or pressure in the vagina with the chorionic and amniotic sacs bulging through the cervix. Cervical incompetence is estimated to cause approximately 15% of all second-trimester losses.

RISK FACTORS

Surgery or other cervical trauma is the most common cause of cervical incompetence (Table 2-3). The other possible cause is a congenital abnormality of the cervix that can sometimes be attributed to di-

TABLE 2-3 Risk Factors for Cervical Incompetence

History of cervical surgery, such as a cone biopsy or dilation of the cervix
History of cervical lacerations with vaginal delivery
Uterine anomalies
History of DES exposure

ethylstilbestrol (DES) exposure in utero. However, many patients who present with cervical incompetence have no known risk factors.

DIAGNOSIS

Patients with incompetent cervix often present with a dilated cervix noted on routine examination, ultrasound, or in the setting of bleeding, vaginal discharge, or rupture of membranes. Occasionally, patients experience mild cramping or pressure in the lower abdomen or vagina. On examination, the cervix is dilated more than expected with the level of contractions experienced. It is often difficult to differentiate between incompetent cervix and PTL. However, patients who present with mild cramping and have advancing cervical dilation on serial examinations and/or an amniotic sac bulging through the cervix (Fig. 2-4) are more likely to have an incompetent cervix, with the cramping being instigated by the dilated cervix and exposed membranes rather than the contractions/cramping leading to cervical change as in the case of PTL.

TREATMENT

Individual obstetric issues should be treated accordingly. If the fetus is previable (i.e., less than 24 weeks' gestational age), expectant management and elective termination are options. Patients with viable pregnancies are treated with betamethasone to decrease the risk of prematurity and are managed expectantly with strict bed rest. If there is a component of preterm contractions or PTL, tocolysis may be used with viable pregnancies.

One alternative course of management for incompetent cervix in a previable pregnancy is the placement of an emergent **cerclage**. The cerclage is a suture placed vaginally around the cervix either at the cervical-vaginal junction (McDonald cerclage) or at the internal os (Shirodkar cerclage). The intent of a cerclage is to close the cervix. Complications include rupture of membranes, PTL, and infection.

If incompetent cervix was the suspected diagnosis in a previous pregnancy, a patient is usually offered an elective cerclage with subsequent pregnancies (Fig. 2-5). Placement of the elective cerclage is similar to that of the emergent cerclage with either the McDonald or Shirodkar methods being used, usually at 12 to 14 weeks' gestation. The cerclage is maintained until 36 to 38 weeks of gestation if possible. At that point it is removed and the patient is fol-

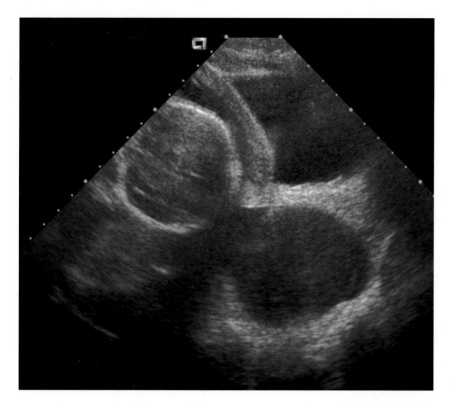

Figure 2-4 • Hourglass membranes.

lowed expectantly until labor ensues. In patients for whom one or both of the vaginal cerclages have failed, a transabdominal cerclage (TAC) is often the next management offered. This is placed around the cervix at the level of the internal os during a laparotomy. This can be placed electively either prior to the pregnancy or at 12 to 14 weeks. Patients with a TAC need to be delivered via cesarean section.

RECURRENT PREGNANCY LOSS

A recurrent or habitual aborter is a woman who has had three or more consecutive SABs. Less than 1% of the population is diagnosed with **recurrent pregnancy loss**. The risk of an SAB after one prior SAB is 20% to 25%; after two consecutive SABs, 25% to 30%; and after three consecutive SABs, 30% to 35%.

PATHOGENESIS

The etiologies of recurrent pregnancy loss are generally similar to those of SABs. These include chromosomal abnormalities, maternal systemic disease, maternal anatomic defects, and infection. Fifteen percent of patients with recurrent pregnancy loss have **antiphospholipid antibody (APA) syndrome**. Another group of patients are thought to have a **luteal phase defect** and lack an adequate level of progesterone to maintain the pregnancy.

DIAGNOSIS

Patients who are habitual aborters should be evaluated for the etiology. Patients with only two consecutive SABs are occasionally assessed as well, particularly those with advancing maternal age or for whom continued fertility may be an issue. Patients are often screened in the following manner. First, a karyotype of both parents is obtained, as well as the karyotypes of the POC from each of the SABs if possible. Second, maternal anatomy should be examined, initially with a hysterosalpingogram (HSG). If the HSG is abnormal or nondiagnostic, a hysteroscopic or laparoscopic exploration may be performed. Third, screening tests for hypothyroidism, diabetes mellitus, antiphospholipid antibody syndrome, hypercoagulability, and systemic lupus erythematosus (SLE) should be performed. These tests should include lupus anticoagulant, factor V Leiden deficiency, prothrombin G20210A mutation, ANA, anticardiolipin antibody, Russell viper venom, antithrombin III, protein S, and protein C. Fourth, a level of serum progesterone should be obtained in the luteal phase of the menstrual cycle. Finally, cultures of the cervix, vagina, and endometrium can be taken to rule out infection. An

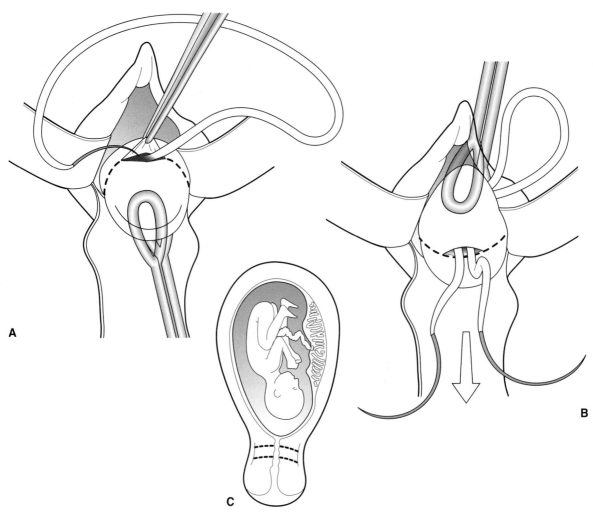

Figure 2-5 • Cervical cerclage (Shirodkar) for incompetent cervix in pregnant patient. **(A)** Placement of the suture.
(B) Cinching the suture down to tie the knot posteriorly. **(C)** The tightened cerclage almost at the internal os.

endometrial biopsy can be done during the luteal phase as well to look for proliferative endometrium.

TREATMENT

Treatment of patients with recurrent pregnancy loss depends on the etiology of the SABs. For many (approximately 30% to 50%), no etiology is ever found. For others, the etiology itself needs to be diagnosed as described above and can often be treated on an individual basis. For patients with chromosomal abnormalities such as balanced translocations, in vitro fertilization can be performed using donor sperm or ova. More recently, such patients may undergo preimplantation diagnosis (PGD) in order to maximize fertilization with their own normal chromosomes. This is where one cell of an embryo harvested through in

vitro fertilization is removed and karyotyped so that abnormal embryos are not implanted. Anatomic abnormalities may or may not be correctable. If incompetent cervix is suspected, a cerclage may be placed. If a luteal phase defect is suspected, progesterone may be given. Patients with APA syndrome are treated with low-dose aspirin. In the presence of a thrombophilia, SQ heparin (either low molecular weight or unfractionated) may be utilized. Maternal diseases should be treated with the appropriate therapy (e.g., hypothyroidism with thyroid hormone, infection with antibiotics). However, with some systemic diseases, treatment may not decrease the risk of SAB. Because even patients with three prior consecutive SABs will have a subsequent normal pregnancy two-thirds of the time, it is difficult to estimate whether certain treatments of recurrent abortions are effective.

KEY POINTS

- Approximately 1% of pregnancies are ectopic; that is, implantation of the pregnancy has occurred outside the uterine cavity.

- Initially, when a pregnant woman presents with vaginal bleeding and abdominal pain, an ectopic pregnancy must be ruled out or diagnosed with physical exam, laboratory assessment, and pelvic ultrasound.

- β-hCG levels double approximately every 48 hours in normal intrauterine pregnancies but not in ectopic pregnancies.

- Treatment of ectopic pregnancies is often surgical and includes stabilizing the patient and removing the pregnancy. Stable, unruptured ectopics can be managed medically with methotrexate therapy.

- The most common cause of first trimester abortions is fetal chromosomal abnormalities.

- Incomplete, inevitable, and missed abortions are usually completed with a D&C or medical management with prostaglandins, although expectant management can also used.

- RhoGAM should be given to all Rh-negative pregnant patients with bleeding.

- Most second-trimester abortions are secondary to uterine or cervical abnormalities, trauma, systemic disease, or infection.

- D&E, prostaglandins, or oxytocic agents can be used for the management of spontaneous abortions in the second trimester that need assistance to completion.

- Incompetent cervix is painless dilation of the cervix. This dilation may lead to infection, rupture of membranes, or preterm labor.

- If the fetus is previable, incompetent cervix is treated with expectant management, elective termination, or emergent cerclage.

- Patients with a history of incompetent cervix should be offered an elective, prophylactic cerclage at 12 to 14 weeks' gestational age.

- Recurrent pregnancy loss is defined as three or more consecutive SABs.

- Despite extensive evaluation to diagnose the etiology of SABs, the cause of recurrent SABs is undiagnosed in greater than one-third of all cases.

- The most common diagnosed causes of recurrent pregnancy loss include antiphospholipid antibody syndrome and luteal phase defects.

- Treatment is specific to the etiology, but efficacy is difficult to measure because two-thirds of subsequent pregnancies will be normal without therapy.

Prenatal Screening, Diagnosis, and Treatment

Prenatal screening, diagnosis, and treatment is a relatively new field within obstetrics. It has been particularly tied to the advent and advancement of real-time ultrasound imaging over the past two decades. Prenatal genetic diagnoses are and will be increasingly available as the association between genes and their phenotypes are discovered. Imperative to understanding prenatal diagnosis is the distinction between screening and diagnostic tests. **Screening** allows high-risk individuals to be selected out of a low-risk population at risk for a given diagnosis or complication. The sensitivity and specificity and resulting false-positive and false-negative rates of screening tests are highly important both because of the number of patients missed by a screen as well as the number of patients who are falsely concerned. **Prenatal diagnosis** is nearly always diagnostic and usually far more specific than screening, but diagnostic procedures such as amniocentesis and chorionic villus sampling (CVS) bear a greater risk of complications.

SCREENING PATIENTS FOR GENETIC DISEASES

Many diseases are passed genetically from parents to their offspring. This is best understood using the principles of Mendelian genetics. **Autosomal dominant** (AD) diseases are usually inherited from one parent with the disease via a single gene defect. Risk of disease and recurrence (if the partners choose to have another child) is usually 50%. **Autosomal recessive** (AR) diseases require two affected alleles. Thus, assuming both parents are carriers, the risk to

the child is 25%. **X-linked disorders** (e.g., hemophilia) are usually carried by the mother who is unaffected and passed only to her sons. The sons have the disease 50% of the time and the daughters are unaffected carriers 50% of the time. Rare **X-linked dominant** syndromes can be passed from either parent to either child similar to that of autosomal dominant syndromes. Phenotypes may vary, however, because of mixed penetrance, X-chromosome lyonization, and genomic imprinting. The first step in determining fetal risk is to screen the mother for the disease, which is usually done in higher risk groups (e.g., by ethnicity or family history). Below, we review several of the common genetic diseases that have prenatal screening and diagnosis.

CYSTIC FIBROSIS

Cystic fibrosis (CF) is an autosomal recessive disease that results from an abnormality in the cystic fibrosis transmembrane conductance regulator (CFTR), which is the gene responsible for chloride channels. Almost all CF patients have chronic lung disease due to recurrent infections, leading eventually to irreversible lung damage and strain on the right ventricle (cor pulmonale). Eighty-five percent of CF patients have pancreatic insufficiency manifested by chronic malabsorption and failure to thrive. Chronic lung disease and its sequelae are the life-limiting factors for most CF patients. Median survival is between 30 to 40 years for CF patients born today in the United States with high phenotypic variability.

In CF, two mutant copies of the CFTR gene are required (homozygosity) for disease, although, for the majority of AR disorders, affected individuals have two different allelic mutations at the same locus (compound heterozygote). For example, ΔF508/G542X are two of the most common mutations in CF. These two specific mutations can be screened for in asymptomatic carrier patients. If the mother has a positive screen, her partner can be screened as well and if he is also positive, then the risk of the fetus being affected is 25%. If desired, amniocentesis or CVS can then be performed to diagnose the fetus. The CF mutations are more common in Caucasians (1:29 is a carrier); but one challenge in screening for cystic fibrosis is that over 1,000 disease-causing mutations have been identified in the CFTR gene. Therefore, even with a negative screen, there remains a small probability that a child could be affected. While the risk of carrier status is less common in other races/ethnicities (e.g., Asian, Hispanic), the number of known mutations is fewer as well, making the screening test less sensitive in these women.

SICKLE-CELL DISEASE

Sickle-cell disease is an autosomal recessive disease caused by a single point mutation in the gene for the beta chain in hemoglobin. The resulting hemoglobin (Hb S) forms polymers that when deoxygenated cause the cells to lose their biconcave shape and become "sickled" in appearance. As a result, patients have a hemolytic anemia, shortened life expectancy, and frequent pain crises secondary to vaso-occlusion by the dysmorphic erythrocytes. Because this disease is more common among African Americans, all persons of African descent should be screened in pregnancy. Individuals with one abnormal sickle-cell allele are known as having sickle-cell trait. It is likely that the increased carrier status in African Americans was selected because of **heterozygote advantage**. This is observed because resistance to malaria in individuals heterozygous for sickle-cell anemia was greater than those without the gene defect. Red blood cells in these individuals function in normal conditions but are inhospitable to *Plasmodium vivax*, the parasitic protozoan responsible for malaria. Interestingly, a recent study demonstrated a lower rate of preterm birth among women who were sickle-cell trait.

The maternal screen is usually accomplished with a hemoglobin electrophoresis. This test distinguishes Hb S from normal Hb A. If the patient is positive,

then her partner can also be screened. If he is also positive, then the fetus carries a 25% chance of being affected, and the couple can choose to undergo invasive fetal diagnosis.

TAY-SACHS DISEASE

Tay-Sachs is an AR disease that is most commonly observed in Eastern European Jews and French Canadians. Approximately 1 in 27 Ashkenazi Jews is a carrier for an abnormal Tay-Sachs allele, resulting in an incidence of Tay-Sachs in this population approximately 100 times greater than in other populations. It is thought that this is due to a **founder effect**, in which the high frequency of a mutant gene in a population is founded by a small ancestral group when one or more individuals is a carrier for the mutation.

Infants with Tay-Sachs develop symptoms approximately 3 to 10 months after birth. These symptoms include a loss of alertness and an excessive reaction to noise (hyperacusis). There is a progressive developmental delay and neurologic degeneration in intellectual and neurologic function. Myoclonic and akinetic seizures can present 1 to 3 months later. One physical exam finding is a cherry-red spot seen on funduscopic eye exam where the prominent red macular fovea centralis is contrasted by the pale macula. These children eventually suffer from paralysis, blindness, and dementia, and typically die by age 4.

Tay-Sachs occurs due to a deficiency of hexosaminidase A (hex A), the enzyme responsible for the degradation of G_{M2} gangliosides. Hex A is a multimeric protein composed of three parts: alpha and beta subunits that comprise the enzyme and an activator protein. The activator protein must associate with both the enzyme and the substrate before the enzyme can cleave the ganglioside between the N-acetyl-α-galactosamine and galactose residues. Gangliosides are continually degraded in lysosomes where multiple degradative enzymes function to sequentially remove the terminal sugars from the gangliosides. The impact of Tay-Sachs is primarily in the brain, which has the highest concentrations of gangliosides, particularly in the gray matter. The deficiency of hex A results in the accumulation of gangliosides in the lysosomes resulting in enlarged neurons containing lipid-filled lysosomes, cellular dysfunction, and ultimately neuronal death.

Similar to other AR syndromes, Tay-Sachs is screened for particularly among high-risk patients (e.g., Ashkenazi Jews) and in their partners if they are positive. Fetal diagnosis can then be performed if both partners are carriers.

THALASSEMIA

The **thalassemias** are a set of hereditary hemolytic anemias that are caused by mutations that result in the reduction in the synthesis of either the α or β chains that make up the hemoglobin molecule. The reduction of a particular chain leads to the imbalance of globin chain synthesis and subsequently a distortion in the α:β ratio. As a result, unpaired globin chains produce insoluble tetramers that precipitate in the cell and cause damage to membranes. The red cells are susceptible to premature red cell destruction by the reticuloendothelial system in the bone marrow, liver, and spleen.

Beta Thalassemia

In **β-thalassemia**, there is an impairment of β-chain production that leads to an excess of alpha chains. These disorders are typically diagnosed several months after birth because the presence of β-chain is only important postnatally when it would normally replace the γ-chain as the major non-α chain. There are multiple mutations that can lead to β-thalassemia. Almost any point mutation that causes a decrease in synthesis of mRNA or protein can cause this disease. β-thalassemia is essentially an AR disorder seen more commonly among patients of Mediterranean descent, as well as Asians and Africans. Because the heterozygotes will have a mild hemolytic anemia and low MCV, they can be screened by getting a CBC. Confirmation can then be made by hemoglobin electrophoresis, which will show an increase in α:β ratio (Hgb A_2).

Alpha Thalassemia

The alpha chain is encoded by four alleles on two chromosomes. Additionally, two out of four mutations can occur cis or trans, with cis being on the same chromosome and trans being on two different chromosomes. Cis mutations are seen more commonly among Asians, whereas trans mutations are seen more commonly among Africans. With α-thalassemia, deletions or alterations of one, two, three, or four genes cause an increasingly severe phenotype. The most severe form of α-thalassemia causes fetal hydrops and is incompatible with life. The infants are pale, premature, hydropic, severely anemic, and have splenomegaly. A hemoglobin electrophoresis would reveal no HbF, no HbA, and approximately 90% to 100% Hbα4 also referred to as **Hb Bart**. **Hemoglobin H disease** (HbH) is due to the deletion of three alpha globin genes resulting in the accumulation of excess beta chains in the red cell. Beta tetramers form, which are unstable and undergo oxidation. Membrane damage results, and these red cells are susceptible to early clearance and destruction. These infants are born with anemia, and the initial hemoglobin electrophoresis shows some Hb Bart and some HbH. Within the following few months, Hb Bart disappears and the hemoglobins detected are HbH and HbA. **Alpha thalassemia trait** (two deletions) carries a milder phenotype with mainly a microcytic anemia and a normal hemoglobin electrophoresis. Patients with only one gene deletion are silent carriers. In that case, diagnosis is confirmed by gene-mapping techniques.

Like beta-thalassemia, alpha-thalassemia is also screened for with a CBC in high-risk groups. Patients can then undergo hemoglobin electrophoresis if they have a microcytic anemia. Sorting out whether patients are cis or trans is particularly important. When both partners have a cis mutation, their child has a 25% chance of getting the most severe variant that usually results in fetal death. If they both have the trans mutation, the child will end up with the trans mutation, as well, and primarily remain an asymptomatic carrier.

CHROMOSOMAL ABNORMALITIES

In addition to genetic disorders caused by single gene mutations, another family of genetic disorders in the fetus is caused by chromosomal abnormalities. Aneuploidy—that is, extra or missing chromosome(s)—is generally the cause of these syndromes. These chromosomal abnormalities are usually accompanied by obvious phenotypic differences and congenital anomalies. However, these may not always be appreciated on prenatal ultrasound. Thus, fetal karyotype remains the only way to achieve a definitive diagnosis of aneuploidy. Screening tests exist for some syndromes, including the expanded maternal serum alpha fetoprotein test, which includes MSAFP, estriol, β-hCG, and inhibin. These four serum analytes are commonly known as the quad screen. While trisomy and monosomy of any of the chromosomes theoretically exist, most result in early miscarriage. In addition, triploidy (i.e., three sets of chromosomes) may also occur and usually results in miscarriage or gestational trophoblastic disease. Despite the high rate of miscarriage, an infant is occasionally born with triploidy and survival for up to 1 year has been described.

DOWN SYNDROME

Trisomy 21, or an extra chromosome 21, is the most common cause of **Down syndrome**. This chromosomal aneuploidy results in higher rates of both miscarriage and stillbirth. However, there are several thousand Down syndrome infants born each year. Because chromosomal abnormalities increase with maternal age, the overall average risk per patient is increasing in the United States as more women delay childbearing. The typical phenotype of Down syndrome is that of a short stature, classic facies, developmental delay, and mental retardation with IQs ranging from 40 to as high as 90. Associated anomalies include cardiac defects, duodenal atresia or stenosis, and short limbs. Some of these anomalies can be seen by ultrasound, but up to 40% to 50% of Down syndrome fetuses will not have diagnosable anomalies by ultrasound, making this a poor screening tool.

Currently, Down syndrome is most commonly screened for using the quad screen (MSAFP, hCG, estriol, and inhibin A) between 15 and 20 weeks' gestation which has a sensitivity of just over 80%. Over the last decade, much research has gone into developing a first trimester screen. The work has produced two types of screens: ultrasound and serum. Ultrasound can be used to perform a nuchal translucency (NT) measurement. This screen provides a sensitivity of approximately 70% when used alone. The serum analytes when used alone, free β-hCG and pregnancy associated plasma protein A (PAPP-A), can achieve a 60% sensitivity. However, when combined, the three tests serve as the first trimester combined screen yielding a sensitivity of 80% or better. First trimester screening has been studied in several large trials and seems to be more effective than second trimester screening as women have the information sooner and make decisions sooner.

TRISOMY 18

Trisomy 18 (**Edward syndrome**) is another common trisomy that can also be screened for using the triple screen. It is not compatible with life beyond age two and commonly results in fetal or neonatal death. This syndrome is associated with multiple congenital anomalies which are typically seen on ultrasound, making this modality a reasonable screening tool. Edward syndrome is classically associated with clenched fists, overlapping digits, and rocker bottom feet. Cardiac defects including ventricular septal defect (VSD) and tetralogy of Fallot, omphalocele, congenital diaphragmatic hernia, neural tube defects, and choroid plexus cysts have also been associated with trisomy 18 (Fig. 3-1).

TRISOMY 13

Trisomy 13 (**Patau syndrome**) has many findings similar to trisomy 18. Eighty-five percent of these newborns will not live past the first year of life. Commonly associated anomalies include holoprosencephaly, cleft lip and palate, cystic hygroma, single nostril or absent nose, omphalocele, cardiac anomalies including hypoplastic left heart, and limb anomalies including clubfoot and -hand, polydactyly, and overlapping fingers. Unfortunately, the serum analytes of the quad screen are variable in these pregnancies making this a poor screening test and thus it is not reported. It is very rare that trisomy 13 fetuses would not have anomalies visible on ultrasound, however, and thus will be commonly diagnosed by routine ultrasound exam.

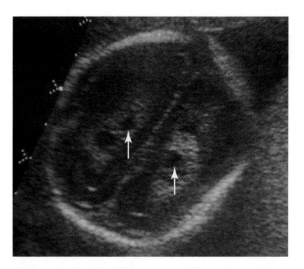

Figure 3-1 • Choroid plexus (CP) cysts located in the lateral ventricles of the brain.
(Image provided by Departments of Radiology and Obstetrics & Gynecology, University of California, San Francisco.)

SEX CHROMOSOMAL ABNORMALITIES

45,X (**Turner syndrome**, or monosomy X) and 47,XXY (**Klinefelter syndrome**) are the most common sex chromosome aneuploidies. This may be because 47,XXX and 47,XYY karyotypes exhibit little variation from standard phenotypes and are not identified as often. Individuals affected by Turner syndrome are phenotypically female and of short stature. They experience primary amenorrhea, sexual infantilism, webbed neck, low-set ears, low posterior hairline, epicanthal folds, wide carrying angle of the arms, shield-like chest, wide-set nipples, short fourth metacarpal, renal anomalies, lymphedema of the extremities at birth, and cardiovascular anomalies—especially coarctation of the aorta. The only anomaly in Turner syndrome commonly seen on ultrasound is cystic hygroma. Unfortunately, no screening test for Turner syndrome is currently available.

Similarly, there is no screening test for Klinefelter syndrome, however, both it and other sex chromosome abnormalities are diagnosed by karyotype when patients undergo amniocentesis or CVS. Testicular development is initially normal in these individuals. However, the presence of at least two X chromosomes causes the germ cells to die off when they enter meiosis, eventually resulting in small, firm testes and hyalinization of the seminiferous tubules. Other classic findings in Klinefelter syndrome include infertility, gynecomastia, mental retardation, and elevated gonadotropin levels due to the decreased levels of circulating androgens.

FETAL CONGENITAL ANOMALIES

Congenital anomalies can occur in any organ system. The affected organ system often depends on which time during gestation a teratogenic insult is received by the fetus. These teratogens can include medications ingested by the mother, infections, particularly viral that the mother contracts and transmits transplacentally, and rarely chemotherapy or radiation. In order to better understand how these anomalies occur, a review of organogenesis is useful.

EARLY EMBRYOGENESIS AND ORGANOGENESIS

After fertilization of the ovum by the sperm, the resulting zygote undergoes a series of cell divisions reaching the 16-cell morula stage by day 4 (Fig. 3-2). After the morula enters the uterine cavity, an influx of fluid separates the morula into the inner and outer cell masses, which forms the blastocyst. This gives rise to the embryo and the trophoblast, respectively. The blastocyst implants into the endometrium by the end of the week 1. By the start of week 2, the trophoblast begins to differentiate into the inner cytotrophoblast and the outer syncytiotrophoblast, and together they eventually give rise to the placenta. Meanwhile, the inner cell mass divides into the bilaminar germ disc composed of the epiblast and the hypoblast.

During week 3 of development, the embryo is primarily preoccupied with the process of gastrulation. This is characterized by the formation of the primitive streak on the epiblast followed by the invagination of

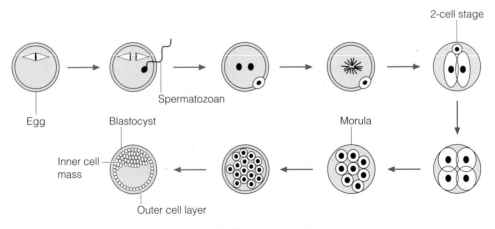

Figure 3-2 • Progression of the ova through fertilization to the blastula phase.

epiblast cells to form the three germ layers of the embryo: the inner endoderm, the middle mesoderm, and the outer ectoderm. The endodermal layer eventually gives rise to the gastrointestinal and respiratory systems. The mesoderm forms the cardiovascular, musculoskeletal, and genitourinary systems. The ectoderm layer will differentiate into the nervous system, skin, and many sensory organs (e.g., hair, eyes, nose, and ears). The period of organogenesis primarily lasts from week 3 to week 8 after conception (i.e., week 5 to 10 gestational age) and is the time when most of the major organ systems are formed.

NEURAL TUBE DEFECTS (NTDS)

The formation of the neural tube begins on days 22 to 23 after conception (week 4) in the region of the fourth and sixth somites. Fusion of the neural folds occurs in cranial and caudal directions. The anterior neuropore (future brain) closes by day 25 and the posterior pore (future spinal cord) closes by day 27. Closure of the neural tube coincides with establishment of its vascular supply. The majority of **neural tube defects** (NTDs) develop as a result of defective closure by week 4 of development (6 weeks gestational age by LMP dating).

NTDs, including spina bifida and anencephaly, are classic examples of multifactorial inheritance, emphasizing the interactions between environmental and genetic factors. Geographic and ethnic variations may reflect environmental and genetic influences on the incidence of NTDs. Decreased levels of maternal folic acid are associated with the development of NTDs. Supplementation with periconceptional folic acid effectively reduces the incidence as well as recurrence of NTDs. The risk of NTDs is doubled in cases of homozygosity for a common mutation in the gene for methyl tetrahydrofolate reductase (MTHFR), the C677T allelic variant that encodes an enzyme with reduced activity. However, even if the association were causal, this MTHFR variant would account for only a small fraction of NTDs prevented by folic acid. The risk of NTDs seen with certain genotypes may vary depending on maternal factors, such as the blood levels of vitamin B_{12} or folate.

Fetuses with **spina bifida** can be identified on ultrasound, which is accomplished not by visualization of the opening of the spinal canal (Fig. 3-3), but by the associated findings. Spina bifida leads to classic ultrasound findings of the "lemon" sign (concave frontal bones), and the "banana" sign (a cerebellum that is pulled caudally and flattened) (Fig. 3-4). Ventriculomegaly and clubfeet are also seen. Prior to the existence of real-time ultrasound, one of the first prenatal screening programs was created using MSAFP to screen for neural tube defects. An open neural tube leads to elevated amniotic fluid α-fetoprotein (AFP) that crosses into the maternal serum.

Function of the infant and child with spina bifida is entirely dependent on the level of the spinal lesion. If the lesion is quite low in the sacral area, bowel and bladder function may be normal, and ambulation can be achieved with crutches. However, in higher lesions,

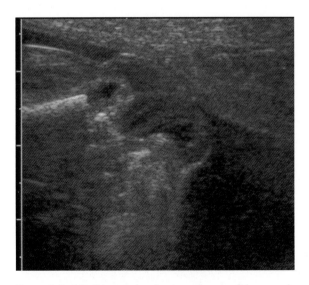

Figure 3-3 • Meningomyelocele—nonclosure of the neural tube at the lower aspect of the spine.
(Image provided by Departments of Radiology and Obstetrics & Gynecology, University of California, San Francisco.)

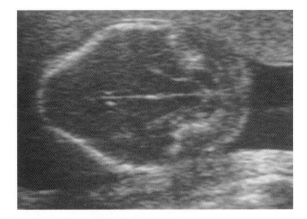

Figure 3-4 • Cerebral findings of the "lemon" and "banana" signs in spina bifida.
(Image provided by Departments of Radiology and Obstetrics & Gynecology, University of California, San Francisco.)

there may be complete disuse of the lower extremities, as well as lack of bowel or bladder control. Currently, there is a trial under way to see if in utero surgical repair can help those who are severely affected.

CARDIAC DEFECTS

Whereas the heart is merely a four-chamber pump, there are a number of ways to change the structure that can lead to some interesting pathophysiology. Cardiac development begins during week 3 after conception when an angiogenic cell cluster forms at the anterior central portion of the embryo. As the embryo folds cephalocaudally, the cardiogenic area also folds into a heart tube. Even at this early stage, the embryonic heart tube is already receiving venous flow from its caudal end and pumping blood through the first aortic arch and into the dorsal aorta. Simultaneously, mesoderm around the endocardial tube forms the three layers of the heart wall composed of an outer epicardium, a muscular wall of myocardium, and the endocardium that is the internal endothelial lining. Between days 23 and 28, the heart tube elongates and bends to create the cardiac loop with a common atrium and a narrow atrioventricular junction connecting it to the primitive ventricle. The bulbus cordis is the caudal section of the heart tube and will eventually form three structures: the proximal third will form the trabeculated part of the right ventricle, the midportion (conus cordis) will form the outflow tracts of the ventricles, and the distal segment (truncus arteriosus) will eventually give rise to the proximal portions of the aorta and pulmonary artery (Fig. 3-5).

Between days 27 and 37, the heart continues to develop through the formation of the major septa. Septum formation is achieved via the formation of tissue, called endocardial cushions, which subdivide the lumen into two cavities. The right and left atria are created by the formation of the septum primum and septum secundum that subdivides the primitive atrium while allowing for an interatrial opening (foramen ovale) to continue the right-to-left shunting of blood. At the end of week 4, endocardial cushions also appear in the atrioventricular canal to form the right and left canals as well as the mitral and tricuspid valves. During this time, the medial walls of the ventricles gradually fuse together to form the muscular interventricular septum. The conus cordis comprises the middle third of the bulbis cordis and, during week 5 of development, cushions subdivide the conus to form the outflow tract of the right and left ventricle as well as the membranous portion of the interventricular septum. Cushions also appear in the truncus arteriosus (distal third of bulbus cordis) and grow in a spiral pattern to form the aorticopulmonary septum and divide the truncus into the aortic and pulmonary tracts.

Any of these points of development can go awry leading to disastrous complications. For example, if the ventricular walls fail to fuse, there is a VSD that, if not repaired, can lead to Eisenmenger physiology;

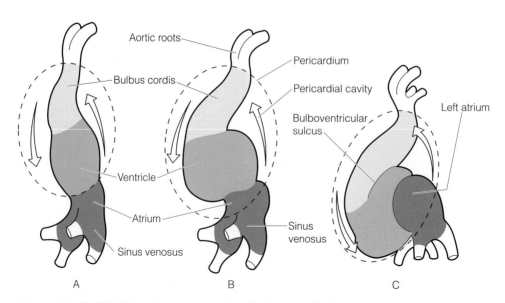

Figure 3-5 • (A–C) Folding of the heart tube into the four-chamber heart.

that is, right ventricular hypertrophy, pulmonary hypertension, and a right-to-left shunt. A commonly seen constellation of cardiac findings is tetralogy of Fallot. This is a VSD with an overriding aorta, pulmonary stenosis (or atresia), and right ventricular hypertrophy. Just as the chambers and valves can be anomalous, so can the great vessels as seen in transposition of the vessels (TOV), where the pulmonary artery and the aorta are connected to the wrong ventricles. Other common anomalies of vessels are coarctation of the aorta, an atretic portion prior to the insertion of the ductus arteriosus; and a patent ductus arteriosus (PDA), which can also lead to Eisenmenger physiology.

Diagnosis of these anomalies varies widely and depends on the lesion and the quality of the sonologist or sonographer imaging the fetal heart. Some of the more common lesions will be identified by the standard four-chamber view of the heart, but many— including coarctation of the aorta, VSD, and ASD—often will not. Outcomes of these congenital anomalies are quite variable. Most of these may be surgically repaired, although hypoplastic left heart, in particular, can have high mortality at a young age.

POTTER SYNDROME

Potter syndrome results from renal failure leading to anhydramnios, which in turn causes pulmonary hypoplasia and contractures in the fetus. Potter disease is bilateral renal agenesis. However, a fetus can also develop renal failure if there is distal obstruction of the urinary system as with posterior urethral valves. To better understand the etiology of this system, we should consider its embryology.

The kidneys are formed from intermediate mesoderm. Kidney development begins in week 4 with the formation of the first of three kidney scaffolds that arise and regress sequentially before the permanent kidney develops. This first scaffold is the pronephros, which is nonfunctional. In week 5 the *meso*nephros develops and functions briefly, creating the *meso*nephric duct (wolffian duct). The ureteric bud is an offshoot of the mesonephric duct that dilates and subdivides to form the urinary collecting system (collecting tubules, calyces, renal pelvis, and ureter) in both males and females. In the presence of testosterone, the mesonephric duct in males also forms the vas deferens, epididymis, ejaculatory duct, and seminal vesicles. In females, it degenerates entirely except for the vestigial Gartner's duct that can form a benign cyst along the broad ligament. The third scaffold—

the *meta*nephros—also appears in week 5 of gestation and becomes the functioning kidney by week 9 of gestation. The ureteric bud from the *meso*nephric duct contacts the *meta*nephros and induces it to form nephrons. If this contact does not occur, renal agenesis results. The adjacent dorsal aorta also sends out collaterals into the *meta*nephros that ultimately develop into glomerular tufts.

Before week 7, the cloaca (the proximal portion of the allantois distally connected to the yolk sac) is divided into the urogenital (UG) sinus and the anorectal canal. During this process, the caudal-most portion of the mesonephric duct is absorbed. Thus, the ureteric bud no longer buds off of the mesonephric duct but enters the UG sinus directly. As such, the UG sinus forms the bladder and the ureteric buds form the ureters. The UG sinus forms the bladder and is continuous with the urethra caudally and the allantois cranially. The urachus is the fibrotic cord that remains when the allantois is obliterated and becomes the median umbilical ligament in the adult.

There are many renal anomalies (e.g., horseshoe kidney, ectopic kidney, double ureter) that go undiagnosed and are without much consequence. Renal agenesis, however, is not one of these. Without kidneys, the fetus can still excrete waste via placental exchange, however, it essentially has anhydramnios. Without amniotic fluid, the fetal lungs do not have constant pressure on them causing them to expand and grow. This leads to pulmonary hypoplasia. Without amniotic fluid, the fetus cannot move much, so develops dramatic contractures of the limbs. There have been attempts to put amniotic fluid into the amniotic cavity via amniocentesis. However, this has been unsuccessful because the fluid is resorbed rapidly. An indwelling catheter has also been considered, but the infectious risks are quite high. At this point in time, there is minimal treatment available for Potter disease. However, in Potter syndrome secondary to bladder outlet obstruction, there have been attempts to place catheters into the bladder or to perform in utero laser ablation of the obstruction. In theory, as long as the fetal kidneys have not been damaged, this idea should work. However, the results thus far are mixed.

PRENATAL SCREENING

Screening for fetal chromosomal and congenital anomalies is dependent on developing screens that are both sensitive and specific for the condition being

■ **TABLE 3-1** Epidemiology		
	Screen Positive (Pos)	**Screen Negative (Neg)**
Affected	a	b
Not affected	c	d

Sensitivity (sens) = a/(a + b); Specificity (spec) = d/(c + d); False negative = b/(a + b); False positive = c/(c + d); Positive predictive value (PPV) = a/(a + c); Negative predictive value (NPV) = d/(b + d); Positive likelihood ratio (LR+) = sens/(1 − spec) = [a/(a+b)]/[c/(c+d)]; Negative likelihood ratio (LR−) = (1 − sens)/spec = [b/(a+b)]/[d/(c+d)].

screened. Before we move on to discuss these modalities, we should quickly review the terms used with screening tests.

EPIDEMIOLOGY

The classic two-by-two table in epidemiology is divided into cases and controls versus exposed and unexposed. In screening tests, the two dimensions are affected/not affected versus screen positive/screen negative (Table 3-1).

As can be seen in Table 3-1, the sensitivity is the proportion of those who are affected and test positive. On the other hand, the specificity is that proportion of individuals who are unaffected and test negative. Sometimes we are more interested in what it means to have a particular test result. In this setting, the positive predictive value (PPV) reports what percentage of patients with a positive screen is af-

fected. The negative predictive value (NPV) is the percentage of people with a negative screen who indeed are not affected. Another set of useful test characteristics are likelihood ratios. The positive likelihood ratio (LR) tells how much to multiply the prior odds to get the posterior odds; that is, if one knows the odds of some event occurring is 1:100, and runs a test with an LR of 5, then the odds after getting a positive result is 5:100. Similarly, the negative likelihood ratio (LR) does the same for a negative result.

FIRST-TRIMESTER SCREENING

First trimester was traditionally the time for the first prenatal visit and to check labs. However, there has recently been increasing interest and research in first-trimester serum and ultrasound screening for aneuploidy for two theoretical benefits. One is to find screening tests that are more sensitive than the current second-trimester tests. The other is that by making the diagnosis sooner, the option of termination is safer. **Nuchal translucency** (NT) appears to be an excellent way to screen for aneuploidy and Down syndrome in particular. NT involves a measurement of the posterior fetal neck taken in profile view (Fig. 3-6). Its sensitivity for Down syndrome has been reported to be between 60% and 90% and is generally assumed to be about 70% or greater.

Several maternal serum analytes have been studied to generate a first-trimester serum screen. Currently, a combination of free β-hCG and PAPP-A (pregnancy-associated plasma protein A) is being studied

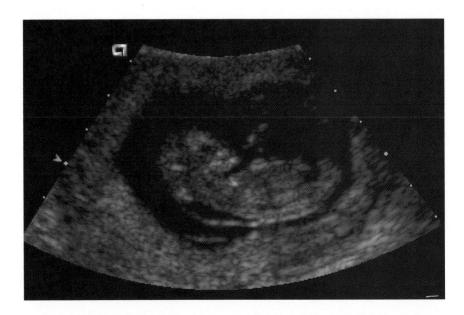

Figure 3-6 • Posterior fetal neck, posterior view.

■ TABLE 3-2 Triple Screen Table			
	Trisomy 21	Trisomy 18	Trisomy 13
MSAFP	Decreased	Decreased	Depends on defects
Estriol	Decreased	Decreased	Depends on defects
β-hCG	Elevated	Decreased	Depends on defects

alone and in combination with NT. Using a 5% false-positive rate, they appear to have a sensitivity of approximately 60% when used alone and, when combined, the two appear to give an approximate sensitivity of 80%. Commonly, thresholds for these tests are established at a 5% false-positive rate, or where the posterior probability of disease is somewhere between 1:190 and 1:300.

SECOND-TRIMESTER SCREENING

The initial second-trimester serum screen was the MSAFP. This was designed to screen for fetuses with neural tube defects (NTDs). When the data from studies was being analyzed it was noted that the cases of Down syndrome had low MSAFP. This has been combined with low serum estriol and high β-hCG as the triple screen (Table 3-2). Overall, the triple screen had only a 60% sensitivity for Down syndrome with a 5% false-positive rate. Maternal age is essentially another screening tool because it has been found that the risk of aneuploidy increases exponentially beyond age 35 (Fig. 3-7). At age 35, the overall risk is about 1:190 of aneuploidy. The triple screen is combined with maternal age to generate an overall risk profile of both Down syndrome and trisomy 18. Among women over 35, the triple screen has a sensitivity of 80%, whereas in women under age 35, the sensitivity drops to about 50%. More recently, a fourth serum analyte, inhibin A, has been added to the triple screen to be used as a quad screen. The quad screen has improved sensitivity approaching 80% at a 5% false-positive rate, and its use is expanding. One advantage of the quad screen over the first trimester screens is that specially trained ultrasound technologists and sonologists are not necessary for performing the test.

Another finding from studies of MSAFP has been in patients whose MSAFP was elevated, but did not have an open NTD. Common reasons for this include inaccurate dating (MSAFP increases with gestation), abdominal wall defects, multiple gestations, and fetal demise. Patients whose MSAFP is elevated without an elevated amniotic fluid AFP or these other etiolo-

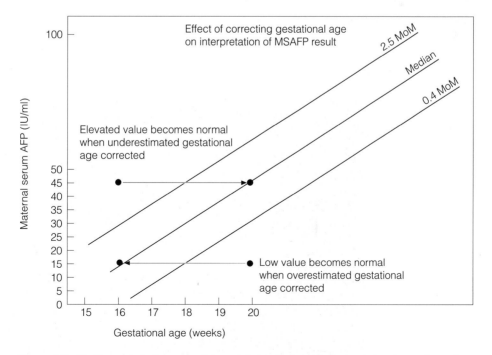

Figure 3-7 • Median maternal serum α-fetoprotein levels throughout gestation. Increasing values with increasing gestational age require accurate dating to interpret low or high MSAFP.

gies have been found to be at greater risk of pregnancy complications associated with the placenta: placental abruption, preeclampsia, IUGR, and possibly IUFD. These problems have been associated with elevated β-hCG as well.

Real-time ultrasound is used to document a singleton, viable gestation and a rudimentary anatomy scan in more than 90% of pregnancies in the United States. The level-I obstetric ultrasound scan is a fair screening tool, but its sensitivity varies between providers. One study showed that there was a two- to threefold difference in the number of anomalies identified between primary and tertiary medical centers. The level-I ultrasound is not designed to be all encompassing and does not look at fetal limbs, identify sex, show the face, or provide extensive views of the heart. These are generally all done in a level-II or targeted ultrasound. A level-II ultrasound is utilized in patients who are at risk for congenital anomalies or who have had an abnormal level-I scan. These tests are generally performed by specially trained perinatologists or radiologists.

There are a number of "soft" findings on obstetric ultrasound that have been associated with aneuploidies. Trisomy 18 has been associated with the finding of a choroid plexus cyst, and Down syndrome has been associated with many ultrasound findings, most notably the **echogenic intracardiac focus** (EIF). Pathologically, the EIF (Fig. 3-8) is a calcification of the papillary muscle without any particular pathophysiology. It is seen in 5% of pregnancies and is more common in the fetuses of Asian women. Unfortunately, the LR for this test is 1.5 to 2.0, so it at most doubles the pretest odds. For example, a young, 25-year-old woman whose Down syndrome risk is 1:1,000 prior to finding the EIF will therefore have an "increased" risk of 1:500 after finding the EIF. Thus, these tests end up needlessly worrying many patients only to identify a few abnormal fetuses.

PRENATAL DIAGNOSIS

In patients who are known carriers of a genetic disease, at high risk for aneuploidy based on age, or who have a positive screening test, the next step is to obtain prenatal diagnosis. This involves obtaining fetal cells in order to perform a karyotype and possibly DNA tests. There are currently three ways that fetal cells are obtained: amniocentesis, CVS, and percutaneous umbilical blood sampling (PUBS).

AMNIOCENTESIS

An amniocentesis may be performed beyond 15 weeks to obtain a fetal karyotype, once the chorion and amnion have fused. Amniocentesis is also offered to any patient of advanced maternal age (AMA). **Amniocentesis** involves placing a needle transabdominally through the uterus into the amniotic sac and withdrawing some of the fluid. The fluid contains sloughed fetal cells that can be cultured. These cultured cells can then be karyotyped and also utilized in DNA tests.

The cultures take about 5 to 7 days to grow, but a newer technique—**fluorescent in-situ hybridization** (FISH)—can be used to identify aneuploidy and gets results in 24 to 48 hours. Generally, the risk of complications secondary to amniocentesis is considered to be about 1:200, but more recent studies indicate a lower risk. The common risks are rupture of membranes, preterm labor, and, rarely, fetal injury. This risk of 1:200 is one of the reasons why the threshold risk for offering patients fetal diagnosis is about 1:200, which is roughly equivalent to age 35. While it is true that the numbers are the same, the outcomes—Down syndrome and miscarriage—are quite different. Thus, there has been a recent push to discard the maternal age 35 threshold in favor of counseling patients regarding their risk and allowing them

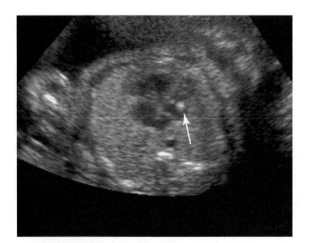

Figure 3-8 • Echogenic intracardiac focus (EIF).
(Image provided by Departments of Radiology and Obstetrics & Gynecology, University of California, San Francisco.)

to make their own decision incorporating risks and benefits of screening and diagnosis.

CHORIONIC VILLUS SAMPLING

Chorionic villus sampling (CVS) can be used to obtain a fetal karyotype sooner than amniocentesis because it can be performed between 9 and 12 weeks. CVS involves placing a catheter into the intrauterine cavity, either transabdominally or transvaginally, and aspirating a small quantity of chorionic villi from the placenta. The risk of complications from CVS is likely higher than the amniocentesis rate of 1:200. Because a greater amount of cells are obtained, CVS results are often faster than those of amniocentesis. However, the cells are from the placenta; therefore, in rare cases of confined placental mosaicism, the cells may be misleading. Complications include preterm labor, premature rupture of membranes, previable delivery, and fetal injury. When performed earlier than 9 weeks of gestation, CVS has been associated with limb anomalies, which is assumed to be secondary to vascular interruption.

FETAL BLOOD SAMPLING

PUBS is performed by placing a needle transabdominally into the uterus and phlebotomizing the umbilical cord. This procedure may be used when a fetal hematocrit needs to be obtained, particularly in the setting of Rh alloimmunization and other causes of fetal anemia. PUBS is also used for rapid karyotype analysis. Because the amount of fetal cells in a PUBS is so high, there is no need to culture the cells prior to analysis. The PUBS needle can also be used to transfuse the fetus in cases of fetal anemia. Intrauterine transfusion (IUT) was performed before the advent of real-time ultrasound by placing needles into the fetal peritoneal cavity and performing intraperitoneal transfusions, but transumbilical transfusions are more effective.

FETAL IMAGING

Currently, ultrasound is used most commonly to image a fetus prenatally. As described above, a level-I ultrasound is commonly performed between 18 and 22 weeks. The fetal anatomy can be difficult to visualize well prior to 18 weeks of gestation, giving the lower threshold. For the upper threshold, if an anomaly is seen, the further workup can take more than a week, giving the patient just a few days prior to 24 weeks of gestation to decide about termination of the pregnancy in the setting of congenital anomalies. A targeted, level-II ultrasound can identify cleft lip, polydactyly, clubfoot (Fig. 3-9), fetal sex, NTDs, abdominal wall defects, and renal anomalies. It can usually identify cardiac and brain anomalies as well, but may not be able to make a specific diagnosis. It is poor at identifying esophageal atresia and tracheoesophageal fistula, in which sometimes the only sign may be a small or nonvisualized stomach in the setting of polyhydramnios.

Fetal echocardiogram is usually used to make specific diagnoses of fetal cardiac anomalies detected on ultrasound. Doppler ultrasound can characterize the blood flow through the chambers of the heart as well as the vessels entering and leaving the heart. Fetal echo is used in some institutions as the first line diagnostic modality in patients at high risk for cardiac anomalies, in particular, pregestational diabetic patients.

Fetal MRI is one of the newest modalities to image a fetus. It is particularly useful in examining the fetal brain and recognizes hypoxic damage sooner than ultrasound. It is also superior in measuring volumes. Another new modality that may be better in measuring volumes is three-dimensional (3-D) ultrasound. While the image provided certainly looks more like an actual fetus than the more common 2-D images, it is unclear whether 3-D ultrasound offers increased diagnostic capabilities.

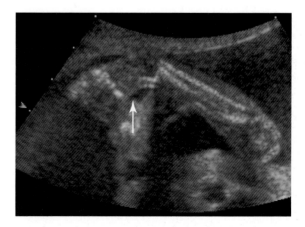

Figure 3-9 • Clubfoot—The fibula and tibia can be seen with the foot at almost a right angle to them.
(Image provided by Departments of Radiology and Obstetrics & Gynecology, University of California, San Francisco.)

KEY POINTS

- Mothers can be asymptomatic carriers of autosomal recessive diseases and can often be screened for carrier status.

- If a mother is a carrier, the father of the baby can be screened as well to determine his carrier status. If the father is negative, there is no risk to the baby; if he is positive, there is a 25% chance of the disease in the fetus.

- Two common ways that AR disorders are introduced and maintained in a population is by the founder effect (Tay-Sachs) and heterozygote advantage (sickle-cell disease).

- Having an abnormal number of chromosomes usually leads to miscarriage. However, several aneuploidies exist that commonly survive until birth and beyond.

- Of all the autosomal trisomies, Down syndrome is the hardiest. While they have foreshortened life expectancies, these individuals commonly survive into their 50s.

- The most common aneuploidies are those of the sex chromosomes. These individuals are less severely affected than the autosomal aneuploidies.

- Fetal congenital anomalies primarily arise during embryogenesis. However, they can progress (as seen in Potter syndrome) as development continues.

- NTDs are associated with folate deficiency and can be screened for by noting an elevated MSAFP.

- Cardiac anomalies that are surgically repaired can often result in minimal impairment, although this is highly lesion dependent.

- Organ systems are often interconnected during development, as in the case of the lungs and kidneys in Potter syndrome.

- The sensitivity of a screening test is that percentage of patients who would be identified by the test.

- Common screening tests for fetal abnormalities include the quad screen and level-I ultrasound.

- Karyotype and DNA tests require fetal or trophoblastic cells for analysis.

- Fetal diagnosis in the first trimester is by CVS, which obtains trophoblastic cells.

- In the second trimester, amniocentesis is used to obtain fetal cells in the amniotic fluid.

- Prenatal diagnosis can also be made by imaging studies, most commonly 2-D ultrasound. Fetal echocardiogram, MRI, and 3-D ultrasound are also used.

Normal Labor and Delivery

LABOR AND DELIVERY

When a patient first presents to the labor floor, a quick initial assessment is made using the history of present pregnancy, obstetric history, and the standard medical and social history. Routinely, patients are queried regarding contractions, vaginal bleeding, leakage of fluid, and fetal movement. Beyond the standard physical examination, the obstetric examination includes maternal abdominal examination for contractions and the fetus (**Leopold maneuvers**), cervical examination, fetal heart tones, and a sterile speculum examination if rupture of membranes is suspected.

OBSTETRIC EXAMINATION

The physical examination includes determination of fetal lie and presentation and a cervical examination. **Fetal lie**, that is, whether the infant is longitudinal or transverse within the uterus, is relatively easy to determine with Leopold maneuvers (Fig. 4-1). The maneuvers involve palpating first at the fundus of the uterus in the maternal upper abdominal quadrants, then on either side of the uterus (maternal left and right), and finally, palpation of the presenting part just above the pubic symphysis. Determination of **fetal presentation**, either breech or vertex (cephalic), can be more difficult, and even the most experienced examiner may require ultrasound to confirm presentation.

RUPTURE OF MEMBRANES

In 10% of pregnancies, the membranes surrounding the fetus rupture at least 1 hour prior to the onset of labor; this is called premature rupture of membranes (PROM). When PROM occurs more than 18 hours before labor, it is considered prolonged PROM and puts both mother and fetus at increased risk for infection. PROM is often confused with PPROM, which is preterm, premature rupture of membranes, with preterm being before 37 weeks of gestation.

Diagnosis

Diagnosis of rupture of membranes (ROM) is suspected with a history of a gush or leaking of fluid from the vagina, although sometimes it is difficult to differentiate between stress incontinence and small leaks of amniotic fluid. Diagnosis can be confirmed by the **pool**, **nitrazine**, and **fern** tests.

Using a sterile speculum to examine the vaginal vault, the pool test is positive if there is a collection of fluid in the vagina. This can be augmented by asking the patient to cough or bear down, potentially allowing one to observe fluid escaping from the cervix. Vaginal secretions are normally acidic, whereas amniotic fluid is alkaline. Thus, when the fluid is placed on nitrazine paper, the paper should immediately turn blue. The estrogens in the amniotic fluid cause crystallization of the salts in the amniotic fluid when it dries. Under low microscopic power, the crystals resemble the blades of a fern, giving the test its name (Fig. 4-2). Caution should be exercised to sample fluid that is not directly from the cervix because cervical mucus also ferns and may result in a false-positive reading. If these tests are equivocal, an ultrasound examination can determine the quantity of fluid around the infant. If fluid volume was previously normal and there is no other

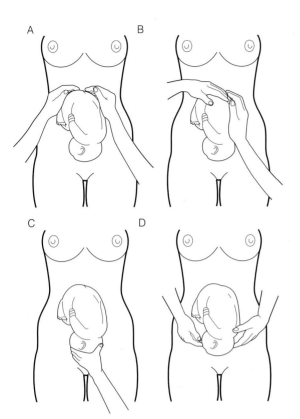

Figure 4-1 • **(A–D)** Leopold maneuvers used to determine fetal presentation, position, and engagement.

reason to suspect low fluid, **oligohydramnios** is indicative of ROM. In situations when an accurate diagnosis is necessary (e.g., PPROM where antibiotic prophylaxis would be indicated), amniocentesis may be used to inject dilute indigo carmine dye into the amniotic sac to look for leakage of fluid from the cervix onto a tampon (the amnio dye test or tampon test). More recently, a rapid test called Amnisure has

been described, which utilizes rapid molecular testing to identify placental alpha-microglobulin-1 via immunoassay, which appears to have a higher sensitivity and specificity than conventional tests for PROM. The clinical utility and cost-effectiveness of utilizing this test require further research.

CERVICAL EXAMINATION

The cervical examination allows the obstetrician to determine whether a patient is in labor, the phase of labor, and how labor is progressing. The five components of the cervical examination are dilation, effacement, fetal station, cervical position, and consistency of the cervix. These five aspects of the examination make up the **Bishop score** (Table 4-1). A Bishop score greater than 8 is consistent with a cervix favorable for both spontaneous labor and, as it is more commonly used, induced labor.

Dilation is assessed by using either one or two fingers of the examining hand to determine how open the cervix is at the level of the **internal os**. The measurements are in centimeters and range from closed, or 0 cm, to fully dilated, or 10 cm. On average, a 10-cm dilation is necessary to accommodate the term infant's biparietal diameter.

Effacement is also a subjective measurement made by the examiner. It determines how much length is left of the cervix and how effaced (i.e., thinned out) it is (Fig. 4-3). Effacement can commonly be reported by percent or by cervical length. The typical cervix is 3 to 5 cm in length; thus, if the cervix feels like it is about 2 cm from external to internal os, it is 50% effaced. Complete or 100% effacement occurs when the cervix is as thin as the adjoining lower uterine segment.

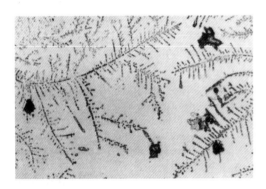

Figure 4-2 • Fern test.
(From Beckmann CRB, Ling LW, Laube DW, et al. *Obstetrics and Gynecology*, 4th ed. Baltimore: Lippincott Williams & Wilkins, 2002.)

■ **TABLE 4-1** The Bishop Score				
Score	**0**	**1**	**2**	**3**
Cervical dilation (cm)	Closed	1 to 2	3 to 4	<5
Cervical effacement (%)	0 to 30	40 to 50	60 to 70	<80
Station	−3	−2	−1, 0	<+1
Cervical consistency	Firm	Medium	Soft	
Cervical position	Posterior	Mid	Anterior	

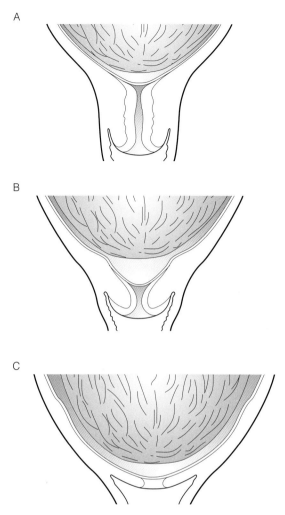

A

B

C

Figure 4-3 • (A) The absence of cervical effacement prior to labor. **(B)** The cervix is approximately 50% effaced. **(C)** The cervix is as thin as the adjoining lower uterine segment, 100% effaced.

The relation of the fetal head to the ischial spines of the female pelvis is known as **station** (Fig. 4-4). When the most descended aspect of the presenting part is at the level of the ischial spines, it is designated 0 station. Station is negative when the presenting part is above the ischial spines and positive when it is below. There are two systems of measuring the distance of the presenting part in relation to the ischial spines. One divides the distance to the pelvic inlet into thirds and thus station is −3 to 0 and then 0 to 3, which is at the level of the introitus. The other system uses centimeters, which gives stations of −5 to +5. Either system is effective and both are widely used among different institutions, however, the American College of Obstetricians and Gynecologists (ACOG)

recommends the usage of the (5) system in its clinical guidelines.

Cervical **consistency** is self-explanatory. Whether the cervix feels firm, soft, or somewhere in between should be noted. Cervical **position** ranges from posterior to mid to anterior. A posterior cervix is high in the pelvis, located behind the fetal head and often quite difficult to reach, let alone examine. The anterior cervix can usually be felt easily on examination and is often lower down in the vagina. During early labor, the cervix often changes its consistency to soft and advances its position from posterior to mid to anterior.

FETAL PRESENTATION AND POSITION

The fetal presentation can be **vertex** (head down), **breech** (buttocks down), or **transverse** (neither down). Although presentation may already be known from the Leopold maneuvers, it can be confirmed by examination of the presenting part during cervical examination. Assuming that the cervix is somewhat dilated, the fetal presenting part may be palpated as well during this examination. In the early stages of labor when the cervix is not very dilated, digital exam of the presenting part can be difficult, leading to inaccurate determination of presentation. However, palpation of hair or sutures on the fetal vertex or the gluteal cleft or anus on the breech usually leaves little doubt. A fetus presenting head-first should actually be designated cephalic rather than vertex, unless the head is flexed and the vertex is truly presenting. If the fetus is cephalic with an extended head, it may be presenting with either the face or brow. If the fetal vertex is presenting along with a fetal extremity such as an arm, this is deemed a compound presentation.

With face presentations, the chin or mentum is the fetal reference point, while with breech presentations the reference is the fetal sacrum (Fig. 4-5). If fetal presentation cannot be determined by physical examination, ultrasound can confirm presentation. Ultrasound is also useful in determining whether a breech presentation is frank, complete, or footling. Breech presentations are discussed further in Chapter 6.

Fetal **position** in the vertex presentation is usually based on the relationship of the fetal occiput to the maternal pelvis. An abnormal fetal position such as OT or OP can lead to prolonged labor and a higher rate of cesarean delivery. Thus, OT or OP position may be suspected with an abnormally long

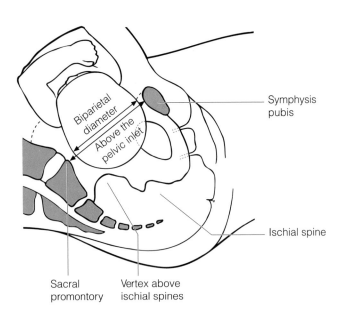

Figure 4-4 • The relationship of the leading edge of the presenting part of the ischial spine determines the station. +1 station is depicted in the frontal view on the left; approximately −2 station is depicted in the lateral view on the right.

labor. Position is determined by palpation of the sutures and fontanelles. The vault, or roof, of the fetal skull is composed of five bones: two frontal, two parietal, and one occipital. The **anterior fontanelle** is the junction between the two frontal bones and two parietal bones and is larger and diamond-shaped. The **posterior fontanelle** is the junction between the two parietal bones and the occipital bone and is smaller and more triangular-shaped. In the setting of extensive molding of the fetal skull or asynclitism, where the sagittal suture is not midline within the maternal pelvis, palpation of the fetal ear can be used to determine position. Ultrasound can also be useful in determining fetal position on labor and delivery and is noted to be more accurate than vaginal exam.

NORMAL LABOR

Labor is defined as contractions that cause cervical change in either effacement or dilation. **Prodromal labor** or "false labor" is common in the differential diagnosis of labor. These patients usually present with irregular contractions that vary in duration, intensity, and intervals and yield little or no cervical change.

The diagnosis of labor strictly defined is regular uterine contractions that cause cervical change. However, clinicians use many other signs of labor, including patient discomfort, bloody show, nausea and vomiting, and palpability of contractions. These signs and symptoms vary from patient to patient; although they can add to the assessment, clinicians should rely on an objective definition.

INDUCTION AND AUGMENTATION OF LABOR

Induction of labor is the attempt to begin labor in a nonlaboring patient, whereas **augmentation of labor** is intervening to increase the already present contractions. Labor is induced with **prostaglandins, oxytocic agents**, mechanical dilation of the cervix, and/or **artificial rupture of membranes**. The indications for induction are based on either maternal, fetal, or fetoplacental reasons. Common indications for induction of labor include postterm pregnancy, preeclampsia, premature ROM, nonreassuring fetal testing, and intrauterine growth restriction. The patient's desire to end the pregnancy is *not* an indication for induction of labor, but would be deemed elective induction of labor.

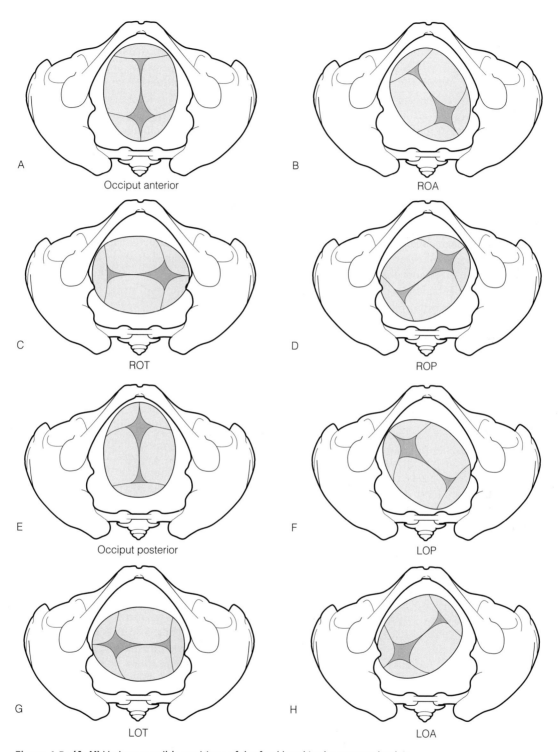

A — Occiput anterior

B — ROA

C — ROT

D — ROP

E — Occiput posterior

F — LOP

G — LOT

H — LOA

Figure 4-5 • (A–H) Various possible positions of the fetal head in the maternal pelvis.

Preparing for Induction

When proper indications for induction exist, the situation should be discussed with the patient and a plan for induction formed. When the indication is more pressing, induction should be started without significant delay. The success of an induction (defined as achieving vaginal delivery) is often correlated with favorable cervical status as defined by the **Bishop score**. A Bishop score of 5 or less may lead to a failed induction as often as 50% of the time. In these patients, prostaglandin E_2 (PGE_2) gel, PGE_2 pessary (cervidil), or PGE_1M (misoprostol) is often used to "ripen" the cervix. The use of cervical ripening agents with prostaglandins or a mechanical means to dilate the cervix can reduce the risk of cesarean delivery.

There are both maternal and obstetric contraindications for the use of prostaglandins. Maternal reasons include asthma and glaucoma. Obstetric reasons include having had more than one prior cesarean section and nonreassuring fetal testing. Because PGE_2 gel cannot be turned off with the ease of oxytocin, there is a risk of uterine hyperstimulation and tetanic contractions. In this setting, a mechanical dilator such as a 30 cc or 60 cc Foley bulb can be used. The Foley is placed inside the cervix adjacent to the amniotic sac, inflated, and placed on gentle traction. It usually dilates the cervix to 2 to 3 cm within 4 to 6 hours.

Induction

Labor may begin with the ripening and dilation of the cervix performed with prostaglandins or mechanical means. However, labor induction is usually formally begun pharmacologically with oxytocin (Pitocin). This is a synthesized, but identical, version of the octapeptide oxytocin normally released from the posterior pituitary that causes uterine contractions. Pitocin is given continuously via IV since it is rapidly metabolized.

Labor may also be induced by **amniotomy**. Amniotomy is performed with an amnio hook that is used to puncture the amniotic sac around the fetus and release some of the amniotic fluid. After the amniotomy is performed, a careful examination should be performed to ensure that prolapse of the umbilical cord has not occurred. When performing amniotomy, it is important not to elevate the fetal head from the pelvis to release more of the amniotic fluid because this may lead to prolapse of the umbilical cord beyond the fetal head.

Augmentation

Pitocin and amniotomy are also used to augment labor. The indications for augmentation of labor include those for induction in addition to inadequate contractions or a prolonged phase of labor. The adequacy of contractions is indirectly assessed by the progress of cervical change. It may also be measured directly using an **intrauterine pressure catheter (IUPC)** that determines the absolute change in pressure during a contraction and thus estimates the strength of contractions. Aggressive augmentation, deemed active management of labor, which involves both ocytocin and amniotomy has been demonstrated to lead to shorter labor courses, but no difference in cesarean delivery rates.

MONITORING OF THE FETUS IN LABOR

It is easy to monitor the mother in labor with vital signs and laboratory studies. Monitoring the infant is indirect and thus more difficult than maternal assessment. Determination of the baseline rate and assessment of fetal heart rate variations with contractions can be done by auscultation. The normal range for the fetal heart rate is between 110 and 160 beats per minute. With baselines above 160, fetal distress secondary to infection, hypoxia, or anemia is of concern. Any bradycardia of greater than 2 minutes' duration with a heart rate less than 90 is of concern and requires immediate action.

External Electronic Monitors

Since the advent of electronic fetal monitoring, auscultation is rarely used. Continuous fetal heart monitors are standard in most hospitals in the United States because they afford several advantages over auscultation. The information gathered is more subtle and includes variations in heart rate. Probably the greatest advantage is that the information is easier to gather and record, thus allowing more time for analyzing the data and has economic advantages as one nurse can readily monitor multiple patients.

The external tocometer has a pressure transducer that is placed against the patient's abdomen, usually near the fundus of the uterus. During uterine contractions, the abdomen becomes firmer, and this pressure is transmitted through the transducer to a tocometer that records the contraction. The relative heights of the tracings on different patients or at different locations on the same patient cannot be used to compare strength of contractions. External tocometers are most useful for measuring the frequency of contractions and comparing to the fetal heart rate tracing to determine the type of decelerations occurring.

A fetal heart rate tracing is examined for several characteristics that are considered reassuring. First, the baseline is determined and should be in the normal range (110 to 160 beats per minute). Then the variations from the baseline should be examined. The moment to moment variation from the baseline is called fetal heart rate variability. Fetal heart rate variability is defined as absent (<3 beats per minute of variation), minimal (3 to 5 beats per minute of variation), moderate (5 to 25 beats per minute of variation), and marked (more than 25 beats per minute of variation). The tracing should be jagged from the beat-to-beat variability of the heart rate.

While a fetal heart rate tracing with minimal variability is not reassuring, this may also occur while the fetus is asleep or inactive. A flat tracing with absent variability is more worrisome and demands that another test to determine fetal well-being be conducted. There should also be at least three to five cycles per minute of the heart rate around the baseline. Finally, a tracing can be considered formally reactive (Fig. 4-6) if there are at least two accelerations of at least 15 beats per minute over the baseline that last for at least 15 seconds within 20 minutes.

Decelerations of the Fetal Heart Rate

The fetal heart rate tracing should also be used to examine decelerations (decels) and can be used along with the tocometer to determine the type and severity. There are three types of decelerations: early, variable, and late. **Early decelerations** begin

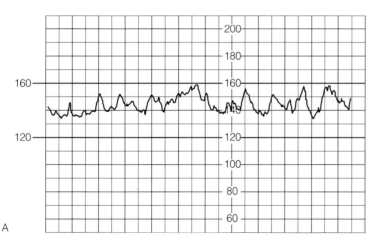

A

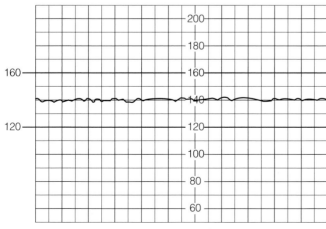

B

Figure 4-6 · **(A)** Normal short- and long-term beat-to-beat variability. **(B)** Reduced variability. This may occur during fetal sleep, following maternal intake of drugs, or with reduced fetal CNS function, as in asphyxia.

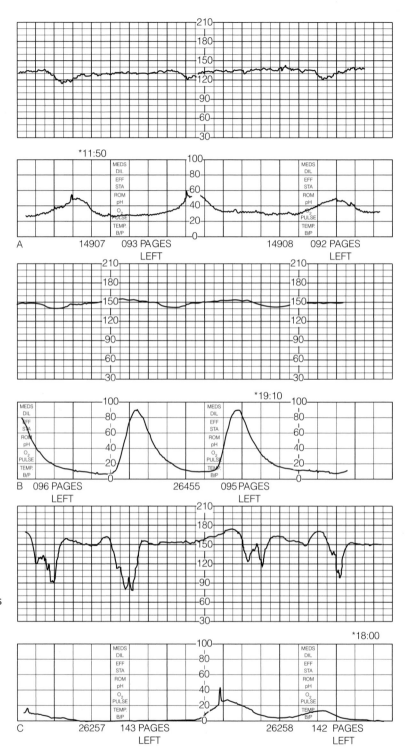

Figure 4-7 • **(A)** An early deceleration pattern is depicted in this FHR tracing. Note that each deceleration returns to baseline before the completion of the contraction. The remainder of the FHR tracing is reassuring. **(B)** Repetitive late decelerations in conjunction with decreased variability. **(C)** Variable decelerations are the most common periodic change of the FHR during labor. Repetitive mild to moderate variable decelerations are present. The baseline is normal.

and end approximately at the same time as contractions (Fig. 4-7A). They are a result of increased vagal tone secondary to head compression during a contraction. **Variable decelerations** can occur at any time and tend to drop more precipitously than either early or late decels (Fig. 4-7C). They are a result of umbilical cord compression. Repetitive variables with contractions can be seen when the cord is entrapped either under a fetal shoulder or around the neck and is compressed with each con-

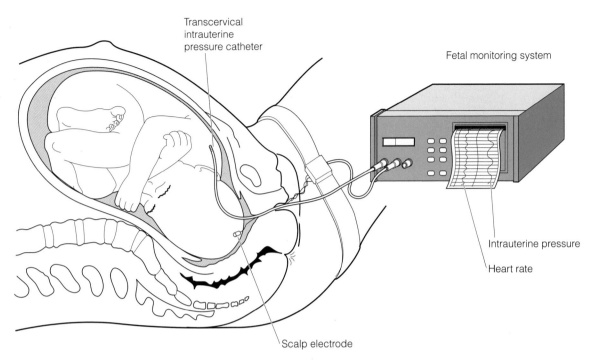

Figure 4-8 • Technique for continuous electronic monitoring of FHR and uterine contractions.

traction. **Late decelerations** begin at the peak of a contraction and slowly return to baseline after the contraction has finished (Fig. 4-7B). These decels are a result of uteroplacental insufficiency and are the most worrisome type. They may degrade into bradycardias as labor progresses, particularly with stronger contractions.

Fetal Scalp Electrode

In the case of repetitive decels or in fetuses who are difficult to trace externally with Doppler, a **fetal scalp electrode** (FSE) is often used. A small electrode is attached to the fetal scalp that senses the potential differences created by the depolarization of the fetal heart. The information obtained from the scalp electrode is more sensitive in terms of the beat-to-beat variability and is in no danger of being lost during contractions as the fetal position changes. Contraindications include a history of maternal hepatitis or human immunodeficiency virus (HIV) or fetal thrombocytopenia.

Intrauterine Pressure Catheter

The external tocometer records the onset and end of contractions. The absolute values of the readings mean little and are entirely position dependent. Further, on some patients—particularly those who are obese—the tocometer does not show much in the way of fluctuation from the baseline. If it is particularly important to determine the timing or strength of contractions, an IUPC may be used (Fig. 4-8). This catheter is threaded past the fetal presenting part into the uterine cavity to measure the pressure changes during contractions. The baseline intrauterine pressure is usually between 10 and 15 mm Hg. Contractions during labor will increase by 20 to 30 mm Hg in early labor and by 40 to 60 mm Hg as labor progresses. The most commonly used measurement of uterine contractions is the **Montevideo unit**, which is an average of the variation of the intrauterine pressure from the baseline multiplied by the number of contractions in a 10-minute period. Some institutions use the Alexandria unit, which multiplies the Montevideo units by the length of each contraction as well.

Fetal Scalp pH and Pulse Oximetry

If a fetal heart rate tracing is nonreassuring, the fetal scalp pH may be obtained to directly assess fetal hypoxia and acidemia (Fig. 4-9). Fetal blood is obtained by making a small nick in the fetal scalp and drawing

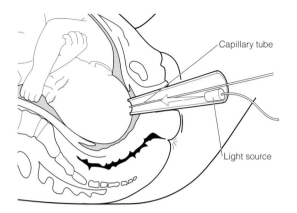

Figure 4-9 • Technique for fetal scalp blood sampling via an amnioscope. After making a small stab incision in the fetal scalp, the blood is drawn off through a capillary tube.

up a small amount of fetal blood into capillary tubes. The results are reassuring when the scalp pH is greater than 7.25, indeterminant between 7.20 and 7.25, and nonreassuring when less than 7.20. Care must be taken to avoid contamination of the blood sample with amniotic fluid, which is basic and will elevate the results falsely. Although this tool is used less frequently now that technology has improved fetal monitoring, it can still provide additional information on fetal well-being.

Another modality for assessing fetal status that is mostly experimental at this point is fetal pulse oximetry. Using technology similar to the monitors placed on ears, fingers, and toes, the fetal pulse oximeter is placed intrauterine along the fetal cheek and measures fetal oxygen saturation. A normal fetal pulse oximeter reading is above 30%. Because fetal variability and decelerations have a poor predictive value of fetal hypoxemia and acidemia, it is theorized that the fetal pulse oximeter would be useful in such patients. An early trial did demonstrate that many of these fetuses with nonreassuring tracings do have normal pulse oximeter readings. However, the use of the pulse oximeter did not have an effect on either the cesarean delivery rate or fetal outcomes. A larger, multicenter study is ongoing.

THE PROGRESSION OF LABOR

Labor is assessed by the progress of cervical effacement, cervical dilation, and descent of the fetal presenting part. To assess the progress of labor, it is important to understand the cardinal movements or mechanisms of labor.

Cardinal Movements of Labor

The cardinal movements are engagement, descent, flexion, internal rotation, extension, and external rotation (also called restitution or resolution) (Fig. 4-10). When the fetal presenting part enters the pelvis, it is said to have undergone **engagement**. The head will then undergo **descent** into the pelvis, followed by **flexion**, which allows the smallest diameter to present to the pelvis. With descent into the midpelvis, the fetal vertex undergoes **internal rotation** from an occiput transverse (OT) position so that the sagittal suture is parallel to the anteroposterior diameter of the pelvis, commonly to the occiput anterior (OA) position. Disruption of the internal rotation or improper rotation can lead to a fetus maintained in OT position or malrotated to the occiput posterior (OP) position. As the vertex passes beneath and beyond the pubic symphysis, it will **extend** to deliver. Once the head delivers, **external rotation** occurs and the shoulders may be delivered.

Stages of Labor

Labor and delivery are divided into three stages. Each stage involves different concerns and considerations. Stage 1 begins with the onset of labor and lasts until dilation and effacement of the cervix are completed. Stage 2 is from the time of full dilation until delivery of the infant. Stage 3 begins after delivery of the infant and ends with delivery of the placenta.

Stage 1

The first stage of labor ranges from the onset of labor until complete dilation of the cervix has occurred. An average first stage of labor lasts approximately 10 to 12 hours in a nulliparous patient and 6 to 8 hours in a multiparous patient. The range of what is considered within normal limits is quite wide, from 6 hours up to 20 hours in a nulliparous patient and from 2 to 12 hours in a multiparous patient. The first stage is divided further into the latent and active phases (Fig. 4-11).

The **latent phase** generally ranges from the onset of labor until 3 or 4 cm of dilation and is characterized by slow cervical change. The **active phase** follows the latent phase and extends until greater than 9 cm of dilation and is defined by the period of time when the slope of cervical change against time increases. A third phase is often delegated at this point called deceleration or transition phase as the cervix completes dilation. During the active phase, at least

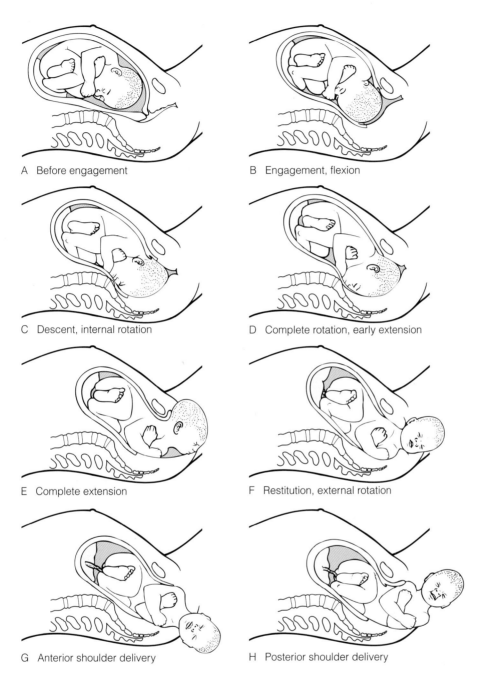

A Before engagement

B Engagement, flexion

C Descent, internal rotation

D Complete rotation, early extension

E Complete extension

F Restitution, external rotation

G Anterior shoulder delivery

H Posterior shoulder delivery

Figure 4-10 • (A–H) Cardinal movements of labor.

1.0 cm/hr of dilation is expected in the nulliparous patient and 1.2 cm/hr in the multiparous patient. This minimal expectation is approximately the fifth percentile of women undergoing labor and the median rates of dilation range from 2.0 to 3.0 cm/hr during the active phase as designated by the Friedman curve. These values of the length of the first stage are primarily derived from studies of labor by Dr. Emmanuel Friedman in the 1950s and 1960s. Studies over the last decade reveal longer first and second stages of labor and variation by maternal race/ethnicity, age, and body habitus.

The three "Ps"—powers, passenger, and pelvis—can all affect the transit time during the active phase of labor. The "powers" are determined by the strength and frequency of uterine contractions. The size and position of the infant affect the duration of the active phase, as do the size and shape of the maternal pelvis. If the "passenger" is too large for the "pelvis" **cephalopelvic disproportion** (CPD) results.

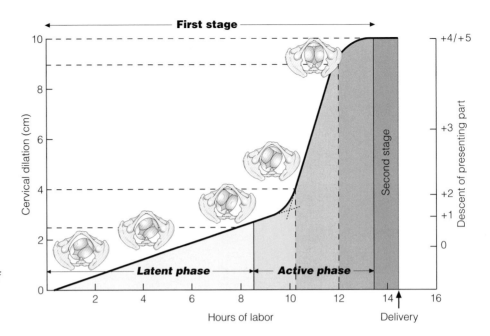

Figure 4-11 • The progress of rotation of OA presentation in the successive stages of labor.

If the rate of change of cervical dilation falls below the fifth percentile (1.0 cm/hr), these three Ps should be assessed to determine whether a vaginal delivery can be expected. Strength of uterine contractions can be measured with an IUPC and is considered adequate with greater than 200 Montevideo units. Signs of CPD include development of fetal caput and extensive molding of the fetal skull with palpable overlapping sutures.

If there is no change in either cervical dilation or station for 2 hours in the setting of adequate Montevideo units during the active phase of labor, this is deemed active phase arrest and is an extremely common indication for cesarean. However, in the past decade, several studies have indicated that if clinicians exhibited more patience in this setting by waiting up to four or more hours to make this diagnosis, that more than half of these women will go on to deliver vaginally. While the issue deserves more research, in a setting with continuous fetal monitoring and no worrisome signs from either the mother or fetus, it appears reasonable to manage such pregnancies expectantly to allow for the possibility of vaginal birth.

Stage 2

When the cervix has completely dilated, stage 2 has begun. Stage 2 is completed with delivery of the infant. Stage 2 is considered prolonged if its duration is longer than 2 hours in a nulliparous patient, although 3 hours are allowed in patients who have epidurals. In multiparous women, stage 2 is prolonged if its duration is longer than 1 hour without an epidural and 2 hours with an epidural. In multiparous women, it is rare for stage 2 to last longer than 30 minutes unless there is fetal macrosomia, persistent occiput posterior or transverse position, compound presentation, or asynclitism. It was commonly perceived that prolonged second stage of labor may lead to worse neonatal outcomes. However, recent studies of the length of the second stage of labor have not actually demonstrated a difference in neonatal outcomes with prolonged second stage of labor in the setting of fetal heart rate monitoring. There remains a concern that prolonged second stage of labor will lead to higher rates of maternal urinary incontinence and pelvic relaxation, but to date, no prospective studies have been performed.

Monitoring

Repetitive early and variable decels are common during the second stage. The clinician can be reassured if these decels resolve quickly after each contraction and there is no loss of variability in the tracing. Repetitive late decels, bradycardias, and loss of variability are all signs of nonreassuring fetal status. With these tracings, the patient should be placed on face mask O_2, turned onto her left side to decrease inferior vena cava (IVC) compression and increase uterine perfusion; if it is being used, the pitocin should be immediately discontinued until the tracing resumes a reassuring pattern. If a bradycardia is felt to be the result of uterine **hypertonus** (a single contraction lasting 2 minutes or longer) or **tachysystole** (greater than five contractions in a 10-minute period), which can be diagnosed by palpation or examination of the tocometer, the patient can be given a dose of terbutaline to help relax the uterus. If a nonreassuring pattern does not resolve with these interventions, the fetal position and station should be assessed to determine whether an operative vaginal delivery can be performed. If fetal station is above 0 station (though many clinicians will require the fetus to be +2 station or lower) or the position cannot be determined, cesarean delivery is the mode of choice.

Vaginal Delivery

As the fetus begins crowning, the delivering clinician should be dressed with goggles, sterile gown, and sterile gloves (for self-protection as much as for prevention of maternal/fetal infection) and have two clamps, scissors, suction bulb, and—when meconium is suspected or confirmed—a DeLee suction trap. Various approaches can be taken to vaginal delivery, but most clinicians would agree that a smooth, controlled delivery leads to less perineal trauma. A modified Ritgen maneuver (Fig. 4-12) using the heel of the delivering hand to exert pressure on the perineum and the fingers below the woman's anus to extend the fetal head to hasten delivery and maintain station between contractions may be performed. Simultaneously, the opposite hand should be used to flex the head to keep it from extending too far and causing periurethral and labial lacerations. This hand can also be used to massage the labia over the head during delivery.

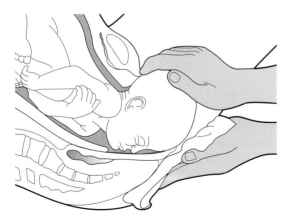

Figure 4-12 • Near completion of the delivery of the fetal head by the modified Ritgen maneuver. Moderate upward pressure is applied to the fetal chin by the posterior hand covered with a sterile towel while the suboccipital region of the fetal head is held against the symphysis.

Once the head of the infant is delivered, the mouth and upper airway are bulb suctioned. If there is meconium in the amniotic fluid, the DeLee suction tube is passed down the infant's nares and mouth and vigorous suctioning is performed before delivery of the shoulders. After suctioning is complete, the infant's neck is checked for a wrapped umbilical cord. If a nuchal cord exists, an attempt is made to reduce the cord over the infant's head. If it is too tight, two options exist. If the clinician is extremely confident that delivery will be accomplished shortly, the cord is clamped and cut at this point. If a shoulder dystocia is suspected, an attempt is made to deliver the infant with the nuchal cord intact.

Delivery of the rest of the infant follows first with delivery of the anterior shoulder by exerting direct downward pressure on the infant's head. Once the anterior shoulder is visualized, a direct upward pressure is exerted to deliver the posterior shoulder (Fig. 4-13). After this, exertion of gentle traction will deliver the torso and the rest of the infant. At this point, the cord is clamped and cut and the infant passed either to the labor nurse and mother or to the waiting pediatricians.

Episiotomy

An **episiotomy** is an incision made in the perineum to facilitate delivery. Indications for episiotomy include need to hasten delivery and impending or ongoing shoulder dystocia. A relative contraindication for episiotomy is the assessment that there will be a large perineal laceration as episiotomies have been associated with higher risk of severe perineal lacerations. Once the episiotomy is cut, great care should be taken to support the perineum around the episiotomy to avoid extension into the rectal sphincter or rectum itself. In the past, episiotomies were used routinely in the setting of spontaneous and operative vaginal deliveries. However, evidence suggests that the rate of third- and fourth-degree lacerations increases with the use of routine midline episiotomy.

There are two common types of episiotomies: median (or midline) and mediolateral (Fig. 4-14). The median episiotomy, the most common type used in the United States, uses a vertical midline incision from the posterior fourchette into the perineal body. The mediolateral episiotomy is an oblique incision made from either the 5 or 7 o'clock position on the perineum and cut laterally. It is used less frequently and reportedly causes more pain and wound infections. However, mediolateral episiotomies are thought to lead to fewer third- and

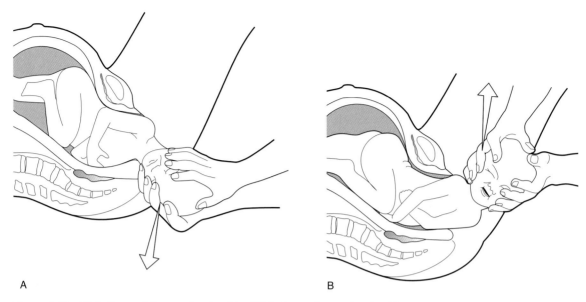

Figure 4-13 • (A) Delivery of the anterior shoulder. **(B)** Delivery of posterior shoulder.

fourth-degree extensions, particularly in patients with short perineums or with operative deliveries.

Operative Vaginal Delivery

In the case of a prolonged second stage, maternal exhaustion, or the need to hasten delivery, an operative vaginal delivery may be indicated. The two possibilities are forceps delivery or vacuum-assisted delivery. Both are effective methods to facilitate

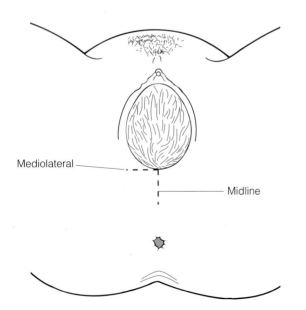

Figure 4-14 • Placement of mediolateral and midline episiotomy.

vaginal delivery and have similar indications. The decision of which method to choose is generally based upon clinician preference and experience, though they carry slightly different risks of maternal and neonatal complications.

Forceps Delivery

Forceps (Fig. 4-15) have blades that are placed around the fetal head and are shaped with a cephalic curve to accommodate the head. In addition, most have a pelvic curve that conforms to the maternal pelvis. The blade of each forcep is at the end of a shank that is connected to a handle. The two forceps are connected at the lock between the shank and the handle. Once the forceps are placed around the fetal head, the operator utilizes varying vector forces on the handles to aid maternal expulsive efforts and guide the fetal head through the curvature of the pelvis (Table 4-2).

The conditions necessary for safe application of forceps include full dilation of the cervix, ruptured membranes, engaged head and at least 2 station, absolute knowledge of fetal position, no evidence of cephalopelvic disproportion, adequate anesthesia, empty bladder, and—most important—an experienced operator. In some institutions mid-forceps applications (fetal station between 0 and 2) and rotational forceps (fetal head more than 45 degrees from either direct OA or OP position) are also used. An experienced operator is, again, the most important component of these deliveries. Use of high forceps

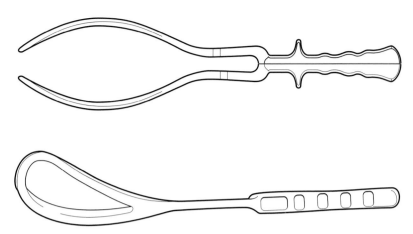

Figure 4-15 • Forceps.

with the fetal vertex above 0 station is no longer considered a safe obstetric procedure. Complications from forceps application include bruising on the face and head, lacerations to the fetal head, cervix, vagina, and perineum, facial nerve palsy, and, rarely, skull fracture and/or intracranial damage.

■ **TABLE 4-2** Classification of Forceps Delivery According to Station and Rotation	
Type of Procedure	**Classification**
Outlet forceps	1. Scalp is visible at the introitus without separating the labia 2. Fetal skull has reached pelvic floor 3. Sagittal suture is in anteroposterior diameter or right or left occiput anterior or posterior position 4. Fetal head is at or on perineum 5. Rotation does not exceed 45 degrees
Low forceps	Leading point of fetal skull is at station 2 or greater, but not on the pelvic floor a. Rotation <45 degrees (left or right occiput anterior to occiput anterior, or left or right occiput posterior to occiput posterior) b. Rotation >45 degrees
Mid forceps	Station above +2 cm but head engaged
High forceps	Not included in classification

From Cunningham FG, Gant NF, Leveno KJ, et al. *Williams Obstetrics*, 19th ed. Norwalk, CT: Appleton & Lange; 1993:557.

Vacuum Extraction

The **vacuum extractor** consists of a vacuum cup that is placed on the fetal scalp and a suction device that is connected to the cup to create the vacuum. Conditions for the safe use of the vacuum extractor are identical to that of forceps. Vacuum should never be chosen because position is unknown or the station is too high. Exertion on the cup and consequently on the fetal scalp is made parallel to the axis of the maternal pelvis concomitant with maternal bearing-down efforts and uterine contractions. The most common complications of use of the vacuum are scalp laceration and cephalohematoma. However, a rare complication from the vacuum extractor is the subgaleal hemorrhage which can be a neonatal emergency.

Forceps vs. Vacuum

There is great debate between clinicians as to which of these forms of operative delivery are safer. In several studies that compare the two modes of operative vaginal delivery the rates of severe neonatal complications such as intracranial hemorrhage are not statistically different. However, vacuums are associated with a higher rate of cephalohematomas and shoulder dystocias, while forceps are associated with a higher rate of facial nerve palsies. With respect to maternal complications, forceps are associated with higher rates of third and fourth degree perineal lacerations. Some of the differences between these instruments are related to design. The forceps are applied around the fetal head and the tips of the blades lie on the fetal cheek, thus are more likely to cause compression of the facial nerve. The vacuum exerts its entire force on the fetal scalp, thus fetal cephalohematomas are a common complication. Because of the higher placement and their rigidity, forceps can be used to generate greater downward force on both the fetus and concomitantly the maternal anatomy. This may lead to a lower rate of shoulder dystocia, but higher rates of maternal lacerations. In the end, the most important factor in the use of these instruments is operator experience. Since either of these instruments may be the tool of choice in different given situations, it is important for obstetricians to be trained in the use of both.

Stage 3

Stage 3 begins once the infant has been delivered. It is completed with delivery of the placenta. Placental separation usually occurs within 5 to 10 minutes of delivery of the infant; however, up to 30 minutes is usually considered within normal limits. With the abrupt decrease in intrauterine cavity size after delivery of the fetus, the placenta is mechanically sheared from the uterine wall with contractions. Classically, the use of oxytocin was contraindicated during stage 3. However, this was established prior to the use of ultrasound out of concern for causing abruption in the case of an undiagnosed twin. If there is no doubt about completion of stage 2, oxytocin can be used during the stage 3 to strengthen uterine contractions to decrease both placental delivery time and blood loss.

The three signs of placental separation include cord lengthening, a gush of blood, and uterine fundal rebound as the placenta detaches from the uterine wall. No attempt to deliver the placenta should be made until all these signs are noted. The placenta is delivered by gentle traction on the cord. It is important not to use too much traction because the cord may avulse or uterine inversion may occur. When the patient begins bearing down for delivery of the placenta, it is imperative that one of the examiner's hands is applying suprapubic pressure to keep the uterus from inverting or prolapsing (Fig. 4-16). When the placenta is evident at the introitus, the delivery should be controlled to avoid both further perineal trauma and tearing of any of the membranes that often trail the placenta at delivery.

Retained Placenta

The diagnosis of retained placenta is made when the placenta does not deliver within 30 minutes after the infant. Retained placenta is common in preterm deliveries, particularly previable deliveries. However, it is also a sign of placenta accreta, where the placenta has invaded into or beyond the endometrial stroma. The retained placenta may be removed by manual extraction. A hand is placed in the intrauterine cavity and the fingers used to shear the placenta from the surface of the uterus (Fig. 4-17). If the placenta cannot be completely extracted manually, a curettage is performed to ensure no products of conception (POC) are retained.

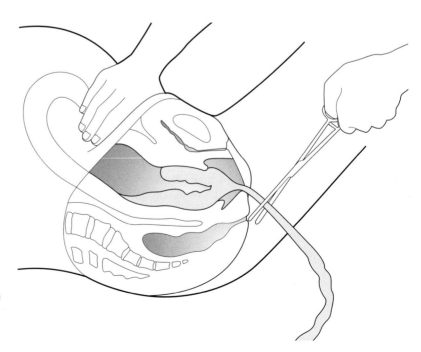

Figure 4-16 • Delivery of the placenta with traction on the cord and suprapubic pressure on the uterus to prevent uterine inversion.

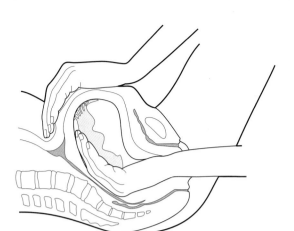

Figure 4-17 • Manual removal of placenta. The fingers are alternately abducted, adducted, and advanced until the placenta is completely detached.

Laceration Repair

Lacerations are usually repaired after placental delivery. A thorough examination of the perineum, labia, periurethral area, vagina, anus, and cervix is performed to assess lacerations. The most common lacerations are perineal lacerations, which are described by the depth of tissues they involve (Fig. 4-18). A first-degree laceration involves the mucosa or skin. Second-degree lacerations extend into the perineal body but do not involve the anal sphincter. Third-degree lacerations extend into or completely through the anal sphincter. A fourth-degree tear occurs if the anal mucosa itself is entered. A rectal exam should always be performed as occasionally a "button-hole" fourth degree laceration will be noted. This is a laceration through the rectal mucosa into the vagina, but with the sphincter still intact.

Repair of any superficial lacerations, including first-degree perineal tears, is usually accomplished with interrupted sutures. A second-degree laceration is repaired in layers. The apex of the laceration, which often lies beyond the hymenal ring, is located and a suture is anchored at the apex. This suture is then run down to the level of the hymenal ring, bringing together the vaginal tissue. This suture is then passed beyond the hymenal ring and used to bring together the perineal body. Sometimes a separate suture is used to place a "crown stitch" that brings together the perineal body. Finally, the skin of the perineum is closed with a subcuticular closure (Fig. 4-19).

Third-degree lacerations require repair of the anal sphincter with several interrupted sutures and then the rest of the repair is completed as in a second-degree repair. Fourth-degree repairs are begun with repair of the anal mucosa. Mucosal repair is performed meticulously to prevent fistula formation. Once the rectum is repaired, a fourth-degree laceration is completed just as a third-degree repair.

Cesarean Delivery

Cesarean delivery or cesarean section has been used effectively throughout the twentieth century and is

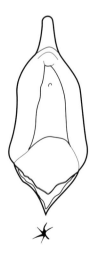
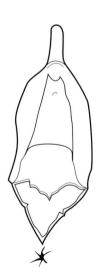
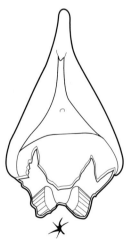
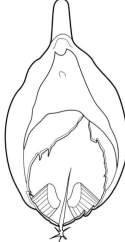

First-degree tear (Superficial)

Second-degree tear (Into the body of the perineum)

Third-degree tear (Into the anal sphincter)

Fourth-degree tear (Into the rectum)

Figure 4-18 • Perineal tears.

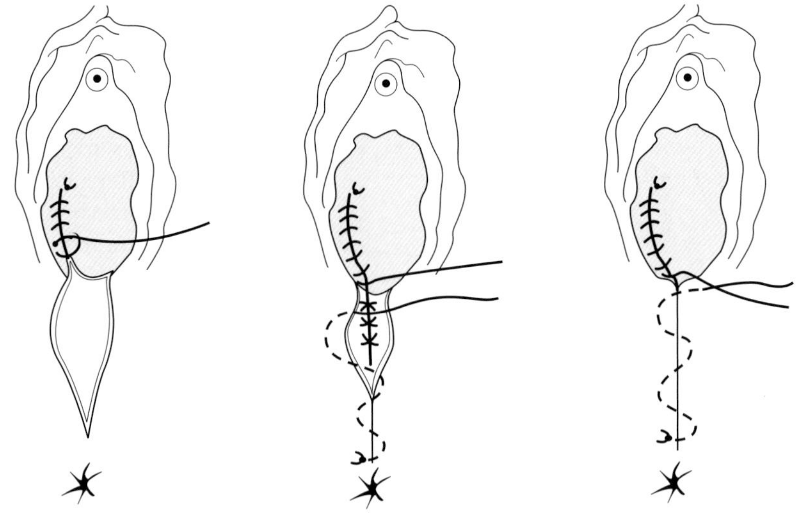

Figure 4-19 • Repair of a second-degree laceration. 1, The vaginal mucosa is repaired down to the level of the hymenal ring. 2, The subcutaneous tissue of the perineum is then brought together. 3, Finally, the skin of the perineum is reapproximated in a subcuticular fashion.

1   2   3

one of the most common operations performed today. The current cesarean rate in the United States is over 31% and it has risen about 1% per year over the last several years. It is not entirely clear why the cesarean delivery rate is rising so rapidly, but it is likely multifactorial including: (i) biologic reasons such as higher rates of multiple gestations, an older population with more medical disorders, and higher rates of overweight and obesity; (ii) patient preferences toward elective cesarean also known as cesarean delivery on maternal request (CDMR); and (iii) clinician preferences related to the escalating medical-legal environment and inadequate economic incentives to encourage clinician patience. Although maternal mortality from cesarean section is low, approximately 0.01% to 0.02%, it is still higher than from vaginal delivery. Further, the morbidity from infections, thrombotic events, wound dehiscence, and recovery time is greater than that of vaginal delivery.

The most common indication for primary cesarean delivery is that of failure to progress in labor. Failure to progress can be caused by problems with any of the three Ps. If the pelvis is too small or the fetus too large (depending on the viewpoint taken), the diagnosis is CPD, which leads to failure to progress. If the uterus simply does not generate enough pressure during contractions, labor can stall and lead to failure to progress. If labor seems to be stalling, there are a number of measures that can be taken to augment it, such as oxytocin or ROM. Commonly, two hours without cervical change in the setting of adequate uterine contractions in the active phase of labor was

deemed failure to progress or active phase arrest often leading to cesarean delivery. However, a recent study suggests that it is reasonable to wait at least four hours for cervical stage in the active phase of labor leading to a vaginal delivery in the majority of these patients.

Other common indications for primary cesarean section (Table 4-3) are breech presentation, transverse lie, shoulder presentation, placenta previa, placental abruption, fetal intolerance of labor, nonreassuring fetal status, cord prolapse, prolonged second stage, failed operative vaginal delivery, or active herpes lesions. The most common indication for cesarean section is a previous cesarean section.

Vaginal Birth after Cesarean

Vaginal birth after cesarean (VBAC) can be attempted if the proper setting exists. This includes an in-house obstetrician, anesthesiologist, and surgical team and informed patient consent. The prior hysterotomy needs to be either a Kerr (low transverse incision) or Kronig (low vertical incision) without any extensions into the cervix or upper uterine segment. The greatest risk during a trial of labor after cesarean (TOLAC) is that of rupture of the prior uterine scar, which occurs approximately 0.5% to 1.0% of the time. Prior classical hysterotomies, or vertical incisions through the thick upper segment of the uterine corpus, are at a higher risk for uterine rupture in labor and women who have had this type of cesarean are not usually allowed to attempt a trial of labor. Similarly, multiple prior ce-

■ TABLE 4-3 Indications for Cesarean Section

Type	Indication
Maternal/fetal	Cephalopelvic disproportion Failed induction of labor
Maternal	Maternal diseases 　Active genital herpes 　Untreated HIV (elevated 　viral load) 　Cervical cancer Prior uterine surgery 　Classical cesarean section 　Full-thickness myomectomy Prior uterine rupture Obstruction to the birth canal 　Fibroids 　Ovarian tumors
Fetal	Nonreassuring fetal testing 　Bradycardia 　Absence of FHR variability 　Scalp pH <7.20 Cord prolapse Fetal malpresentations 　Breech, transverse lie, brow Multiple gestations 　Nonvertex first twin 　Higher-order multiples Fetal anomalies 　Hydrocephalus 　Osteogenesis imperfecta
Placental	Placenta previa Vasa previa Abruptio placentae

■ TABLE 4-4 Risk Factors for Uterine Rupture and Success or Failure in a TOLAC

Increased Success of TOLAC	Increased Risk of Uterine Rupture
Prior vaginal birth	More than one prior cesarean delivery
Prior VBAC	Prior classical cesarean
Nonrecurring indication for prior C/S (herpes, previa, breech)	Induction of labor Use of prostaglandins Use of high amounts of oxytocin
Presentation in labor at: 　>3 cm dilated 　>75% effaced	Time from last cesarean <18 months
	Uterine infection at time of last cesarean

Decreased Success of TOLAC	Decreased Risk of Uterine Rupture
Prior C/S for cephalopelvic disproportion	Prior vaginal birth
Induction of labor	

sarean deliveries increases the risk of uterine rupture and are a relative contraindication. Unfortunately, induction of labor has been associated with higher rates of uterine rupture, thus women with a medical indication for induction of labor need to be counseled and consented again regarding the risks and benefits of a trial of labor when they present for an induction. Other factors associated with success or failure of a TOLAC and with uterine rupture are listed in Table 4-4. Common signs of rupture include abdominal pain, FHR decelerations or bradycardia, sudden decrease of pressure on an IUPC, and maternal sensation of a "pop." Therefore, the patient needs to be monitored closely in labor and delivered emergently if uterine rupture is suspected. Over the last decade, the rate of VBAC in the United States has plummeted from as high as 40% to 50% in some populations to below 15%. Because of medical-legal issues, many smaller hospitals no longer sanction trial of labor after cesarean. These trends have contributed to the overall rising cesarean delivery rate.

OBSTETRIC ANALGESIA AND ANESTHESIA

Natural Childbirth

Certainly a component of the discomfort during labor comes from the anticipation of pain and the apprehension that accompanies this event. The concept behind natural childbirth is to educate patients regarding the experiences of labor and delivery in order to prepare them for the event. In addition, a variety of relaxation techniques, showers, and massage are used to help patients cope with the pain from uterine contractions. These techniques have been formalized in the Lamaze method, which involves a series of classes for both the patient and a birthing coach that teach relaxation and breathing techniques.

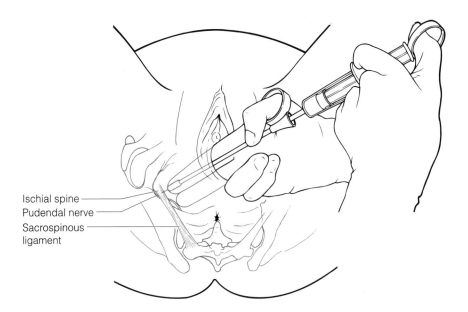

Ischial spine
Pudendal nerve
Sacrospinous
ligament

Figure 4-20 • Technique for transvaginal pudendal block.

Systemic Pharmacologic Intervention

Either narcotics or sedatives can be useful in the first
stage of labor to relax patients and decrease pain.
These commonly include fentanyl, Nubain, and
Stadol. Early in labor, IM morphine sulfate is commonly used to achieve patient pain relief and rest.
Because they cross the placenta, sedating medications
should not be used close to the time of expected delivery because they may result in a depressed infant.
Other complications of these medications are respiratory depression and increased risk of aspiration.

Pudendal Block

The pudendal nerve travels just posterior to the ischial spine at its juncture with the sacrospinous
ligament. With the pudendal block, anesthetic is injected at that site, bilaterally, to give perineal anesthesia. A pudendal block is commonly used in the
case of operative vaginal delivery with either forceps
or vacuum. It may be combined with local infiltration of the perineum to ensure perineal anesthesia
(Fig. 4-20).

Local Anesthesia

In patients without anesthesia who are going to
require an episiotomy, local infiltration with an anesthetic is used. Local anesthetic is also used before repair of vaginal, perineal, and periurethral lacerations.

Epidural and Spinal Anesthesia

Epidurals are commonly administered to patients
who wish to have anesthesia throughout the active
phase and delivery of the infant. Many patients worry
about nerve damage and the pain of the epidural itself. An early consult with an anesthesiologist to help
answer questions about the epidural can be reassuring. The epidural catheter is placed in the L3–L4
interspace when the patient requires analgesia, although usually not until labor is deemed to be in the
active phase. Once the catheter is placed, an initial
bolus of anesthetic is given and a continuous infusion
is started. Again, the epidural does not commonly remove all sensation and can actually be detrimental to
the stage 2 if it does so. However, if the patient requires cesarean delivery, the epidural can be bolused
and usually provides adequate anesthesia.

Spinal anesthesia provides anesthesia over a region
similar to that of an epidural, but differs in that it is
given in a one-time dose directly into the spinal canal
leading to more rapid onset of anesthesia. It is used
more commonly for cesarean section than vaginal delivery. A common complication of both forms of
anesthesia is maternal hypotension secondary to decreased systemic vascular resistance, which can lead
to decreased placental perfusion and fetal bradycardia. A more serious complication can be maternal
respiratory depression if the anesthetic reaches a level
high enough to affect diaphragmatic innervation. A
spinal headache due to the loss of cerebrospinal fluid

is a postpartum complication seen in less than 1% of patients.

General Anesthesia

Although general anesthesia is rarely used for vaginal delivery, it may be used for cesarean delivery, particularly in the emergent setting. For less urgent cesarean sections, epidural or spinal anesthesia is usu-ally preferred. The two principal concerns of general anesthesia are the risk of maternal aspiration and the risk of hypoxia to mother and fetus during induction. Thus, when choosing the route of anesthesia for a cesarean section, the urgency of the delivery must be assessed. Common reasons for an emergent cesarean section are abruption, fetal bradycardia, umbilical cord prolapse, uterine rupture, and hemorrhage from a placenta previa.

 KEY POINTS

- The physical exam of a pregnant woman in labor and delivery often includes Leopold maneuvers, a sterile speculum exam, and a cervical exam.

- It is important to determine both the presentation of the fetus and status of the cervix. The cervical exam includes dilation, effacement, station, consistency, and position.

- Labor can be induced or augmented with prostaglandins, oxytocin, laminaria, Foley bulb, and artificial rupture of membranes.

- The fetus can be monitored in labor with external fetal monitoring, fetal scalp electrode, ultrasound, and fetal scalp pH.

- Labor is divided into stages: stage 1 extends until complete cervical dilation, stage 2 until delivery of the infant, and stage 3 until delivery of the placenta.

- Forceps delivery and vacuum extraction are two forms of operative vaginal delivery that are used to expedite vaginal delivery.

- Cesarean delivery has multiple indications and is the most common operation performed in the United States.

- Because the most common indication for cesarean delivery is a prior cesarean delivery, attempts should be made to achieve vaginal delivery in the first pregnancy.

- Obstetric anesthesia allows for more patient comfort throughout labor.

- Epidurals are commonly used during labor, whereas spinals are used more often for cesarean section.

- Epidural anesthesia leads to a longer stage 2 of labor, but offers better control during crowning.

- Occasionally, general anesthesia is used in the emergent setting.

Antepartum Hemorrhage

Obstetric hemorrhage is a leading cause of maternal death in the United States and one of the leading causes of perinatal morbidity and mortality. Bleeding during pregnancy has different etiologies depending on the trimester. As discussed in Chapter 2, first-trimester bleeding is associated with spontaneous abortion, ectopic pregnancy, and even normal pregnancies. Third-trimester vaginal bleeding occurs in 3% to 4% of pregnancies and may be obstetric or nonobstetric (Table 5-1). Hemorrhage can occur antepartum or postpartum (Chapter 12), with the major causes of antepartum hemorrhage including placenta previa (20%) and placental abruption (30%).

PLACENTA PREVIA

PATHOGENESIS

Placenta previa is defined as abnormal implantation of the placenta over the internal cervical os (Fig. 5-1). **Complete previa** occurs when the placenta completely covers the internal os. **Partial previa** occurs when the placenta covers a portion of the internal os. **Marginal previa** occurs when the edge of the placenta reaches the margin of the os. A low-lying placenta is implanted in the lower uterine segment in close proximity but not extending to the internal os. Rarely, a fetal vessel may lie over the cervix known as a **vasa previa**, discussed later in this chapter.

Bleeding from a placenta previa results from small disruptions in the placental attachment during normal development and thinning of the lower uterine segment during the third trimester. As a result, profuse hemorrhage and shock can occur, leading to significant maternal and fetal mortality and morbidity. Although the maternal and perinatal mortality from placenta previa has dropped rapidly in the United States over the past few decades, the perinatal mortality rate is still 10 times higher than in the general population. Most risk to the fetus comes from premature delivery, which is responsible for 60% of perinatal deaths. Other fetal risks associated with placenta previa are listed in Table 5-2.

Placenta previa may also be complicated by an associated placenta accreta (placenta previa accreta). **Placenta accreta** is defined as the abnormal invasion of the placenta into the uterine wall. An **accreta** is defined as the superficial invasion of the placenta into the uterine myometrium. An **increta** occurs when the placenta invades the myometrium. A **percreta** occurs when the placenta invades through the myometrium to the uterine serosa.

Placenta accreta causes an inability of the placenta to properly separate from the uterine wall after delivery of the fetus. This can result in profuse hemorrhage and shock with substantial maternal morbidity and mortality. Two-thirds of women with both a placenta previa and an associated accreta require a hysterectomy at the time of delivery (puerperal hysterectomy). Table 5-3 summarizes the abnormalities of placentation.

■ **TABLE 5-1** Differential Diagnosis of Antepartum Bleeding	
Obstetric causes	
Placental	Placenta previa, placental abruption, vasa previa
Maternal	Uterine rupture
Fetal	Fetal vessel rupture
Nonobstetric causes	
Cervical	Severe cervicitis, polyps, cervical cancer
Vaginal/vulvar	Lacerations, varices, cancer
Other	Hemorrhoids, congenital bleeding disorder, abdominal or pelvic trauma, hematuria

Adapted from Hacker N and Moore JG. *Essentials of Obstetrics and Gynecology*. Philadelphia: WB Saunders, 1992:155.

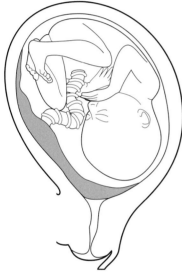

Complete placenta previa

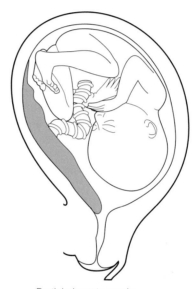

Partial placenta previa

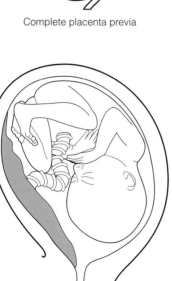

Marginal placenta previa

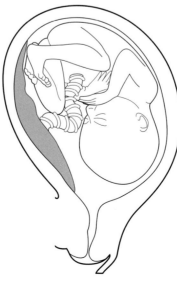

Low implantation or low-lying placenta

Figure 5-1 • Classifications of placenta previa.

■ **TABLE 5-2** Fetal Complications Associated with Placenta Previa

Preterm delivery and its complications
Preterm premature rupture of membranes
Intrauterine growth restriction
Malpresentation
Vasa previa
Congenital abnormalities

Adapted from Hacker N and Moore JG. *Essentials of Obstetrics and Gynecology.* Philadelphia: WB Saunders, 1992:155.

EPIDEMIOLOGY

Placenta previa occurs in 0.5% of pregnancies (1:200 births) and accounts for nearly 20% of all antepartum hemorrhage. Because a bleeding previa often results in delivery and this may occur preterm, it is a common cause of indicated preterm delivery. Previa occurs in as many as 1% to 4% of women with a prior cesarean section. Placenta previa can also be complicated by an associated placenta accreta (placenta previa accreta) in approximately 5% of cases. The risk of accreta is increased in women with placenta previa in the setting of prior cesarean delivery and in 15% to 30% of women with one prior cesarean section, 25% to 50% in women with two prior cesareans, and in 29% to 65% of women with three or more prior cesarean sections.

Abnormalities in placentation are the result of events that prevent normal migration of the placenta during normal progressive development of the lower uterine segment during pregnancy (Table 5-4). Previous placental implantations and prior uterine scars are thought to contribute to abnormal placentation in subsequent pregnancies. Thus, the risk of placenta previa is increased in patients with other prior uterine surgery such as myomectomy, uterine anomalies, multiple gestations, multiparity, advanced maternal age, smoking, and previous placenta previa. Of note, because many patients receive a routine obstetric ultrasound, marginal previa or low-lying placenta is not uncommonly diagnosed in the second trimester. Most resolve on repeat ultrasound by moving up and away from the cervix during the third trimester as the lower uterine segment develops.

CLINICAL MANIFESTATIONS

History

Patients with placenta previa classically present with sudden and profuse **painless vaginal bleeding**. The first episode of bleeding—the "sentinel" bleed—usually occurs after 28 weeks of gestation. During this

■ **TABLE 5-3** Abnormalities of Placentation

Circumvallate placenta	Occurs when the membranes double back over the edge of the placenta, forming a dense ring around the periphery of the placenta. Often considered a variant of placental abruption, it is a major cause of second-trimester hemorrhage.
Placenta previa	Occurs when the placenta develops over the internal cervical os. Types include complete, partial, and marginal.
Placenta accreta	Abnormal adherence of part or all of the placenta to the uterine wall. May be associated with a placenta in normal locations, but incidence increases in placenta previa.
Placenta increta	Abnormal placentation in which the placenta invades the myometrium.
Placenta percreta	Abnormal placentation in which the placenta invades through the myometrium to the uterine serosa. Occasionally, placentas may invade into adjacent organs such as the bladder or rectum.
Vasa previa	Occurs when a velamentous cord insertion causes the fetal vessels to pass over the internal cervical os. Seen also with velamentous and succenturiate placenta.
Velamentous placenta	Occurs when the blood vessels insert between the amnion and the chorion, away from the margin of the placenta. This leaves the vessels largely unprotected and vulnerable to compression or injury.
Succenturiate placenta	An extra lobe of the placenta that is implanted at some distance away from the rest of the placenta. Fetal vessels may course between the two lobes, possibly over the cervix, leaving these blood vessels unprotected and at risk for rupture.

■ **TABLE 5-4** Predisposing Factors for Placenta Previa
Prior cesarean section, uterine surgery such as myomectomy
Multiparity
Multiple gestation
Erythroblastosis
Smoking
History of placenta previa
Increasing maternal age

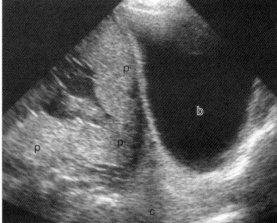

Figure 5-2 • Complete placenta previa. (p, placenta; c, cervix; b, bladder)

time, the lower uterine segment develops and thins, disrupting the placental attachment and resulting in bleeding. Placenta accreta is usually asymptomatic. On rare occasions, however, a patient with a percreta into the bladder or rectum may present with hematuria or rectal bleeding.

Physical Examination

Vaginal examination is contraindicated in placenta previa because the digital examination can cause further separation of the placenta and trigger catastrophic hemorrhage. Because many patients have an ultrasound exam that can diagnose placenta previa, diagnosis by digital examination of the placenta previa is uncommon today; the cervical exam may reveal soft, spongy tissue just inside the cervix. Because of the increased vascularity, there may be notable varices in the lower uterine segment or cervix that can be visualized on speculum exam or palpated. A marginal previa can be palpated at the edge of, or quite near, the internal os.

DIAGNOSTIC EVALUATION

The diagnosis of placenta previa can be made via ultrasonography with a sensitivity of greater than 95% (Fig. 5-2). If made before the third trimester in pregnancy, a follow-up ultrasound is often obtained in the third trimester to determine if the previa has resolved. In patients with a known or suspected previa, transvaginal sonography is usually avoided. Transabdominal or translabial views can usually be used to determine the extent of placentation. If the ultrasound is performed with a full maternal bladder, placenta previa may be overdiagnosed secondary to compression of the lower uterine segment, resem-

bling a longer cervix. It is therefore important to have the bladder entirely emptied before this portion of the ultrasound is performed if a previa is a possibility.

TREATMENT

Management of patients with placenta previa varies between providers. Commonly, antepartum patients with a placenta previa are managed with strict pelvic rest (i.e., no intercourse) and modified bed rest. However, some clinicians will not institute this conservative management until the patient presents with the sentinel bleed. Similarly, hospitalized bed rest is sometimes prescribed after the sentinel bleed by some clinicians, whereas others wait until the patient has a large bleed by history, exam, or drop in hematocrit of at least 3 points.

Unstoppable labor, fetal distress, and life-threatening hemorrhage are all indications for immediate cesarean delivery regardless of gestational age. In the case of preterm pregnancy, if the bleeding is not profuse, fetal survival can be enhanced by aggressive expectant management. However, 70% of patients with placenta previa have a recurring bleeding episode and will require delivery before week 36. For patients who make it to week 36, typical management involves amniocentesis to determine fetal lung maturity and delivery by cesarean section between 36 and 37 weeks after confirmation of fetal lung maturity.

The following should be done in the case of vaginal bleeding and suspected placenta previa.

1. **Stabilize the patient.** Every patient with vaginal bleeding and a known or suspected previa should be hospitalized with continuous fetal monitoring and

have IV access established. If the patient presents with a particularly large bleed, two large bore IVs will commonly be placed. Laboratory evaluation includes hematocrit, type and cross, and, if considerable bleeding or coagulopathy is suspected, PT, PTT, D-dimer or fibrin split products, and fibrinogen. For an Rh-negative woman, a Kleihauer-Betke test should be performed to determine the extent of any fetomaternal transfusion so that the appropriate amount of RhoGAM can be administered to prevent alloimmunization.

2. **Prepare for catastrophic hemorrhage.** Expectant management in the stabilized patient includes hospitalization, bed rest, hematocrit monitoring, and consideration of limiting any oral intake. Two or more units of blood should be typed, cross-matched, and made available. Transfusions are usually given to maintain a hematocrit of 25% or greater.

3. **Prepare for preterm delivery.** Prior to 34 weeks of gestation, betamethasone is administered to promote fetal lung maturity. Tocolysis is also used to assist in prolonging the pregnancy up to 34 weeks of gestation. Occasionally, tocolysis is used past week 34 to help control the bleeding.

PLACENTAL ABRUPTION

PATHOGENESIS

Placental abruption (abruptio placentae) is the premature separation of the normally implanted placenta from the uterine wall, resulting in hemorrhage between the uterine wall and the placenta. Fifty percent of abruptions occur before labor and after 30 weeks of gestation, 15% occur during labor, and 30% are identified only on placental inspection after delivery. Large placental separations may result in premature delivery, uterine tetany, disseminated intravascular coagulation (DIC), and hypovolemic shock.

The primary cause of placental abruption is unknown, although it is associated with a variety of predisposing and precipitating factors (Table 5-5). These factors include maternal hypertension, prior history of placental abruption, maternal cocaine use, external maternal trauma, and rapid decompression of the overdistended uterus.

At the initial point of separation, nonclotted blood courses from the injury site. The enlarging collection

TABLE 5-5 Predisposing and Precipitating Factors for Placental Abruption
Predisposing factors
Hypertension
Previous placental abruption
Advanced maternal age
Multiparity
Uterine distension
Multiple pregnancy
Hydramnios
Vascular deficiency
Diabetes mellitus
Collagen vascular disease
Cocaine use
Cigarette smoking
Alcohol use (>14 drinks/wk)
Circumvallate placenta
Short umbilical cord
Precipitating factors
Trauma
External/internal version
Motor vehicle accident
Abdominal trauma
Sudden uterine volume loss
Delivery of first twin
Rupture of membranes with polyhydramnios
Preterm premature rupture of membranes

of blood may cause further separation of the placenta. In 20% of placental separations, bleeding is confined within the uterine cavity and is referred to as a **concealed hemorrhage** (Fig. 5-3). In the remaining 80% of placental separations, the blood dissects downward toward the cervix, resulting in a **revealed** or **external hemorrhage.** Because there is an egress for the blood, revealed hemorrhages are less likely to result in larger retroplacental clots, which are associated with fetal demise. The result of hemorrhage from torn placental vessels can vary from maternal anemia in mild cases to shock, acute renal failure, and maternal death in severe cases.

Global maternal mortality from placental abruption varies from 0.5% to 5.0%. Most deaths are due

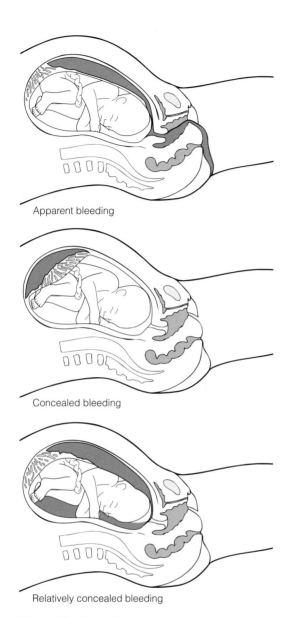

Apparent bleeding

Concealed bleeding

Relatively concealed bleeding

Figure 5-3 • Types of placental separation.

to hemorrhage, cardiac failure, or renal failure. Fetal mortality occurs in about 35% of all clinically relevant antepartum placental abruptions and can be as high as 50% to 80% in cases of severe placental abruption. The cause of demise is due to hypoxia resulting from decreased placental surface area and maternal hemorrhage.

EPIDEMIOLOGY

Placental abruption occurs in about 0.5% to 1.5% of pregnancies and is responsible for 30% of cases of third-trimester bleeding and 15% of perinatal mortal-ity. The predisposing and precipitating factors for placental abruption are listed in Table 5-5. The most common factor associated with increased incidence of abruption is hypertension, whether it is chronic, the result of preeclampsia, or maternal ingestion of cocaine or methamphetamine. In cases of abruptions that are severe enough to cause fetal death, 50% are due to hypertension: 25% of these are from chronic hypertension and 25% are from preeclampsia. The risk of abruption in future pregnancy is 10% after one abruption and 25% after two prior abruptions.

CLINICAL MANIFESTATIONS

History

The classic presentation of placental abruption is third-trimester vaginal bleeding associated with severe abdominal pain and/or frequent, strong contractions. However, about 30% of placental separations are small with few or no symptoms and are identified only after inspection of the placenta at delivery. The symptoms of abruption and their rate of occurrence are listed in Table 5-6.

Physical Examination

On physical examination, a patient with placental abruption will often have vaginal bleeding and a firm, tender uterus. On tocometer, small frequent contractions are usually seen as well as tetanic contractions. On fetal monitoring, nonreassuring fetal heart tracing may be seen secondary to hypoxia. A classic sign of placental abruption that can only be seen at the time of cesarean delivery is the Couvelaire uterus. If enough blood from the abruption penetrates into the uterine musculature, it can be seen subserosally when the uterus is removed from the abdomen during repair of the hysterotomy.

■ **TABLE 5-6** Presentation of Abruptio Placentae	
Symptom	**Occurrence (%)**
Vaginal bleeding	80
Uterine tenderness/abdominal or back pain	67
Abnormal contractions/increased uterine tone	34
Fetal distress	50
Fetal demise	15

DIAGNOSTIC EVALUATION

The diagnosis of placental abruption is primarily clinical. Only 2% of abruptions are picked up by ultrasound (evidenced by a retroplacental clot). However, because abruption can present similarly to placenta previa, ultrasonography is routinely performed to rule out previa in cases of suspected abruption. The diagnosis of abruption may be confirmed by inspection of the placenta at delivery. The presence of a retroplacental clot with overlying placental destruction confirms the diagnosis.

TREATMENT

The potential for rapid deterioration (e.g., hemorrhage, DIC, fetal hypoxia) necessitates delivery in some cases of placental abruption. However, most abruptions are small and noncatastrophic, and do not therefore necessitate immediate delivery.

The following should be done in the case of suspected placental abruption.

1. **Stabilize the patient.** When placental abruption is known or suspected, the patient should be hospitalized with continuous fetal monitoring and IV access gained. Laboratory evaluation should include CBC, type and cross, PT/PTT, and D-dimer or fibrin split products. For an Rh-negative woman, RhoGAM should be administered to prevent alloimmunization.
2. **Prepare for the possibility of future hemorrhage.** Standard antishock measures should be taken, including placement of large-bore intravenous catheters, infusion of lactated Ringer's solution, and preparation of units of crossed-matched blood (whole or packed red blood cells). Blood loss due to placental abruption is commonly grossly underestimated due to concealed bleeding.
3. **Prepare for preterm delivery.** In the preterm pregnancy, betamethasone may be given to promote fetal lung maturity and tocolysis may be given to assist in prolonging the pregnancy to week 34.
4. **Deliver if bleeding is life threatening or fetal testing is nonreassuring.** Delivery should be performed in patients with a life-threatening hemorrhage. This is a clinical determination, but any patient whose vital signs are unstable or has a coagulopathy should be delivered. Vaginal delivery is preferred as long as bleeding is controlled and there are no signs of fetal distress. Because the uterus is typically hyperactive in patients with an abruption, a rapid labor and delivery should be expected. If the fetal heart rate (FHR) tracing is nonreassuring, delivery should occur for fetal indications.

UTERINE RUPTURE

PATHOGENESIS

Uterine rupture represents a potential obstetric catastrophe and can lead to both maternal and fetal death. Most complete uterine ruptures occur during the course of labor. Over 90% of all uterine ruptures are associated with a prior uterine scar either from cesarean section or other uterine surgery. In the remaining cases (<10%), no prior scarring is present. Uterine ruptures without a prior uterine scar may be related to an abdominal trauma (e.g., auto accidents, external or internal version procedures), associated with labor or delivery (e.g., improper oxytocin use or excessive fundal pressure), or spontaneously initiated (e.g., placenta percreta, multiple gestation, grand multiparity, invasive mole, or choriocarcinoma).

The primary maternal complications from a ruptured uterus include hemorrhage and hypovolemic shock. The overall maternal mortality for uterine rupture is less than 1%, but if rupture occurs in the antepartum patient at home, it is likely to be higher. The perinatal mortality for uterine rupture ranges from 1% to 15%, again depending on where the patient is when the uterine rupture occurs.

EPIDEMIOLOGY

Uterine rupture is rare, occurring in an estimated 1:15,000 deliveries of patients with no prior uterine surgery. In women with a prior cesarean delivery, it is estimated to occur in 0.5% to 0.1% of deliveries. Risk factors for uterine rupture are conditions that predispose to a weakened uterine wall, including uterine scars, overdistension, inappropriately aggressive use of uterotonic agents, maternal congenital uterine anomalies, and abnormal placentation (Table 5-7).

CLINICAL MANIFESTATIONS

The presentation of uterine rupture is highly variable. Typically, it is characterized by the sudden onset of intense abdominal pain. Vaginal bleeding, if present, may vary from spotting to severe hemorrhage. Nonreassuring fetal testing, abnormal abdominal contour, cessation of uterine contractions, disappearance of fetal heart tones, and regression of the presenting part are other signs of uterine rupture.

■ **TABLE 5-7** Risk Factors for Uterine Rupture
Prior uterine scarring
Injudicious use of oxytocin
Grand multiparity
Marked uterine distension
Abnormal fetal lie
Large fetus
External version
Trauma

TREATMENT

Management of uterine rupture requires immediate laparotomy and delivery of the fetus. If feasible, the rupture site should be repaired and hemostasis obtained. In cases of large rupture extensions, repair may not be feasible and the patient may require a hysterectomy. Patients are usually discouraged to attempt future pregnancies given the high risk of recurrent rupture. Trial of labor would be avoided in any subsequent pregnancy, and the patient would commonly be delivered via repeat cesarean section at week 36 with documentation of fetal lung maturity.

FETAL VESSEL RUPTURE

PATHOGENESIS

Most pregnancies complicated by rupture of a fetal vessel are due to **velamentous cord insertion** where the blood vessels insert between the amnion and chorion away from the placenta instead of inserting directly into the chorionic plate (Table 5-3). Because the vessels course unprotected through the membranes before inserting on the placental margin, they are vulnerable to rupture, shearing, or laceration. In addition, these unprotected vessels may cross over the internal cervical os (**vasa previa**), making them vulnerable to compression by the presenting fetal part or to being torn when the membranes are ruptured. Although vasa previa is rare, perinatal mortality is high and increases if the membranes are also ruptured.

Unprotected fetal vessels and vasa previa may occur with a **succenturiate placenta** or accessory placental lobe. In this case, the bulk of the placenta is implanted in one portion of the uterine wall, but a small lobe of the placenta is implanted in another location. The vessels that connect these two portions of the placenta are unprotected and may course over the cervix and present as a vasa previa.

EPIDEMIOLOGY

Only 0.1% to 0.8% of pregnancies are complicated by the rupture of a fetal vessel. The incidence of vasa previa is 1:5,000 pregnancies. Risk factors for fetal vessel rupture include abnormal placentation leading to a succenturiate lobe as well as multiple gestations that increases the risk of velamentous insertion. Although the rate of velamentous insertion is only 1% in singleton gestations, it increases to 10% for twin gestations and 50% for triplet gestations.

CLINICAL MANIFESTATIONS

In fortunate cases, the fetal vessels are palpated and recognized through the dilated cervix. More commonly, the presentation of a fetal vessel rupture is vaginal bleeding associated with a sinusoidal variation of the FHR indicative of fetal anemia.

DIAGNOSIS

Unfortunately, diagnosis is often made after a large bleed and fetal compromise have already occurred. With advancing capabilities of ultrasound, velamentous insertion of the umbilical cord and succenturiate placental lobes can be diagnosed in the antepartum period. Further, with the use of color Doppler, vasa previa may also be diagnosed antepartum, but the sensitivity and specificity of these diagnoses have not as yet been determined and is likely related to the experience of the sonographer and/or sonologist and ultrasound equipment available. Diagnosis at the time of vaginal bleeding can be accomplished by the **Apt test** or examination of the blood for nucleated (fetal) red blood cells. The Apt test, involves diluting the blood with water, collecting the supernatant and combining it with 1% NaOH. If the resulting mixture is pink it indicates fetal blood, a yellow-brown color is seen with maternal blood.

TREATMENT

Given the high risk of fetal exsanguination and death (the vascular volume of the term fetus is less than 250 mL), the treatment for a ruptured fetal vessel is emergent cesarean delivery. Now that vasa previa can occasionally be diagnosed antepartum, these patients are often given the option of elective cesarean delivery, although there are few data as to the fetal risk. If they elect to undergo a trial of labor, artificial rupture of membranes (AROM) is contraindicated.

NONOBSTETRIC CAUSES OF ANTEPARTUM HEMORRHAGE

Nonobstetric causes of antepartum hemorrhage are listed in Table 5-1. Patients with these conditions usually present with spotting rather than frank bleeding. Typically, there are no uterine contractions or abdominal pain. The diagnosis is usually made by speculum examination, Pap smear, cultures, or colposcopy as indicated. Other than advanced maternal neoplasia, which is associated with poor maternal outcome, most nonobstetric causes of antepartum hemorrhage require relatively simple management and have good outcomes. Vaginal lacerations and varices can be located and repaired. Infections may be treated with appropriate agents, cervical polyps can be removed, and benign neoplasms usually require simple treatment.

 KEY POINTS

- Placenta previa accounts for 20% of antepartum hemorrhage and is associated with placenta accreta in up to 5% of cases and 25% to 50% of cases with a prior cesarean delivery.
- Previa occurs more often in patients with prior placenta previa, uterine scars, or multiple gestations.
- The classic presentation of placenta previa is painless vaginal bleeding in the third trimester, but is usually diagnosed via ultrasound today.
- Placenta previa is associated with antepartum hemorrhage, preterm delivery, preterm premature rupture of membranes (PPROM), and intrauterine growth restriction (IUGR) and increases the risk of puerperal hysterectomy.
- Patients are delivered by cesarean section in the case of unstoppable preterm labor, large hemorrhage, or nonreassuring fetal testing, or at week 36 with mature lung indices.
- Placenta accreta is the abnormal attachment of the placenta to the uterus. Invasion into the myometrium is placenta increta, whereas invasion through the myometrium and to the serosa is placenta percreta.
- Placental abruption accounts for 30% of all third-trimester hemorrhages and is seen more often in women with chronic hypertension, preeclampsia, use of cocaine or methamphetamines, or a history of abruption.
- Women with placental abruption usually present with vaginal bleeding, painful contractions, and a firm, tender uterus; 20% of cases present with no bleeding (concealed hemorrhages).

- Placental abruption can be complicated by hypovolemic shock, DIC, and preterm delivery. Women can be delivered vaginally if they are stable; cesarean delivery is necessary in the unstable patient or when fetal testing is nonreassuring.
- Uterine rupture is a rare obstetric catastrophe, but seen in 1 in 200 laboring women with a prior cesarean delivery.
- Maternal and fetal morbidity and mortality are increased in the setting of uterine rupture.
- Uterine rupture requires immediate laparotomy, delivery of the fetus, and either repair of the rupture site or hysterectomy.
- Fetal vessel rupture is a rare obstetric complication, usually associated with multiple gestation and a velamentous cord insertion.
- Fetal vessel rupture is associated with a perinatal mortality of up to 50% of cases.
- Patients may present with vaginal bleeding and a sinusoidal FHR pattern which requires emergent cesarean delivery.
- Nonobstetric causes of antepartum hemorrhage include cervical and vaginal lacerations, hemorrhoids, infections, and neoplasms.
- Nonobstetric causes of antepartum hemorrhage generally require simple management and have good outcomes.

Complications of Labor and Delivery

PRETERM LABOR

Labor that occurs before week 37 is called **preterm labor** (PTL). Many patients present with preterm contractions, but only those who have changes in the cervix are diagnosed as having preterm labor. PTL differs from **cervical insufficiency**, which is a silent, painless dilation of the cervix. Both can result in preterm delivery, which is the leading cause of fetal morbidity and mortality in the United States. The incidence of preterm delivery increased to over 12% of all births in 2005 from approximately 11% in 2003.

PRETERM DELIVERY

Infants born before 37 weeks of gestation are termed preterm and have higher rates of morbidity and mortality. Infants are also at risk when they are born weighing less than 2,500 g, and are termed **low birth weight** (LBW) infants. Infants who have not grown appropriately for their gestational age have **intrauterine growth restriction** (IUGR) or are **small for gestational age** (SGA). Thus, an IUGR infant can be born after week 37 but still be LBW. Prematurity puts infants at increased risk of respiratory distress syndrome (RDS) or hyaline membrane disease, intraventricular hemorrhage, sepsis, and necrotizing enterocolitis. Morbidity and mortality of preterm infants are dramatically affected by gestational age and birth weight. Infants born on the cusp of viability at 24 weeks' gestation have a greater than 50% mortality rate, whereas infants born after week 34 have a mortality rate similar to that of full-term infants.

ETIOLOGY AND RISK FACTORS

The defining physiologic mechanism that causes the onset of labor is unknown. However, various risk factors have been associated with PTL. These include preterm rupture of membranes (PROM); chorioamnionitis; multiple gestations; uterine anomalies such as a bicornuate uterus; previous preterm delivery; maternal prepregnancy weight less than 50 kg; placental abruption; maternal disease including preeclampsia, infections, intra-abdominal disease or surgery; and low socioeconomic status.

TOCOLYSIS

Tocolysis is the attempt to prevent contractions and the progression of labor. Many tocolytics are used in the United States, but only ritodrine—a beta-mimetic agent—is FDA approved for this purpose. Because most patients and clinicians are unwilling to allow contractions to proceed without some tocolytic therapy, it is difficult to conduct placebo-controlled studies of new tocolytics. Thus, many of the current trials compare currently used tocolytics to other tocolytics. Many of the tocolytics used have only been demonstrated to make a difference in prolonging gestation for 48 hours.

The principal benefit from gaining 48 hours in a pregnancy is to allow treatment with steroids to enhance fetal lung maturity and reduce the risk of complications associated with preterm delivery. **Betamethasone**, a glucocorticoid, has been shown to reduce the incidence of RDS and other complications from preterm delivery. Thus, prior to 34 weeks of gestation, the advantage of treating with steroids needs to be weighed against the risk of prolonging the pregnancy. In fact, there are many situations in which preterm labor should be allowed to progress. Chorioamnionitis, nonreassuring fetal testing, and significant placental abruption are absolute indications to allow labor to progress, and often to hasten delivery. With many other issues such as maternal disease—particularly preeclampsia or poor placental perfusion—an assessment of the severity of the situation, the precipitous nature of the complication, and the risks from prematurity all contribute to the decision of whether or not to tocolyze. In addition, because evidence for the efficacy of tocolytics is unclear, institutions and practitioners vary widely in practice.

TOCOLYTICS

The goal of a tocolytic is to decrease or halt the cervical change resulting from contractions. In the case of preterm contractions without cervical change, hydration can often decrease the number and strength of the contractions. This operates along the principle that a dehydrated patient has increased levels of vasopressin or **antidiuretic hormone** (ADH), the octapeptide synthesized in the hypothalamus along with oxytocin. As it differs from oxytocin by only one amino acid, ADH may bind with oxytocin receptors and lead to contractions. Thus, hydration, which decreases the level of ADH, may also decrease the number of contractions. For patients who do not respond to hydration or whose cervices are actively changing, a variety of tocolytics may be used.

Beta-mimetics

Uterine myometrium is composed of smooth muscle fibers. The contraction of these fibers is regulated by myosin light chain kinase that is activated by calcium ions through their interaction with calmodulin (Fig. 6-1). Thus, by increasing the level of cAMP, the level of free calcium ions decreases, likely by sequestration in the sarcoplasmic reticulum, and uterine contractions may be decreased. Conversion of ATP to cAMP is increased by β-agonists that bind and activate β_2 receptors on myometrial cells.

The two **beta-mimetics** commonly used for preterm labor are **ritodrine** and **terbutaline**. Although both are certainly effective in halting preterm contractions, in randomized controlled studies in which patients were truly in preterm labor, β-agonists gained an average of only 24 to 48 hours' further gestation over hydration and bed rest alone. Side effects of these drugs include tachycardia, headaches, and anxiety. More seriously, pulmonary edema may occur and, in rare cases, maternal death. Ritodrine is given as continuous IV therapy, whereas terbutaline is usually given as 0.25 mg SC, loaded Q 20 min × 3 dosages and then Q 3 to 4 hr maintenance.

Magnesium Sulfate

Magnesium decreases uterine tone and contractions by acting as a calcium antagonist and a membrane stabilizer. Although magnesium can stop contractions, in small placebo-controlled trials it has not been shown to change gestational age of delivery. In larger trials, the efficacy of magnesium did not vary significantly from that of beta-mimetics. Side effects such as flushing, headaches, fatigue, and diplopia are seen, but they are generally considered to be less severe than those seen with ritodrine and terbutaline. At toxic levels of magnesium (>10 mg/dL), respiratory depression, hypoxia, and cardiac arrest have been seen. Since deep tendon reflexes (DTR) are depressed and then lost at levels <10 mg/dL, the best way to rule out magnesium toxicity is with serial reflex checks rather than serum levels. Pulmonary edema has also been seen in women treated with magnesium sulfate, although it may be secondary to the concomitant fluid given to patients in preterm labor. Generally, magnesium sulfate should be loaded as a 6 g bolus over 15 to 30 minutes, then maintained with a 2 to 3 g/hr continuous infusion. Because magnesium is cleared via the kidneys, a slower infusion should be used in the case of renal insufficiency.

Calcium Channel Blockers

Calcium channel blockers decrease the influx of calcium into smooth muscle cells thereby diminishing uterine contractions. These have definitely been shown to decrease myometrial contractions in vitro. In clinical studies, **nifedipine** has been the principal drug studied and seems to have comparable efficacy to that of ritodrine and magnesium. Side effects include headaches, flushing, and dizziness. Nifedipine is given orally and, as with other tocolytics, should be loaded. A 10 mg dose Q 15 min for the first hour or until contractions have ceased is typical. This is followed by a maintenance dosage of 10 to 30 mg Q 4 to 6 hr as tolerated according to the patient's blood pressure. Long-acting preparations of nifedipine in small studies seem

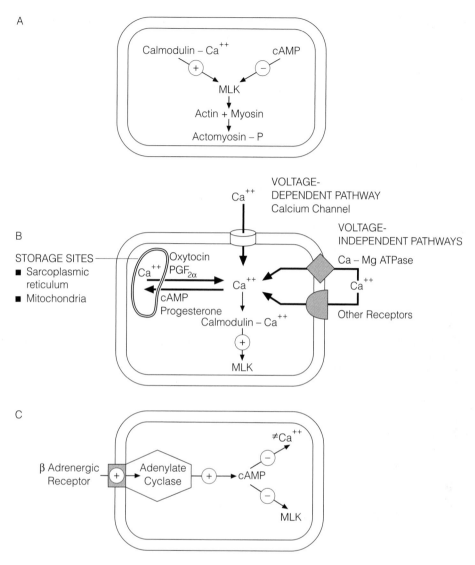

Figure 6-1 • Control of myometrial contractility: myosin light-chain kinase (MLK) is the key enzyme.

to have similar efficacy to the quick-release doses and can be used for long-term therapy to increase compliance and decrease side effects.

Prostaglandin Inhibitors

Prostaglandins increase the intracellular levels of calcium, thereby increasing myometrial contractions. Further, these have been shown to enhance myometrial gap junction formation and are commonly used to induce labor and to heighten contractions in postpartum patients with uterine atony. Thus, antiprostaglandin agents should theoretically inhibit contractions and possibly halt labor. **Indomethacin**—a nonsteroidal anti-inflammatory drug (NSAID) that blocks the enzyme cyclooxygenase and decreases the level of prostaglandins—is used as a tocolytic. In clinical trials, it has been shown to effectively decrease contractions and forestall labor with minimal maternal side effects. However, it has been associated with a variety of fetal complications. These include premature constriction of the ductus arteriosus, pulmonary hypertension, and oligohydramnios secondary to fetal renal failure. Furthermore, in one study, extremely premature fetuses that had been exposed to indomethacin within 48 hours of delivery had an increased risk of necrotizing enterocolitis and intraventricular hemorrhage. Therefore, even though indomethacin is a promising tocolytic, many practitioners shy away from its use.

Oxytocin Antagonists

Currently, oxytocin antagonists (e.g., atosiban) are being studied as tocolytics. These have been shown to decrease uterine myometrial contractions, but clinical studies have been small thus far. In theory, these seem to be an obvious choice for an effective tocolytic and should have minimal side effects. Current clinical use has been limited to experimental trials that have shown no difference from the other commonly used tocolytics.

PRETERM AND PREMATURE RUPTURE OF MEMBRANES

Rupture of membranes (ROM) occurring before week 37 is considered **preterm rupture of the membranes**, whereas rupture of membranes occurring before the onset of labor is termed **premature rupture of the membranes** (PROM). If the two occur together it is termed **preterm premature rupture of the membranes** (PPROM). Anytime rupture of membranes lasts longer than 18 hours before delivery, it is described as **prolonged rupture of membranes**.

PRETERM RUPTURE OF MEMBRANES

Spontaneous rupture of the fetal membranes before week 37 is a common cause of preterm labor, preterm delivery, and chorioamnionitis. Without intervention, approximately 50% of patients who have ROM will go into labor within 24 hours, and up to 75% will do so within 48 hours. These rates are inversely correlated to gestational age at ROM; thus, patients with ROM prior to 26 weeks' gestational age are more likely to gain an additional week than those greater than 30 weeks' gestational age. While maintaining the pregnancy to gain further fetal maturity would seem beneficial, prolonged PPROM has been associated with increased risk of chorioamnionitis, abruption, and cord prolapse.

Diagnosis

Commonly, a patient complains of a gush of fluid from the vagina. However, any increased vaginal discharge or complaints of stress incontinence should be evaluated to rule out ROM. The diagnosis is made by obtaining a history of leaking vaginal fluid, pooling on speculum examination, and positive nitrazine and fern tests. If these tests are equivocal, an ultrasound can be performed to examine the level of amniotic fluid, and some providers and hospitals will use the Amnisure test as noted in Chapter 4. If the diagnosis is still unconfirmed, an amniocentesis dye test can be performed with injection of a dye via amniocentesis and observation of whether or not the dye leaks into the vagina. This is also known as the **tampon test** because the dye is usually identified by its absorption into a tampon. If there is concern for chorioamnionitis, maternal temperature and white blood count, uterine tenderness, and the fetal heart tracing should all be checked for signs of infection.

Treatment

The management of PROM varies depending on the gestational age of the fetus. The rationale for the management of PPROM is that at some gestational age, the risk from prematurity is equal to the risk of infection. That point is somewhere between 32 and 36 weeks; thus, up to this point, the risk of prematurity drives management, whereas after it the risk of infection motivates delivery. There is debate regarding the exact gestational age at which the risk of infection is greater. Some practitioners prefer to wait until week 36, whereas others prefer to test for fetal lung maturity starting at week 32 and deliver when mature, while still others would deliver at 32 to 34 weeks' gestation without fetal lung maturity testing. Of note, depending on the population being cared for, the optimal week of gestation to deliver probably varies.

There is strong evidence that the use of antibiotics in PPROM leads to a longer latency period prior to the onset of labor. Thus, ampicillin with or without erythromycin is recommended in the setting of PPROM. There is debate surrounding the use of tocolysis and corticosteroids in the setting of PPROM. Tocolysis seems to add little, if any, benefit in PPROM and may even be harmful in the setting of chorioamnionitis. However, at many institutions tocolysis is used for 48 hours, particularly at earlier gestational ages, in order to gain time to administer a course of corticosteroids. Currently, the recommendation is to use corticosteroids in the setting of PPROM despite any concern regarding immunosuppression because of the fetal benefits.

PREMATURE RUPTURE OF THE MEMBRANES

The most common concern of PROM is that of chorioamnionitis, the risk of which increases with the length of ROM. If ROM is expected to last beyond 18 hours, it is termed prolonged rupture of the membranes and if the GBS status is unknown maternal administration of antibiotics is recommended during the remainder of labor. Commonly, if ROM occurs anytime after 34 to 36 weeks, labor is induced/augmented. Some patients may elect to bear the risk of increased infection to await the onset of spontaneous labor. However, the risks of infection with prolonged PROM should be discussed with patients before any decision is made. One large, randomized, controlled trial demonstrated that there is no difference in length of labor or mode of delivery with immediate augmentation/induction of PROM, but the rate of chorioamnionitis is higher among those with expectant management.

OBSTRUCTION, MALPRESENTATION, AND MALPOSITION

Although the most common form of delivery is the spontaneous vertex vaginal delivery, other presentations and deliveries also occur. Many of the malpresentations lead to cesarean delivery.

CEPHALOPELVIC DISPROPORTION

One of the most common indications for cesarean section is failure to progress (FTP) in labor, most often caused by **cephalopelvic disproportion** (CPD). The three "Ps"—pelvis, passenger, and power—are primarily responsible for a vaginal delivery. If the pelvis is too small, the fetal presenting part is too large, or the contractions are inadequate, there will be FTP. The strength of uterine contractions can be measured with an intrauterine pressure catheter (IUPC) and augmented with oxytocin, but little can be done about the other two factors that contribute to CPD.

Diagnosis

The maternal pelvis is described as one of four dominant types: **gynecoid**, **android**, **anthropoid**, and **platypelloid** (Fig. 6-2). Further, many pelves have characteristics from more than one of these types. Common measurements of the pelvis include those of the pelvic inlet, the midpelvis, and the pelvic outlet. The **obstetric conjugate**, which is the distance between the sacral promontory and the midpoint of the symphysis pubis, is the shortest anteroposterior

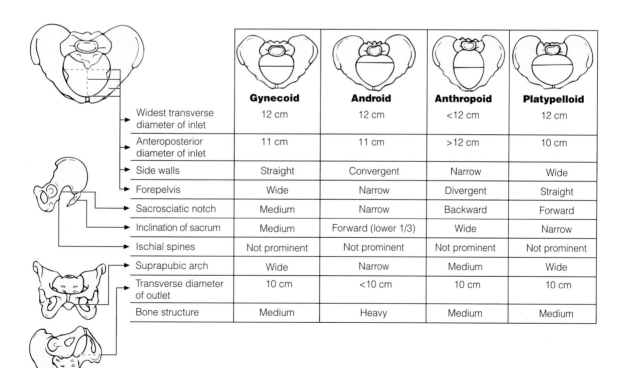

	Gynecoid	Android	Anthropoid	Platypelloid
Widest transverse diameter of inlet	12 cm	12 cm	<12 cm	12 cm
Anteroposterior diameter of inlet	11 cm	11 cm	>12 cm	10 cm
Side walls	Straight	Convergent	Narrow	Wide
Forepelvis	Wide	Narrow	Divergent	Straight
Sacrosciatic notch	Medium	Narrow	Backward	Forward
Inclination of sacrum	Medium	Forward (lower 1/3)	Wide	Narrow
Ischial spines	Not prominent	Not prominent	Not prominent	Not prominent
Suprapubic arch	Wide	Narrow	Medium	Wide
Transverse diameter of outlet	10 cm	<10 cm	10 cm	10 cm
Bone structure	Medium	Heavy	Medium	Medium

Figure 6-2 • Characteristics of four types of pelvises.

diameter of the pelvic inlet. The anteroposterior diameter of the pelvic outlet, which measures from the tip of the sacrum to the inferior margin of the pubic symphysis, ranges from 9.5 to 11.5 cm. These measurements are performed with both clinical and x-ray pelvimetry, but it is rare to assume CPD based on measurements alone.

The fetal skull is composed of the face, the base, and the vault. The face and base are composed of fused bones that do not change during labor; however, the bones of the vault are not fused and can undergo molding to conform to the maternal pelvis. The vault is composed of five bones: two frontal, two parietal, and one occipital. The spaces between the bones are known as sutures; the two places where the sutures intersect are the **anterior** and **posterior fontanelles**. How the fetal head presents to the maternal pelvis is important in accomplishing a vaginal delivery. There is great variation in the diameter of the skull at various levels and with various inclinations. When the fetal skull is properly flexed, the suboccipitobregmatic diameter presenting to the pelvis averages 9.5 cm in a term infant. When the sagittal suture is not located midline in the pelvis (asynclitism), the diameter of the skull being accommodated is effectively increased.

Treatment

Even if cephalopelvic disproportion is suspected, it is still often worthwhile to attempt a trial of labor. In the case of fetal macrosomia, elective induction of labor may be chosen before the opportunity for vaginal delivery passes. This practice leads to a similar rate of cesarean delivery but as a result of failed induction rather than CPD.

BREECH PRESENTATION

Breech presentation, or buttocks first, occurs in 3% to 4% of all singleton deliveries. Factors associated with breech presentation include previous breech delivery, uterine anomalies, polyhydramnios, oligohydramnios, multiple gestation, PPROM, hydrocephaly, and anencephaly. Persistent breech presentation is also associated with placenta previa and fetal anomalies. Complications of a vaginal breech delivery include prolapsed cord and entrapment of the head.

Types of Breech

There are three categories of the breech presentation (Fig. 6-3): **frank**, **complete**, and **incomplete** or **footling**. The frank breech has flexed hips and extended knees and thus the feet are near the fetal head. The complete breech has flexed hips, but one or both knees are flexed as well, with at least one foot near the breech. The incomplete or footling breech has one or both of the hips not flexed so that the foot or knee lies below the breech in the birth canal.

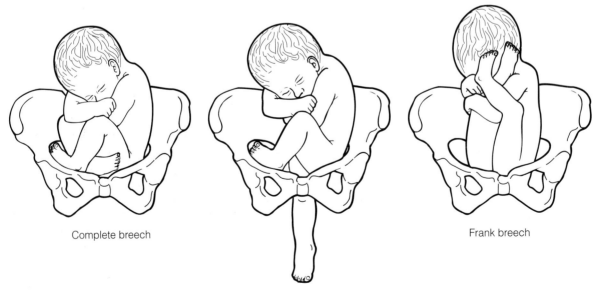

Complete breech

Footling breech

Frank breech

Figure 6-3 • Types of breech presentations.

Diagnosis

The breech presentation may be diagnosed in several ways. With abdominal examination using the Leopold maneuvers, the fetal head can be palpated near the fundus while the breech is palpated in the pelvis. With vaginal examination, the breech can be palpated, the common landmarks being the gluteal cleft and the anus or, in the case of an incomplete breech, the fetal lower extremity. Diagnosis is often made or confirmed with ultrasound. On ultrasound, it is easy to confirm breech and then to determine the type of breech.

Treatment

How a breech presentation is managed depends on the experience of the obstetrician and the patient's wishes. The three options are external cephalic version of the breech, trial of breech vaginal delivery, and elective cesarean delivery. External version consists of manipulation of the breech infant into a vertex presentation. It is rarely performed before 36 to 37 weeks' gestation because of the potential for spontaneous version before this point and the risk of delivery after version secondary to abruption or rupture of membranes. External version is usually attempted without anesthesia and if successful, the patient can continue the pregnancy to go into spontaneous labor, though the risk of the fetus reverting back to breech presentation is about 5% to 10%. If the version is not successful, often it is rescheduled under epidural anesthesia at 39 weeks of gestation. If successful, then either labor can be induced or the patient can continue the pregnancy. If it fails, often the patient will then have cesarean delivery.

Trial of breech vaginal delivery can be attempted in the proper setting, but is becoming increasingly rare in the United States, particularly since a prospective randomized trial found higher rate of neonatal morbidity and mortality with trial of labor. Complications of breech deliveries include cord prolapse, entrapment of the fetal head, and fetal neurologic injury. A favorable pelvis (by clinical or CT pelvimetry), a flexed head, estimated fetal weight between 2,000 and 3,800 g, and frank or complete breech are common criteria used for trial of labor of breech presentation. Relative contraindications include nulliparity, incomplete breech presentation, and estimated fetal weight greater than 3,800 g. Patients with these contraindications are usually recommended to undergo cesarean delivery. However, if a patient wishes to attempt vaginal delivery, careful monitoring of the fetus and progress of labor is imperative.

MALPRESENTATION OF VERTEX

Malpresentation can occur even in the setting of a cephalic or vertex presentation. The face, brow, persistent occiput posterior (OP), or a compound presentation with a fetal upper extremity can complicate the cephalic presentation. In addition, the shoulder can present in the setting of a transverse lie.

Face

The diagnosis of face presentation (Fig. 6-4) can be made with vaginal examination and palpation of the nose, mouth, eyes, or chin (mentum). If the fetus is mentum anterior, vaginal delivery will often ensue. However, with a mentum posterior or transverse, the fetus must rotate to mentum anterior to deliver vaginally. Of note, many anencephalic fetuses have a face presentation. Augmentation is used only sparingly with a face presentation as the pressure on the face leads to edema.

Brow

Brow presentation (Fig. 6-5) occurs when the portion of the fetal skull just above the orbital ridge presents. With the brow presenting, a larger diameter must pass through the pelvis. Therefore, unless the fetal head is particularly small (e.g., preterm) or the pelvis is particularly large, the brow presentation must convert to vertex or face to deliver.

Shoulder

If the fetus is in a transverse lie, often the shoulder is presenting to the pelvic inlet. Diagnosis of this malpresentation can be made with abdominal or vaginal examination and ultrasound confirmation. Unless there is spontaneous conversion to vertex, shoulder presentations are delivered via cesarean section because of the increased risk of cord prolapse, increased risk for uterine rupture, and the difficulty of vaginal delivery.

Compound Presentation

A fetal extremity presenting alongside the vertex or breech is considered a compound presentation

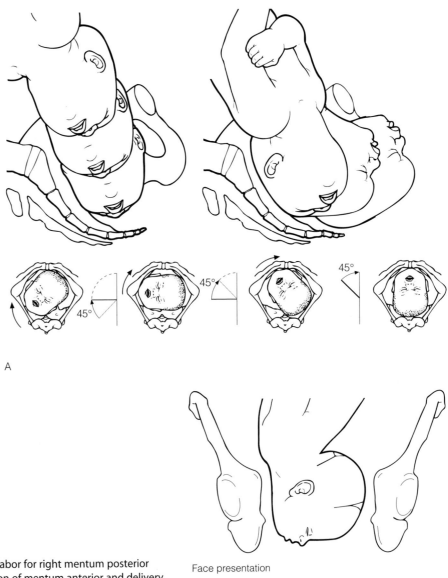

A

Figure 6-4 • (A) Mechanisms of labor for right mentum posterior position with subsequent rotation of mentum anterior and delivery. **(B)** Face presentation. Well engaged in the mentolateral position.

Face presentation

B

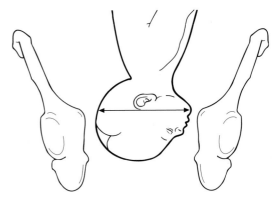

Figure 6-5 • Brow presentation with mentovertex diameter presenting.

Brow presentation

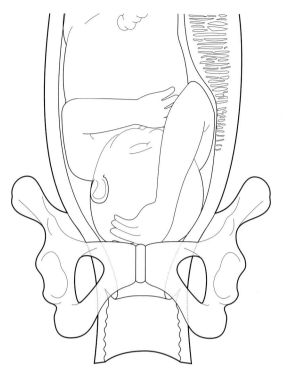

Figure 6-6 • Compound presentation. The left hand is lying in front of the vertex. With further labor, the hand and arm may retract from the birth canal and the head may then descend normally.

(Fig. 6-6). This occurs in less than 1:1,000 pregnancies. The rate increases with prematurity, multiple gestations, polyhydramnios, and CPD. A common complication of compound presentation is umbilical cord prolapse. The diagnosis is often made with vaginal examination when the fetal extremity is palpated alongside the presenting part. At this point it should be determined whether the prolapsed fetal part is a hand or foot. Ultrasound may be used to determine the type of extremity presenting.

Treatment

Often, if an upper extremity is presenting alongside the vertex, the part may be gently reduced. However, prolapse of a lower extremity in vertex presentation is far less likely to deliver vaginally. Compound presentation of a lower extremity with a breech is considered a footling or incomplete breech presentation and calls for cesarean section. In all cases of compound presentation, umbilical cord prolapse should be suspected and careful monitoring with continuous fetal heart tracings and frequent vaginal examinations should ensue.

Persistent Occiput Transverse and Posterior Position

The most common position of the fetus at the onset of labor is either left occiput transverse (LOT) or right occiput transverse (ROT). From the transverse position, the cardinal movement of internal rotation usually converts the fetus to the occiput anterior (OA) position. However, it is not uncommon for the fetus to stay in the occiput transverse (OT) position, or rotate to the occiput posterior (OP) position. If this occurs, the progress of labor may be arrested. Diagnosis is made by palpation of the fetal sutures and fontanelles and following the progress of labor.

A persistent OT position leading to transverse arrest of labor is more common in women with a platypelloid pelvis. If the cervix is not fully dilated, an attempt may be made at manual rotation to the OA position. If the cervix is fully dilated, rotation to the OA position can be attempted manually or with forceps. Additionally, in the setting of full dilation, an attempt at vacuum delivery may be effective as the traction on the fetal scalp may lead to autorotation to the OA position.

During descent, OP positions may rotate to OA, although this does not always occur and can slow progress in labor. The management is similar to that for OA position: patiently watch and wait. However, spontaneous vaginal delivery occurs less often. In the setting of OP or OT position and active phase arrest, manual rotation prior to complete cervical dilation has been described, though it may be associated with injury to the cervix. If the second stage of labor is prolonged, the options include delivery of the fetus with forceps or vacuum in the OP position, rotation with forceps, or manual rotation. In either the OT or OP position, if the attempt at rotation or operative vaginal delivery fails, cesarean delivery is required.

OBSTETRIC EMERGENCIES

FETAL BRADYCARDIA

One of the most common events in labor and delivery that leads to anxiety among both the practitioners and the patients is fetal heart rate (FHR) bradycardia. Any time the fetal heart rate is below 100 to 110 for longer than 2 minutes it is called a prolonged deceleration. Longer than 10 minutes is termed bradycardia. Older terminology deemed a deceleration lasting longer than 2 minutes a bradycardia, so this is commonly used in labor and delivery in the setting of prolonged decelerations. Either way, these FHR decelerations are associated with a number of other complications such as placental abruption, cord prolapse, tetanic contraction, uterine rupture, pulmonary embolus (PE), amniotic fluid embolus (AFE), and seizure. They have also been associated with poor fetal outcome.

The etiology of prolonged FHR decelerations can be considered to be preuterine, uteroplacental, or postplacental. Pre-uterine issues would be any event leading to maternal hypotension or hypoxia. These would include seizure, amniotic fluid embolus (AFE), PE, MI, respiratory failure, or recent epidural or spinal placement with hypotension. Uteroplacental issues include placental abruption, infarction, and hemorrhaging previa, as well as uterine hyperstimulation. Postplacental etiologies include cord prolapse, cord compression, and rupture of a fetal vessel.

Diagnosis

FHR decelerations are usually not subtle. However, the FHR should be differentiated from the maternal heart rate, which is commonly in the 60s to 100s. This can be done by placing a fetal scalp electrode (FSE) on the fetal scalp and concomitantly an O_2 saturation monitor on the mother. In facilities without access to these tools, palpation of the maternal pulse while listening to the FHR can usually differentiate between the two.

Diagnosis of the etiology of the bradycardia is often more important than the diagnosis of bradycardia, which is relatively straightforward in the era of continuous fetal monitoring. A simple algorithm follows.

1. *Look at the mother for signs of respiratory compromise or change in mental status.* This should commonly diagnose seizures, PE, and AFE.
2. *While putting on a glove for a cervical examination, assess the maternal blood pressure and heart rate.* This will diagnose maternal hypotension, commonly seen after epidural placement and a potential cause of FHR decelerations. This will also aid in determining whether the FHR being recorded could be maternal.
3. *Immediately before the examination look to see how much vaginal blood is passing.* With increased vaginal bleeding, placental abruption and uterine rupture should be considered. If placentation is unknown, placenta previa is also a possibility. Rarely,

vaginal bleeding is secondary to rupture of a fetal vessel as in vasa previa.

4. *Examine the patient with one hand on the maternal abdomen and one hand vaginally feeling for cervical dilation, fetal station, and prolapsed umbilical cord.* The abdominal hand should feel for uterine tetany and fetal parts outside the uterus. If the fetal station is dramatically lower than expected, then the prolonged FHR deceleration may be due to rapid descent and vagal stimulation. If the fetal station is much higher than expected, uterine rupture should be suspected. If the cervix is fully dilated and the fetus in the pelvis, operative vaginal delivery can be performed if the FHR deceleration does not resolve in a timely fashion.

Treatment

In the setting of prolonged FHR deceleration, the initial management is standardized. The patient is moved to left or right lateral decubitus to resolve a FHR deceleration secondary to compression of the inferior vena cava (IVC) leading to decreased preload or more commonly a compressed umbilical cord by the fetus. Oxygen by face mask is commonly administered to the mother in case hypoxia is an issue. The examination is performed as described above, and the individual etiologies are diagnosed and treated appropriately. In the setting of maternal hypotension, the patient can be given aggressive IV hydration and ephedrine. The management of seizure, AFE, uterine rupture, and PE are discussed elsewhere. Tetanic uterine contraction is treated with nitroglycerin, usually administered via a sublingual spray, and/or terbutaline a β-agonist tocolytic. If umbilical cord prolapse is identified, there have been case reports of replacement into the uterus, but most commonly this requires an emergent cesarean delivery, performed with the examining clinician lifting the fetal head to avoid compression of the prolapsed cord. In the setting of previa, cesarean delivery should be expedited as well. If abruption is suspected, and the patient is remote from delivery, cesarean section may be necessary.

It is imperative that the timing of these events is followed very closely. Further, clinicians need to know the capabilities of their labor and delivery units and the rapidity of response of the anesthesiologists. Commonly, a patient is moved from the labor room to the OR after 4 to 5 minutes of FHR deceleration. If the FHR is checked in the OR (at this time, usually 8 minutes) and the bradycardia persists, plans for emergent cesarean delivery should proceed. The rapidity of this delivery may allow all of the most common sterile techniques typically employed because delivery of the fetus within the next 2 to 4 minutes is the goal.

SHOULDER DYSTOCIA

Once the head of the fetus is delivered, difficulty in delivering the shoulders, particularly because of impaction of the anterior shoulder behind the pubic symphysis, is termed **shoulder dystocia**. Risk factors for shoulder dystocia include fetal macrosomia, preconceptional and gestational diabetes, previous shoulder dystocia, maternal obesity, postterm pregnancy, prolonged second stage of labor, and operative vaginal delivery. Increased morbidity and mortality are associated with shoulder dystocia. Fetal complications include fractures of the humerus and clavicle, brachial plexus nerve injuries (Erb palsy), phrenic nerve palsy, hypoxic brain injury, and death.

Diagnosis

The actual diagnosis of a shoulder dystocia is made when routine obstetric maneuvers fail to deliver the fetus. When antepartum risk factors are present, shoulder dystocia can be predicted, prepared for, and possibly even prevented. Preparation for a shoulder dystocia includes placing the patient in the dorsal lithotomy position, having adequate anesthesia, cutting a generous episiotomy, and having several experienced clinicians present at the birth. At the time of delivery, suspicion is increased with prolonged crowning of the head and then with the "turtle" sign of either incomplete delivery of the head or the chin tucking up against the maternal perineum.

Treatment

As with any obstetric emergency, it is important to have a team of clinicians providing care, so once a shoulder dystocia is identified, the labor and delivery alert should be sounded. Similar to a code, someone needs to be running the shoulder dystocia emergency; in a teaching hospital this is usually the attending or chief resident, in a private hospital, this is usually the delivering obstetrician. Someone should be assigned to keep track of time as a shoulder dystocia can lead

to entrapment and complete compression of the umbilical cord, so delivery in less than 5 minutes is imperative. Two individuals should be assigned to hold the patient's legs and one person assigned to do suprapubic pressure. The pediatric team should be called.

The specific series of maneuvers for delivering an infant with a shoulder dystocia are as follows.

- **McRoberts maneuver:** Sharp flexion of the maternal hips that decreases the inclination of the pelvis increasing the AP diameter can free the anterior shoulder (Fig. 6-7).
- **Suprapubic pressure:** This is to dislodge the anterior shoulder from behind the pubic symphysis and should be directed at an oblique angle (Fig. 6-8).
- **Rubin maneuver:** Place pressure on an accessible shoulder to push it toward the anterior chest wall of the fetus to decrease the bisacromial diameter and free the impacted shoulder (Fig. 6-9).
- **Wood's corkscrew maneuver:** Apply pressure behind the posterior shoulder to rotate the infant and dislodge the anterior shoulder.
- **Delivery of the posterior arm/shoulder:** By sweeping the posterior arm across the chest and delivering it, the bisacromial diameter can then be rotated to an oblique diameter of the pelvis and the anterior shoulder is freed.

If these maneuvers are unsuccessful, they may be performed again. If the infant is still undelivered, there are several other maneuvers that can be performed. Cutting or fracturing the fetal clavicle or cutting the maternal pubic symphysis will often release the infant. Symphysiotomy is a morbid procedure often complicated by infection, healing difficulties, and chronic pain, and thus should be reserved for the true emergency. If none of these maneuvers is successful, the **Zavanelli** maneuver, which involves placing the infant's head back into the pelvis and performing cesarean delivery, can be attempted.

UTERINE RUPTURE

Uterine rupture is seen in one in 10,000 to 20,000 deliveries in patients with unscarred uteri. Associated complications in these patients include uterine fibroids, uterine malformations, obstructed labor, and the use of uterotonic agents such as oxytocin and prostaglandins. In patients who have had a prior uterine scar from myomectomy or cesarean delivery, the

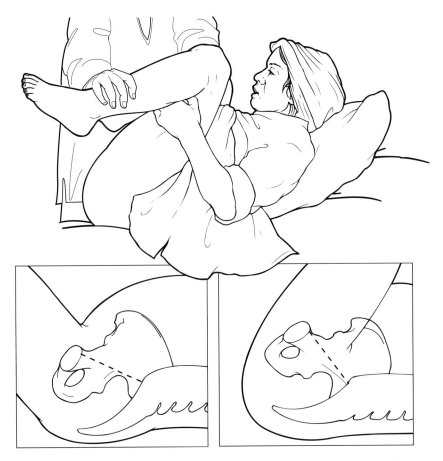

Figure 6-7 • Sharp ventral rotation of both maternal hips (McRoberts maneuver) brings the pelvic inlet and outlet into a more vertical alignment, facilitating delivery of the fetal shoulders.

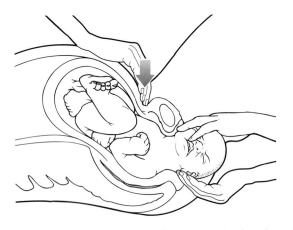

Figure 6-8 • Moderate suprapubic pressure is often the only additional maneuver necessary to free the anterior fetal shoulder.

risk of uterine rupture is theoretically 0.5% to 1.0%. The risk is increased in patients who have more than one cesarean scar, have a "classical" or high vertical scar, undergo labor induction, and/or are treated with uterotonic agents.

Uterine rupture is suspected in the setting of FHR decelerations in patients with prior scars on their uterus. Patients may feel a "popping" sensation or experience sudden abdominal pain. On physical examination, the fetus may be palpable in the extrauterine space, there may be vaginal bleeding, and commonly the fetal presenting part is suddenly much higher than previously. If a uterine rupture is strongly suspected, the patient should be taken to the OR for immediate cesarean delivery and exploratory laparotomy.

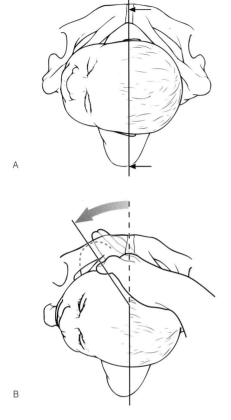

A

B

Figure 6-9 • Rubin maneuver. **(A)** The shoulder-to-shoulder diameter is shown as the distance between the two small arrows. **(B)** The most easily accessible fetal shoulder (the anterior is shown here) is pushed toward the anterior chest wall of the fetus. Most often, this results in abduction of both shoulders, reducing the shoulder-to-shoulder diameter and freeing the impacted anterior shoulder.

MATERNAL HYPOTENSION

Pregnant patients commonly have blood pressures around 90/50. BPs much lower than the 80/40 range is unusual and can lead to poor maternal and uterine perfusion. Common etiologies of maternal hypotension include vasovagal events, regional anesthesia, overtreatment with antihypertensive drugs, hemorrhage, anaphylaxis, and amniotic fluid embolus (AFE). Most of these events can be differentiated from each other quickly and by the clinical scenario.

Treatment of maternal hypotension may vary based on the etiology, but the mainstays are aggressive IV hydration and adrenergic medications to constrict peripheral vessels and increase both the

preload and the afterload. If the event does occur in close proximity to medication administration, Benadryl and even epinephrine should be considered for a possible anaphylactic reaction. If the patient has an AFE, the mortality rate is quite high. The definitive diagnosis of AFE is the finding of fetal cells in the pulmonary vasculature at autopsy.

SEIZURE

Seizures on labor and delivery are usually quite startling and can be dangerous. In patients with a history of a seizure disorder as well as those with preeclampsia, careful observation for particular seizure precursors is maintained. However, many patients who seize on labor and delivery have no history and may be normotensive.

Many vasovagal events are misdiagnosed as a seizure because the patient may have several tonic-clonic movements. One of the key ways to differentiate between the two is the presence of a postictal period after the event. To help sort out the etiology, patients should have a full preeclamptic workup and, when it is safe for the patient to leave the floor, obtain a head CT. A neurology consult is also indicated. Acutely, the patients should be managed with the ABCs of resuscitation and with antiseizure medications (Table 6-1). In pregnancy, magnesium sulfate is the antiseizure medication of choice.

■ **TABLE 6-1** Management of a Pregnant Patient with Seizures or in Status Epilepticus
Assess and establish airway and vital signs including oxygenation
Assess FHR or fetal status
Bolus magnesium sulfate, or give 10 g IM
Bolus with lorazepam 0.1 mg/kg, 5.0 to 10.0 mg at no more than 2.0 mg/min
Load phenytoin 20 mg/kg, usually 1 to 2 g at no more than 50 mg/min
If not successful, load phenobarbital 20 mg/kg, usually 1 to 2 g at no more than 100 mg/min
Labs include electrolytes, AED levels, glucose, and toxicology screen
If fetal testing is not reassuring, move to emergent delivery

KEY POINTS

- Preterm delivery occurs in greater than 10% of all pregnancies.

- PTL is treated with tocolytics including beta-agonists, magnesium, calcium channel blockers, and NSAIDs.

- Current tocolytics are only marginally effective, but may buy time for a course of betamethasone to accelerate fetal lung maturity.

- Preterm rupture of membranes is when ROM occurs before 37 weeks of gestation; premature rupture of membranes (PROM) is ROM that occurs before the onset of labor.

- The latency period prior to the onset of labor is inversely correlated with gestational age in PPROM.

- Once ROM is confirmed, the therapeutic course depends on gestational age, risk of infection, and fetal lung maturity; any patient who shows signs of infection or fetal distress needs delivery.

- If the fetal head is too large to pass through the maternal pelvis, it is deemed cephalopelvic disproportion (CPD).

- Unless ultrasound and CT have been used to document a fetal head larger than the maternal pelvis, in the case of suspected CPD, a trial of labor is often attempted.

- There are three types of breech: frank, complete, and incomplete or footling.

- Breech presentations may be managed by external version to vertex, cesarean delivery, and less frequently a trial of labor. The complications of labor and delivery of breech presentation include cord prolapse and entrapment of the fetal head.

- Vertex malpresentations include face, brow, compound, and persistent OP. These presentations will often deliver vaginally but need closer monitoring and sometimes require different maneuvers.

- Prolonged fetal heart rate decelerations may have a variety of etiologies and can be thought of as pre-uterine, uteroplacental, and postplacental.

- A quick examination and verification of vital signs will often determine the etiology of a prolonged deceleration.

- If there is no sign of resolution of the FHR deceleration in 4 to 5 minutes, the patient should either be delivered vaginally or moved to the OR for cesarean.

- Shoulder dystocias can result in fetal fractures, nerve damage, and hypoxia.

- Risk factors for shoulder dystocia include fetal macrosomia, diabetes, previous dystocia, maternal obesity, postterm deliveries, and prolonged stage 2 of labor.

- The maneuvers to reduce a shoulder dystocia include suprapubic pressure, McRoberts maneuver, Rubin maneuver, Wood's corkscrew, delivery of posterior arm, fracture or cutting the clavicle or pubic symphysis, and the Zavanelli maneuver.

- Uterine rupture is uncommon in patients with no prior uterine scar; it is seen in 0.5% to 1.0% of patients who labor with a prior cesarean delivery.

- Maternal hypotension may have a variety of etiologies including regional anesthesia, hemorrhage, vasovagal events, AFE, and anaphylaxis.

- Patients with seizures in pregnancy are managed first line with IV or IM magnesium sulfate.

Fetal Complications of Pregnancy

DISORDERS OF FETAL GROWTH

Newborns with birth weight less than the 10th percentile or greater than the 90th percentile are easily identified. However, the accuracy of antepartum estimates of fetal weight can vary. Ultrasound is the most commonly used modality to estimate fetal weight. Fetuses whose estimated fetal weight (EFW) is less than the 10th percentile are termed **small for gestational age** (SGA). Those whose EFW is greater than the 90th percentile are termed **large for gestational age** (LGA). SGA fetuses are further described as either symmetric or asymmetric. *Symmetric* implies that the fetus is proportionally small. *Asymmetric* implies that certain organs of the fetus are disproportionately small. Classically, an asymmetric infant will have wasting of the torso and extremities while preserving the brain. Thus, the skull will be at a greater percentile than the rest of the body. Screening for disorders of fetal growth is done during routine prenatal care. Once the fetus is at or greater than 20 weeks' gestational age, the uterine fundal height (in centimeters) should be approximately equal to the gestational age (in weeks). Fetal growth can therefore be followed by serial examinations of the fundal height. Before making the diagnosis of either SGA or LGA, it is imperative that accurate dating of the pregnancy is ascertained. If the fundal height varies by more than 3 cm from the gestational age, ultrasound is usually obtained.

SMALL FOR GESTATIONAL AGE

Small for gestational age (SGA) infants are associated with higher rates of mortality and morbidity for their gestational age. However, even within the SGA category, infants, <5th percentile or even <3rd percentile have even worse outcomes. Of note, SGA infants do better than infants with the same weight delivered at earlier gestational ages. For example, SGA babies born at 34 weeks that weigh the same as 28-week infants will have lower morbidity and mortality rates. Factors that can result in infants being SGA can be divided into those that lead to **decreased growth potential** and those that lead to **intrauterine growth restriction** (IUGR) (Table 7-1).

Decreased Growth Potential

Congenital abnormalities account for approximately 10% to 15% of SGA infants. Trisomy 21 (Down syndrome), trisomy 18 (Edward syndrome), and trisomy 13 (Patau syndrome) all lead to SGA babies. Turner syndrome (45,XO) leads to a decrease in birth weight. Infants with osteogenesis imperfecta, achondroplasia, neural tube defects, anencephaly, and a variety of autosomal recessive syndromes may all be SGA.

All intrauterine infections—particularly **cytomegalovirus** (CMV) and **rubella**—lead to SGA infants. These probably account for 10% to 15% of all SGA babies. Exposure to **teratogens**, most chemotherapeutic agents, and other drugs during pregnancy can also lead to decreased growth potential. The two most common teratogens causing SGA are alcohol and cigarettes. Up to 10% of SGA fetuses are constitutionally small based purely on parental stature.

Intrauterine Growth Restriction (IUGR)

Fetal growth can be divided into two phases. Prior to 20 weeks of gestation, growth is primarily hyperplastic

■ TABLE 7-1 Risk Factors for SGA Infants
Decreased growth potential
Genetic and chromosomal abnormalities
Intrauterine infections
Teratogenic exposure
Substance abuse
Radiation exposure
Small maternal stature
Pregnancy at high altitudes
Female fetus
Intrauterine growth restricted (IUGR)
Maternal factors including hypertension, anemia, chronic renal disease, malnutrition, and severe diabetes
Placental factors including placenta previa, chronic abruption, placental infarction, multiple gestations

(increasing number of cells); after 20 weeks, it is primarily hypertrophic. Because of this, an insult leading to growth restriction occurring prior to 20 weeks will most likely result in symmetric growth restriction, whereas insults occurring after 20 weeks in a prolonged fashion result in asymmetric growth. Asymmetric growth most likely results from decreased nutrition and oxygen being transmitted across the placenta, which is then shunted to the fetal brain. Two-thirds of the time, growth restriction is asymmetric and can be identified by increased head to abdominal measurements.

Maternal risk factors include baseline hypertension, anemia, chronic renal disease, antiphospholipid antibody syndrome, systemic lupus erythematosus (SLE), and severe malnutrition. Severe diabetes with extensive vascular disease may also lead to IUGR. Placental factors leading to diminished placental blood flow may lead to IUGR. These factors include placenta previa, marginal cord insertion, and placental thrombosis with

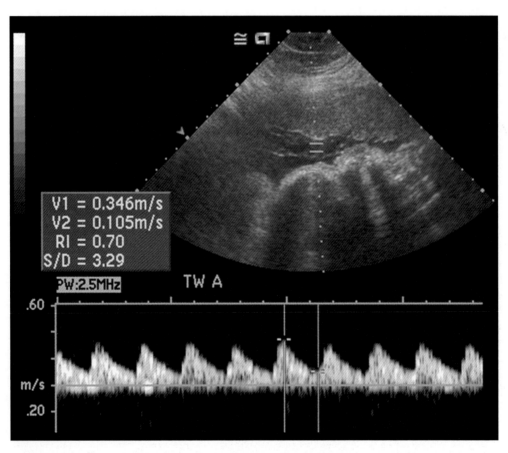

Figure 7-1 • Normal umbilical artery Doppler: Note the ratio between systolic peak and diastolic trough is 3.29:1.

or without infarction. Multiple gestations often lead to lower birth weights because of earlier delivery and SGA infants. In twins, SGA infants are seen particularly in the twin-twin transfusion syndrome.

Diagnosis

The risk of having an SGA baby increases in mothers with a previous SGA baby or with any of the above etiologies. These fetuses should be followed carefully for intrauterine growth. Fundal height is measured at each prenatal visit. Oligohydramnios and SGA fetuses have fundal heights less than expected. Anytime a fundal height is 3 cm less than expected, fetal growth should be estimated via ultrasound. Of note, the use of fundal height as a screening tool for either SGA or LGA is quite poor with sensitivities well below 50% and positive predictive values below 50% as well.

If SGA is suspected, the accuracy of the pregnancy's dating should be verified. Any infant at risk for IUGR or being SGA is followed with serial ultrasound scans for growth every 2 to 3 weeks. A fetus with decreased growth potential will usually start small and stay small, whereas one with IUGR will progressively fall off the growth curve. Another test to differentiate IUGR fetuses is Doppler investigation of the umbilical artery. The normal flow through the umbilical artery is higher during systole, but only decreases 50% to 80% during diastole (Fig. 7-1). The flow during diastole should never be absent or reversed (Fig. 7-2). However, in the setting of increased placental resistance which can be seen with a thrombosed or calcified placenta, diastolic flow decreases or even becomes absent or reversed. Reversed diastolic flow is particularly concerning and is associated with a high risk of intrauterine fetal demise.

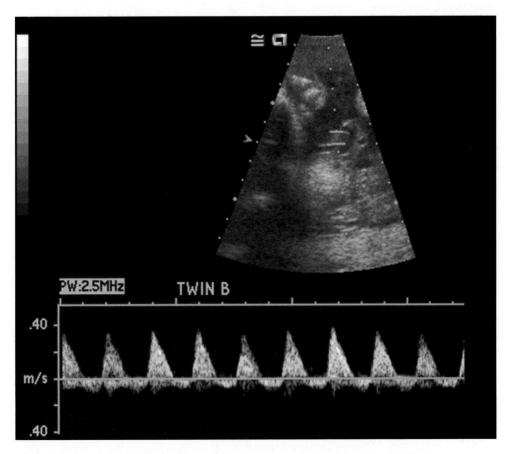

Figure 7-2 • Reversed diastolic flow on umbilical artery Doppler in the setting of IUGR.

Treatment

For patients with a history of SGA infants, the underlying etiology should be explored. If malnutrition or drugs like alcohol or cigarettes were issues in a prior pregnancy, these should be dealt with at each prenatal visit. Patients with a history of placental insufficiency, preeclampsia, collagen vascular disorders, or vascular disease are often treated with low-dose aspirin. Patients with prior placental thrombosis, thrombophilias, or antiphospholipid antibody syndrome have been treated with heparin and corticosteroids as well, with mixed results.

There is no indication to expedite delivery in SGA fetuses who have consistently been small throughout the pregnancy. However, the risk of prematurity is likely to be lower than that of remaining in the intrauterine environment for SGA fetuses near term who have fallen off the growth curve. This is assessed with fetal testing such as a nonstress test (NST), oxytocin challenge test (OCT), biophysical profile (BPP), and/or umbilical Doppler velocimetry. With increasing placental resistance due to calcifications or thromboses, the umbilical arterial diastolic flow will decrease, halt, and occasionally reverse. Doppler investigation of the fetal umbilical cord is particularly useful because of the high predictive value of poor outcomes in the setting of absent or reversed end diastolic flow. If fetal testing is nonreassuring, the fetus should be delivered. The decision of whether to deliver SGA fetuses remote from term is based on how the infant will do in a neonatal intensive care unit versus how it will be maintained in the intrauterine environment. For those left undelivered, frequent antenatal testing with NSTs, OCTs, and BPPs; weekly ultrasounds for fetal growth; antenatal corticosteroids to accelerate pulmonary maturity; and, possibly, admission to the hospital for continuous monitoring may be indicated.

LARGE FOR GESTATIONAL AGE AND FETAL MACROSOMIA

A large for gestational age (LGA) fetus is defined as having an EFW greater than the 90th percentile. However, while LGA speaks to the increased growth at a particular gestational age, in terms of identifying fetuses at higher risk for birth trauma or cesarean delivery, it is considered less important than the diagnosis of fetal macrosomia. Although definitions of macrosomia vary, the American College of Obstetricians and Gynecologists uses **a birth weight greater than 4,500 g**. Birth weights of greater than 4,000 g or 4,200 g are also used by many clinicians and researchers to define macrosomia. Macrosomic fetuses have a higher risk of shoulder dystocia and birth trauma with resultant brachial plexus injuries with vaginal deliveries. Other neonatal risks include low Apgar scores, hypoglycemia, polycythemia, hypocalcemia, and jaundice. LGA infants are at a higher risk for childhood leukemia, Wilms tumor, and osteosarcoma.

Mothers with LGA or macrosomic fetuses are at increased risk for cesarean delivery, perineal trauma, and postpartum hemorrhage. There is a higher rate of cesarean delivery for macrosomic infants due to failure to progress in labor and electively because of suspected increased risk for shoulder dystocia.

Etiology

The most classically associated risk factor for fetal macrosomia is gestational or preexisting diabetes. **Maternal obesity**, with a BMI >30 or weight greater than 90 kg, is also correlated with an increased risk for fetal macrosomia as is increased maternal weight gain in pregnancy. This association is seemingly independent of maternal stature and gestational diabetes. Any woman who has previously delivered an LGA infant is at increased risk in ensuing pregnancies for fetal macrosomia. **Postterm pregnancies** have an increased rate of macrosomic infants. **Multiparity** and **advanced maternal age** are also risk factors (Table 7-2), but these are mostly secondary to the increased prevalence of diabetes and obesity.

■ TABLE 7-2 Risk Factors for Macrosomic Infants
Diabetes
Maternal obesity
Postterm pregnancy
Previous LGA or macrosomic infant
Maternal stature
Multiparity
AMA
Male infant
Beckwith-Wiedemann syndrome (pancreatic islet-cell hyperplasia)

Diagnosis

Upon routine prenatal care, patients with macrosomic infants will often be of a size greater than dates on measurement of the fundal height and, by the late third trimester, Leopold's examination reveals a fetus that seems large. Patients whose fetuses are a size greater than dates by 3 cm or more are referred to ultrasound for EFW. Again, as noted under the SGA section, such fundal height screening has a relatively poor sensitivity and specificity for fetal growth disorders. Ultrasound uses the biparietal diameter, femur length, and abdominal circumference to estimate fetal weight. These estimates are usually accurate to within 10% to 15%. As with SGA fetuses, pregnancy dating should be verified. At many institutions, any patient with diabetes or a previous LGA infant merits an estimated fetal weight by ultrasound in the late third trimester.

Treatment

Management of LGA and macrosomic infants includes prevention, surveillance, and—in some cases—induction of labor before the attainment of macrosomia. Patients with type 1 and 2 diabetes require tight control of blood glucose during pregnancy. Well-controlled sugars are thought to decrease the incidence of macrosomic infants in this population, although this has not been confirmed by large randomized studies. Studies of gestational diabetes have demonstrated a decrease in birth weight when women maintained good control of blood glucose.

Obese patients can be counseled to lose weight before conception. Once pregnant, these patients are advised to gain less weight (but never to lose weight) than the average patient and should be referred to a nutritionist for assistance in maintaining adequate nutrition with some control of caloric intake.

Because of the risk for birth trauma and failure to progress in labor secondary to cephalopelvic disproportion, LGA pregnancies are often induced before the fetus can attain macrosomic status. The risks of this course of action are increased rate of cesarean section for failed induction and prematurity in a poorly dated pregnancy. Thus, induction should be used primarily when there is either excellent dating or lung maturity as assessed via amniocentesis. Induction in the setting of an unfavorable cervix should utilize prostaglandins and mechanical means for cervical ripening, which can often take several days to accomplish. Prospective studies of the practice of induction for impending macrosomia have not shown to decrease cesarean delivery rates, but it does appear to lead to lower rates of macrosomia. Vaginal delivery of the suspected macrosomic infant involves preparing for a shoulder dystocia. Operative vaginal delivery with forceps or vacuum is generally not advised because such a delivery increases the risk of shoulder dystocia.

DISORDERS OF AMNIOTIC FLUID

The amniotic fluid reaches its maximum volume of about 800 mL at about 28 weeks. This volume is maintained until close to term when it begins to fall to about 500 mL at week 40. The balance of fluid is maintained by production of the fetal kidneys and lungs and resorption by fetal swallowing and the interface between the membranes and the placenta. A disturbance in any of these functions may lead to a pathologic change in amniotic fluid volume.

Ultrasound can be used to evaluate the amniotic fluid volume. The classic measure of amniotic fluid is the **amniotic fluid index** (AFI). The AFI is calculated by dividing the maternal abdomen into quadrants, measuring the largest vertical pocket of fluid in each quadrant in centimeters, and summing them. An AFI of less than 5 is considered **oligohydramnios**. An AFI greater than 20 or 25 is used to diagnose **polyhydramnios**, depending on gestational age.

OLIGOHYDRAMNIOS

Oligohydramnios in the absence of rupture of membranes is associated with a 40-fold increase in perinatal mortality. This is partially because without the amniotic fluid to cushion it, the umbilical cord is more susceptible to compression leading to fetal asphyxiation. It is also associated with congenital anomalies, particularly of the genitourinary system, and growth restriction. In labor, nonreactive nonstress tests, fetal heart rate (FHR) decelerations, meconium, and cesarean section due to nonreassuring fetal testing are all associated with an AFI of less than 5.

Etiology

The cause of oligohydramnios can be thought of as either decreased production or increased withdrawal. Amniotic fluid is produced by the fetal kidneys and lungs. It can be resorbed by the placenta, swallowed by the fetus, or leaked out into the vagina. Chronic uteroplacental insufficiency (UPI) can lead to oligohydramnios because the fetus likely does not have the nutrients or blood volume to maintain an adequate glomerular filtration rate. UPI is commonly associated with growth-restricted infants.

Congenital abnormalities of the genitourinary tract can lead to decreased urine production. These malformations include renal agenesis (Potter syndrome), polycystic kidney disease, or obstruction of the genitourinary system. The most common cause of oligohydramnios is rupture of membranes. Even without a history of leaking fluid, the patient should be examined to rule out this possibility.

Diagnosis

Diagnosis of oligohydramnios is made by AFI less than 5 as measured by ultrasound. Patients screened for oligohydramnios include those measuring size less than dates, with a history of ruptured membranes, with suspicion of IUGR, and who have a postterm pregnancy. Once the diagnosis of oligohydramnios is made, the etiology also needs to be determined prior to creating a management plan.

Treatment

Management of oligohydramnios is entirely dependent on the underlying etiology. In pregnancies that are IUGR, a host of other data needs consideration, including the rest of the biophysical profile (BPP), umbilical artery Doppler flow, gestational age, and the cause of the IUGR. Labor is usually induced in the case of a pregnancy at term or postdate. In the case of a fetus with congenital abnormalities, the patient should be referred to genetic counseling. A plan for delivery should be made in coordination with the pediatricians and pediatric surgeons. Severely preterm patients with no other etiology are usually managed expectantly with frequent antenatal fetal testing.

Labor is induced in patients with rupture of membranes at term if they are not already in labor. If there is meconium or frequent decelerations in the FHR, an amnio infusion may be performed to increase the AFI. Amnioinfusion is performed to dilute any meconium present in the amniotic fluid and theoretically to decrease the number of variable decelerations caused by cord compression. Preterm premature rupture of membranes (PPROM) was discussed in Chapter 6.

POLYHYDRAMNIOS

Polyhydramnios, defined by an AFI greater than 20 or 25, is present in 2% to 3% of pregnancies. Fetal structural and chromosomal abnormalities are more common in polyhydramnios. It is associated with maternal diabetes and malformations such as neural tube defects, obstruction of the fetal alimentary canal, and hydrops.

Etiology

Polyhydramnios is not as ominous a sign as oligohydramnios. However, it is associated with an increase in congenital anomalies. It is also more common in pregnancies complicated by diabetes, hydrops, and multiple gestation. An obstruction of the gastrointestinal tract may render the fetus unable to swallow the amniotic fluid, leading to polyhydramnios. Just as in other diabetic patients, the increased levels of circulating glucose can act as an osmotic diuretic in the fetus leading to polyhydramnios. Hydrops secondary to high output cardiac failure is generally associated with polyhydramnios. Monozygotic multiple gestations can lead to twin-to-twin transfusion syndrome with polyhydramnios around one fetus and oligohydramnios around the other.

Diagnosis

Polyhydramnios is diagnosed by ultrasound in patients being scanned for size greater than dates, routine screening of diabetic or multiple gestation pregnancies, or as an unsuspected finding on an ultrasound performed for other reasons.

Treatment

As in oligohydramnios, the particular setting of polyhydramnios dictates the management of the pregnancy. Patients with polyhydramnios are at risk for malpresentation and should be carefully evaluated during labor. There is an increased risk of cord prolapse with polyhydramnios. Thus, rupture of membranes should be performed in a controlled setting if possible and only if the head is truly engaged in the pelvis. Upon spontaneous rupture of membranes, a sterile vaginal examination should be performed to verify fetal presentation and rule out cord prolapse.

RH INCOMPATIBILITY AND ALLOIMMUNIZATION

If a woman is Rh negative and her fetus is Rh positive, she may be sensitized to the Rh antigen and develop antibodies. These IgG antibodies cross the placenta and cause hemolysis of fetal red blood cells. The incidence of Rh negativity varies among race (Table 7-3), with the highest incidence of 30% seen among individuals in the Basque region of Spain. Commonly, most individuals only become sensitized during pregnancy and blood transfusion. In the United States, the incidence of sensitization is decreasing from both causes due to careful management of transfusions and the use of Rh immunoglobulin (RhoGAM) in pregnancy. Interestingly, because there is some transplacental passage of fetal cells in all pregnancies, ABO incompatibility actually decreases the risk of Rh sensitization because of destruction of these fetal cells by anti-A or anti-B antibodies.

In sensitized patients with Rh-positive fetuses, the antibodies cross the placenta and cause hemolysis leading to disastrous complications in the fetus. The anemia caused by hemolysis leads to increased extramedullary production of fetal red cells. **Erythroblastosis fetalis**, or fetal hydrops (see Color Plate 1), a syndrome that includes a hyperdynamic state, heart failure, diffuse edema (Fig. 7-3), ascites (Fig. 7-4), and pericardial effusion, is the result of serious anemia. Bilirubin, a breakdown product of red blood cells, is cleared by the placenta before birth but can lead to jaundice and neurotoxic effects in the neonate.

THE UNSENSITIZED RH NEGATIVE PATIENT

If a patient is Rh negative but has a negative antibody screen, the goal during pregnancy is to keep her from

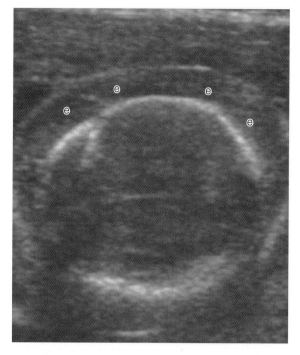

Figure 7-3 • Scalp edema (*e*).

becoming sensitized. Any time during the pregnancy that there is a possibility that a patient may be exposed to fetal blood, such as during amniocentesis, miscarriage, vaginal bleeding, abruption, and delivery, she should be given RhoGAM, an anti-D immunoglobulin (Rh IgG). An antibody screen is

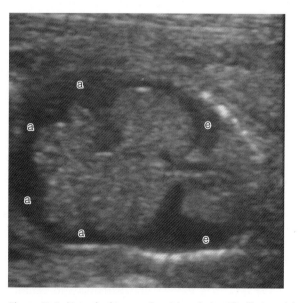

Figure 7-4 • Note the large ascites (*a*) and pleural effusions (*e*) in this fetus with hydrops.

■ **TABLE 7-3** Prevalence of Rh Negativity by Race and Ethnicity

Race and Ethnicity	Percent Rh Negative
Caucasian	15
African American	8
African	4
Native American	1
Asian	<1

performed at the initial visit to detect prior sensitization. RhoGAM should be administered at 28 weeks and postpartum if the neonate is Rh positive.

A standard dose of RhoGAM, 0.3 mg of Rh IgG, will eradicate 15 mL of fetal red blood cells (30 mL of fetal blood with a hematocrit of 50). This dose is adequate for a routine pregnancy. However, in the setting of placental abruption or any antepartum bleeding, a Kleihauer-Betke test for amount of fetal red blood cells in the maternal circulation can be sent. If the amount of fetal red blood cells is more than can be eliminated by the single RhoGAM dose, additional dosages can be given.

THE SENSITIZED RH-NEGATIVE PATIENT

If the antibody screen for Rh comes back positive during the initial prenatal visit, the titer is checked as well. Antibody titers of 1:16 and greater have been associated with fetal hydrops. If paternity is not in question, blood type can be performed on the father of the baby to determine whether the fetus is at risk. However, because approximately 5% of all pregnancies have unknown or incorrect paternity, the safest course is to treat all pregnancies as if the fetus is at risk.

Throughout pregnancy, the antibody titer is followed approximately every 4 weeks. As long as it remains less than 1:16, the pregnancy can be managed expectantly. However, if it becomes 1:16 or greater, serial amniocentesis is begun as early as 16 to 20 weeks. At the first amniocentesis, fetal cells can be collected and analyzed for the Rh antigen. If negative, the pregnancy can be followed expectantly. However, if the fetus is Rh positive, serial amniocenteses are done and the amniotic fluid is analyzed by a spectrophotometer that measures the light absorption (ΔOD_{450}) by bilirubin, which will accumulate in the amniotic fluid with increasing fetal hemolysis. These measurements are plotted on the Liley curve (Fig. 7-5), which predicts the severity of disease. The curve is divided into three zones.

Zone 1 is suggestive of a mildly affected fetus, and follow-up amniocentesis can be performed approximately every 2 to 3 weeks. Zone 2 is suggestive of a moderately affected fetus, and amniocentesis should be repeated every 1 to 2 weeks. The severely affected fetus will fall into zone 3. Once in zone 3, it is likely that the fetus has anemia, and percutaneous umbilical blood sampling (PUBS) is usually the next step. PUBS can be used to obtain a fetal hematocrit and to

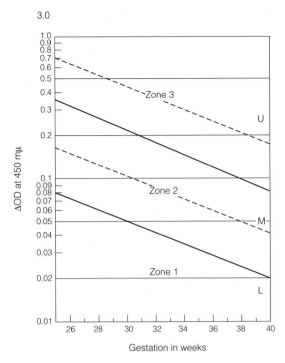

Figure 7-5 • Liley curve used to predict severity of fetal hemolysis with red cell isoimmunization.

perform an intrauterine transfusion (IUT). If a PUBS or IUT cannot be performed, fetal intraperitoneal transfusion has also been utilized.

More recently, fetal anemia has been screened for with middle cerebral artery Doppler measurements of blood flow. The basis for this is that with fetal anemia, in order to achieve improved oxygenation of the fetal brain in the setting of fetal anemia, there will be increased flow, measured by the peak systolic velocity. There are several studies of this testing modality that suggest it may have sensitivities for fetal anemia as high or even higher than the use of amniocentesis for ΔOD_{450}. Currently, many institutions utilize both modalities and act in the setting of a positive screen on either test because of the high morbidity and mortality in the setting of fetal anemia.

OTHER CAUSES OF IMMUNE HYDROPS

There are a variety of other red blood cell antigens including the **ABO** blood type, antigens **CDE** in which D is the Rh antigen, **Kell**, **Duffy**, and **Lewis**. Some may cause fetal hydrops (e.g., Kell and Duffy), whereas others may lead to a mild hemolysis but not severe immune hydrops (e.g., ABO, Lewis). With the advent of treatment with RhoGAM, the incidence of Rh isoimmunization has decreased and the other causes of immune-related fetal hydrops now account for a greater percentage of cases. Sensitized patients are managed similarly to Rh negative patients with antibody titers, amniocentesis, PUBS, and transfusions.

FETAL DEMISE

Intrauterine fetal demise (IUFD) is a rare but disastrous occurrence, occurring in approximately 1:1,000 births. It is increased with a variety of medical and obstetric complications of pregnancy including abruption, congenital abnormalities, and postterm pregnancy. Chronic placental insufficiency secondary to rheumatologic, vascular, or hypertensive disease may lead to IUGR and eventually IUFD. When there is no explanation for a fetal demise, it is usually attributed to a "cord accident." A retained IUFD greater than 3 to 4 weeks can lead to hypofibrinogenemia secondary to the release of thromboplastic substances from the decomposing fetus. In some cases, full-blown disseminated intravascular coagulation (DIC) can result.

DIAGNOSIS

Early in pregnancy, before 20 weeks, the diagnosis of fetal death (missed abortion) is suspected by lack of uterine growth or cessation of symptoms of pregnancy. Diagnosis is confirmed with serially falling human chorionic gonadotropin (hCG) and ultrasound documentation. After week 20, fetal death is suspected with absence of fetal movement noted by the mother and absence of uterine growth. Diagnosis can be confirmed by ultrasound.

TREATMENT

Because of the risk of DIC with retained IUFD, the best treatment is delivery. Early gestations can be terminated by dilation and evacuation. After 20 weeks, the pregnancy is usually terminated by induction of labor with prostaglandins or high-dose oxytocin. Helping patients understand what may have caused the fetal death is imperative to helping them cope with the situation. Tests for causes of fetal death include screening for collagen vascular disease or hypercoagulable state, fetal karyotype, and often TORCH titers (i.e., toxoplasmosis, RPR, CMV, and HSV). It is

extremely important to get an autopsy on the fetus, which can contribute valuable information. Despite this extensive battery of tests, the etiology of fetal demise will likely remain unknown greater than 90% of the time.

POSTTERM PREGNANCY

A postterm pregnancy is defined as one that goes beyond 42 weeks' gestational age or greater than 294 days past the last menstrual period (LMP). It is estimated that 3% to 10% of all pregnancies will go postterm. This is an important obstetric issue because of the increased risk of macrosomic infants, oligohydramnios, meconium aspiration, intrauterine fetal death, and dysmaturity syndrome. There is also greater risk to the mother because of a greater rate of cesarean delivery (approximately doubled) and delivery of large infants. With improved dating, there are an increasing number of studies that show these complications of pregnancy may increase after 40 or 41 weeks of gestation.

ETIOLOGY

The most common reason for the diagnosis of postterm pregnancy is inaccurate dating; accurate dating is therefore imperative. Because the physiologic basis for the onset of labor is poorly understood, the mechanisms for preterm or postterm labor are also unclear. There are a few rare conditions of the fetus associated with postterm pregnancy. These include anencephaly, fetal adrenal hypoplasia, and absent fetal pituitary. All are notable for diminished levels of circulating estrogens.

DIAGNOSIS

Again, the diagnosis is made by accurate dating. Because ultrasound can be off by as much as 3 weeks near term, this cannot be used to confirm dating. Accurate dating is made by a certain LMP consistent with a bimanual examination in the first trimester or a first or second trimester ultrasound. Dating by a third trimester ultrasound or unsure LMP is more suspect.

TREATMENT

The varying approaches to the postterm pregnancy generally involve more frequent visits, increased fetal testing, and plans for eventual induction. A typical plan for following a postterm pregnancy is outlined below.

Patients whose pregnancies go past 40 weeks of gestation usually receive an NST during the 41st week of pregnancy. Induction is indicated with nonreassuring fetal testing. During the 42nd week (between 41 and 42 weeks of gestation), the patient should be seen twice and receive a BPP at one of the visits and an NST at the other. Alternatively, many practitioners use the modified BPP (an NST and AFI) for fetal testing at each visit past the due date. Induction is indicated with nonreassuring fetal testing or electively with an inducible cervix (Bishop score >6). After 42 weeks of gestation, the patient is induced regardless of cervical examination.

Increasingly, patients are induced between 41 and 42 weeks, as a result of improved dating by ultrasound, patient demand, as well as the risk-averse environment of obstetrics. Several randomized trials have demonstrated that induction of labor at 41 weeks of gestation as compared to expectant management leads to lower rates of cesarean delivery as well as lower rates of meconium aspiration syndrome in the neonate. However, in the face of this evidence, 42 weeks of gestation is still utilized by ACOG as the definition of postterm.

MULTIPLE GESTATIONS

If a fertilized ovum divides into two separate ova, monozygotic, or "identical," twins result. If ovulation produces two ova and both are fertilized, dizygotic twins result. Without assisted fertility, the rate of twinning is approximately 1:80 pregnancies, with 30% of those monozygotic. The rate of naturally occurring triplets is approximately 1:7,000 to 8,000 pregnancies. However, with ovulation-enhancing drugs and in vitro fertilization (IVF), the incidence of multiple gestations is increasing.

COMPLICATIONS OF MULTIPLE GESTATION

Multiple gestations result in an increase in a variety of obstetric complications including preterm labor, placenta previa, cord prolapse, postpartum hemorrhage, cervical incompetence, gestational diabetes, and preeclampsia. The fetuses are at increased risk for preterm delivery, congenital abnormalities, SGA, and malpresentation. The average gestational age of delivery for twins is between 36 and 37 weeks; for triplets it is 33 to 34 weeks. Monochorionic (one placenta), diamnionic (two amniotic sacs) twins, also referred to as MoDi twins, often have placental vascular communications and can develop **twin-to-twin transfusion syndrome** (TTTS). Monochorionic, monoamnionic (Mo-Mo) twins have an extremely high mortality rate (40% to 60%) secondary to cord accidents from entanglement.

Pathogenesis

Monozygotic twinning results from division of the fertilized ovum or cells in the embryonic disk. If separation occurs before the differentiation of the trophoblast, two chorions and two amnions (Di-Di) result (Fig. 7-6). After trophoblast differentiation and before amnion formation (days 3 to 8), separation leads to a single placenta, one chorion, and two amnions (Mo-Di). Division after amnion formation leads to a single placenta, one chorion, and one amnion (Mo-Mo) (days 8 to 13) and rarely, conjoined or "Siamese" twins (days 13 to 15). Division of cells beyond day 15 or 16 will result in a singleton fetus. Monozygotic twinning does not follow any inheritable pattern and, historically, the only risk factor ever identified is a slight increase with advancing maternal age. In the 1990s it was determined that assisted reproductive techniques, while increasing the risk of dizygotic twins, also increases the risk of monozygotic twins to as high as 5%.

Dizygotic twins primarily result from fertilization of two ova by two sperm. There are varying risk factors associated with dizygotic twinning. Dizygotic twins tend to run in families and are more common in people of African descent. Globally, the rate of dizygotic twins ranges from 1:1,000 in Japan to 1:20 in several Nigerian tribes. The rate of all multiple gestations has increased sharply since the onset of medical treatment of infertility. Clomiphene citrate, a fertility-enhancing drug, increases the rate of dizygotic twinning up to 8%. However, the utilization of multiple embryos in the setting of IVF in order to improve the pregnancy rates leads to rates of twinning and higher order multiple gestations in 30% to 50% of these pregnancies.

Diagnosis

Multiple gestations are usually diagnosed by ultrasound. Multiple gestations are indicated by rapid uterine growth, excessive maternal weight gain, or

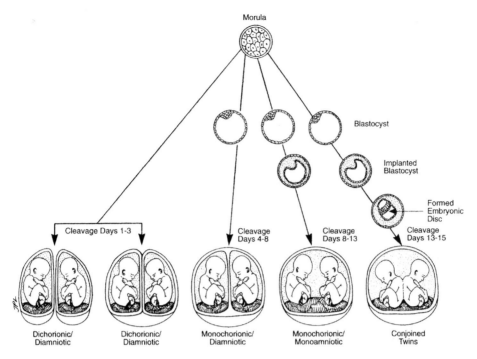

Figure 7-6 • The relationship between the timing of cleavage and the resulting amnionicity/chorionicity in monozygotic twinning.
(From LifeART image copyright © 2006 Lippincott Williams & Wilkins. All rights reserved.)

palpation of three or more fetal large parts (cranium and breech) on Leopold's. The level of β-hCG, human placental lactogen (HPL), and maternal serum α-fetoprotein (MSAFP) are all elevated for gestational age. Rarely, diagnosis will be made after delivery of the first fetus with palpation of the after-coming fetus(es). Differentiation between Di-Di and Mo-Di twins is easier the earlier the ultrasound is performed. For example, quite early in pregnancy, one can see a single chorion and two amniotic sacks (Fig. 7-7) indicative of Mo-Di twins. Later in pregnancy, sonologists rely on the thickness of the membrane and the "twin peak" sign (Fig 7-8), which is formed by the two placentae fusing together in the setting of Di-Di twins. Mo-Mo twins are usually easiest as they should have no intertwin membrane.

Treatment

Because of the increased risk of complications, multiple-gestation pregnancies are managed as high-risk pregnancies, usually in conjunction with a perinatologist. Aside from the antenatal management of the complications, the principal issue in twin gestations is mode of delivery. With higher order multiple gestations, triplets and above, selective reduction down to twins or even a singleton, is commonly recommended. While there is a chance of losing the entire pregnancy in the setting of selective reduction, if successful, the chances of delivering a severely premature infant is also dramatically reduced. However, the question of the risks and benefits of selective reduction from twins to a singleton gestation is unanswered at this time.

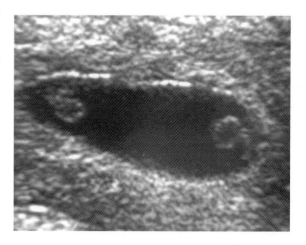

Figure 7-7 • Monochorionic-diamniotic (Mo-Di) twins: Note the single chorion, but two developing amniotic sacs.

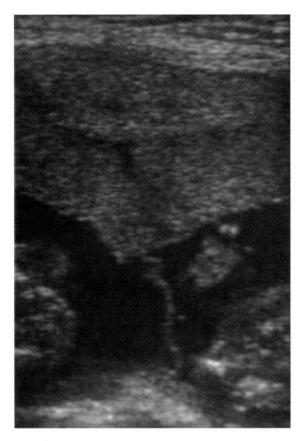

Figure 7-8 • The fused chorionic and amniotic membranes lead to the "twin peak" sign in the middle of image in Di-Di twins.

TWIN-TO-TWIN TRANSFUSION SYNDROME (TTTS)

Polyhydramnios-oligohydramnios (poly-oli) sequence or TTTS has been described for several centuries and results in a small, anemic twin and a large, plethoric, polycythemic, and occasionally hydropic twin. The etiology of TTTS appears to be secondary to unequal flow within vascular communications between the twins in their shared placenta leading to one twin becoming a donor and the other a recipient of this unequal blood flow. This can result in one fetus with hypervolemia, cardiomegaly, glomerulotubal hypertrophy, edema, and ascites and the other with hypovolemia, growth restriction, and oligohydramnios. Because of the risk of this syndrome in Mo-Di twins, serial ultrasounds examining the amniotic fluid and fetal growth should be obtained every 2 weeks after diagnosis.

TTTS has historically been managed with serial amnioreduction, which can reduce preterm contractions secondary to uterine distension and maternal symptoms, but only occasionally actually cures the fetal syndrome. More recently, as these vascular connections have been identified as the etiology of the syndrome, coagulating these vessels has been proposed as the treatment of choice in more severe cases. This is accomplished by fetal surgeons using a fetoscopically placed laser to coagulate the vessels. While this procedure carries risks both to the mother and of losing the pregnancy entirely or eventual preterm delivery, TTTS itself almost inevitably will lead to extremely poor pregnancy outcomes, so it appears to be, on balance, beneficial to these patients. However, because of the potential risks, pregnancy termination should always be offered as an option as well in the setting of TTTS.

MO-MO TWINS

Because of the risk of cord entanglement and IUFD, Mo-Mo twins are often managed with frequent antenatal testing and early delivery. Unfortunately, frequent antenatal testing has not in and of itself appeared to make a difference in the rate of IUFD in these cases. Because of this, some patients are offered admission to the hospital and continuous electronic fetal monitoring from weeks 28 to 34, at which time delivery is performed via cesarean section. Mo-Mo and conjoined twins are almost always delivered via cesarean section.

DELIVERY OF TWINS

There are four possibilities for twin presentation: both vertex (40%), both breech, vertex then breech (40%), and breech then vertex. When deciding mode of delivery, all breech-presenting twins (20%) are considered together.

Vertex/vertex twins should undergo a trial of labor with cesarean section reserved for the usual indications. Vertex/nonvertex twins can also undergo a trial of labor if the twins are concordant or the presenting twin is larger. Generally, the twins should be between 1,500 g and 3,500 g, though there is scant data that breech extraction between 500 g and 1,500 g leads to any worse outcomes. Breech extraction for delivery of the second twin has advantages over a vertex second twin because the twin B's lower extremity can be grasped and delivery expedited quickly. In the setting of a vertex second twin, occasionally, placental abruption occurs necessitating a rapid delivery. But if the cervix is no longer fully dilated or the fetal vertex is above 0 station, a cesarean delivery may be necessary. External cephalic version and internal podalic version have also been used for delivery of the second twin, but in small studies lower Apgar scores have been found as compared to breech extraction. Further, the chances of failure of such maneuvers is higher. Nonvertex presenting twins are usually delivered via cesarean.

DELIVERY OF TRIPLETS

Most triplet gestations are delivered via cesarean section. Rarely, triplets will be concordant, with vertex presenting, all greater than 1,500 g to 2,000 g and a vaginal delivery can be attempted. Multiple gestations beyond triplets are all delivered via cesarean.

 KEY POINTS

- Fetuses whose EFW is less than the 10th percentile are considered small for gestational age (SGA), though the rate of poor neonatal outcomes rises significantly below the 5th and 3rd percentiles.
- Common causes of decreased growth potential include congenital abnormalities, drugs, infections, radiation, and small maternal stature.
- IUGR infants are commonly born to women with systemic diseases leading to poor placental blood flow.
- An LGA fetus has an EFW greater than the 90th percentile at any particular gestational age.
- Both 4,000 g and 4,500 g have been used as the threshold for defining fetal macrosomia.
- LGA and macrosomic fetuses are at greater risk for birth trauma, hypoglycemia, jaundice, lower Apgar scores, and childhood tumors.
- Increased size in the fetus is seen with maternal diabetes, maternal obesity, increased maternal height, postterm pregnancies, multiparity, advanced maternal age, and male sex.
- Oligohydramnios is defined by an AFI of less than 5 and can be caused by decreased placental perfusion, decreased fluid production by the fetus, and rupture of membranes.
- Pregnancies at term complicated by oligohydramnios should be delivered.
- Polyhydramnios is diagnosed by an AFI greater than 20 on ultrasound and is associated with diabetes, multiple gestations, hydrops, and congenital abnormalities.
- Obstetric management of polyhydramnios should include careful verification of presentation and close observation for cord prolapse.
- Rh sensitized women with Rh-positive fetuses have antibodies that cross the placenta, leading to hemolysis and anemia in the fetuses. If the anemia is severe enough, hydrops develops with edema, ascites, and heart failure.
- Rh-negative patients who are not sensitized should be treated with antepartum RhoGAM to prevent sensitization. Postpartum, they should receive another dose of RhoGAM if the fetus is Rh positive.
- Rh-negative patients undergoing miscarriage, abruption, amniocentesis, ectopic pregnancy, and vaginal bleeding should also be given RhoGAM.
- Rh-negative patients who are sensitized are followed closely with serial ultrasounds and amniocentesis. The amniocentesis is done to measure the amount of bilirubin in the fluid, which is indicative of the amount of hemolysis.
- While IUFD is more common with disorders of the placenta the actual cause of most IUFDs is usually unknown and is often attributed to cord accidents.
- Retained IUFD can lead to DIC; thus, delivery soon after diagnosis is indicated.
- Postterm pregnancy is defined as greater than 42 weeks' gestational age.
- Postterm pregnancies are at increased risk for fetal demise, macrosomia, meconium aspiration, and oligohydramnios.
- Increased fetal surveillance and labor induction are the most common management options for postterm pregnancies.
- Monozygotic twins carry identical genetic material, whereas dizygotic twins are from separate ova and sperm.
- Multiple gestations are at increased risk for preterm labor and delivery, placenta previa, postpartum hemorrhage, preeclampsia, cord prolapse, malpresentation, and congenital abnormalities.
- There is a genetic predisposition for dizygotic twinning, whereas the rate of monozygotic twinning is the same throughout all races and families.
- Monozygotic twins are at risk for TTTS, and should have frequent ultrasound examinations to diagnose this early.
- Vaginal delivery of vertex/vertex presenting twins is preferred and is possible with vertex/nonvertex twins under the right circumstances. Nonvertex presenting twins are delivered by cesarean section.

Hypertension and Pregnancy

Blood pressure in pregnancy is usually decreased. As a result of decreased vascular resistance, the blood pressure decreases in the latter half of the first trimester reaching its nadir in the mid-second trimester. During the third trimester, blood pressure will usually increase, but should not be higher than prepregnancy. Hypertension may be present before pregnancy—as with chronic hypertension, or may be induced by pregnancy—as with gestational hypertension (GH), preeclampsia, and eclampsia (Table 8-1). Liver injury is seen in a small percentage of patients with preeclampsia and is associated with two diseases in pregnancy with high morbidity and mortality: HELLP syndrome (hemolysis, elevated liver enzymes, low platelets) and acute fatty liver of pregnancy. Complications from these disorders are consistently among the leading causes of maternal death in developed countries. Because treatment is delivery, these disorders are also leading causes of premature delivery.

PREECLAMPSIA

PATHOGENESIS

Preeclampsia is the presence of nondependent edema, hypertension, and proteinuria in the pregnant woman. While this triad is typically how women present, nondependent edema is no longer a component of the diagnosis. The classic presentation is of a nulliparous woman in her third trimester. Although no definitive cause for preeclampsia has been determined, it is well accepted that the underlying pathophysiology involves a **generalized arteriolar constriction** (vasospasm) and intravascular depletion secondary to a generalized

transudative edema that can produce symptoms related to ischemia, necrosis, and hemorrhage of organs. Thus, one of the fundamental aspects of the disease is vascular damage and an imbalance in the relative concentrations of prostacyclin and thromboxane. It is theorized that this is primarily related to circulating antibodies or antigen-antibody complexes (not unlike systemic lupus erythematosus) that damage the lining of vessel walls leading to exposure of the underlying collagen structure. The hyperdynamic state of pregnancy has also been proposed to cause this underlying vascular injury rather than an immunogenic phenomenon.

As outlined in Table 8-2, major fetal complications of preeclampsia are due to prematurity. Also, the generalized vasoconstriction of preeclampsia can result in decreased blood flow to the placenta. This may manifest as acute uteroplacental insufficiency, resulting in abruption or fetal distress. The uteroplacental insufficiency may also be chronic in nature and result in an intrauterine growth restricted (IUGR) fetus.

Maternal complications associated with preeclampsia (Table 8-3) are related to the generalized arteriolar vasoconstriction that affects the brain (seizure and stroke), kidneys (oliguria and renal failure), lungs (pulmonary edema), liver (edema and subcapsular hematoma), and small blood vessels (thrombocytopenia and disseminated intravascular coagulation [DIC]). Severe preeclampsia is diagnosed with severely elevated blood pressures, defined as SBP >160 or DBP >110 or the presence of any of the above clinical findings.

About 10% of patients with severe preeclampsia develop HELLP syndrome. **HELLP syndrome** is a subcategory of preeclampsia in which the patient presents with hemolysis, elevated liver enzymes, and low platelets. Hypertension and proteinuria may be

■ TABLE 8-1 Hypertensive States of Pregnancy

| Pregnancy-induced (or gestational) hypertension |
| Preeclampsia |
| Severe preeclampsia |
| Chronic hypertension |
| Chronic hypertension w/superimposed preeclampsia |
| HELLP syndrome |
| AFLP |

■ TABLE 8-3 Maternal Complications of Preeclampsia

| *Medical manifestations* |
| Seizure |
| Cerebral hemorrhage |
| DIC and thrombocytopenia |
| Renal failure |
| Hepatic rupture or failure |
| Pulmonary edema |
| *Obstetric complications* |
| Uteroplacental insufficiency |
| Placental abruption |
| Increased premature deliveries |
| Increased cesarean section deliveries |

minimal in these patients. HELLP syndrome is uncommon, but patients who experience it decline rapidly, resulting in poor maternal and fetal outcomes. Despite careful management, HELLP syndrome results in a high rate of stillbirth (10% to 15%) and neonatal death (20% to 25%).

EPIDEMIOLOGY

Preeclampsia occurs in 5% to 6% of all live births and can develop any time after the 20th week, but is most commonly seen in the third trimester near term. When hypertension is seen early in the second trimester (14 to 20 weeks), a hydatidiform mole or previously undiagnosed chronic hypertension should be considered. Unlike other preeclamptic patients, the patient with HELLP is more likely to be less than 36 weeks' gestation at the time of presentation.

■ TABLE 8-2 Fetal Complications of Preeclampsia

| *Complications related to prematurity (if early delivery is necessary)* |
| Acute uteroplacental insufficiency |
| Placental infarct and/or abruption |
| Intrapartum fetal distress |
| Stillbirth (in severe cases) |
| Chronic uteroplacental insufficiency |
| Asymmetric and symmetric SGA fetuses |
| IUGR |
| Oligohydramnios |

Although 80% of patients develop HELLP after being diagnosed with preeclampsia (30% with mild preeclampsia; 50% with severe preeclampsia), 20% of patients with HELLP have no previous history of hypertension before their diagnosis, and will present merely with the symptom of right upper-quadrant pain.

RISK FACTORS

Risk factors for preeclampsia fall essentially into two categories: those related to the manifestations of the disease (like chronic hypertension or renal disease), and those related to the immunogenic nature of preeclampsia (Table 8-4). These latter risk factors are quite interesting. For example, it has been shown that in addition to a family history in the parturient, if the mother of the father of her baby (mother-in-law) had preeclampsia, the patient is at greater risk of developing preeclampsia. Further, it has been demonstrated that parental ethnic discordance slightly increases the risk of developing preeclampsia. While multiparous women who have not had preeclampsia in the past have a decreased risk, if a woman conceives with a new father of her baby, her risk increases back to that of a nullipara. A tolerance effect is seen in women who cohabitate with the father of the baby longer than 1 year prior to conceiving in comparison to women who conceive sooner. These risk factors

■ **TABLE 8-4** Risk Factors for Preeclampsia
Primarily disease related
Chronic hypertension
Chronic renal disease
Collagen vascular disease (e.g., SLE)
Pregestational diabetes
African American
Maternal age (<20 or >35)
Primarily immunogenic related
Nulliparity
Previous preeclampsia
Multiple gestation
Abnormal placentation
New paternity
Family history
Female relatives of parturient
Mother-in-law
Cohabitation less than 1 year

support the theory that preeclampsia has an alloimmunogenic pathophysiology.

CLINICAL MANIFESTATIONS AND DIAGNOSES

Gestational Hypertension

Blood pressures elevated above 140/90 are necessary to diagnose GH (formerly known as pregnancy-induced hypertension [PIH]). Blood pressures should be elevated on at least two occasions 4 to 6 hours apart and taken while the patient is seated. In the past an increase of 30 mm Hg above prepregnancy systolic BP or 15 mm Hg above prepregnancy diastolic BP had been utilized as well to identify GH. Currently, these changes are not recognized as diagnostic, but should still be noted clinically. If the patient's 24-hour urinary protein total is <300 mg, then preeclampsia is ruled out and the patient can be managed expectantly. Because it is believed that preeclampsia is a continuum from GH through severe disease, these patients are at risk for developing preeclampsia and should be followed closely with frequent blood pressure checks, laboratory tests, and antenatal fetal testing.

Mild Preeclampsia

As shown in Table 8-5, mild preeclampsia is classically defined as a third-trimester **blood pressure** greater than 140 mm Hg systolic or 90 mm Hg diastolic on two occasions at least 6 hours apart accompanied by **proteinuria** greater than 300 mg/24 hr and **nondependent edema** (face and/or hands). It has been determined that edema is not essential to the diagnosis of preeclampsia, but the occurrence of hypertension and proteinuria is diagnostic. If a diagnosis is being made in the acute setting, proteinuria of 1 or greater on two occasions has also been used to diagnose proteinuria. Of note, women with 2+ or greater have been demonstrated to have significant proteinuria, >300 mg/24 hr, well above 90% of the

■ **TABLE 8-5** Criteria for Diagnosis of Gestational Hypertension, Preeclampsia, and Eclampsia
Gestational hypertension
Blood Pressure: SBP >140 OR DBP >90
Mild preeclampsia
Blood Pressure: SBP >140 OR DBP >90
Proteinuria: >300 mg/24 hr or >1 to 2 plus on dipstick
Severe preeclampsia (by systems)
Neuro: Severe headache (not relieved by acetaminophen)
Visual changes; scotomata
Cardiovascular: SBP >160 OR DBP >110
Pulmonary: Pulmonary edema
Renal: Acute renal failure with rising creatinine
Oliguria <400 mL/24 hr or <30 mL/hr
Proteinuria: 24 hr urine protein of ≥5 gm or >3+ on dipstick
GI: Right upper-quadrant pain
Elevation of transaminases, AST and ALT
Heme: Hemolytic anemia
Thrombocytopenia
DIC
Fetal: IUGR, abnormal umbilical Dopplers
Eclampsia
Seizure

time. While an abnormal urine dip for protein is concerning, a negative urine dip should be less reassuring in the setting of hypertension. In one study, more than two-thirds of patients with elevated blood pressures and negative or trace on urine dip had greater than 300 mg/24 hr of urine protein and all patients with 3+ and 4+ protein had significant proteinuria. A better predictor of significant proteinuria is the urine protein to creatinine ratio. Because creatinine excretion is relatively constant, this ratio gives a rough estimate of the amount of protein that will be excreted over a 24-hour period. Ratios from 0.2 to 0.3 have been used as thresholds.

Severe Preeclampsia

Criteria for severe preeclampsia (Table 8-5) include blood pressure greater than 160 mm Hg systolic or 110 mm Hg diastolic on two occasions at least 6 hours apart, accompanied by proteinuria greater than 5 g/24 hr (or 3 to 4+ protein on dipstick on two occasions). A woman with mild preeclampsia by blood pressure and proteinuria parameters would be diagnosed with severe preeclampsia if she also developed certain associated conditions. These include altered consciousness, headache or visual changes, epigastric or right upper-quadrant pain, significantly impaired liver function (>2 times normal), oliguria (<400 mL in 24 hr), pulmonary edema, and significant thrombocytopenia (<100,000/mm^3). Many clinical manifestations of preeclampsia are explained by vasospasm leading to necrosis and hemorrhage of organs.

HELLP Syndrome

The disorder is characterized by rapidly deteriorating liver function and thrombocytopenia. In addition, a number of patients will develop DIC. The criteria for diagnosis and relevant laboratory tests are outlined in Table 8-6. Liver capsule distension produces epigastric pain, often with progressive nausea and vomiting, and can lead to hepatic rupture. Patients with HELLP syndrome who present with frank hepatic failure should be screened for acute fatty liver of pregnancy (AFLP).

Acute Fatty Liver of Pregnancy (AFLP)

It is unclear whether AFLP is truly in the spectrum of preeclamptic syndromes or an entirely separate entity with similar signs and symptoms. More than 50% of patients with AFLP will also have hypertension

■ TABLE 8-6 Diagnosis of HELLP Syndrome
Hemolytic anemia
Schistocytes on peripheral blood smear
Elevated lactate dehydrogenase
Elevated total bilirubin
Elevated liver enzymes
Increase in aspartate aminotransferase
Increase in alanine aminotransferase
Low platelets
Thrombocytopenia

and proteinuria. It presents in approximately 1:10,000 pregnancies and has a high mortality rate. Interestingly, it has been found that a number of AFLP patients will have fetuses with long-chain hydroxyacyl-CoA dehydrogenase (LCHAD) deficiency.

To differentiate AFLP from HELLP, labs associated with liver failure such as an elevated ammonia level, blood glucose less than 50, and markedly reduced fibrinogen and antithrombin III levels have been associated with AFLP. Management of these patients is supportive and, while liver transplant has been used, in some studies, it appears that the disease will resolve in many patients without this aggressive intervention.

TREATMENT

Mild Preeclampsia

Because delivery is the ultimate treatment for preeclampsia, induction of labor is the treatment of choice for pregnancies at term, unstable preterm pregnancies, or pregnancies where there is evidence of fetal lung maturity. In these cases, vaginal delivery may be attempted with the assistance of prostaglandins, oxytocin, or amniotomy as needed. Cesarean delivery need only be performed for obstetric indications. For stable preterm patients, bed rest and expectant management, commonly in the hospital, are used. Betamethasone is given to enhance fetal lung maturity.

Patients with mild preeclampsia are often started on magnesium sulfate therapy for seizure prophylaxis (4 g load and 2 g/hr maintenance) during labor and delivery and should be continued for 12 to 24 hours after delivery.

Severe Preeclampsia

The goals of treatment in severe preeclampsia are to prevent eclampsia, control maternal blood pressure, and deliver the fetus. However, management varies based on gestational age. Initially, patients with severe preeclampsia should be stabilized using magnesium sulfate for seizure prophylaxis and hydralazine (a direct arteriolar dilator) or labetalol (beta and alpha blockade) for blood pressure control. Once the patient is stabilized, if the gestational age is between 24 and 32 weeks, expectant management to gain treatment with betamethasone and further fetal maturity is often used. Beyond 32 weeks of gestation or in a severe preeclamptic with signs of renal failure, pulmonary edema, hepatic injury, HELLP syndrome, or DIC, delivery should ensue immediately.

Even though delivery is the cure for preeclampsia, patients can have lingering effects for up to several weeks. In fact, some patients will worsen acutely in the immediate postpartum period, possibly related to the increased placental antigen exposure during labor and delivery. Because of this, seizure prophylaxis is usually continued 24 hours postpartum, or until the patient improves markedly. In the setting of chronically elevated blood pressures, antihypertensive medications (most commonly labetalol and nifedipine) should be used and, in some cases, patients may need to continue medications for several weeks after release to home. Patients with HELLP syndrome may have worsening thrombocytopenia, and it has been shown that corticosteroid treatment can decrease the amount of time until the nadir and return to normal levels.

Follow-Up

Women who develop preeclampsia during their first pregnancy will have a 25% to 33% recurrence rate in subsequent pregnancies. In patients with both chronic hypertension and preeclampsia, the risk of recurrence is 70%. Low doses of aspirin prior to and during subsequent pregnancies to decrease the risk of preeclampsia, IUGR, and preterm deliveries have been studied. While this appeared to be a promising treatment in smaller, nonrandomized studies, larger studies have shown mixed outcomes. Calcium supplementation has also been associated with decreased rates of subsequent preeclampsia, but one large randomized controlled trial found no difference between calcium and placebo.

ECLAMPSIA

Eclampsia is the occurrence of grand mal seizures in the preeclamptic patient not attributed to other causes (Table 8-5). Although patients with severe preeclampsia are at greater risk for developing seizures, 25% of women with eclampsia were originally found to have only mild preeclampsia before the onset of seizures. Of note, eclampsia may also occur without proteinuria. Complications of eclampsia include cerebral hemorrhage, aspiration pneumonia, hypoxic encephalopathy, and thromboembolic events.

CLINICAL MANIFESTATIONS

Seizures in the eclamptic patient are tonic-clonic in nature and may or may not be preceded by an aura. These seizures may develop before labor (25%), during labor (50%), or after delivery (25%). Most postpartum seizures occur within the first 48 hours after delivery, but will occasionally occur as late as several weeks after delivery.

TREATMENT

Treatment strategy for eclamptic patients includes seizure management, blood pressure control, and prophylaxis against further convulsions. Seizure management should always start with the ABCs (airway, breathing, circulation), though the majority of seizures are unwitnessed by clinicians and will resolve spontaneously without major morbidity. Hypertension management can usually be achieved using hydralazine to lower the blood pressure. For seizure control and prophylaxis, eclamptic patients are treated with magnesium sulfate ($MgSO_4$) to decrease hyperreflexia and prevent further seizures by raising the seizure threshold. In prospective, randomized studies, magnesium has been found to be as good as or better than phenytoin, carbamazepine, and phenobarbital in the prevention of recurrent seizures in eclamptic patients.

In eclampsia, $MgSO_4$ therapy is initiated at the time of diagnosis and continued for 12 to 24 hours after delivery. The goal of magnesium sulfate therapy is to reach a therapeutic level while avoiding toxicity through careful clinical monitoring (Table 8-7). In the case of overdose, 10 mL 10% calcium chloride or calcium gluconate should be rapidly administered intravenously for cardiac protection.

■ **TABLE 8-7** Clinical Response to Serum Magnesium Sulfate Concentrations

Serum Concentration MgSO$_4$ (mg/mL)	Clinical Response
4.8 to 8.4	Therapeutic seizure prophylaxis
8	Central nervous system depression
10	Loss of deep tendon reflexes
15	Respiratory depression/paralysis
17	Coma
20 to 25	Cardiac arrest

Delivery should only be initiated after the eclamptic patient has been stabilized and convulsions have been controlled. It is common for prolonged fetal heart rate decelerations to occur in the setting of an eclamptic seizure. The best way to treat the fetus is to stabilize the mother, establishing adequate maternal oxygenation and cardiac output. Occasionally the fetal heart rate abnormalities will not resolve and emergent cesarean delivery will be necessary. Otherwise, cesarean delivery should be reserved for obstetric indications and such patients can undergo an induction of labor.

CHRONIC HYPERTENSION

PATHOGENESIS

Chronic hypertension is defined as hypertension present before conception, before 20 weeks' gestation, or persisting more than 6 weeks' postpartum. For women who present without prenatal care prior to 20 weeks of gestation, this can be difficult to differentiate from gestational hypertension. Approximately one-third of patients with chronic hypertension in pregnancy will develop superimposed preeclampsia. Because of poor vascular development, the fetus may suffer from IUGR and the mother is at increased risk for superimposed preeclampsia, premature delivery, and abruptio placentae.

TREATMENT

Treatment of mild chronic hypertension is controversial. However, mothers with controlled blood pressures tend to have fewer problems. Patients with chronic hypertension whose blood pressures in early pregnancy are consistently 140/90 and less can be managed expectantly. Antihypertensives are used in patients with persistently elevated blood pressures or in those who were already on medications prior to pregnancy. The two most common medications used are labetalol (a beta-blocker with concomitant alpha blockade) and nifedipine (a peripheral calcium channel blocker). In retrospective studies, beta-blocker use has been associated with decreased birth weight. However, these studies are likely biased by the severity of disease. Methyldopa (a central alpha-adrenergic agonist) has been the drug of choice in these patients for several decades. It has not been shown to effectively manage blood pressure or change outcomes, so its usage has therefore decreased.

Because these patients are at risk for other complications of chronic hypertension, a baseline ECG and 24-hour urine collection for creatinine clearance and protein should be obtained. This will also help differentiate superimposed preeclampsia from chronic renal disease later in pregnancy. Low-dose aspirin may decrease the risk of developing superimposed preeclampsia and is used by some practitioners.

Superimposed Preeclampsia

One-third or more of patients with chronic hypertension will develop superimposed preeclampsia. Because the hypertension is longstanding, complications such as IUGR and placental abruption are also more common. The diagnosis can sometimes be difficult to make because many of these patients will have concomitant renal disease at baseline. An increase in the systolic BP of 30 mm Hg or in the diastolic BP of 15 mm Hg over prepregnancy blood pressure is also indicative of superimposed preeclampsia, but experts disagree on how to use blood pressure changes in the diagnosis of superimposed preeclampsia. If a 24-hour urine protein is now elevated, the diagnosis is made; if not, then the blood pressure can be managed with increasing dosages of medications. In patients who have baseline renal disease as well, an elevated uric acid above 6.0 to 6.5 has been used to differentiate preeclampsia from exacerbation of hypertension. Of course, any of the severe preeclampsia signs and symptoms can be utilized to diagnose severe superimposed preeclampsia.

KEY POINTS

- Preeclampsia is the presence of hypertension (>140/90 mm Hg) and proteinuria (>300 mg/day).

- It has an incidence of 5% to 6% of all live births and occurs most commonly in nulliparous women in their third trimester.

- Preeclampsia is characterized by a generalized multi-organ vasospasm that can lead to seizure, stroke, renal failure, liver damage, DIC, or fetal demise.

- Risk factors include nulliparity, multiple gestation, and chronic hypertension.

- Preeclampsia is ultimately treated with delivery, but seizures can be prevented with magnesium sulfate and blood pressures controlled with antihypertensive medications.

- Eclampsia is the occurrence of grand mal seizures in the preeclamptic patient that cannot be attributed to other causes.

- Patients present with seizures occurring before labor (25%), during labor (50%), or after delivery (25%).

- Eclampsia is treated with seizure management and prophylaxis with magnesium sulfate, hypertension management with hydralazine, and vaginal delivery only after the patient has been stabilized.

- Chronic hypertension is defined as hypertension occurring before conception, before 20 weeks' gestation, or persisting more than 6 weeks' postpartum.

- Chronic hypertension leads to superimposed preeclampsia in one-third of patients.

- Chronic hypertension is generally treated with anti-hypertensives, commonly nifedipine or labetalol.

- A baseline ECG and 24-hour urine collection for protein and creatinine should be performed.

Diabetes During Pregnancy

Diabetes during pregnancy encompasses a range of disease entities that include gestational diabetes and overt diabetes mellitus (Table 9-1). In the nonpregnant state, diabetics are subgrouped into two types based on the pathophysiology of their disease, whereas during pregnancy, diabetes is usually characterized as pregestational or gestational diabetes. Pregestational diabetics include all patients with type 1 and type 2 diabetes diagnosed prior to pregnancy. Gestational diabetics are those diagnosed with carbohydrate intolerance during pregnancy. Due to a lack of routine screening for diabetes in many nonpregnant women, this latter group may occasionally include women with undiagnosed pregestational diabetes mellitus.

GESTATIONAL DIABETES MELLITUS

True **gestational diabetes mellitus** (GDM) is an impairment in carbohydrate metabolism that first manifests during pregnancy. These patients may have borderline carbohydrate metabolism impairment at baseline or be entirely normal in the nonpregnant state. However, during pregnancy, human chorionic somatomammotropin (a.k.a. human placental lactogen) and other hormones produced by the placenta act as anti-insulin agents leading to increased insulin resistance and generalized carbohydrate intolerance. Because these hormones increase in volume with the size and function of the placenta, the carbohydrate metabolism abnormalities usually are not apparent until the late second trimester or early third trimester. Thus, women with gestational diabetes

generally are not at increased risk for congenital anomalies like women with pregestational diabetes. They do, however, carry an increased risk of fetal macrosomia and birth injuries as well as neonatal hypoglycemia, hypocalcemia, hyperbilirubinemia, and polycythemia like those with pregestational diabetes. Further, these women have a four- to tenfold increased risk of developing type 2 diabetes during their lifetime.

EPIDEMIOLOGY

The incidence of GDM ranges from 1% to 12% of pregnant women depending on the population. In the United States, it often has been reported to range between 5% and 8%. Gestational diabetes is seen at higher rates in women of Hispanic/Latina, Asian/Pacific Islander, and Native American descent, increasing maternal age, obesity, family history of diabetes, history of a previous infant weighing more than 4,000 g, and previous stillborn infant. Initial studies had found higher rates of GDM among African American women. However, subsequent studies controlling for maternal body mass index (BMI) have found little difference in incidence between African-Americans and Caucasians.

DIAGNOSTIC EVALUATION

The best time to screen for diabetes during pregnancy is at the end of the second trimester between 24 and 28 weeks' gestation in women with low risk for GDM. Patients with one or more risk factors for

■ **TABLE 9-1** White Classification for Diabetes During Pregnancy

Classification	Description
Class A₁	Gestational diabetes; diet controlled
Class A₂	Gestational diabetes; insulin controlled
Class B	Onset: age 20 or older Duration: less than 10 years
Class C	Onset: age 10 to 19 Duration: 10 to 19 years
Class D	Onset: before age 10 Duration: greater than 20 years
Class F	Diabetic nephropathy
Class R	Proliferative retinopathy
Class RF	Retinopathy and nephropathy
Class H	Ischemic heart disease
Class T	Prior renal transplantation

■ **TABLE 9-3** Three-Hour Glucose Tolerance Test: Venous and Plasma Criteria for GDM*

Timing of Glucose Measurement	Normal Venous Blood Glucose (mg/dL)	Normal Whole Plasma Glucose (mg/dL)
Fasting	90	105
1 h	165	190
2 h	145	165
3 h	125	145

*Results reflect upper limits of normal. Diagnosis of gestational diabetes is made if fasting value or any two values are exceeded.

developing gestational diabetes should be screened at their first prenatal visit and, if negative, again in the early third trimester.

There are a variety of proposed methods of screening for diabetes during pregnancy (Table 9-2). In the United States, the most common laboratory screening test consists of giving a 50-g glucose load and then measuring the plasma glucose 1 hour later. If the 1-hour glucose level is greater than 130 or 140 mg/dL, then the test is considered positive and a glucose tolerance test, which often consists of a 100-g glucose load, is indicated. Recently, screening thresholds of 130 mg/dL or 135 mg/dL have been proposed that would increase the sensitivity of the test but at a cost of a larger proportion of women who will screen positive and thus need subsequent confirmatory testing. Thus, the optimal screen-positive threshold that maximizes sensitivity and costs is still under intense research and requires further elucidation.

Women with a positive screening test are diagnosed with a 100-g, 3-hour oral glucose tolerance test (GTT) to evaluate their carbohydrate metabolism (Table 9-3). The GTT involves the administration of 100 gm of oral glucose given after an 8-hour overnight fast preceded by a 3-day special carbohydrate diet. Glucose levels are measured immediately before glucose administration (fasting) and again at 1, 2, and 3 hours after the load. If two or more of the four values are elevated, a diagnosis of gestational diabetes is made. The values shown in Table 9-3 reflect recently lowered values that will increase the number of women diagnosed with gestational diabetes.

TREATMENT

Once the diagnosis of gestational diabetes is made, the patient is usually started on a diabetic diet. An American Diabetic Association (ADA) diet of 2,200 calories per day is recommended for all patients with diabetes during pregnancy, although the total carbohydrate intake is more important. The recommended intake is approximately 200 to 220 g of carbohydrates per day. In addition, both the timing and content of meals are important; therefore, a meal plan based on intake of 30 to 35 kcal/kg of ideal body weight is suggested. Patients are taught to count carbohydrates and meals are designed to contain between 30 to 45 g of carbohydrates at breakfast, with 45 to 60 g of carbohydrates for lunch and dinner, and

■ **TABLE 9-2** Glucose Screening Tests During Pregnancy

Test	Normal Glucose Level (mg/dL)
Fasting	<105
1 h after a 50-g glucose load	<140

15 g for snacks. While on this diet, the patient also monitors her blood glucose levels four times per day, which includes a fasting and three postprandial values. In addition to diet, mild exercise, usually walking, is encouraged as well. The best way for the walking to enhance postprandial blood sugar control is to have the woman walk for 15 minutes about 30 to 40 minutes after the meal.

If the diabetic diet plus exercise controls the blood sugar levels within target range (fasting values <90 and 1 hour postprandial values <140 mg/dL or 2 hour postprandial values <120 mg/dL), then this management is continued throughout the pregnancy. These patients are classified as class A_1 or diet-controlled gestational diabetics in the **White classification of gestational diabetes**. This classification is used as a prognostic tool to determine the likely severity of a woman's diabetes and its interaction with pregnancy; it was originally designed to predict perinatal survival. However, if more than 25% to 30% of a patient's blood sugar values are elevated, medication—usually insulin or an oral hypoglycemic agent—is indicated. These individuals are then considered class A_2 or medication-controlled gestational diabetics.

In true gestational diabetics, fasting values are commonly normal while postprandial values are elevated. This is because the pathophysiology is related to metabolism of large carbohydrate boluses rather than carbohydrate intolerance at baseline. These patients can be started on short-acting insulin in combination with an intermediate-acting insulin in the morning (to cover breakfast and lunch) and a short-acting insulin at dinner. Commonly, the short-acting insulin is humalog (Lispro) or novalog and the intermediate-acting insulin is NPH. Regular insulin had long been the mainstay of diabetic management. However, its use has been replaced by humalog insulin due to its faster onset of action and shorter length of action. Humalog's profile better represents normal physiology and leads to better control of postprandial blood sugars with less hypoglycemia.

Historically, the oral hypoglycemic agents were not used in pregnancy due to concerns regarding fetal hypoglycemia. However, recent studies indicate that in some patients, adequate blood glucose control can be achieved without particular harm to the fetus. One study, in fact, demonstrated that glyburide crossed the placenta in undetectable levels. Because of the ease of patient administration and possibly improved compliance, oral agents such as glyburide or metformin are now being used by some clinicians. With respect to glyburide, there is only one small randomized prospective trial that did not have adequate statistical power to examine neonatal outcomes, and long-term results are not yet available. A recent randomized trial comparing metformin and insulin recently demonstrated no differences in outcomes. At this time, ACOG still considers the use of oral hypoglycemic agents during pregnancy to be experimental.

FETAL MONITORING

In A_2 GDM patients who are started on insulin or an oral hypoglycemic agent, fetal monitoring via nonstress test (NST) or modified biophysical profile (BPP) is typically begun between 32 and 36 weeks' gestation and continued until delivery on a weekly or biweekly basis. Because of the increased risk of macrosomia, these patients commonly receive an obstetric ultrasound for an estimated fetal weight (EFW) between 34 and 37 weeks. It is not common to offer fetal monitoring to A_1 GDM patients who are well controlled on diet alone. The decision to offer these patients an ultrasound for EFW varies among practitioners.

DELIVERY MANAGEMENT

The intrapartum management of diet-controlled gestational diabetics does not differ from that of nondiabetic women, provided that a random glucose check on admission does not reveal significant hyperglycemia that requires correction to avoid neonatal hypoglycemia. It is unclear whether well-controlled gestational diabetics have any particular increased risk for peripartum complications other than the theoretical risk of macrosomia. A closer evaluation of fetal weight at term may be prudent in patients whose pregnancy extends beyond their due date.

Scheduled delivery (typically via induction of labor) at 39 weeks of gestation is common in patients on insulin or a hypoglycemic agent (class A_2 gestational diabetes). One concern about allowing their pregnancies to proceed is that there may be an increased risk of hypoglycemia as their placental function decreases toward the end of pregnancy. These patients are commonly brought in to labor and delivery at 39 weeks for induction, where their long-acting hypoglycemic agents are discontinued and blood sugars monitored every hour. Dextrose and insulin drips are used if necessary to maintain blood sugars within normal limits (<120 mg/dL). Patients with poor glycemic control are offered delivery between weeks 37 and 39 after verification of fetal lung maturity. Patients who have an estimated fetal weight above 4,000 gm have increased risks of shoulder dystocia and their labor curves should be followed closely. Some clinicians offer these patients an elective cesarean birth but, more commonly, elective cesarean delivery is offered to those with an EFW greater than 4,500 gm.

At the time of delivery, forceps and vacuum are generally not used if macrosomia is suspected because of the increased risk of shoulder dystocia, except in the case of true outlet forceps for nonreassuring fetal monitoring. To prepare for a possible shoulder dystocia, there should be at least one experienced obstetrician in the delivery room and usually several extra nurses/assistants. This allows one individual to perform suprapubic pressure, two others to perform McRobert's maneuver, while another can be available to time events and function as an assistant.

FOLLOW-UP

Among patients who develop GDM during pregnancy, over 50% will experience GDM in subsequent pregnancies and 25% to 35% will go on to develop overt diabetes within 5 years. Women with gestational diabetes should be screened for type 2 DM at the postpartum visit and every year thereafter, most commonly with a fasting serum blood glucose or a 75 g, 2-hour GTT. The infants of patients with GDM have an increased incidence of childhood obesity and type 2 diabetes during early adulthood and later in life.

PREGESTATIONAL DIABETES

Diabetes during pregnancy can have devastating effects on both the mother (Table 9-4) and the fetus (Table 9-5). Women with diabetes are four times more likely to develop preeclampsia or eclampsia than women without diabetes. They are also twice as likely to have a spontaneous abortion. In addition, the risks of infection, polyhydramnios, postpartum hemorrhage, and cesarean delivery are all increased for diabetic mothers. Similarly, diabetes can have adverse effect on the fetus, including a fivefold increase in perinatal death and a two- to threefold increase in the risk of congenital malformations, depending on glycemic control.

■ TABLE 9-4 Maternal Complications of Diabetes During Pregnancy
Obstetric complications
Polyhydramnios
Preeclampsia
Miscarriage
Infection
Postpartum hemorrhage
Increased cesarean section
Diabetic emergencies
Hypoglycemia
Ketoacidosis
Diabetic coma
Vascular and end organ involvement
Cardiac
Renal
Ophthalmic
Peripheral vascular
Neurologic
Peripheral neuropathy
Gastrointestinal disturbance

Control of maternal glucose levels in overtly diabetic women is a particularly important factor in determining fetal outcome. In older studies, with minimal glycemic management in gravid diabetic women, the perinatal mortality was as high as 30%. However, with careful management by specialists, this risk can be reduced to less than 1%. The fetuses of diabetic mothers are more likely to develop congenital anomalies, including both cardiac anomalies and neural tube defects, and most dramatically, caudal regression syndrome. The fetus is also at risk for fetal growth abnormalities and sudden intrauterine fetal demise (IUFD).

EPIDEMIOLOGY

Less than 1% of pregnant women have pregestational diabetes. However, with improved management of type 1 diabetics and increased rates of type 2 diabetics, the number of women with pregestational diabetes who become pregnant is increasing.

■ **TABLE 9-5** Fetal Complications of Diabetes Mellitus

Macrosomia
Traumatic delivery
Shoulder dystocia
Erb palsy
Delayed organ maturity
Pulmonary
Hepatic
Neurologic
Pituitary-thyroid axis
Congenital malformations
Cardiovascular defects
Neural tube defects
Caudal regression syndrome
Situs inversus
Duplex renal ureter
IUGR
Intrauterine death

RISK FACTORS

The White classification system was originally designed to prognosticate perinatal survival; with changing management of diabetes as a chronic disease, it has, however, become less applicable. The length of illness used to differentiate classes B, C, and D has little predictive value at this point because there are likely some class B patients with poor control and many class D patients with excellent control, and thus less likely to be at risk of perinatal complications. However, the severity of illness as reflected by classes R (retinopathy), F (nephropathy), and H (heart disease) is certainly predictive of worsened perinatal outcomes in these patients. Along with the White classification, other prognostic factors include hypertension, pyelonephritis, ketoacidosis, and poor glycemic control. Glycemic control is often measured by a HgbA$_1$c, which gives an estimate of the average blood glucose control over the prior 8 to 12 weeks. Patients with an HgbA$_1$c <6.5% generally have good outcomes, whereas patients with an HgbA$_1$c of 12% or greater are estimated to have a 25% rate of congenital anomalies.

TREATMENT

The goals of managing the diabetic patient include thorough patient education, control of maternal glucose, as well as careful maternal and fetal monitoring and testing. To achieve these goals, tight glycemic control should be maintained prior to conception and throughout pregnancy. Studies now show that stricter control of serum glucose levels during pregnancy can decrease the rate of maternal and neonatal complications. To achieve euglycemia, diet, insulin, and exercise must all be regulated.

Diabetic patients have become increasingly aware of the differences that tight control can make as well as the importance of this management during pregnancy. Ideally, these patients should be seen prior to conception to discuss the risks and benefits of pregnancy. In these visits, a diabetic woman can be counseled regarding the risks to her health, particularly in the setting of chronic renal disease that has been shown to worsen during pregnancy. The patient can also be counseled about the risk of congenital anomalies in the fetus based on her HgbA$_1$c. If she is not in optimal control, this can be tightened to prepare for pregnancy. Because these patients are at higher risk of neural tube defects, they are also placed on 4 mg of folate daily.

It has been standard for patients to use the American Diabetic Association diet of 2,200 calories per day. More recently, however, the focus on diabetic diet management has focused on total carbohydrate intake rather than caloric intake. Generally, patients keep their carbohydrate intake at 30 to 45 g for breakfast and 45 to 60 g for lunch and dinner with 15 g for snacks. Patients can increase or decrease protein and fat based on whether they need more or fewer calories to gain or maintain weight. These carbohydrate-focused diets should be maintained during pregnancy, although the total caloric intake is usually about 300 kcal higher than in nonpregnant patients.

TYPE 1 DIABETES

Historically, these patients had extremely poor maternal and perinatal outcomes, many of which can be attributed to long-standing disease and difficulty in maintaining euglycemia. Currently, many type 1 diabetics are checking their blood sugars seven or more times per day, doing carbohydrate counting, and maintaining their HgbA$_1$c below 6.0% to 6.5%.

When patients are able to maintain tight control prior to and during their pregnancies, the risks of microvascular disease, renal disease, and hypertension are significantly decreased. These lower rates of baseline disease lead to fewer complications during pregnancy.

Because of the correlation of outcome with prepregnant disease, patients are extensively screened at their first visit (if not preconceptionally). Routinely, patients should obtain an electrocardiogram (ECG), particularly those with long-standing disease, hypertension, advanced maternal age (AMA), or renal disease. A 24-hour urine collection for creatinine clearance and protein should be sent to assess baseline renal function. An HgbA$_1$c is ordered to assess baseline glucose management as well as thyroid function tests (TSH and free T4) since these patients are at risk for other autoimmune endocrinopathies. In addition, a referral to an ophthalmologist should be made to check for baseline retinopathy.

Because type 1 diabetics require insulin, they are usually very experienced at managing their disease. However, this experience may not be applicable during pregnancy, during which glycemic control can be dramatically different. During the first half of pregnancy, the patient's prior dosing regimen is usually increased slightly, but can increase substantially during the latter half of pregnancy as insulin resistance increases. If patients have been managed on an insulin pump, this practice should be continued. In fact, because an insulin pump can help maintain patients in tight control, it is often begun either preconception for patients planning to conceive or after the first trimester in patients who are becoming increasingly difficult to manage with NPH and humalog insulin shots. Some patients will have had excellent control prepregnant with Lantes, glargine insulin. This insulin is a slow-release insulin that gives a very flat steady state level of insulin for 24 hours. Unfortunately, the experience in pregnancy is minimal. Though it is generally not recommended during pregnancy at this time, it is being used increasingly by clinicians who care for preconceptional diabetics during pregnancy.

Table 9-6 demonstrates the relationship between the time of insulin dose, the time of glucose testing, and the target blood glucose levels. When adjusting a patient's dosing schedule, it is important to consider other factors that may alter insulin require-

■ **TABLE 9-6** Glucose Monitoring and Insulin Dosing During Pregnancy		
Insulin Type and Dose Time	**Time Impact Seen**	**Target Glucose Level (mg/dL)**
Evening NPH	Fasting	70 to 90
Morning Humalog	Post breakfast	100 to 139
Morning NPH	Post lunch	100 to 139
Evening Humalog	Post dinner	100 to 139

ments, such as diet, exercise, stress, and infection. When insulin changes become necessary, there are a few simple rules that aid in the process (Table 9-7). In addition to the schedules given in Table 9-6 and Table 9-7, patients on insulin pumps should also check premeal glucose values throughout the day to get a sense of how well blood sugars are being managed at baseline.

Because the level of physical activity affects the plasma glucose level, consistent levels of physical activity are suggested. Keep in mind that a hospitalized patient who achieves euglycemia in the context of relatively low activity may encounter bouts of hypoglycemia when discharged home on the same insulin regime because her physical activity level increases at home, thus lowering the need for insulin. Physical activity can also be used to help manage blood glucose. If a patient consistently has an elevated postmeal blood glucose, the premeal insulin or postmeal activity can be increased. It is also important to consider differences between weekday and weekend activity. Some patients will require entirely different insulin regimens on the weekends.

■ **TABLE 9-7** Instructions for Adjusting Insulin Dosage
1. Establish a fasting glucose level between 70 and 90 mg/dL.
2. Only adjust one dosing level at a time.
3. Do not change any dosage by more than 20% per day.
4. Wait 24 h between dosage changes to evaluate the response.

TYPE 2 DIABETES

The pathophysiology of type 2 diabetes differs from type 1 diabetes. Type 1 diabetics have had autoimmune destruction of their pancreatic islet cells resulting in diminished or absent insulin production, whereas type 2 diabetics have peripheral insulin resistance. Many type 2 diabetics are managed prior to pregnancy with oral hypoglycemic agents or diet alone. However, in pregnancy, most will require insulin. Oral hypoglycemic agents have not generally been used during pregnancy because of concerns regarding fetal hypoglycemia or potential teratogenicity, but recent studies have not demonstrated any particular association with congenital anomalies, and patients are often initially maintained on these medications during pregnancy. However, eventually, most of these patients will be hyperglycemic even on the maximum doses of the oral agents and need to be switched to insulin.

When oral hypoglycemic agents do not adequately maintain glucose control during pregnancy, insulin can be substituted or supplemented. In general, insulin is started as NPH at bedtime to control fasting blood sugars and in the AM to provide a longer-acting substrate throughout the day. A short-acting insulin, usually humalog or Lispro, is used at meals to control immediate carbohydrate intake. Once patients are started on insulin, management is very similar to that of type 1 diabetics, although the doses are often higher depending on the patient's degree of insulin resistance. Again, although regular insulin has been used traditionally, it is a poor substitute for the newer fast-acting insulins for postprandial blood sugar control.

Fetal Testing and Delivery

In the patient with pregestational diabetes, antenatal testing to evaluate the growth and well-being of the fetus usually begins at 32 weeks. Earlier testing is recommended in the setting of poor glycemic control. Testing regimens vary, but may resemble the following: antenatal fetal assessment consisting of weekly NSTs until 36 weeks, at which time biweekly testing is implemented, which includes weekly NST alternating with weekly modified BPP to assess amniotic fluid measurement as well. In addition to the weekly testing, an ultrasound to assess fetal growth is usually obtained between 32 and 36 weeks' gestation.

In general, well-controlled pregestational insulin-dependent diabetics with no complications are offered fetal lung maturity testing at 37 weeks' gestation and delivered if mature. Many patients may decline this management, and are instead offered induction of labor at 38 or 39 weeks' gestation without fetal lung maturity testing. Indications for earlier delivery include nonreassuring fetal testing, poor glycemic control, worsening or uncontrolled hypertension, worsening renal disease, or poor fetal growth.

Blood sugars can be extremely difficult to manage in the laboring diabetic woman. The physical effort of labor and delivery decreases the overall insulin requirements. Patients are usually begun on dextrose and insulin drips to maintain blood sugars between 100 and 120 mg/dL. If the blood sugar increases above 120, the insulin can be increased. Conversely, if the blood sugar drops to between 80 and 100, an infusion of dextrose can be started or increased.

After delivery, maternal insulin requirements decrease significantly because of the removal of the placenta, which contains many insulin antagonists. In fact, insulin requirements may go below prepregnant levels during the puerperium, particularly in breast-feeding women. Type 2 diabetics may require no insulin during this period. However, type 1 diabetics should always be maintained on at least a small amount of insulin because they do not produce any endogenously.

Follow-Up

In the puerperal period, pregestational diabetics should resume their prepregnancy regimens. Patients who were on oral hypoglycemic agents, however, are generally not advised to resume their use if breast-feeding because of concerns regarding neonatal hypoglycemia. This complication is more theoretical as it has not been documented in any large case series or cohort studies. In patients with preexisting renal disease, a 24-hour urine collection for creatinine clearance and protein is usually done at 6 weeks postpartum to assess worsening of disease. In addition, an ophthalmologic appointment is usually scheduled 12 to 14 weeks postpartum. After 6 to 8 weeks postpartum, management of the patient's diabetes should be transferred back to her primary provider or endocrinologist.

KEY POINTS

- Gestational diabetes occurs in 1% to 12% of pregnant women.
- Risk factors for gestational diabetes include Hispanic, Asian American, Native American, and African American ethnicity, obesity, family history of diabetes, and prior pregnancy complicated by gestational diabetes, macrosomia, shoulder dystocia, or fetal death.
- All pregnant women should be screened for diabetes between weeks 24 and 28. High-risk women should also be screened at their first prenatal visit.
- Fetal complications of gestational diabetes include macrosomia, shoulder dystocia, and neonatal hypoglycemia.
- Pregnancy management should include frequent healthcare visits, thorough patient education, American Diabetic Association diet, glucose monitoring, fetal monitoring, and insulin or an oral hypoglycemic agent as indicated.
- Patients should generally be induced between 39 and 40 weeks' gestation. Intrapartum insulin and dextrose are used to maintain tight control during delivery. Cesarean section is offered if fetal weight is over 4,500 g.
- Maternal complications of diabetes during pregnancy include hyperglycemia, hypoglycemia, urinary tract infection, worsening renal disease, hypertension, and retinopathy.
- Fetal complications of diabetes during pregnancy include spontaneous abortion, congenital anomalies, macrosomia, IUGR, neonatal hypoglycemia, respiratory distress syndrome, and perinatal death.
- Pregnancy management is optimized by a preconceptional visit, early prenatal care, thorough patient education, tight glucose monitoring and management with insulin, fetal monitoring, and thoughtful plan for delivery.
- Motivated type 1 diabetics can usually maintain tighter control on an insulin pump. Management in labor and delivery usually requires an insulin drip; however, insulin requirements decrease dramatically postpartum.

Infectious Diseases in Pregnancy

As with other diseases in pregnancy, one must think about the effect of an infectious disease on the pregnant woman and the fetus, as well as the pregnancy outcome. In this chapter we discuss common infections that increase or whose complications increase in pregnancy, infections specific to pregnancy, and infections that can affect the fetus (Table 10-1). The infectious complications that are common to the puerperium (postpartum period), such as endomyometritis and wound infections, are discussed in Chapter 12.

URINARY TRACT INFECTIONS (UTIs)

The incidence of **urinary tract infections** (UTIs) increases during pregnancy. Multiple studies show that asymptomatic bacteriuria with greater than 100,000 colonies on culture occurs in approximately 5% of all pregnancies. Although this prevalence is similar to that in the nonpregnant population, it can lead to episodes of cystitis and pyelonephritis at higher rates in pregnant women. Bacteriuria in pregnancy is further associated with preterm birth and low birth-weight infants. Untreated asymptomatic bacteriuria will progress to cystitis or pyelonephritis in 25% to 40% of pregnant patients. Of the cases of pyelonephritis, up to 15% may be complicated by bacteremia, sepsis, or adult respiratory distress syndrome (ARDS). Furthermore, in pregnant sickle-cell patients, the rate of asymptomatic bacteriuria doubles to 10%.

PATHOGENESIS

A number of factors can contribute to a higher incidence of cystitis and pyelonephritis in pregnancy.

During pregnancy, the smooth muscle relaxation effects of progesterone decrease bladder tone and cause ureteral dilation. In addition, mechanical compression from the enlarged uterus can cause obstruction of the ureters, leading to stasis. Both cystitis and vesicoureteral reflux are increased, leading to more ascending infections.

DIAGNOSIS

UTIs are diagnosed with clinical signs and symptoms of dysuria, urinary frequency, and urinary urgency in conjunction with a positive urine culture. Because urine cultures may take 3 to 4 days to become positive, a urinalysis is often used as a proxy during initial evaluation. The urinalysis may be positive for leukocyte esterase, nitrates, or hematuria, and the urine sediment will have elevated white blood cells and bacteria. Cystitis is diagnosed with suprapubic tenderness upon palpation and complaints of lower abdominal pain in the setting of a UTI.

TREATMENT

Escherichia coli accounts for greater than 70% of all UTIs. The remainder are usually due to *Klebsiella*, *Enterococcus*, *Proteus*, coagulase-negative *Staphylococcus*, and group B *Streptococcus*. Because most UTIs are caused by *E. coli*, initial treatment of asymptomatic bacteriuria is usually with amoxicillin, nitrofurantoin (Macrodantin), trimethoprim/sulfamethoxazole (Bactrim), or cephalexin. Treatment duration consists of a 3- to 7-day course of antibiotics although many authorities prefer 7-day treatment course for pregnant women. Symptomatic UTIs and cystitis are

■ TABLE 10-1 Infectious Diseases in Pregnancy

Infections whose complications increase during pregnancy
UTIs
Bacterial vaginosis
Surgical wound
Group B *Strep*
Infections more common in pregnancy and the puerperium
Pyelonephritis
Endomyometritis
Mastitis
Toxic shock syndrome (TSS)
Infections specific to pregnancy
Chorioamnionitis
Septic pelvic thrombophlebitis
Episiotomy or perineal lacerations
Infections that affect the fetus
Neonatal sepsis (e.g., Group B *Strep*, *E. coli*)
HSV
VZV
Parvovirus B19
CMV
Rubella
HIV
Hepatitis B & C
Gonorrhea
Chlamydia
Syphilis
Toxoplasmosis

also treated in this fashion, with adjustment of medication based on culture-sensitivity results. Because an asymptomatic bacteriuria may persist, a test of cure culture should be obtained 1 to 2 weeks after completion of therapy. In addition to treating the infection, in patients with dysuria or bladder pain, phenazopyridine (Pyridium), which is concentrated in the urine and acts as a local anesthetic to reduce the pain, is commonly used for symptomatic relief. Of note, patients should be counseled that Pyridium may cause the urine to turn bright orange.

PYELONEPHRITIS

The most common complication of a lower UTI is an ascending infection to the kidneys, or **pyelonephritis**. Pyelonephritis is estimated to complicate as many as 1% to 2% of pregnancies and has particularly serious associated complications including septic shock and ARDS. Because of these risks, pyelonephritis during pregnancy is usually treated aggressively with hospital admission, intravenous (IV) hydration, and IV antibiotics—often cephalosporins (cefazolin, cefotetan, or ceftriaxone) or ampicillin and gentamicin—until the patient is afebrile and asymptomatic for 24 to 48 hours. The patient is then transitioned to an oral antibiotic regimen. Small trials have examined the possibility of treating these patients with a single dose of IV or IM antibiotics, such as ceftriaxone, followed by outpatient oral antibiotic regimen. While these treatments seem to be effective in certain groups, consideration of appropriate patient criteria, including absence of signs of sepsis, compliance, ability to tolerate oral medications, and gestational age, is imperative. Treatment duration for pyelonephritis consists of a total of 10 to 14 days of combined IV and oral antibiotics. Pregnant patients with one episode of pyelonephritis or two or more episodes of asymptomatic bacteriuria and/or cystitis are generally placed on antimicrobial prophylaxis for the duration of the pregnancy.

BACTERIAL VAGINOSIS IN PREGNANCY

Studies have demonstrated that **bacterial vaginosis** (BV) increases the risk for preterm premature rupture of membranes (PPROM), preterm delivery, and puerperal infections. Because of this, it has been proposed that patients with BV be treated and followed up with a test of cure to decrease their risk of preterm delivery. Several studies have also demonstrated a reduction of preterm births when high-risk asymptomatic pregnant women (those with prior preterm delivery or PPROM) were treated for BV with an oral agent. Therefore, screening and treatment of BV may be considered in this subgroup of pregnant women.

DIAGNOSIS AND TREATMENT

Common symptoms of BV include a malodorous discharge or vaginal irritation, although many patients with BV may be asymptomatic. Diagnosis can be made with three of the following findings: presence of thin, white, homogeneous discharge coating the vaginal walls; an amine odor noted with addition of 10% KOH ("whiff" test); pH of >4.5; of presence of clue cells on microscopic examination. Gram's stain with examination of bacteria in the vaginal discharge is considered the gold standard for BV diagnosis. Common BV organisms include *Gardnerella vaginosis*, *Bacteroides*, and *Mycoplasma hominis*. Oral metronidazole (Flagyl) is the treatment of choice for treatment of BV in pregnancy. Clindamycin oral form may also be used. Because a majority of studies have demonstrated adverse perinatal events when intravaginal forms of clindamycin were used for treatment of BV, an oral form is preferred for use in pregnant women. In pregnancy, because of high rates of asymptomatic infection and because treatment of high-risk patients may prevent adverse perinatal outcomes, a test of cure may be considered 1 month after treatment completion.

GROUP B STREPTOCOCCUS

Group B *Streptococcus* is commonly responsible for UTIs, chorioamnionitis, and endomyometritis during pregnancy. It is also a major pathogen in neonatal sepsis, which has severe implications. Although early-onset neonatal sepsis occurs in two to three per 1,000 live births, the mortality rate with group B streptococcal sepsis ranges from 5% to 50%, depending on gestational age at time of delivery. Various studies have demonstrated a wide range of asymptomatic colonization in pregnant women, from 10% to 35%. To protect infants from group B *Streptococcus* infections, widespread screening programs have been implemented utilizing a rectovaginal culture for group B *Strep* colonization between 35 and 37 weeks. Large prospective studies have demonstrated that these screening programs do decrease the rate of neonatal sepsis from group B *Strep*. Of note, there are concerns that the increase in prophylactic antibiotics given to these patients will increase widespread antibiotic resistance. Another concern is that by focusing clinical attention on GBS, the incidence of *E. coli* sepsis, which has an even higher mortality rate, will increase.

DIAGNOSIS AND TREATMENT

Group B *Strep* screening is performed by a culture of the vagina and rectum between 35 and 37 weeks of gestation. Women with positive group B *Strep* cultures are subsequently treated with IV penicillin G in labor. Women with an unknown group B *Strep* status experiencing labor before 37 weeks of gestation or those with an unknown status who have rupture of membranes greater than 18 hours are also treated with penicillin G until delivery based on risk factor criteria. Because of the difficulty of obtaining the correct dosage of penicillin G, ampicillin is commonly used instead. However, because ampicillin is a broader spectrum antibiotic than penicillin, some authorities feel that its use should be discouraged because of the development of resistance. For GBS colonized women with rash allergies, cefazolin is used for prophylaxis during labor. In women with a significant penicillin allergy, sensitivities for the GBS culture should be obtained and treatment should be guided by these results. Clindamycin is a common antibiotic alternative in this setting.

CHORIOAMNIONITIS

Chorioamnionitis is an infection of the membranes and amniotic fluid surrounding the fetus. It is frequently associated with preterm and prolonged rupture of membranes (ROM) but can also occur without ROM. It is the most common precursor of neonatal sepsis, which has a high rate of fetal mortality. It has maternal sequelae of endomyometritis and septic shock.

DIAGNOSIS

The common signs of chorioamnionitis are maternal fever, elevated maternal white blood count, uterine tenderness, and fetal tachycardia. Because chorioamnionitis is of such great concern with need for delivery, other physiologic events that may have similar signs and symptoms should be excluded. Other loci of maternal infection may cause maternal fever and elevated white blood cell count as well as fetal tachycardia. Elevations in maternal temperature have also been seen in patients undergoing labor induction with prostaglandins as well as those with epidurals. Fetal tachycardia may be congenital. Thus, a prior baseline fetal heart rate (FHR) can be useful. Fetal tachycardia can also be caused by medications administered to the mother, such as β-agonist tocolytic agents. The maternal white blood cell count is elevated in pregnancy and further elevated with the onset of labor. The white blood cell count is also increased by the administration of corticosteroids.

In patients at term, if the constellation of the above signs exists without any other etiology, the diagnosis of chorioamnionitis should be presumed and treatment started. In preterm patients whose fetuses would benefit from remaining in utero for more time, a more aggressive means to reach the diagnosis can be taken if there is any doubt. The gold standard for diagnosis of chorioamnionitis is a culture of the amniotic fluid, which can be obtained via amniocentesis. At the same time, the amniotic fluid can be sent for glucose, white blood cell count, protein, and Gram's stain. Unfortunately, these tests have a sensitivity that ranges from 40% to 70%. The infected fetus has been described to experience a fetal immune response syndrome (FIRS), which results in the release of cytokines. This has led to research that shows that the most sensitive screening test for chorioamnionitis appears to be IL-6 levels in the amniotic fluid that rise prior to changes in many of the other screening tests. This screening test is still used only in experimental protocols at most institutions.

TREATMENT

When chorioamnionitis is suspected, intravenous antibiotics should be started. Commonly, the causative organisms are those that colonize the vagina and rectum. Thus, broad-spectrum coverage should be used, most commonly a second- or third-generation cephalosporin or ampicillin and gentamicin. In addition to antibiotics, delivery should be hastened with induction and augmentation by vaginal delivery, or, in the case of a nonreassuring fetal tracing, by cesarean delivery.

INFECTIONS THAT AFFECT THE FETUS

HERPES SIMPLEX VIRUS (HSV)

Herpes simplex virus (HSV) is a DNA virus that has two subtypes: HSV-1 and HSV-2. Genital herpes infections are primarily caused by HSV-2; however, there are extragenital HSV-2 infections and genital HSV-1 infections. Patients with a history of herpes should have thorough perineal examination for lesions when presenting in labor because of the risk of vertical transmission of HSV to the fetus during vaginal delivery. If lesions are present, cesarean delivery is the recommended mode of delivery for prevention of vertical

transmission by leading authorities, although data demonstrating a clear benefit of cesarean delivery in prevention of neonatal HSV during a recurrent maternal infection is limited. Patients with an HSV genital outbreak during their pregnancies are offered acyclovir prophylaxis from week 36 until delivery to prevent recurrent lesions. Women with a history of genital HSV, but without an outbreak in pregnancy are more controversial, with some clinicians also recommending acyclovir prophylaxis beyond 36 weeks of gestation. Additionally, since a large proportion of women who are infected with HSV are unaware of their status, universal screening for HSV in pregnancy has been proposed as well. Currently this practice is dissuaded as it is an expensive venture with no demonstrated benefit and may lead to anxiety in a great many women and their partners.

Primary herpes infections in pregnancy have a much higher fetal and neonatal attack rate than secondary lesions. This virus can even be transmitted across the placenta during the viremic segment of the illness. A primary infection can be differentiated from a secondary one by checking antibody titers. A previously infected person will have circulating IgG antibodies. A primary infection transmitted late in the third trimester—particularly close to delivery—is far more dangerous because of the lack of maternal antibodies transmitted to the fetus. Thus, to determine whether an HSV lesion is primary or secondary, IgM and type-specific IgG HSV antibodies may be ordered. Of note, while this does not specifically change management or outcomes, it does change the patient's prognosis and is useful in counseling.

HSV can cause severe infections in the neonate. Risk of transmission to infant is up to 50% in a primary maternal infection and less than 1% to 5% in a recurrent maternal infection. Additionally, primary infection acquired near the time of labor is associated with the highest risk of transmission to the neonate during delivery. Infection in the neonate can be diagnosed by viral cultures of the herpetic lesions, oropharynx, or eyes. The infection in the neonate can progress to a viral sepsis, pneumonia, and herpes encephalitis, which can lead to neurologic devastation and death (see Color Plate 2). Infected infants are treated with IV acyclovir as soon as infection is suspected.

VARICELLA ZOSTER VIRUS (VZV)

Varicella zoster virus (VZV) is a DNA herpes virus that causes chickenpox and can reactivate to cause herpes zoster or shingles. Because it is primarily a disease of childhood, more than 90% of adults are immune to VZV infection. The infection in adults tends to be more serious than in children, with a higher rate of varicella pneumonia. Varicella titers may be evaluated during pregnancy for those patients who are unsure about exposure history. Women who present preconceptionally can be screened for VZV titers and, if negative, be immunized prior to conceiving.

Vertical transmission occurs transplacentally. More recent large studies do not demonstrate an increased risk of spontaneous abortion during maternal VZV infection in the first trimester. However, VZV is associated with congenital malformations characterized as congenital varicella syndrome (see Color Plate 3) in approximately 0.5% to 2% of cases, resulting predominantly when mothers are infected between 8 and 20 weeks of gestation. Infections near term may lead to a postnatal infection that may range from a benign course (like chickenpox) to a fulminant disseminated infection, leading to death. Other infants may show no signs of infection at birth; however, they will develop shingles at some point later in childhood. Of note, maternal herpes zoster is not associated with congenital anomalies.

Varicella zoster immune globulin (VZIG) may ameliorate maternal disease but does not prevent transmission of the disease to the fetus. Therefore, any patient without a history of chickenpox with an exposure in pregnancy should receive VZIG within 96 hours of exposure. Infants of mothers who develop varicella disease within 5 days before delivery or 2 days after should also receive VZIG.

PARVOVIRUS

Parvovirus B19 causes erythema infectiosum (fifth disease). Classically, this mild infection presents with a red macular rash giving the slapped cheek appearance, and usually resolves with minimal intervention. In pregnancy, however, there is concern for maternal-fetal transmission, which has been noted to cause fetal infection and death. First trimester infections have been associated with miscarriage, but midtrimester and later infections are associated with fetal hydrops. The parvovirus B19 attacks fetal erythrocytes leading to a hemolytic anemia, hydrops, and death.

If parvovirus exposure is suspected in the mother, acute infection can be diagnosed by checking parvovirus IgM and IgG levels. If studies indicate an acute parvovirus infection (positive IgM and positive or negative IgG) beyond 20 weeks of gestation, then the fetus should undergo serial ultrasounds, up to 8 to 10 weeks after maternal infection. Because of the risk of fetal anemia, serial ultrasounds, and management with fetal transfusion when there is evidence of hydrops have been recommended by some perinatologists. This intervention has not been studied in large populations, however, and is of unclear benefit. More recently, the use of Doppler ultrasound to examine the peak systolic velocity of the middle cerebral artery has been described to identify fetal anemia. Because the fetal anemia in the setting of parvovirus is due to marrow suppression rather than hemolysis, this screening test offers the ability to identify patients at risk prior to the development of hydrops.

CYTOMEGALOVIRUS (CMV)

Cytomegalovirus (CMV) infections in the mother usually cause either a subclinical or mild viral illness. Only rarely will it lead to hepatitis or a mononucleosis-like syndrome. Thus, maternal infections are rarely diagnosed. CMV causes in utero infections in approximately 1% of all newborns. Of these infected infants, approximately 10% will be symptomatic at birth.

Infants who are symptomatic can develop cytomegalic inclusion disease manifested by a constellation of findings including hepatomegaly, splenomegaly, thrombocytopenia, jaundice, cerebral calcifications, chorioretinitis, and interstitial pneumonitis (see Color Plate 4). Affected infants have a high mortality rate of up to 30% and may develop mental retardation, sensorineural hearing loss, and neuromuscular disorders. Of the remaining 90% of asymptomatic infants, 15% will go on to develop late disabilities, while 85% will have no sequelae of the infection.

Currently, there is no treatment or prophylaxis for the disease. Studies reporting use of intravenous hyperimmune globulin and antiviral medications have been published, but large randomized trials demonstrating decrease in fetal infection are still lacking. A vaccine for the prevention of disease in the mother is also being investigated.

RUBELLA VIRUS

Rubella infection in adults leads to a mild illness with a maculopapular rash, arthritis, arthralgias, and a diffuse lymphadenopathy that lasts 2 to 4 days. The infection can be transmitted to the fetus and cause congenital rubella infection, which may lead to **congenital rubella syndrome** (CRS). The maternal–fetal transmission rate is highest during the first trimester, as are the rates of congenital abnormalities. However, transmission may occur at any time during pregnancy.

The congenital abnormalities associated with CRS include deafness, cardiac abnormalities, cataracts, and mental retardation. Specifically, if maternal rubella infection occurs during the period of organogenesis, any fetal organ system may be affected. There are a variety of latent sequelae including the delayed onset of diabetes, thyroid disease, deafness, ocular disease, and growth hormone deficiency. The diagnosis of rubella infection is made with serology studies. IgM titers will result from primary infection and reinfection with rubella. Because IgM does not cross the placenta, IgM titers in the infant are indicative of infection. IgG titers that are elevated over time support the diagnosis of CRS in an infant as well.

Currently, there is no treatment for rubella once acquired. However, the institution of rubella immunization has decreased the number of CRS cases to less than 20 per year. In pregnancy, the rubella titer is checked during the first trimester. Because of theoretic risk of transmission of the live virus in the vaccine, patients do not receive the measles, mumps, and rubella vaccine until postpartum, and patients are advised to avoid pregnancy for 1 month following vaccination. Women who are known to have low or nonexistent titers should be advised to avoid anyone with possible rubella infections.

HUMAN IMMUNODEFICIENCY VIRUS

In the United States approximately 7,000 infants are born annually to mothers who are infected with **human immunodeficiency virus** (HIV). With no treatment, approximately 25% of infants born to HIV-infected mothers will become infected with HIV. Increased transmission can be seen with higher viral burden or advanced disease in the mother, rupture of the membranes, and invasive procedures during labor and delivery that increase neonatal exposure to maternal blood. Transmission occurs in-utero (1/3) generally late in pregnancy or during labor and delivery (2/3). In 1994, Pediatric AIDS Clinical Trials Group (PACTG) protocol 076 demonstrated that a three-part regimen of zidovudine (ZDV) administered during pregnancy and labor and to the newborn could reduce the risk of perinatal transmission by two-thirds. Additionally, with the use of highly active antiretroviral therapy (HAART) to further decrease viral load with potent regimens, the rate of transmission can be further decreased to less than 1% to 2% with an undetectable viral load. Currently, antiretroviral therapy in pregnancy includes a 3-drug regimen generally started in the second trimester with a goal of viral suppression by the third trimester, regardless of need for antiretrovirals for maternal health indication. Cesarean delivery has been shown to lower transmission rates by roughly two-thirds compared to vaginal delivery in patients on no therapy and particularly without onset of labor or rupture of membranes or in the setting of high viral load. However, in women with viral loads of <1,000 copies/mL, there is no additional benefit of cesarean delivery versus vaginal delivery in HIV perinatal transmission. Therefore, cesarean delivery should be considered in HIV-infected pregnant women with viral loads >1,000 copies/mL and without long-standing onset of labor or rupture of membranes. Because of the effective interventions in HIV-positive women to decrease vertical transmission, it is recommended that HIV screening be offered to all pregnant women at their first prenatal visit and again in the third trimester if the woman has specified risk factors for HIV infection. Furthermore, in resource-rich nations where safe bottle-feeding alternatives are available, breastfeeding is contraindicated in HIV-infected woman as virus is found in breast milk and responsible for HIV transmission to the infant. Postnatal HIV transmission from breast milk at 2 years may be as high as 15%. Furthermore, studies are lacking regarding the efficacy of maternal antiretroviral therapy for prevention of transmission of HIV through breast milk and the toxicity of antiretroviral exposure of the infant via breast milk.

NEISSERIA GONORRHOEAE

Gonococcal infections are associated with pelvic inflammatory disease in early pregnancy, as well as preterm delivery, PPROM, and puerperal infections throughout pregnancy duration. The infection is transmitted during passage of the neonate through the birth canal. Neonatal infection can affect the eye, oropharynx, external ear, and anorectal mucosa. These infections can furthermore become disseminated, causing arthritis and meningitis.

Screening for gonorrhea should be performed for pregnant women with risk factors in the first prenatal visit and again in the third trimester. The diagnosis is made by nucleic acid amplification tests (NAAT) or culture. Treatment can be with IM ceftriaxone, oral cefixime, or IM spectinomycin in cases where cephalosporins cannot be tolerated. Patients should be treated with azithromycin or amoxicillin for presumed *Chlamydial* infection as well, since the two diseases often co-occur.

CHLAMYDIA TRACHOMATIS

Chlamydial infections in the newborn can lead to serious sequelae. The infection is transmitted during delivery from the genital tract to the infant. In infected patients with vaginal deliveries, 40% of infants will develop conjunctivitis and greater than 10% will develop *Chlamydia* pneumonia.

Asymptomatic infection is common. Therefore many authorities recommend that all pregnant women should be screened in the first prenatal visit and if deemed as high risk again in the third trimester. Because tetracycline and doxycycline are not advised in pregnancy, the treatment of choice for *Chlamydia* in pregnancy is azithromycin, amoxicillin, or erythromycin.

HEPATITIS B

Viral hepatitis caused by the **hepatitis B** DNA virus can be acquired from sexual contact, exposure to blood products, and transplacentally. The clinical manifestations of the disease range from mild hepatic dysfunction to fulminant liver failure and death. It can be diagnosed using a variety of antibody and antigenic markers.

During the prenatal period, all patients are screened for hepatitis B surface antigen (HBsAg). Those with HBsAg are likely to have chronic disease and are at risk for transmission to the fetus. If pregnant patients are exposed to HBV during pregnancy, postexposure prophylaxis with one dose of hepatitis B immunoglobulin and a complete hepatitis B vaccination series is recommended, which may be protective. Neonates of mothers who are HBsAg positive or have unknown status should be given HepB immunoglobulin at birth (preferably within 12 hours of birth) and should undergo HepB vaccination at birth (preferably within 12 hours of birth), 1 month, and 6 months. All infants are routinely immunized with the hepatitis B vaccine.

SYPHILIS

Syphilis is caused by infection with the spirochete *Treponema pallidum* and is usually transmitted via sexual contact or transplacentally to the fetus. Although vertical transmission can occur at any time during pregnancy and during any stage of disease, because there must be spirochetemia for vertical transmission to occur, approximately half of prenatal transmission occurs in pregnant women with primary or secondary syphilis. More than 70% of infants born to mothers with untreated syphilis will be infected, compared with 1% to 2% of infants born to women who received adequate treatment during pregnancy. Despite prenatal screening and readily available treatment, there are still several hundred cases of congenital syphilis annually in the United States.

Syphilis in pregnancy that results in vertical transmission may lead to a late abortion, intrauterine fetal demise, or a congenitally infected infant. Patients with early congenital syphilis present with a systemic illness accompanied by a maculopapular rash, snuffles, hepatomegaly, splenomegaly, hemolysis, lymphadenopathy, and jaundice. Diagnosis can be made by identification of IgM antitreponemal antibodies, which do not cross the placenta. Penicillin remains the only treatment with sufficient evidence demonstrating efficacy for preventing maternal syphilis transmission to the fetus and for treating fetal infection. If early congenital syphilis is untreated, manifestations of late congenital syphilis can develop, including eighth nerve deafness, saber shins, mulberry molar (see Color Plate 5), Hutchinson's teeth, and a saddle nose.

TOXOPLASMOSIS

Toxoplasma gondii is a common protozoan parasite that can be found in humans and domestic animals. The infections in immunocompetent hosts are often subclinical. Occasionally, a patient will develop fevers, malaise, lymphadenopathy, and a rash as with most viral infections. A pregnant woman who is infected can transmit the disease transplacentally to the fetus. Transmission is more common when the disease is acquired in the third trimester, although neonatal manifestations are usually mild or subclinical. Infections acquired in the first trimester are transmitted less commonly; however, the infection has far more serious consequences in the fetus. Severe congenital infection can involve fevers, seizures, chorioretinitis, hydro- or microcephaly, hepatosplenomegaly, and jaundice (see Color Plate 6). Thus, the differential diagnosis for this infection includes nearly all other commonly acquired intrauterine infections. Diagnosis of toxoplasmosis in the neonate can be made with detection of IgM antibodies, but lack of the antibodies does not necessarily rule out infection.

Because women with previous *Toxoplasma* exposure are likely to be protected from further infections, high-risk patients can be screened with titers for IgG to ascertain whether or not they are at risk for infection. Pregnant women have been advised to avoid contact with cat litter boxes and significant gardening without glove and mask protection during pregnancy, as the organism is found in cat feces and soil that may be contaminated with animal feces. Toxoplasmosis in pregnancy can be diagnosed maternally with IgM and IgG titers. Because IgM may persist for years, presence of IgM antibody cannot confirm acute infection. Given the wide variability of IgM assays, diagnosis of acute infection should be confirmed by a reference laboratory. If maternal diagnosis is made or suspected early in pregnancy, evaluation of amniotic fluid with DNA PCR for *T. gondi* per amniocentesis at least 4 weeks after maternal infection is the recommended procedure for evaluation of fetal infection. Fetal blood evaluation via percutaneous umbilical blood sampling is discouraged given the low sensitivity, as absence of fetal IgM does not completely rule out fetal infection and in turn has the potential of transplacental fetal infection. Diagnosis may influence the decision of whether to terminate a pregnancy in the first two trimesters. Maternal disease can be treated with spiramycin. Spiramycin is preferable in pregnant women because no teratogenic effects are known. However, because spiramycin does not cross the placenta, it is not effective in treatment of fetal infection. Therefore, pyrimethamine and sulfadiazine are recommended for treatment of documented fetal infection. Folic acid is concurrently administered due to the bone marrow suppression effects of pyrimethamine and sulfadiazine, given their folate antagonist effects.

 KEY POINTS

- Five percent of pregnant women have asymptomatic bacteriuria and are at increased risk for cystitis and pyelonephritis.
- Lower UTIs can be treated with oral antibiotics, whereas pyelonephritis in pregnancy is usually treated initially with IV antibiotics, with change to oral regimen once afebrile for 24 to 48 hours.
- Pyelonephritis may be complicated by septic shock and ARDS.
- Symptomatic BV is associated with preterm delivery.
- BV treatment in pregnancy consists of oral metronidazole for 7 days.
- Screening and treatment of BV in asymptomatic high-risk pregnant women may be considered.
- Group B *Strep* has traditionally been a leading cause of neonatal sepsis.
- Screening for group B *Strep* and using prophylactic antibiotics in labor has been shown to decrease group B *Strep* neonatal sepsis.
- Group B *Strep* screening is performed between 35 and 37 weeks of gestation.
- Chorioamnionitis is diagnosed by maternal fever, uterine tenderness, elevated maternal white blood cell count, and fetal tachycardia.
- Although the infection is often polymicrobial, group B *Strep* colonization has a high correlation with both chorioamnionitis and neonatal sepsis.
- Chorioamnionitis is treated by IV antibiotics and delivery.
- It is important to differentiate between infections that are transmitted transplacentally and those that are acquired from passage through the birth canal.
- Infections during the first trimester during organogenesis are more likely to cause congenital abnormalities and spontaneous abortions.
- Congenital infections can lead to serious infections in the neonatal period, often with severe long-term sequelae, including mental retardation, blindness, and deafness.

Other Medical Complications of Pregnancy

The previous three chapters discussed hypertension, diabetes, and infectious disease in the context of the pregnant patient. In this chapter, a variety of the other common medical complications of pregnancy are discussed. Pregnancy affects every physiologic system in the body as well as many disease states. When considering disease management in pregnancy, the potential teratogenic effects of any treatment or imaging modality must also be taken into consideration.

HYPEREMESIS GRAVIDARUM

Nausea and vomiting in pregnancy, or "morning sickness," are common. Seen in 88% of pregnancies, this usually resolves by week 16. Various etiologies have been proposed, including elevated levels of human chorionic gonadotropin, thyroid hormone, or the intrinsic hormones of the gut. There seems to be a disordered motility of the upper gastrointestinal tract that contributes to the problem. Despite the nausea and vomiting, patients are usually able to maintain adequate nutrition. However, patients will occasionally become dehydrated and potentially develop electrolyte abnormalities. When this occurs, the diagnosis of **hyperemesis gravidarum** is given. In particular, hyperemesis is common in the setting of molar pregnancies (likely since HCG levels can be very high) and a viable IUP should always be documented in patients with hyperemesis.

TREATMENT AND PROGNOSIS

For patients with true hyperemesis gravidarum, symptoms may persist into the third trimester and, rarely, until term. The goal of therapy is to maintain adequate nutrition. Upon presentation with dehydration, patients should be rehydrated and electrolyte abnormalities corrected. Since a hypochloremic alkalosis often results from extensive vomiting, normal saline with 5% dextrose is commonly used for intravenous hydration. The nausea and vomiting may respond to antiemetics. Compazine, Phenergan, Tigan, and Reglan are commonly used. If these fail, droperidol and Zofran can also be used safely in pregnancy. In the acute setting, antiemetics should be given intravenously, intramuscularly, or as suppositories because oral medications may be regurgitated prior to systemic absorption. In addition to antiemetics, ginger and supplementation with vitamin B12 have been utilized.

Long-term management of hyperemesis includes maintaining hydration, adequate nutrition, and symptomatic relief from the nausea and vomiting. Many patients respond to antiemetics and IV hydration. Once they are rehydrated, they will be able to use the antiemetic to control their nausea so that they are able to maintain oral intake. In addition, since hypoglycemia may contribute to the symptom of nausea, frequent small meals can help maintain more stable blood sugar and decrease nausea.

Rarely, patients will not respond to antiemetics and recurrent rehydration, but treatment with corticosteroids has been shown to decrease symptoms. Further, alternative treatment with acupuncture, acupressure, and nerve stimulation replicating such treatments has been demonstrated to decrease nausea as well. Even with these therapies, a small percentage of patients will require feeding tubes or even parenteral nutrition for the course of the pregnancy. As long as hydration and adequate nutrition are maintained, pregnancy outcomes are usually good.

SEIZURE DISORDERS

Approximately 20,000 women with seizure disorders give birth each year. Concerns during these pregnancies include risk of fetal malformations, miscarriage, perinatal death, and increased seizure frequency. Women with epilepsy appear to have a greater baseline risk of fetal malformations that is further increased with the use of antiepileptic drugs (AEDs). During pregnancy, there is both increased volume of distribution (V_D) as well as increased hepatic metabolism of the AEDs. Coupled with decreased compliance of AEDs due to concerns regarding fetal effects, these factors lead to an increase in seizure frequency seen in 17% to 33% of pregnancies. When managing these women in pregnancy the risks of increased seizures versus use of AEDs need to be weighed carefully.

SEIZURE FREQUENCY

There are a variety of possible etiologies proposed for the increase in seizure frequency that may be seen in pregnancy. Increased levels of circulating estrogen during pregnancy in turn increase the function of the P_{450} enzymes, which leads to more rapid hepatic metabolism of the AEDs. In addition, renal function increases during pregnancy with a 50% rise in creatinine clearance that impacts on the metabolism of carbamazepine, primidone, and the benzodiazepines. The increase in total blood volume and concomitant rise in the V_D leads to decreased levels of circulating AEDs. The increased stress, hormonal changes, and decreased sleep during pregnancy likely lower seizure threshold and have been shown to increase seizure frequency in nonpregnant patients. Finally, many women may have decreased compliance with AEDs because of concerns regarding fetal effects.

The increased levels of estrogen and progesterone may both have direct impact on seizure activity during pregnancy. Estrogen has been shown to be epileptogenic, decreasing seizure threshold. Thus, the rising estrogen levels in pregnancy that peak in the third trimester may have some impact on the observed increase in seizure frequency. Conversely, progesterone seems to have an antiepileptic effect. It has been observed that women with seizure disorders have fewer seizures during the luteal phase of the menstrual cycle.

FETAL CONGENITAL ABNORMALITIES AND ADVERSE OUTCOMES

The earliest reports of congenital malformations associated with AEDs occurred in the 1960s. Since then, unique malformations and syndromes have been ascribed to phenytoin, phenobarbital, primidone, valproate, carbamazepine, and trimethadione. However, there are similarities between most of the congenital abnormalities caused by the AEDs (Table 11-1). There is evidence that epileptic women have an increased risk of fetal malformations even without AED use. Further, while some studies suggest monotherapy does not increase that baseline risk, there are other studies that do show evidence of an increase in fetal malformations with AED polytherapy.

Specific increases in congenital abnormalities seen in infants born to epileptic mothers include a fourfold increase in cleft lip and palate, and a three- to fourfold increase in cardiac anomalies. There is also an increase in the rate of neural tube defects (NTDs) seen in the offspring of epileptic patients who are using carbamazepine or valproic acid. Long-term studies on neurodevelopment show higher rates of abnormal EEG findings, higher rates of developmentally delayed children, and lower IQ scores. There are specific findings that are attributed to particular AEDs.

MECHANISMS OF TERATOGENICITY

The mechanisms of teratogenicity of the AEDs have not been fully characterized. Phenobarbital, primidone, and phenytoin act as folate antagonists. Certainly, it appears that folate deficiency can lead to an increase in congenital malformations, particularly NTDs. Folate prior to conception has therefore been recommended for prophylaxis. Since the AEDs all have a similar central mechanism to control seizures, there may be a common pathway—disrupted during embryogenesis—that leads to the similarities in the syndromes described and this may explain why there is an additive effect in polytherapy.

Recent studies in teratogenesis—particularly in the fetal hydantoin syndrome—point to a genetic predilection for the generation of epoxides. These anomalies have been seen at an increased rate in children where the enzyme activity of epoxide hydrolase is one-third

■ TABLE 11-1 Fetal Anomalies Associated with Antiepileptic Drugs

Fetal Anomaly	Phenytoin	Pheno-barbital	Primidone	Valproate	Carbamaz-epine	Trimetha-dione
NTD				X	X	
IUGR	X					X
Microcephaly					X	X
Low IQ	X		X			
Distal digital hypoplasia	X	X	X			
Low-set ears	X	X				X
Epicanthal fold	X	X		X	X	X
Short nose	X	X		X	X	
Long philtrum			X		X	
Lip abnormalities	X	X	X	X		
Hypertelorism	X	X				
Developmental delay		X			X	X
Other	Ptosis	Ptosis	Hirsutism of forehead		Hypoplastic nails	Cardiac anomalies

less than normal. Anomalies have also been observed in children with low epoxide hydrolase activity in carbamazepine exposure.

CLINICAL MANAGEMENT

Because exposure to multiple AEDs seems to be more teratogenic than monotherapy, patients are advised to switch to a single AED prior to conception and taper down to the lowest possible dose. Patients who have been seizure-free for 2 to 5 years may wish to attempt complete withdrawal from AEDs prior to conception. Because there is evidence that high peak plasma levels of valproic acid may be more teratogenic, it should be dosaged 2 to 4 times per day rather than the standard twice per day dosing. However, epileptic patients should be counseled that they are still at a greater risk (4% to 6% vs. 2% to 3%) for fetal anomalies than the baseline population. Folate has been shown to decrease NTDs in patients without epilepsy. Therefore patients should be advised to take supplemental folate prior to conception, particularly those using either valproic acid or

carbamazepine. There are a number of new AEDs (levetiracetam, lamotrigine, felbamate, topiramate, and oxcarbazepine) that have not demonstrated the same frequency of congenital anomalies as the older AEDs, but these medications have not been formally studied beyond small case series, so it is difficult to truly determine the safety at this time.

Because of the increased risk of anomalies a level II fetal survey at 19 to 20 weeks of gestation should be performed with careful attention to the face, central nervous system, and heart (Table 11-2). Due to the increased risk of NTDs, a maternal serum α-fetoprotein (MSAFP) screening test should be offered. The decision to perform an amniocentesis routinely for AFP and acetylcholinesterase is controversial. Many practitioners recommend it in the setting of a family history of NTDs or with use of valproic acid or carbamazepine since the sensitivity of amniocentesis is higher than either MSAFP or ultrasound for NTDs.

Recent studies of seizure frequency show less of an increase than older studies, which suggests that the practice of closer monitoring of AED dosing and levels may have some impact on the number of seizures

■ **TABLE 11-2** Management of Women with Epilepsy During Pregnancy
Check total and free levels of antiepileptic drugs on a monthly basis
Consider early genetic counseling
Check MSAFP
Level II ultrasound for fetal survey at 19 to 20 weeks' gestation
Consider amniocentesis for α-fetoprotein and acetyl-cholinesterase
Supplement with oral vitamin K 20 mg QD starting at 37 weeks until delivery

during pregnancy. A recent study shows that 38% of pregnant patients with epilepsy require changes in their AED dosing to achieve seizure control. Assuming that monotherapy with one of the AEDs has been achieved preconceptionally, total and free levels of the AED that keep the patient seizure-free should be obtained on a monthly basis (see Table 11-2).

LABOR AND DELIVERY

Management of the epileptic patient on labor and delivery should involve preparation and close monitoring. All care providers—obstetricians, neurology, nursing, anesthesia, and pediatrics—should be informed about an epileptic patient in labor and delivery. AED levels should be checked upon admission. If the level is low, patients may be given extra dosing or switched to intravenous benzodiazepines or phenytoin, bearing in mind that benzodiazepines can cause respiratory depression in both the mother and newborn. Since trauma and hypoxia from a seizure can put both the mother and fetus at risk, treatment of seizures should be discussed a priori with the group of practitioners caring for the patient. Management of seizures on labor and delivery is discussed in Chapter 6. One difference is that the drug of choice in patients with a known seizure disorder is usually phenytoin compared to magnesium used in preeclamptic patients.

There have been reports of increased risk of spontaneous hemorrhage in newborns because of the inhibition of vitamin K–dependent clotting factors (i.e., II, VII, IX, X) secondary to increased vitamin K metabolism and inhibition of placental transport of vitamin K by AEDs. While the risk is small, conservative management is to overcome this theoretical vitamin K deficiency by aggressive supplementation with vitamin K toward the end of pregnancy. Upon delivery, clotting studies can be performed on the cord blood and vitamin K administered to the infant. If the cord blood is deficient in clotting factors, fresh frozen plasma may be required to protect the newborn.

MATERNAL CARDIAC DISEASE

The cardiovascular system undergoes a number of dramatic changes in pregnancy with a 50% increase in blood volume, decrease in systemic vascular resistance, increase in cardiac stroke volume, and actual remodeling of the myocardium to accommodate some of these changes. When caring for patients with cardiac disease preconceptionally or during pregnancy, these changes are paramount when counseling them regarding their options and managing their disease. In particular, patients with primary pulmonary hypertension, Eisenmenger physiology, severe mitral or aortic stenosis, and Marfan syndrome are at a high risk of maternal mortality in pregnancy reportedly ranging from 15% to 70% in small case series. In cardiac patients with an increased risk of maternal mortality, the option to terminate the pregnancy should always be offered and discussed at length with the patient. Unfortunately, since such women often may not be able to adopt because of their illness, they may think of their own pregnancy as the only way to have children.

PRINCIPLES OF MANAGEMENT

Cardiac diseases vary widely but the principles of management are similar. Many of the diseases are stable prior to pregnancy with medical management, but during pregnancy can become quite unstable in response to the physiologic changes. One reason is that the medications being used may be different. In particular, many of the newest antihypertensives and antiarrhythmics have had little experience in pregnancy, and are thus commonly avoided. Of the more common agents, ACE inhibitors, diuretics, and Coumadin have all been associated with congenital anomalies and other fetal effects and are usually discontinued in pregnancy. Other aspects of medical management may include rest. However, even when resting, the cardiac output is increased in pregnancy, leading to increased stress on the heart. In patients with cardiac anomalies, SBE prophylaxis should be used during labor.

In patients who would benefit from surgical repair of a lesion as in mitral or aortic stenosis, it is often best to recommend that the surgical repair is performed a year or more prior to becoming pregnant. In the high-risk patients listed above, recommending a termination of pregnancy because of the high risk to them is the first line of management. For patients who decline, preparing them and their families for the possibilities of disabling morbidity and mortality is important. In most cardiac patients, the stress of labor and delivery is minimized with an early epidural to diminish pain response, and possibly an assisted vaginal delivery (using forceps or vacuum) to diminish the effects from valsalva. In addition, careful fluid monitoring should be maintained, often with a central venous pressure monitor and arterial line. The immediate postpartum period gives rise to massive fluid shifts and can be a particularly dangerous period for women with congenital heart disease. These fluid shifts are due both to increased venous return as the pregnant uterus is now off the vena cava and because the uterus clamps down, leading to an autotransfusion of its blood supply (approximately 500 cc).

CARDIOVASCULAR DISEASE

Because of the rising average maternal age in pregnancy, there will be an increasing number of patients with a history of a myocardial infarction (MI) who become pregnant. If these patients have been optimally managed, there are small case series that show they do relatively well in pregnancy. A baseline ECG and adjustment of medications, if necessary, should be performed at the initial visit. Throughout pregnancy and on labor and delivery, it is important to diminish the workload on the heart.

EISENMENGER SYNDROME AND PULMONARY HYPERTENSION

Patients with right-to-left shunts and pulmonary hypertension (PH) are among the sickest in pregnancy, with mortality rates estimated at 50% and higher. The most common causes of right-to-left shunts are patent ductus arteriosus (PDA) and ventricular septal defect (VSD). These result from Eisenmenger physiology that occurs when the initial left-to-right shunt leads to right ventricular hypertrophy and pulmonary hypertension and eventually a right-to-left shunt.

These patients are chronically hypoxic secondary to the mixing of deoxygenated blood and are encouraged to terminate their pregnancies. Patients who elect to continue are followed with serial echocardiograms to measure the pulmonary pressures and cardiac function. Some have been managed with inhaled nitric oxide, but this has not been shown to significantly improve the measured clinical indicators of disease or the outcomes. These patients often decompensate in the third trimester of pregnancy. Delivery via labor and assisted delivery is preferable to elective cesarean delivery. Perhaps the greatest concentrated risk of morbidity and mortality is in the postpartum period for to 2 to 4 weeks. It has been hypothesized that this risk is secondary to the sudden changes in hormones. Unfortunately, attempts to counter this with progesterone and estrogen supplementation have been tried with little success.

VALVULAR DISEASE

While the manifestations of the different valvular diseases vary, one similarity is that, with moderate or severe disease that may increase maternal mortality, it is better to surgically treat or repair the lesion prior to becoming pregnant. Aortic stenosis and aortic insufficiency patients require a decreased afterload to maintain cardiac output, so initially may have diminished symptoms in response to the decreased systemic vascular resistance seen in pregnancy. Patients with mitral stenosis may be unable to meet the increased demands of pregnancy and experience a backup into the pulmonary system leading to congestive heart failure (CHF). Patients with pulmonary stenosis who elect to continue their pregnancy may actually undergo valvuloplasty during the pregnancy if they have severe disease.

MARFAN SYNDROME

Patients with Marfan syndrome have a deficiency in their elastin that leads to a number of valvular cardiac complications as well as dilation of the aortic root. During pregnancy, the hyperdynamic state can increase the risk of aortic dissection and/or rupture, particularly in those patients with an aortic root diameter greater than 4 cm. In order to decrease some of the pressure on the aorta, patients are advised to maintain a sedentary lifestyle and are often placed on beta-blockers to decrease cardiac output.

PERIPARTUM CARDIOMYOPATHY (PPCM)

A small percentage of patients will be found to have heart failure secondary to a dilated cardiomyopathy, immediately before, during, or after delivery. Some of these patients likely have a baseline mild cardiomyopathy, whereas others have a postinfectious dilated cardiomyopathy. However, the epidemiology supports the idea that, at least in some cases, PPCM is specifically caused by pregnancy. Patients present with classic signs and symptoms of heart failure and on echocardiogram have a dilated heart with an ejection fraction far below normal in the 20% to 40% range.

Patients with PPCM should be managed according the gestational age of the fetus. Beyond 34 weeks' gestational age, the risks to the mother of remaining pregnant are usually greater than those of premature delivery of the fetus. At earlier gestational ages, however, betamethasone should be administered to promote fetal lung maturity, and the patient delivered accordingly. The patient's heart failure is managed similarly to other patients with heart failure using diuretics, digoxin, and vasodilators. Well over half of the patients with PPCM have excellent return to baseline of their cardiac activity within several months of delivery.

MATERNAL RENAL DISEASE

Chronic renal disease can be divided into mild (Cr <1.5), moderate (Cr from 1.5 to 2.8), and severe (Cr >2.8), although other thresholds have been used. Renal blood flow and creatinine clearance increase during pregnancy in patients without renal disease, and this is also true initially in patients with renal disease. In fact, patients with mild renal disease will usually experience improvement in renal function throughout much of pregnancy. Moderate and severe patients, however, may experience decreasing renal function in the latter half of pregnancy that may persist postpartum in as many as half of pregnancies. Because of this, it is important to counsel these patients preconceptionally regarding the risks to them

from pregnancy—in particular, the increased risk of requiring dialysis and its concomitant morbidities.

Patients with chronic renal disease have increased risk of preeclampsia, preterm delivery, and intrauterine growth restriction (IUGR) in addition to worsening renal disease. Because of this, they should be screened at least once per trimester with a 24-hour urine for creatinine clearance and protein. Patients who present in early pregnancy should be counseled regarding these risks and offered termination of pregnancy, particularly for the mother's health. Because of the risk to the fetus, antenatal fetal testing usually begins at 32 to 34 weeks' gestation. For patients who have baseline proteinuria and hypertension, the diagnosis of preeclampsia can be difficult to make. In these patients, a baseline uric acid is assessed and, if normal at baseline, can be used in the setting of worsening blood pressures to help diagnose preeclampsia. An increase in blood pressure of 30/15 mm Hg above prepregnancy blood pressures can also be used, though experts disagree on its utility.

An interesting subgroup of women are those who are status post renal transplant. It seems that such women will have outcomes similar to women with similar creatinine clearance. However, there are several issues. Commonly, these women will be on immunosuppressants such as prednisone and Imuran. Because of increased metabolism and volume of distribution, dosages of these medications may need to be increased during pregnancy. If they are not, the risk of acute rejection increases due to undertreatment. Similarly, because women may be concerned about the effects of these medications on the developing fetus, they may stop taking the medications and be at increased risk for rejection. Medication levels, creatinine, and creatinine clearance are commonly checked monthly in such women.

COAGULATION DISORDERS

Pregnancy is generally considered a "hypercoagulable" state. The pathogenesis of this state has not been elucidated, but several mechanisms have been proposed, including increased coagulation factors, endothelial damage, and venous stasis (Virchow's triad). The risk for superficial vein thrombosis (SVT), deep vein thrombosis (DVT), and pulmonary embolus (PE) is further increased postpartum, and pulmonary embolus remains one of the leading causes of maternal mortality. Additionally, women with a preexisting thrombophilia may get pregnant. These women, in particular, are at high risk for developing a DVT or PE.

PATHOGENESIS

No single cause of the hypercoagulability of pregnancy has been found, but there are several possible mechanisms hypothesized. The first is that there is an intrinsic increase in coagulability of the serum itself. In pregnancy, the production of clotting factors is increased and levels of all the clotting factors except XI and XIII are noted. Also noted in pregnancy is that the turnover time for fibrinogen is decreased and that there are increased levels of fibrinopeptide A, which is cleaved from fibrinogen to make fibrin. Additionally, there are increased levels of circulating fibrin monomer complexes. These levels increase further at the time of delivery and immediately postpartum. Finally, it has been hypothesized that the placenta synthesizes a factor that decreases fibrinolysis, but there is minimal evidence for this.

Another proposed source of hypercoagulability is increased exposure to subendothelial collagen secondary to increased endothelial damage during pregnancy, although no mechanism has been proposed. It has also been hypothesized that endothelial damage in the venous system during parturition increases the amount of thrombogenesis postpartum. This seems feasible, particularly as the etiology of pelvic vein thrombosis, but it does not account for the hypercoagulability throughout pregnancy.

Venous stasis may also account for some of the increase in venous thromboses during and after pregnancy. There are two principal causes for venous stasis in pregnancy. The first is decreased venous tone during pregnancy, which may be related to the smooth muscle relaxant properties of this high progesterone state. Second, the uterus, as it enlarges, compresses the inferior vena cava, the iliac, and pelvic veins. This compression, in particular, likely contributes to the increase in pelvic vein thromboses.

SUPERFICIAL VEIN THROMBOSIS

Although **superficial vein thrombosis** is a painful complication of hypercoagulability, it is believed to be unlikely to lead to emboli. The diagnosis is usually obvious with a palpable, usually visible, venous cord that is quite tender, with local erythema and edema. Because of the low risk of emboli from SVT, it is not routinely treated other than symptomatically with warm compresses and analgesics. However, the patient should be informed of the signs and symptoms of DVTs and PEs because she may be at an increased risk for either.

DEEP VEIN THROMBOSIS

Diagnosis of **deep vein thrombosis** is often made clinically with confirmation by Doppler studies or venography. The usual patient presents with unilateral lower extremity pain and swelling. On examination patients will often have edema, local erythema, tenderness, venous distension, and a palpable cord underlying the region of pain and tenderness. When clinical suspicion is high, the patient is usually sent for noninvasive lower extremity studies with the Doppler ultrasound for confirmation of a venous obstruction. Rarely, venography, the gold standard, will be used.

Treatment of DVT during pregnancy involves the use of heparin. Initially, the treatment is with IV heparin that is often continued with subcutaneous heparin throughout the remainder of the pregnancy and postpartum. Recently, low molecular weight heparin has been studied and found to be effective for both prophylaxis and treatment in pregnancy. Coumadin therapy is contraindicated in pregnancy secondary to evidence of fetal abnormalities caused by Coumadin. When given in the first trimester, it causes warfarin embryopathy that involves nasal hypoplasia and skeletal abnormalities. In addition, Coumadin appears to cause diffuse central nervous system (CNS) abnormalities, including optic atrophy, when given during pregnancy.

PULMONARY EMBOLUS

Pulmonary embolus (PE) results when emboli from DVTs travel to the right side of the heart and then lodge in the pulmonary arterial system, leading to **pulmonary hypertension, hypoxia**, and, depending on the extent of the emboli, **right-sided heart failure** and **death**. Clinical suspicion of pulmonary embolus is raised whenever a patient presents with acute onset of shortness of breath, simultaneous onset of pleuritic chest pain, hemoptysis, and/or concomitant signs of DVT.

The diagnosis of PE usually involves the clinical picture correlated with a variety of diagnostic tests. A chest x-ray may be entirely normal. However, two common signs are the abrupt termination of a vessel as it is traced distally and an area of radiolucency in the area of the lung beyond the PE. An electrocardiogram may also be entirely normal or simply show sinus

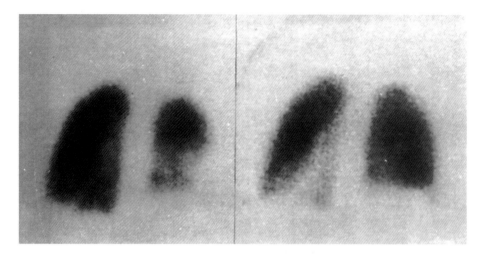

Figure 11-1 • In these posterior views, the perfusion lung scan (left) reveals segmental defects that are not matched in the normal ventilation scan (right). This is consistent with a high probability of pulmonary embolism.
(Reproduced with permission from Clark SL, et al. *Critical Care Obstetrics*, 2nd ed. Cambridge: Blackwell Science, 1991:162.)

tachycardia. On occasion, however, it will show signs of right-heart strain with right-axis deviation, nonspecific ST changes, and peaked T-waves. Spiral CT scan is becoming the most common diagnostic tool for pulmonary embolism in both the pregnant and nonpregnant patient. The risk of radiation exposure must be weighed against the suspected risk of a PE and the dangers that this poses to a pregnant woman's health. As with other life-threatening medical conditions, the woman's health should be considered first and foremost and she should be worked up and treated just as any nonpregnant patient would be in a similar condition. The old standby of a ventilation/perfusion (V/Q) scan is decreasingly utilized nowadays. The V/Q scan is a radionuclide scan that first examines the perfusion of the lungs by detecting a radioisotope in the pulmonary circulation (Fig. 11-1). An entirely normal perfusion scan rules out PE. However, if there is a defect in perfusion, a ventilation scan is performed. Mismatched defects in the ventilation and perfusion scans are suggestive of PE. Pulmonary angiography is the gold standard for diagnosis of PE. The pulmonary artery is catheterized and a radiopaque dye is injected. Diagnosis is made if there are intraluminal filling defects or if sharp vessel cutoffs are seen (Fig. 11-2).

Treatment of mild PE is similar to treatment of DVT with IV heparin and, eventually, subcutaneous heparin therapy or low molecular weight heparin (e.g., Lovenox). If Lovenox is used, because of its long half-life, it is commonly switched to unfractionated heparin at 36 weeks of gestation so that when a woman presents in labor, she can have regional anesthesia (e.g., epidural) without an increased risk for epidural hematoma. Massive PE leading to an unstable hypoxic patient is often treated with streptokinase for thrombolysis in addition to supportive measures.

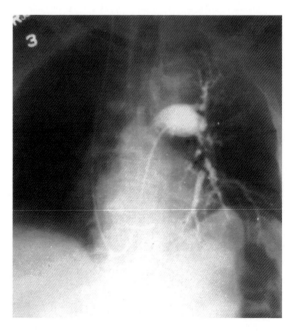

Figure 11-2 • Arteriogram of the left pulmonary artery showing filling defects and an unperfused segment of lung as demonstrated by the absence of contrast dye.
(Reproduced with permission from Clark SL, et al. *Critical Care Obstetrics*, 2nd ed. Cambridge: Blackwell Science, 1991:162.)

In the postpartum period, Coumadin can be used as well, though some women will choose to simply remain on Lovenox because of the need for serial blood draws to check PT/PTT and INR on Coumadin. Patients are usually treated for a minimum of 6 months.

MATERNAL THYROID DISEASE IN PREGNANCY

Management of thyroid disease changes in pregnancy because of the V_D, increased circulating thyroid binding globulin, and sex hormone binding globulin (SHBG), which is secondary to estrogen stimulation of hepatic enzymes. Additionally, because metabolic demands increase in pregnancy, thyroid-stimulating hormone (TSH) and FT4 levels are commonly followed every 6 to 8 weeks.

HYPERTHYROIDISM

The most common cause of hyperthyroidism is **Graves disease**. Patients with medically managed Graves disease can continue their **propylthiouracil** (PTU) or methimazole, which decrease production of the T4 moiety and in the case of PTU, block its peripheral conversion to T3. Since Graves disease is the result of thyroid-stimulating immunoglobulins (TSI), levels are checked and, if elevated, the fetus is at risk of developing a fetal goiter. Thus, the fetus should undergo a fetal survey at 18 to 20 weeks of gestation as well as an ultrasound in the third trimester to look for fetal goiter. The fetus can also develop fetal hyperthyroidism, which can be diagnosed with fetal tachycardia. Thus, antenatal testing of such pregnancies with serial NSTs is indicated. Finally, PTU and methimazole can cross the placenta and can lead to fetal goiter as well. Thus, during pregnancy, it is best to use the minimum dosage possible. Occasionally, patients with Graves disease can be tapered off of their medications.

Given these issues, it is important to follow both symptoms of hyperthyroidism and the thyroid function labs closely. In general, TSH should be kept between 0.5 and 2.5, but in pregnancy, it should be kept closer to 0.5 than 2.5 if possible.

HYPOTHYROIDISM

In patients with hypothyroidism, the most common etiology is **Hashimoto thyroiditis**, and the second is

ablation or removal of the thyroid after Graves disease or cancer. Because the demands on thyroid hormone are all going to increase in pregnancy due to increased volume of distribution, increased binding globulin (in particular, SHBG), increased clearance, and increased need due to increased basal metabolic rate, all women on levothyroxine (Synthroid) supplementation should have their dosage increased 25% to 30%. The levels of TSH mentioned above should be kept low normal by increasing levothyroxine supplementation throughout pregnancy and following the TSH level. In the setting of women with a history of thyroid cancer, their TSH levels should be kept below the normal range of TSH to prevent recurrence of disease.

SYSTEMIC LUPUS ERYTHEMATOSUS

Systemic lupus erythematosus (SLE) and other associated collagen vascular disorders (CVD) such as Sjögren syndrome, scleroderma, and antiphospholipid antibody syndrome can be particularly worrisome in pregnancy. There is particular concern in patients with concomitant hypertension or renal disease because these patients bear an even greater risk of developing preeclampsia, IUGR, and having preterm deliveries. The natural history of SLE in pregnancy tends to the one-third rule; that is, one-third improve, one-third worsen, and one-third remain unchanged. In general, it seems also that patients who are without flares immediately prior to pregnancy have a better course. Medications such as aspirin and corticosteroids are continued in pregnancy, whereas cyclophosphamide and methotrexate are not.

EARLY PREGNANCY COMPLICATIONS

Patients with SLE and, in particular, antiphospholipid antibody syndrome, have a high risk of early pregnancy loss both in the first and second trimester. The pathophysiology of these losses is placental thrombosis. The high rate of second trimester losses is a hallmark of these diseases, and they will often show symmetric IUGR by 18 to 20 weeks' gestation. Treatment and prophylaxis with low-dose aspirin, heparin, and corticosteroids have been tried with some improvement.

LATER PREGNANCY COMPLICATIONS

Just as in the early pregnancy losses, the placenta can become thrombosed in the third trimester as well, leading to IUGR and intrauterine fetal demise (IUFD). Because of this, frequent antenatal testing is performed, usually starting at week 32. Because of this risk of thrombosis, SQ heparin prophylaxis and low-dose aspirin have been used, both exhibiting some improvement. However, even on these agents, the risks are still quite higher than those of the baseline population. Patients are also at increased risk of developing preeclampsia.

LUPUS FLARES VERSUS PREECLAMPSIA

One of the most difficult differential diagnoses to sort out is that of a lupus flare versus preeclampsia in the pregnant lupus patient. Both diseases are likely mediated by circulating antigen-antibody complexes or tissue-specific antibodies that cause a vasculitis. The similarity between the two diseases is remarkable (Table 11-3). One method of differentiating between the two is checking complement levels. Patients having a lupus flare will have reduced C3 and C4, whereas preeclamptics should have normal levels. In addition, lupus flares are often accompanied by an active urine sediment whereas preeclampsia is not. Differentiating between the two conditions is important because the management for each highly differs.

A lupus flare is managed with high-dose corticosteroids and, if unresponsive, cyclophosphamide. Worsening preeclampsia, on the other hand, is managed by delivery.

NEONATAL LUPUS

As with other maternal diseases, lupus can affect the fetus and neonate. There are two complications of interest. The first is a lupus syndrome related to maternal antigen-antibody complexes that have crossed the placenta and cause lupus in the neonate. These flares can be quite severe. The other complication seen is that of irreversible congenital heart block. SLE patients (and more commonly Sjögren disease patients) can produce antibodies called anti-Ro (SSA) and anti-La (SSB) that are tissue-specific to the fetal cardiac conduction system. Anti-Ro seems much more likely to cause the congenital heart block that is seen in 1 in 20 patients with the antibody. Patients are screened for these antibodies at the first prenatal visit, and several interventions utilizing corticosteroids, plasmapheresis, and IVIG have been used. It is unclear whether any of these interventions improves outcomes.

SUBSTANCE ABUSE IN PREGNANCY

Substance abuse in pregnancy contributes to maternal and fetal morbidity and mortality in both the antepartum and postpartum periods. The most commonly used substances are alcohol and cigarettes, both of which contribute to poor outcomes of pregnancy. The two most common illicit drugs used in pregnancy are cocaine and opiates, each of which has associated problems for the infant. Finally, even when infants are born with minimal effects from the intrapartum insult, substance abuse is an indicator for other social problems that may contribute to a poor environment for child rearing.

ALCOHOL

A constellation of abnormalities in the infants born to women who abuse alcohol during pregnancy have been included in the diagnosis of **fetal alcohol syndrome** (FAS). The syndrome has a spectrum of increasing severity in children of women who drink more heavily (2 to 5 drinks/day) during pregnancy. FAS, which includes growth retardation, CNS effects, and abnormal facies, is estimated to occur in

■ TABLE 11-3 Lupus Flare Versus Severe Preeclampsia		
Organ System	**Lupus Complication**	**Severe Preeclampsia**
Neuro	Lupus cerebritis, seizures	Seizures, visual changes
CV	Hypertension	Hypertension
Pulmonary	Pulmonary edema	Pulmonary edema
Renal	Worsening renal disease	Significant proteinuria, oliguria, renal failure
GI	Hepatitis	Liver dysfunction, ↑ transaminases, hepatic edema
Heme	Thrombocytopenia	Thrombocytopenia, hemolytic anemia
	Hemolytic anemia	DIC

approximately 1 in 2,000 live births. However, many milder cases may go unrecognized. Diagnosis is made by a history of alcohol abuse in the mother combined with the constellation of infant abnormalities. Other teratogenic effects of alcohol include almost every organ system. Cardiac defects are particularly associated with alcohol abuse.

Treatment

Several studies show that aggressive counseling programs for expectant mothers have led to a significant decrease in alcohol intake in greater than 50% of the participants. For patients who are at risk for alcohol withdrawal, barbiturates are often used for withdrawal symptoms because of the potential teratogenicity of benzodiazepines. Because alcoholics are at higher risk for nutritional deficiencies, special care should be taken to ensure adequate nutrition during pregnancy.

CAFFEINE

Caffeine is found in coffee (30 to 170 mg/cup), tea (10 to 100 mg/cup), and caffeinated soft drinks (30 to 60 mg/12 oz). It is the most commonly used drug during pregnancy, with almost 80% of all pregnant women being exposed in the first trimester. Studies on rats show teratogenicity at high levels of caffeine exposure. However, these studies have not been duplicated with humans. There does appear to be an increased risk of first and second trimester miscarriages with consumption of greater than 150 mg/day of caffeine. Patients should be advised of this risk and to reduce caffeine consumption during pregnancy to less than 150 mg/day.

CIGARETTES

Cigarette smoking in pregnancy has been correlated with increased risk of spontaneous abortions, preterm births, abruptio placentae, and decreased birth weight. Further, infants exposed to cigarette smoking in the womb are at an increased risk for sudden infant death syndrome (SIDS) and respiratory illnesses of childhood. A dose-response effect has been noted for many of these outcomes. In the Ontario Perinatal Mortality Study, smokers were divided into less than 1 pack per day (PPD) and more than 1 PPD. A 20% increase in the risk of fetal death was found in those pregnancies in which patients smoked less than 1 PPD and a 35% increase in the more than 1 PPD group.

Treatment

Because of the demonstrated dose-response effect of smoking, patients should be counseled as to the increased risks for the fetus and advised at the very minimum to decrease cigarette use, although there is no demonstrated safe amount of smoking. Several studies show that smoking cessation programs targeting pregnant patients are more effective than those for nonpregnant patients. Further, primary care providers of women of childbearing age should begin this counseling prior to pregnancy.

COCAINE

Cocaine use in pregnancy is correlated with abruptio placentae, IUGR, and an increased risk for preterm labor and delivery. There has been a reported delivery of an infant with a massive cerebral infarction born to a woman who took a large dose of cocaine within 72 hours of delivery. The physiologic effects of cocaine, which causes vasoconstriction and hypertension, are consistent with this event, as well as the increased risk for abruption. Increasing amounts of evidence show that children who were exposed to cocaine in utero are at increased risk for CNS complications, including developmental delay.

Treatment

Patients who admit to cocaine use should be advised of its risks to themselves and their infants. Social services should be involved in prenatal care, and patients who continue to abuse the drug should be encouraged to enter a detoxification center.

OPIATES

The two most common narcotics used in pregnancy are heroin and methadone. There are no known teratogenic effects of narcotics. In fact, there is likely to be more danger to fetuses from heroin withdrawal syndrome, including miscarriage, preterm delivery, and fetal death, than from chronic narcotic use. Patients using heroin in pregnancy should therefore be enrolled in methadone programs rather than advised to quit outright. Once infants are delivered, they will need careful monitoring and slow withdrawal from their narcotic addiction using tincture of opium. An aggressive effort should be made to taper their methadone postpartum.

KEY POINTS

- Nausea and vomiting in pregnancy are common; however, patients with hyperemesis gravidarum (HG) will not be able to maintain adequate hydration and nutrition.

- Acute management of HG involves IV hydration, electrolyte repletion, and antiemetics; chronic management utilizes antiemetics and occasionally tube feeding or parenteral nutrition.

- The increase in seizure frequency may be related to increased metabolism of AEDs, decreased patient compliance, lower seizure threshold, and/or hormonal changes in pregnancy; patients should be followed frequently in pregnancy with monthly AED level.

- Whereas patients with seizure disorders have an increased baseline risk for congenital anomalies, this risk is likely increased with the use of AEDs, particularly in cases of polytherapy. Because of the risk for congenital anomalies, all patients should have a targeted ultrasound/fetal survey.

- The changes in cardiac physiology during pregnancy can have an enormous impact on cardiac disease. Common aspects of management include offering termination of pregnancy, medical stabilization, surgical or valvuloplasty repair if necessary, and consideration of the changes of pregnancy.

- On labor and delivery, cardiac patients are commonly given prophylactic antibiotics, an early epidural, careful fluid monitoring, and an assisted vaginal delivery to minimize maternal stress and strain. The most risky period of time for cardiac patients is during labor, delivery, and the puerperium.

- Patients with mild renal disease suffer minimal effects, but may carry an increased risk of preeclampsia and IUGR, which is associated with the underlying diagnosis.

- Patients with moderate or severe renal disease are at risk for preeclampsia and IUGR, as well as worsening renal disease during and after the pregnancy. Careful monitoring of the patient's renal function and of fetal status are hallmarks of the management of these patients during pregnancy.

- Pregnancy is a hypercoagulable state with increased clotting factors, endothelial damage, and venous stasis.

- Pulmonary embolus is the leading cause of maternal death. DVT and PE may be treated with unfractionated heparin or Lovenox. Thrombolysis may be necessary for the unstable patient.

- In pregnancy, there are particular changes to the thyroid system including increased VD and metabolism.

- In hyperthyroidism, TSIs should be screened for and, if elevated, fetal surveillance initiated to screen for fetal goiter and IUGR.

- In hypothyroidism, increased Synthroid requirements are common.

- Patients with SLE are at risk of developing complications throughout pregnancy. Prophylaxis against pregnancy loss, preeclampsia, and IUGR has been tried with low-dose aspirin, heparin, and corticosteroids, all of which have some possible benefit.

- Lupus flares and preeclampsia can be differentiated on the basis of complement levels.

- Mothers with anti-Ro and anti-La antibodies are at risk of having a fetus with congenital heart block.

- Heavy alcohol abuse is correlated with FAS, which includes a constellation of growth restriction, CNS effects, and abnormal facies. Alcohol has also been correlated with other teratogenic effects, particularly cardiac defects.

- Caffeine use greater than 150 mg/day has been correlated with an increased risk of spontaneous abortions.

- Cigarette use during pregnancy has been correlated with growth restriction, abruptions, preterm delivery, and fetal death. Patients should be strongly encouraged to forgo use during pregnancy.

- Cocaine use has been correlated with abruptio placentae and CNS effects in children. Patients should be advised to quit outright.

- Narcotic abusers should be enrolled in methadone programs because the acute withdrawal effects of narcotics are more dangerous to the fetus than chronic use.

Postpartum Care and Complications

ROUTINE POSTPARTUM CARE

The puerperium, or postpartum period, is defined as the first 6 weeks after delivery. While still in the hospital, the patient often needs instruction about care of the neonate, breastfeeding, and her limitations, if any, during the ensuing weeks. In addition, the patient needs emotional support during the period of adjustment to the new member of the family and to her own physiologic changes.

VAGINAL DELIVERY

Routine medical issues in patients after vaginal delivery include pain control and perineal care. Usually, pain can be reduced with nonsteroidal anti-inflammatory drugs (NSAIDs) or acetaminophen. Low-dose opioids are occasionally required for adequate patient comfort, particularly at the hour of sleep. For patients with vaginal deliveries that involved either episiotomies or lacerations, perineal care is particularly important. Ice packs around the clock for the first 24 hours can be beneficial for both pain and edema in the perineum and labia. When inspecting the perineum of a postpartum patient, it is important to ensure that the perineal repair is intact and that no hematomas have developed. It is also important to note whether the patient has hemorrhoids, which are common in pregnancy and postpartum, particularly after a long second stage of labor. These should resolve with time, but patients' symptoms may be ameliorated with over-the-counter hemorrhoidal medications, stool softeners, and ice packs.

CESAREAN DELIVERY

As more than 30% of deliveries are now by cesarean, wound care and pain management in these women are a common component of postpartum care. Local wound care and observation for signs of wound infection or separation are part of routine care. Wound infections include cellulitis or a wound abscess. Wound separations can be at the level of the skin or subcutaneous tissue or deeper at the level of the rectus fascia known as a *wound dehiscence*. Pain is usually managed with opioids that can contribute to a postoperative ileus or constipation. Patients on opioids should therefore be prescribed stool softeners and occasionally laxatives. NSAIDs should be used concomitantly for the cramping pain caused by uterine involution. Patients have usually received a first- or second-generation cephalosporin during the cesarean section as prophylaxis against infection. Although it is routine in many institutions to give additional dosages, this has never been shown to further decrease the risk of infection.

BREASTFEEDING AND BREAST CARE

While there are rare contraindications such as infections that may lead to an increase in vertical transmission to the infant or in the case of mothers on medications that could be dangerous to a newborn, the vast majority of new mothers should be encouraged to breastfeed. There are various beliefs and racial/cultural differences regarding the practice of breastfeeding, but regardless, the health benefits to babies and mothers are being increasingly identified. Numerous studies have demonstrated a decrease in childhood infectious diseases in newborns and infants of breastfeeding mothers attributed to the passive immunity via immunoglobulin in the breast milk. Additionally, women who breastfeed are more likely to lose the weight they have gained during pregnancy. Further, women who have breastfed appear to have a lower long-term risk of developing type 2 diabetes and its associated morbidities.

Despite all of these benefits, breastfeeding is challenging, particularly for the primipara, first-time mother. Historically, women would have likely learned about breastfeeding from female relatives and family, but in today's society in the United States, many women have not had such experiences. Thus, while they may be interested in breastfeeding, many women don't recognize the inherent difficulties and discomfort. A number of barriers to breastfeeding, both iatrogenic and natural, can be introduced in the birthing process and initial postpartum period. In a variety of complicated births such as a preterm birth, emergency birth, or simply a cesarean delivery, the initial skin-to-skin contact that has been shown to initiate breastfeeding in the neonate is interrupted. Further, while breastfeeding is natural, it is often not instinctive or intuitive to many women. Since they have expectations that breastfeeding should be easier, they end up feeling like a failure. This misalignment of expectations and reality coupled with concerns about providing adequate nutrition of the neonate leads many women to give up breastfeeding only a few days postpartum. Reassurance that breastfeeding can be challenging and uncomfortable (even painful) but that it should become easier and less uncomfortable can help women to get through the initial weeks of breastfeeding.

All postpartum patients need breast care, regardless of whether or not they are breastfeeding. Patients usually experience the onset of lactation, engorgement or "letdown," approximately 24 to 72 hours postpartum. When this occurs, the breasts usually become uniformly warmer, firmer, and tender. Patients often complain of pain or warmth in the breasts and may experience a fever. For patients not breastfeeding, ice packs, a tight bra, analgesics, and anti-inflammatory medications are all useful. Patients who are breastfeeding obtain relief from the breastfeeding itself, although this can lead to its own difficulties, such as tenderness and erosions around the nipple.

POSTPARTUM CONTRACEPTION

Most patients are advised to have pelvic rest until the 6-week follow-up visit. However, many women resume sexual activity prior to this time. Thus, contraception is an important issue to begin addressing during the prenatal period and continue while patients are still in the hospital postpartum. Because most states require women to consent to a postpartum tubal ligation (PPTL) at least 30 days prior to their EDD, this should be brought up early in the third trimester. For women who desire permanent sterilization, PPTL is an extremely effective form of sterilization.

For those women who have not undergone PPTL, counseling regarding other options is important. For patients interested in hormonal modes of contraception and who are breastfeeding, the progesterone-only mini-pill, Depo-Provera, or implantable progestogenic agents are the usual recommended options. Combination estrogen-progesterone OCPs in some studies have been shown to decrease milk production so are usually recommended only to those patients who are not interested in breastfeeding or have excellent milk production (not usually known during first week postpartum). Progesterone-only contraceptives may decrease milk production as well, but this has not been demonstrated to be clinically significant. They are therefore preferable to combination OCPs for patients who are dedicated to breastfeeding and interested in hormonal forms of birth control. An alternative course of action for those women who are interested in using combination OCPs is to establish breastfeeding and then begin the combination OCPs at 4 to 6 weeks postpartum. If their milk production is adequate, they can then continue on this form of contraception.

For patients interested in nonhormonal methods, condoms are particularly good because of the prevention against sexually transmitted infections. The other barrier methods—the diaphragm and cervical cap—should be avoided until 6 weeks postpartum when the cervix has returned to its normal shape and size. Intrauterine devices (IUDs) may be inserted postpartum. With the introduction of the progesterone-eluting IUD (Mirena), this form of contraception has increased over the past decade. Prior concerns about infections from IUDs in the 1970s or the increased volume and length of menses from the copper IUD are alleviated by the Mirena. Because of the low release of local progesterone, the use of the Mirena can actually lead to lighter, shorter menses and even amenorrhea in 15% to 20% of users. However, the IUD has a higher rate of expulsion in the immediate postpartum period. Because of the dilated cervix, placement usually is done at the 6-week postpartum appointment. In women who are less likely to follow up or for whom contraception is paramount, placement postpartum with several follow-up visits to verify that it is still in situ may be used.

DISCHARGE INSTRUCTIONS

Hospital stay after delivery is short, and while it has been mandated that insurance companies must cover up to 2 days after a vaginal delivery and 4 days after a cesarean delivery, many hospitals still discharge patients after 1 and 3 days, respectively. After a vaginal delivery, the above issues of perineal care, contraception, and breast care are discussed with the patient. Further, a discussion regarding how common the postpartum "blues" can be as well as the availability of professionals to talk the patient through any problems as she transitions to home can be of help. Patients who have a cesarean delivery should be counseled regarding wound care and activity in addition to the above. With Pfannenstiel incisions that were stapled closed, the staples can be removed prior to discharge. Patients are often advised to avoid heavy lifting ("nothing heavier than your baby") and vigorous activities including driving. Before patients drive, it is recommended that they try to slam on the brakes as an experiment to be sure they are comfortable enough to drive.

POSTPARTUM COMPLICATIONS

The primary complications that arise postpartum include postpartum hemorrhage, endomyometritis, wound infections and separations, mastitis, and postpartum depression (Table 12-1). Postpartum hemorrhage usually occurs during the first 24 hours, while the patient is still in the hospital. However, it can also occur in patients with retained products of conception (POCs) for up to several weeks postpartum. Endomyometritis and wound complications typically occur in the first week to 10 days postpartum, and mastitis typically occurs 1 to 2 weeks after delivery but may present anytime during breastfeeding. Postpartum depression can occur at any time during the puerperium and beyond and is probably grossly underdiagnosed.

POSTPARTUM HEMORRHAGE

Postpartum hemorrhage is defined as blood loss exceeding 500 mL in a vaginal delivery and greater than 1,000 mL in a cesarean section. If the hemorrhage occurs within the first 24 hours, it is deemed early postpartum hemorrhage; after 24 hours, it is considered late or delayed postpartum hemorrhage. Common causes of postpartum bleeding include uterine atony, retained POCs, placenta accreta, cervical lacerations, and vaginal lacerations (Tables 12-2 and 12-3). While the cause of the hemorrhage is being investigated, the patient is simultaneously started on fluid resuscitation and preparations are made for blood transfusions. With blood loss greater than 2 to 3 L, patients may develop a consumptive

■ **TABLE 12-1** Complications of Vaginal and Cesarean Deliveries		
	Vaginal Delivery	**Cesarean Delivery**
Common complications	Postpartum hemorrhage Vaginal hematoma Cervical laceration Retained POCs Mastitis Postpartum depression	Postpartum hemorrhage Surgical blood loss Wound infection Endomyometritis Mastitis Postpartum depression
Rare complications	Endomyometritis Episiotomy infections Episiotomy breakdown	Wound separation Wound dehiscence

■ TABLE 12-2 Risk Factors for Postpartum Hemorrhage

Prior Postpartum Hemorrhage
Abnormal placentation
Placenta previa
Placenta accreta
Hydatidiform mole
Trauma during labor and delivery
Episiotomy
Complicated vaginal delivery
Low- or midforceps delivery
Sulcal or sidewall laceration
Uterine rupture
Cesarean delivery or hysterectomy
Cervical laceration
Uterine atony
Uterine inversion
Overdistended uterus
Macrosomic fetus
Multiple gestation
Polyhydramnios
Exhausted myometrium
Rapid labor
Prolonged labor
Oxytocin or prostaglandin stimulation
Chorioamnionitis
Coagulation defects—intensify other causes
Placental abruption
Prolonged retention of dead fetus
Amnionic fluid embolism
Severe intravascular hemolysis
Severe preeclampsia and eclampsia
Congenital coagulopathies
Anticoagulant treatment

■ TABLE 12-3 Etiology of Postpartum Hemorrhage in Vaginal and Cesarean Deliveries

Vaginal Delivery	Cesarean Delivery
Vaginal lacerations	Uterine atony
Cervical lacerations	Surgical blood loss
Uterine atony	Placenta accreta
Placenta accreta	Uterine rupture
Vaginal hematoma	
Retained POCs	
Uterine inversion	
Uterine rupture	

Each of the etiologies of postpartum hemorrhage is discussed sequentially; the obstetrician often has to consider and/or attempt to treat several etiologies simultaneously.

Vaginal Lacerations and Hematomas

Vaginal lacerations with uncontrolled bleeding should be considered in the case of postpartum hemorrhage. Initially after a delivery, the perineum, labia, periurethral area, and deeper aspects of the vagina are examined for lacerations. These should be repaired at that time. However, deep sulcal tears or vaginal lacerations behind the cervix may be quite difficult to visualize without careful retraction. Occasionally, these lacerations will involve arteries and arterioles and lead to a significant postpartum hemorrhage. Adequate anesthesia, an experienced obstetrician, and assistance with retraction are all necessary to perform an adequate exploration and repair of these lacerations.

Occasionally, the trauma of delivery will injure a blood vessel without disrupting the epithelium above it. This leads to the development of a hematoma. If a patient has a larger than expected drop in hematocrit, an examination should be performed to rule out a vaginal wall hematoma. A hematoma can be managed expectantly unless it is tense or expanding, in which case it should be opened, the bleeding vessel ligated, and the vaginal wall closed. Rarely, a patient will develop a retroperitoneal hematoma that can lead to a large blood loss into this space. Patients usually complain of low back or rectal pain and there will be a large drop in hematocrit. Diagnosis is made via ultrasound or CT. If the patient is stable without a falling

coagulopathy and require coagulation factors and platelets. In rare cases, if patients become hypovolemic and hypotensive, Sheehan syndrome, or pituitary infarction, may occur. Sheehan syndrome may manifest with the absence of lactation secondary to the lack of prolactin or failure to re-start menstruation secondary to the absence of gonadotropins.

hematocrit, expectant management may be utilized. However, if the patient demonstrates continued bleeding with evidence of expansion of the hematoma or a further drop in hematocrit, interventional radiology can utilize embolization techniques in order to treat such bleeding. Because these clinicians are rarely in house, early notification of the potential for such an intervention is necessary. If the patient becomes unstable, surgical exploration and ligation of the disrupted vessels may be required.

Cervical Lacerations

Cervical lacerations can cause a brisk postpartum hemorrhage. Commonly, they are a result of rapid dilation of the cervix during the stage 1 of labor or maternal expulsive efforts prior to complete dilation of the cervix. If a patient is bleeding at the level of the cervix or above, a careful exploration of the cervix should be performed. The patient should have adequate anesthesia via epidural, spinal, or pudendal block. The walls of the vagina are retracted so the cervix can be well visualized. When the anterior lip of the cervix is seen, it is grasped with a ring forcep. Then another ring forcep can be used to grasp beyond the first and in this fashion the cervix should be "walked" around its entirety so that no lacerations, particularly on the posterior aspect, are missed. If any lacerations are seen, they are usually repaired with either interrupted or running absorbable sutures.

Uterine Atony

Uterine atony is the leading cause of postpartum hemorrhage. Patients are at a higher risk for uterine atony if they have chorioamnionitis, exposure to magnesium sulfate, multiple gestations, a macrosomic fetus, polyhydramnios, prolonged labor, a history of atony with any prior pregnancies, or if they are multiparous, particularly a grand multipara (more than five deliveries). Uterine abnormalities or fibroids may also interfere with uterine contractions leading to and increasing bleeding. The diagnosis of atony is made by palpation of the uterus, which is soft, enlarged, and boggy. Occasionally the uterine fundus is well contracted, but the lower uterine segment, which has less contractile tissue, will be less so.

Atony is initially treated with IV oxytocin (Pitocin), which is usually given prophylactically after delivery of the infant. While the oxytocin is being administered, strong uterine massage should be performed to assist the uterus in contracting. If atony continues, the next step is methylergonovine (Methergine), which is contraindicated in hypertensive patients. If the uterus is still atonic, the next step is to give Hemabate (also known as Prostin or PGF$_{2\alpha}$), which is contraindicated in asthmatics. The prostaglandin is thought to be more effective if injected directly into the uterine musculature, either transabdominally or transcervically, although this has not been demonstrated in studies. If atony continues despite maximal medical management, the patient is brought to the OR for a **dilation and curettage** (D&C) to rule out possible retained POCs. Patients with uterine atony unresponsive to these conservative measures, but bleeding at a rate that can tolerate some watchful waiting, may benefit from uterine packing with an inflatable balloon or occlusion of pelvic vessels (uterine artery embolization) by interventional radiology to prevent the necessity of a hysterectomy. If this is unsuccessful, exploratory laparotomy with ligation of pelvic vessels and possible hysterectomy is required.

Retained Products of Conception

Careful inspection of the placenta should always be performed. However, with vaginal delivery, it can often be difficult to determine whether a small piece of the placenta has been left behind in the uterus. Usually the retained fetal membranes or placental tissue pass in the lochia. However, they occasionally lead to endomyometritis and postpartum hemorrhage. If the suspicion is high for retained POCs, the uterus should be explored either manually if the cervix has not contracted down or by ultrasound. If there is evidence of a normal uterine stripe, the probability of retained products is much lower. However, if clinical suspicion is high, a D&C would be next for both diagnostic and therapeutic measures. If hemorrhage continues once it has been ascertained that there are no further POCs via exploration, placenta accreta should be suspected.

Accreta

Placenta accreta, increta, and percreta are discussed briefly in Chapter 5 with antepartum hemorrhage. These conditions are the result of abnormal attachment of placental tissue to the uterus that may invade into or beyond the uterine myometrium, leading to incomplete separation of the placenta postpartum and postpartum hemorrhage. Risk factors for developing placenta accreta include placenta previa and prior uterine surgery, including cesarean delivery and myomectomy. Often the third stage will have been longer than usual and the placenta may have delivered in fragments. Accreta involves bleeding that is unresponsive to uterine massage and contractile agents such as oxytocin, ergonovines, and prostaglandins. Patients with accreta are taken to the operating room for surgical management via exploratory laparotomy.

Uterine Rupture

Uterine rupture is estimated to occur in 0.5% to 1.0% of patients with prior uterine scars and about 1:15,000 to 20,000 women with an unscarred uterus. It is an intrapartum complication but may lead to postpartum bleeding. It is rare for rupture to occur in a nulliparous patient. Risk factors include previous uterine surgery, breech extraction, obstructed labor, and high parity. Symptoms usually include abdominal pain and a popping sensation intra-abdominally. Treatment involves laparotomy and repair of the ruptured uterus. If hemorrhage cannot be controlled, hysterectomy may be indicated.

Uterine Inversion

Uterine inversion may occur in 1:2,500 deliveries. Risk factors include fundal implantation of the placenta, uterine atony, placenta accreta, and excessive traction on the cord during the third stage. Diagnosis is made by witnessing the fundus of the uterus attached to the placenta on placental delivery. Uterine inversion can be an obstetric emergency if hemorrhage occurs. Additionally, patients often experience an intense vasovagal response from the inversion and may require stabilization with the aid of an anesthesiologist before manual replacement of the uterus can be attempted, which should be the first step in treatment (Fig. 12-1). Uterine relaxants such as nitroglycerin or general anesthesia with halogenated agents may be given to aid uterine relaxation and replacement. If this is unsuccessful, laparotomy is required to surgically replace the uterus.

Operative Management of Postpartum Hemorrhage

In the case of vaginal delivery, the management of postpartum hemorrhage is as described above. A differential diagnosis is created and a rapid physical exam is performed to establish the likely etiology. If vaginal and cervical lacerations have been ruled out and the patient is unresponsive to uterotonic agents

and massage, the patient should be moved to an operating room and a D&C performed. If this fails to stop the bleeding, placement of an inflatable balloon in the uterine cavity may limit further hemorrhage; if these measures fail, a laparotomy is performed.

On entering the abdomen, the surgeon should note whether there is blood in the abdomen, which would indicate a uterine rupture. Unless the patient is unstable and coagulopathic secondary to excessive blood loss, the first surgical procedure is usually bilateral O'Leary sutures to tie off the uterine arteries. The second is ligation of the hypogastric, or internal iliac, arteries, which requires considerable skill and experience. If uterine atony is the cause of hemorrhage, B-Lynch sutures can be placed in an attempt to compress the uterus and achieve hemostasis. A uterine incision must first be made, through which a suture is looped around the uterus and used to tamp it back into place. If these measures fail to provide hemostasis, often the patient requires a puerperal hysterectomy (known as cesarean hysterectomy if that has been the mode of delivery).

If the patient has been delivered via cesarean section and there is evidence of accreta, the first step is usually to place hemostatic sutures in the placental bed. If these fail, or the patient has no focal site of bleeding, O'Leary sutures can be placed next with

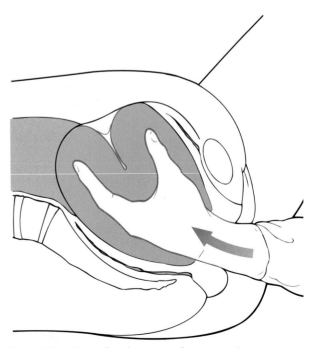

Figure 12-1 • Manual replacement of an inverted uterus.

the uterus still open to watch the bleeding. If this fails, often the next step is to close the uterus with or without packing it and proceed to hypogastric artery ligation. If this fails, hysterectomy is the definitive procedure.

If a patient is not bleeding too briskly, with either vaginal or cesarean delivery, packing the uterus and obtaining an interventional radiology consult for uterine artery embolization is possible. This is reserved for those patients who are truly stable and desire future fertility.

ENDOMYOMETRITIS

Endomyometritis is a polymicrobial infection of the uterine lining that often invades the underlying wall. It is most common after cesarean section but may occur after vaginal deliveries as well, particularly if manual removal of the placenta was performed. It is increased in patients with meconium, chorioamnionitis, and prolonged rupture of membranes.

Diagnosis is made in the setting of fever, elevated white blood count, and uterine tenderness, with a higher suspicion after cesarean. Endomyometritis commonly occurs 5 to 10 days after delivery but may be suspected when all other sources of infection have been ruled out for several weeks after delivery. Because retained POCs can be the etiology of infection, an ultrasound is often obtained to examine the intrauterine contents.

Endomyometritis is usually treated with broad-spectrum intravenous antibiotics, or triple antibiotics, though in some institutions a second-generation cephalosporin is utilized. If retained POCs are identified on ultrasound, a D&C is performed. Because the postpartum uterus is at greater risk for perforation, great care should be taken during dilation using blunt rather than sharp curettage and ultrasound guidance to limit complications. Antibiotics are continued until the patient is afebrile for 48 hours, uterine pain and tenderness are absent, and the white blood cell count normalizes.

WOUND COMPLICATIONS

Wound Infections

Wound infections include cellulitis and abscess. While such infections of the cesarean skin incision are seen in 1% to 5% of cases, such infections can also be seen in the perineal laceration or episiotomy site. Cellulitis is suspected with local erythema around the surgical site. If the erythema is tender and particularly warm, the level of suspicion is usually high enough to diagnose cellulitis. If these two symptoms are not present, often a line is drawn around the erythema and if it expands over 12 to 24 hours, this also makes a diagnosis of cellulitis. Cellulitis can be treated with broad-spectrum antibiotics with a focus on covering skin flora. In the case of a cellulitis not responding to antibiotics with increasing fever, evidence of pus from the wound, or a palpable collection within the incision, an abscess should be suspected. Wound abscesses need to be treated with I&D and wound cleaning and packing. Often, antibiotics are continued until 48 hours afebrile as well. Anytime a wound abscess is suspected, it should either be ruled out with an imaging study or definitively by opening the wound as delay in treating a wound abscess may lead to necrotizing fasciitis. One hallmark sign of necrotizing fasciitis is that the initial pain of a cellulitis goes away due to nerve injury despite no change in the visual appearance of the cellulitis. Necrotizing fasciitis requires surgical resection of the necrotic tissue and often repair of the fascia with grafts.

Perineal cellulitis or abscesses are treated similarly to abdominal wound infections. However, the diagnosis is often more difficult to make as the area can be more difficult to readily inspect and women can confuse the infection with normal postpartum perineal pain. Similar treatment with broad-spectrum antibiotics for cellulitis and opening the wound in the setting of an abscess is performed. If such an abscess occurs in the setting of third- or fourth-degree perineal laceration, usually the infection is treated and a long-delayed closure by a specialist such as a urogynecologist or rectal surgeon is performed. Of note, perineal infections in the setting of third- and fourth-degree lacerations may be decreased by the use of prophylactic antibiotics.

Wound Separations

Even in the absence of an infection, wounds may not heal by primary intention after their first closure. Fluid collections of either serum (seroma) or blood (hematoma) can increase the chances of wound separation by preventing tissue apposition. Thus, continued leaking of either fluid or blood from a wound can signal a seroma or hematoma. Usually the skin of a transverse incision has adequately healed to remove staples on postoperative day 3 and for a vertical incision by postoperative day 6 or 7. If, when the staples are removed, the skin separates, this is considered a wound separation. In this setting, it is important to make sure it is just a superficial separation and the wound should be probed to verify that the fascia is still intact. If the fascia is also separated, this is termed a *wound dehiscence*.

With a superficial wound separation, there are two options. The first is to simply let the wound heal by secondary intention. The wound may be packed with gauze or Sorbsan and changed once to twice per day. More recently, wounds are treated with a wound vacuum, which is placed over the wound and applies negative pressure to the wound, decreasing wound healing time. However, an alternative is that if the wound is not infected to simply attempt to close the wound by primary intention again. As many postcesarean wounds are complicated by seromas due to the surrounding tissue edema, these reattempts at primary closure will often be successful. For a complete wound dehiscence, the fascia is usually closed and the skin incision above can be treated in either fashion detailed above.

MASTITIS

Mastitis is a regional infection of the breast, commonly caused by the patient's skin flora or the oral flora of breastfeeding infants. The organisms enter an erosion or cracked nipple and proliferate, leading to infection. Lactating women will often have warm, diffusely tender, and firm breasts, particularly at the time of engorgement or milk letdown. This should be differentiated from focal tenderness, erythema, and differences in temperature from one region of the breast to another, which are classic signs of mastitis. The diagnosis can be made with physical examination, a fever, and an elevated white blood count. Mastitis can be complicated by formation of an abscess, which then requires treatment by incision and drainage (I&D).

Mastitis can be treated with oral antibiotics; Dicloxacillin is the treatment of choice. In addition, patients should also continue to breastfeed, which prevents intraductal accumulation of infected material. Those who are not breastfeeding should breast pump in the acute phase of the infection. Women who are unresponsive to oral antibiotics are admitted for intravenous antibiotics until they remain afebrile for 48 hours. If there is no response to intravenous antibiotics, a breast abscess should be suspected and an imaging study obtained.

POSTPARTUM DEPRESSION

Many patients have the postpartum blues with mood swings and changes in appetite and sleep, if not frank postpartum depression. The pathophysiology of depression is poorly understood, but may be due to the rapid changes in estrogen, progesterone, and prolactin in postpartum patients. It also may be related to the lack of sleep in the postpartum period, as well as the psychosocial stress of caring for a newborn. Greater than 50% of postpartum patients experience postpartum blues, whereas postpartum depression complicates greater than 5% of pregnancies. While these events are common, they are seen in higher rates in patients with a history of depression or other mental illness as well as in patients with poor support networks.

Diagnosis

Most patients have normal changes in appetite, energy level, and sleep patterns in the initial postpartum period that do not necessarily indicate frank depression. However, patients who experience low energy level, anorexia, insomnia, hypersomnolence, extreme sadness, and other depressive symptoms for greater than a few weeks may have postpartum depression. These patients often feel incapable of caring for their infants. Occasionally, depressed patients have suicidal or homicidal ideation, which is a much clearer marker for depression and merits close observation.

Therapy and Prognosis

In patients with transient postpartum depression, symptoms are usually self-limited with support and encouragement. However, these symptoms can occasionally progress to a more severe postpartum depression or even psychosis. In these situations, the caregiver needs to determine whether the patient is having suicidal or homicidal ideation. A social worker and professional counselor should be involved, as should the immediate family and any other individuals who are close to the patient and can provide support. Antidepressant medications are commonly used. While an episode of postpartum blues may resolve quite readily, depression and psychosis should be treated with medications. SSRIs have been used for postpartum depression with good efficacy and appear to be safe for breastfeeding mothers. Most patients without a history of depression or other mental illness improve, usually to their prepregnant state.

KEY POINTS

- Two central issues in the immediate postpartum period, regardless of the mode of delivery, are pain management and wound care.

- Condoms with a spermicidal foam or gel can be used by anyone postpartum.

- Diaphragms and cervical caps need to be refitted at 6 weeks. IUDs are best placed at 6 weeks as well.

- Depo-Provera, Norplant, or the progesterone-only mini-pill are the hormonal contraceptives of choice in the puerperium because they are less likely to decrease milk production in breastfeeding patients.

- Discharge instructions should include discussion of medical issues such as contraception and wound care. Instructions on social issues, such as the transition to home with the newborn, how to deal with some of the changes related to the delivery, and care of the baby are also needed.

- Causes of postpartum hemorrhage include uterine atony, uterine rupture, uterine inversion, retained POCs, placenta accreta, and cervical or vaginal lacerations.

- Treatment of PPH may require use of blood products including fresh frozen plasma, cryoprecipitate, and platelets in patients who develop a consumptive coagulopathy.

- Surgical management of PPH ranges from D&C to exploratory laparotomy, uterine artery ligation, hypogastric artery ligation, and, if these fail, hysterectomy.

- In PPH patients for whom there is enough time, an alternative to exploratory laparotomy is uterine artery embolization by interventional radiology.

- Endomyometritis is more common in patients with cesarean section than vaginal delivery, although patients with manual removal of the placenta are also at increased risk.

- Diagnosis of endomyometritis is clinical with fever, elevated white blood cell count, and uterine tenderness, and treatment is with broad-spectrum antibiotics and D&C for retained POCs.

- Cesarean incisions may be complicated by cellulitis, wound abscess, wound separation, or frank dehiscence.

- Mastitis is differentiated from engorgement by focal tenderness, erythema, and edema, and treatment is usually with oral antibiotics and breast pumping or feeding.

- Changes in appetite, sleep patterns, and energy level are common in the first few weeks postpartum.

- Postpartum depression is common and probably underdiagnosed. In most patients, the depressive symptoms resolve on their own, but occasionally antidepressants are required.

Part 2

Gynecology

BENIGN LESIONS OF THE VULVA, VAGINA, AND CERVIX

This chapter encompasses an overview of the many congenital anomalies, epithelial disorders, and benign cysts and tumors of the vulva, vagina, and cervix. Infections of these structures are covered in Chapter 16, and premalignant and malignant lesions are covered in Chapter 27 (vulva and vagina) and Chapter 28 (cervix).

CONGENITAL ANOMALIES OF THE VULVA AND VAGINA

A variety of congenital defects occur in the external genitalia, vagina, and cervix including but not limited to labial fusion, imperforate hymen, transverse vaginal septum, vaginal atresia, and vaginal agenesis. Congenital anomalies of the female genital tract are associated with concomitant **anomalies in the upper reproductive tract** as well as **anomalies in the genital urinary (GU) tract** (unilateral renal agenesis, pelvic or horseshoe kidneys, or irregularities in the collecting system).

LABIAL FUSION

Labial fusion is associated with excess androgens. Most commonly, the etiology is the result of **exogenous androgen exposure** but may also be due to an enzymatic error leading to increased androgen production. The most common form of enzymatic deficiency is **21-hydroxylase deficiency** (Chapter 23) leading to **congenital adrenal hyperplasia**. This may be phenotypically demonstrated in the neonate with **ambiguous genitalia**, hyperandrogenism with salt wasting, hypotension, hyperkalemia, and hypoglycemia. The neonates often present in adrenal crisis with salt wasting seen approximately 75% of the time. This autosomal recessive trait occurs in roughly 1 in 40,000 to 50,000 pregnancies. The diagnosis is made by elevated **17α-hydroxyprogesterone** or urine 17-ketosteroid with decreased serum cortisol.

Treatment of this defect is with **cortisol**, which is not being produced by the adrenal cortex. The exogenous cortisol then negatively feeds back on the pituitary to decrease the release of adrenocorticotropic hormone (ACTH), thus inhibiting the stimulation of the adrenal gland that is shunting all steroid precursors into androgens. If salt wasting is documented, a mineralocorticoid (usually fludrocortisone acetate) is also given. The labial fusion and other ambiguous genitalia often require **reconstructive surgery**.

IMPERFORATE HYMEN

The hymen is at the junction between the urogenital sinus and the sinovaginal bulbs (Fig. 13-1). Before birth, the epithelial cells in the central portion of the hymenal membrane degenerate, leaving a thin rim of mucous membrane at the vaginal introitus. This is known as the **hymenal ring**. When this degeneration fails to occur, the hymen remains intact. This is known as an imperforate hymen. It occurs in 1 in 1,000 female births. Other congenital abnormalities of the hymen are shown in Figure 13-2. These can result from incomplete degeneration of the central portion of hymen.

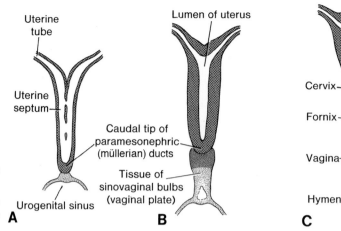

Figure 13-1 • Embryonic formation of the vagina and uterus.
(From Sadler T. *Langman's Medical Embryology*, 9th ed. Baltimore: Lippincott Williams & Wilkins, 2003.)

An **imperforate hymen** results in an obstruction to the outflow tract of the reproductive system. This can lead to a buildup of secretions in the vagina behind the hymen (hydrocolpos or **mucocolpos**) similar to that seen with a transverse vaginal septum (Fig. 13-3). If not identified at birth, an imperforate hymen is often diagnosed at puberty in adolescents who present with **primary amenorrhea** and **cyclic pelvic pain**. These symptoms are due to the accumulation of menstrual flow behind the hymen in the vagina (**hematocolpos**) and uterus (**hematometria**). In these patients, the physical exam may be notable for the absence of an identifiable vaginal lumen, a tense bulging hymen, and possibly increasing lower abdominal girth. Treatment of imperforate hymen and other hymenal abnormalities is with **surgery** to excise the extra tissue, evacuate any obstructed material, and create a normal-sized vaginal opening (Color Plate 7).

TRANSVERSE VAGINAL SEPTUM

The **upper vagina** is formed as the paramesonephric (müllerian) ducts elongate and meet in the midline. The internal portion of each duct is canalized and the remaining septum between them dissolves (Fig. 13-1A). The caudal portion of the müllerian ducts develop into the uterus and upper vagina (Fig. 13-1B,C). The **lower vagina** is formed as the urogenital sinus evaginates to form the sinovaginal bulbs (Fig. 13-1B). These then proliferate to form the vaginal plate. The lumen of the lower vagina is then formed as the central portion of this solid vaginal plate degenerates (Fig. 13-1C). This process is known as canalization or vacuolization.

The vagina is formed as the müllerian system from above joins the sinovaginal bulb–derived system from below. This takes place at the **müllerian tubercle** (Fig.

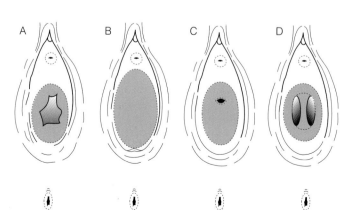

Figure 13-2 • Congenital abnormalities of the hymen. **(A)** Normal. **(B)** Imperforate. **(C)** Microperforate. **(D)** Septate.

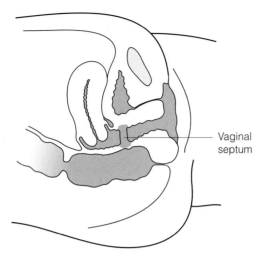

Figure 13-3 • Transverse vaginal septum.

13-1B). The müllerian tubercle must be canalized for a normal vagina to form. If this does not occur, this tissue may be left as a **transverse vaginal septum**. These septa often lie near the junction between the lower two-thirds and upper one-third of the vagina (Fig. 13-3) but can be found at various levels in the vagina. This occurs in approximately 1 in 30,000 to 1 in 80,000 females. Similar to the imperforate hymen, diagnosis is usually made at the time of puberty in adolescents who present with **primary amenorrhea and cyclic pelvic pain** accompanied by menstrual symptoms. On physical exam, patients typically have normal external female genitalia and a short vagina that appears to end in a blind pouch. The transverse vaginal septa are usually less than 1 cm thick and may have a central perforation. **Ultrasound and MRI** can be used to characterize the thickness and location of the septum and to confirm the presence of other parts of the reproductive tract. **Surgical correction** is the only form of treatment.

VAGINAL ATRESIA

Vaginal atresia (also known as agenesis of the lower vagina) is often confused with imperforate hymen or transverse vaginal septum. It occurs when the **lower vagina fails to develop** and is replaced by fibrous tissue. The ovaries, uterus, cervix, and upper vagina are all normal. Developmentally, vaginal atresia results when the urogenital sinus fails to contribute the lower portion of the vagina (Fig. 13-1). It presents during adolescence with **primary amenorrhea and cyclic pelvic pain**. Physical examination reveals the absence of an introitus and the presence of a **vaginal dimple**. Pelvic imaging with ultrasound and/or MRI may show a large **hematocolpos** and confirm the presence of a normal upper reproductive tract. **Surgical correction** can be achieved by incising the fibrous tissue and dissecting it until the normal upper vagina is identified. Any accumulated blood or materials can be evacuated and the normal upper vaginal mucosa is then brought down to the introitus and sutured to the hymenal ring. This is known as a **vaginal pull-through procedure**.

VAGINAL AGENESIS

Vaginal agenesis, also known as **Mayer-Rokitansky-Kuster-Hauser** syndrome (MRKH), occurs in 1 to 2.5 per 10,000 female births. It is characterized by the congenital **absence of the vagina** (Color Plate 8) and the absence or hypoplasia of all or part of the cervix, uterus, and fallopian tubes. These patients typically have normal external genitalia, normal secondary sexual characteristics (breast development, axillary, and pubic hair), and normal ovarian function. These patients are **phenotypically and genotypically female** with normal 46,XX karyotypes. These patients typically present in adolescence with primary amenorrhea. Pelvic imaging with **ultrasound and MRI** can be used to assess the vagina, uterus, ovaries, and kidneys since these patients will often have associated urologic and skeletal anomalies.

Treatment for patients with vaginal agenesis involves a combination of **psychosocial support**, counseling, and **nonsurgical and surgical correction** individualized to the patient. In motivated patients, a vagina can be created using **serial vaginal dilators** pressed into the perineal body (Frank and Ingram procedures). This can take 4 months to several years depending on the patient. If this nonsurgical approach fails, a variety of vaginal, laparoscopic, and abdominal procedures are available to **create a neovagina**. The most commonly used is the **McIndoe** procedure, which utilizes a split-thickness skin graft taken from the buttocks. The graft is placed over a silicone mold to create a tube with one closed end (Fig. 13-4). A transverse incision is then made at the vaginal dimple and the fibrous tissue replacing the vagina is dissected to the level of the peritoneum. The mold and graft are inserted into the vagina. Once the mold is removed, dilators must still be used for several months to maintain vaginal patency. While **normal sexual intercourse** is possible after these surgical and

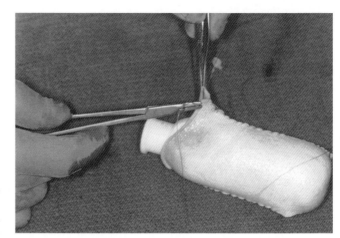

Figure 13-4 • McIndoe procedure to make a neovagina. The skin graft is sewn around a mold.
(Image from Emans, J. *Pediatric & Adolescent Gynecology*, 5th ed. Philadelphia: Lippincott Williams & Wilkins, 2004.)

nonsurgical procedures, the patient will be unable to carry a pregnancy. She can, however, have her eggs harvested for use with a gestational surrogate.

BENIGN EPITHELIAL DISORDERS OF THE VULVA AND VAGINA

Benign lesions of the mucosa of the vulva and vagina come under this broad category. The **nonneoplastic epithelial disorders** of the vulva (lichen sclerosis, squamous cell hyperplasia, lichen planus, and lichen simplex chronicus) were formerly known as the vulvar dystrophies. Along with vulvar psoriasis they represent a broad spectrum of atrophic and hypertrophic conditions characterized by vulvar skin changes due to a variety of etiologic agents (Table 13-1). These lesions and the most common benign vaginal epithelial lesion, vaginal adenosis, **require histologic examination** to identify and treat the disorder and to differentiate the lesion from vulvar and vaginal intraepithelial neoplasia and cancer (Chapter 27).

Pathogenesis

Lichen sclerosis can be found on the vulva of females of all age groups, but has major significance in **postmenopausal women**, where it is associated with a 5% to 15% risk of cancer. The etiology is unknown, but several mechanisms have been proposed including genetic, immunologic, hormonal, and infectious mechanisms. The resulting atrophy can cause labial fusion, contracture of the vaginal introitus, thinning of the vulvar skin, and skin fragility (Fig. 13-5).

Squamous cell hyperplasia (also known as atopic dermatitis or **atopic eczema**) is the histologic result of scratching and rubbing due to **chronic vulvar irritation**. Patients often complain of vulvar itching with localized thickening of the vulvar skin. This presents histologically as **hyperkeratotic changes**.

Lichen simplex chronicus similarly involves a chronic inflammatory process associated with vulvar pruritis, but involves **reactive changes** to chronic scratching and rubbing, rather than hyperkeratotic changes.

Lichen planus is an atrophic inflammatory condition that results in chronic eruption of shiny **purple papules** with white striae on the flexor surfaces, mucous membranes, and vulva. Lichen planus can cause **vaginal adhesions** and can even develop into an erosive vaginitis. Lichen planus generally occurs in women age 30 to 60 and has two forms: drug-induced and spontaneous.

Vulvar psoriasis (seborrheic dermatitis) is secondary to **chronic inflammation** in areas rich in sebaceous glands (scalp, face, axilla, groin, and upper trunk). The etiology is unknown, but it may be secondary to a skin saprophyte called Malassezia furfur.

Vaginal adenosis is a benign lesion of the vaginal mucosa involving red granular spots and patches that can be palpated and occasionally seen on the vaginal wall. It typically and most frequently involves the upper third of the vagina and the anterior vaginal wall. Adenosis is found in 30% to 90% of women who have been exposed to **diethylstilbestrol (DES) in utero**. This epithelium usually contains various cell types, resembling müllerian structures such as the endocervix, endometrium, and fallopian tubes. Because vaginal adenocarcinomas arise from the tuboendometrial cells, biopsy should therefore always be performed when vaginal adenosis is suspected.

	Physical Findings	Symptoms	Treatment Options
Lichen sclerosis	Symmetric white, thinned skin on labia, perineum, and perianal region. Shrinkage and agglutination of labia minora	Usually asymptomatic Occasional pruritis or dyspareunia	High potency topical steroids (clobetasol or halobetasol 0.05%) 1 to 2×/day for 6 to 12 weeks
Squamous cell hyperplasia	Localized thickening of the vulvar skin from edema Raised white lesion usually on the labia majora and clitoris	Chronic pruritis and thickened skin	Medium potency topical steroids 2×/day for 4 to 6 weeks
Lichen planus	Multiple shiny, flat, purple papules usually on the inner aspects of the labia minora, vagina, and vestibule. Often erosive. May have vaginal adhesions resulting in vaginal stenosis	Pruritis with mild inflammation to severe erosion	Vaginal hydrocortisone suppositories. Surgical excision or vaginal dilators for vaginal adhesions. Vaginal estrogen for patients with vaginal atrophy
Lichen simplex chronicus	Thickened white epithelium, slight scaling, usually unilateral and circumscribed	Vulvar pruritis	Medium potency topical steroids 2×/day for 4 to 6 weeks
Vulvar psoriasis	Red moist lesions, sometimes scaly. May also be found on the scalp, axilla, groin and trunk	Asymptomatic or occasional pruritis	Ultraviolet light or topical steroids
Vaginal adenosis	Palpable red glandular spots and patches in the upper third of the vagina on the anterior wall	None	Follow with serial exams

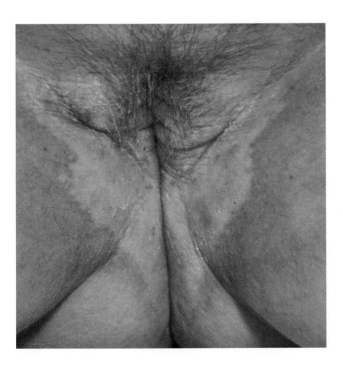

Figure 13-5 • A late case of lichen sclerosis. Note the thin, white, atrophic epithelium and labial fusion.
(From Rubin E, Farber JL. *Pathology*, 3rd ed. Philadelphia: Lippincott Williams & Wilkins, 1999.)

Clinical Manifestations

History

Patients with benign lesions of the vulva and vagina present with a variety of complaints including vulvar itching, irritation, and burning. They may also report dysuria, dyspareunia and vulvodynia and feel that the skin of their vulva is tender, bumpy, or thickened.

Physical Examination

These disorders range in appearance from erythematous plaques to hyperkeratotic white plaques (Table 13-1). Occasionally petechiae and/or ecchymoses are present as a result of trauma from scratching.

Diagnostic Evaluation

Diagnosis is made histologically; therefore, all vulvar lesions should be biopsied (Fig. 13-6) for identification purposes and to rule or premalignant and malignant disease. Indications for **definite biopsy** include ulceration, unifocal lesions, suspicion of lichen sclerosus, unidentifiable lesions, and lesions or symptoms that recur or persist after conventional therapy. Vaginal lesions can be biopsied and evaluated via **colposcopy**.

Differential Diagnosis

The differential diagnosis of benign lesions of the vulva and vagina includes disorders such as Behçet syndrome, Crohn disease, erythema multiforme, bullous pemphigoid, and plasma cell vulvitis. The differential diagnosis also includes carcinomas such as squamous

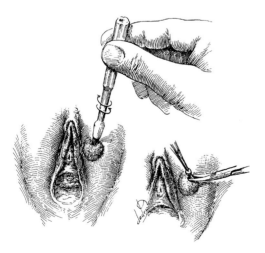

Figure 13-6 • Vulvar biopsy.
(From Beckman CRB, Ling FW, Laube DW, et al. *Obstetrics and Gynecology*, 4th ed. Baltimore: Lippincott Williams & Wilkins, 2002.)

cell, basal cell, melanoma, sarcoma, and Paget disease. Biopsies should therefore be performed and clinical correlations made.

Treatment

The histologic diagnosis is the basis for treatment. For all of these lesions, **healthy vulvar and vaginal hygiene practices** are of utmost importance. Patients should avoid tight-fitting clothes; pantyhose; panty liners; scented soaps and detergents; bubble baths; washcloths; and feminine sprays, douches, and powders. Patients should wear loose-fitting cotton underwear and **loose-fitting clothing**. They should use **unscented detergents and soaps** such as Neutrogena or Dove, and take morning and evening tub baths without additives.

High-potency **topical steroids** such as clobetasol can be used to treat lichen sclerosus or planus, and low- to medium-potency steroids should be used for mild cases of dermatoses (atopic eczema, lichen simplex chronicus). The duration of use ranges from one to two times a day for 2 to 4 weeks for dermatoses, to 6 to 12 weeks for lichen sclerosus. In most cases, patients benefit from a maintenance dosage of one to three times per week to avoid recurrence.

In general, there is **no role for topical estrogens or testosterone** in the treatment of these disorders; however, estrogen is an effective treatment for postmenopausal vulvovaginal atrophy. Similarly, surgical management is generally not indicated in treatment of these disorders. The exception is in the case of lichen planus where postinflammatory sequelae can include vaginal adhesions and introital stenosis.

BENIGN CYSTS AND TUMORS OF THE VULVA AND VAGINA

A variety of cysts and tumors can arise on the vulva and vagina. Cysts can originate from occlusion of pilosebaceous ducts, sebaceous ducts, and apocrine sweat glands. Treatment of benign cystic and solid tumors is only needed if the lesions become symptomatic or infected.

EPIDERMAL INCLUSION CYSTS

Epidermal inclusion cysts are the **most common tumor found on the vulva**. These cysts usually result from occlusion of a pilosebaceous duct or a blocked hair follicle. They are lined with squamous epithelium and contain tissue that would normally be exfoliated. These solitary lesions are normally small and asymptomatic; however, if these become superinfected and develop into abscesses, incision and drainage or complete excision is the treatment.

SEBACEOUS CYSTS

When the duct of a sebaceous gland becomes blocked, a sebaceous cyst forms. The normally secreted sebum accumulates in this cyst. Cysts are often multiple and asymptomatic. As with any cyst, these can become superinfected with local flora and require treatment with incision and drainage.

APOCRINE SWEAT GLAND CYSTS

These sweat glands are found throughout the mons pubis and labia majora. They can become occluded and form cysts. **Fox-Fordyce disease** is a pruritic microcystic disease that results from occlusion of these sweat glands. As in the axillary region, if these cysts become infected and form multiple abscesses, **hidradenitis suppurativa** can result. Excision or incision and drainage are the treatments of choice. If an overlying cellulitis is present, antibiotics are often used as well.

SKENE'S GLAND CYSTS

Skene's glands, or **paraurethral glands**, are located next to the urethra meatus (Fig. 13-7). Chronic inflammation of the Skene's glands can cause obstruction of the ducts and result in cystic dilation of the glands.

BARTHOLIN'S DUCT CYST AND ABSCESS

The Bartholin's glands are located bilaterally at approximately **4 o'clock and 8 o'clock** on the posterior-lateral aspect of the vaginal orifice (Fig. 13-7). They are mucus-secreting glands with ducts that open just external to the hymenal ring. Obstruction of these ducts leads to **cystic dilation of the Bartholin's duct** while the gland itself is unchanged (Fig. 13-8). If the cyst remains small (1 to 2 cm) and is not causing any symptoms, it can be left untreated and will often resolve on its own or with sitz baths. When a Bartholin's duct cyst first presents in a woman over age 40, a biopsy should be performed to rule out the rare possibility of **Bartholin's gland carcinoma**.

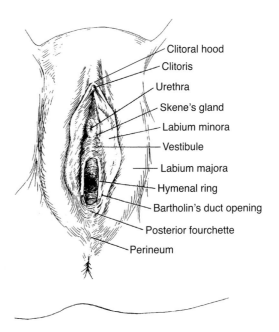

Figure 13-7 • Vulvar and perineal anatomy.
(From Beckman CRB, Ling FW, Laube DW, et al. *Obstetrics and Gynecology*, 4th ed. Baltimore: Lippincott Williams & Wilkins, 2002.)

While many Bartholin's cysts will resolve with minimal treatment, some cysts can become quite large and cause pressure symptoms such as local pain, dyspareunia, and difficulty walking. If these cysts do not resolve, they can become infected and lead to a

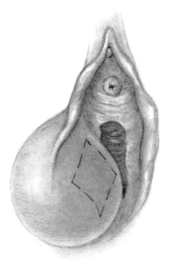

Figure 13-8 • Gross appearance of a Bartholin's cyst of the vulva.
(From LifeART image copyright © 2006 Lippincott Williams & Wilkins. All rights reserved.)

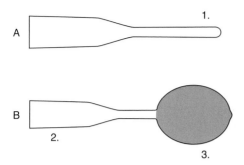

Figure 13-9 • Word catheter before inflation **(A)** and after inflation **(B)**. 1. The balloon-tipped end is placed into the incision site on the Bartholin's cyst. 2. A small-gauge needle is inserted into the opposite end and 2 to 4 mL of water is injected. 3. The inflated balloon remains inside the cyst for 4 to 6 weeks until an epithelialized tract is formed to prevent blockage of the duct to recur.

Bartholin's gland abscess. These abscesses are the result of polymicrobial infections, but they are also occasionally associated with sexually transmitted diseases. These abscesses can become quite large, causing exquisite pain and tenderness, and associated cellulitis. Bartholin's abscesses or symptomatic cysts should be treated like any other abscess: by **incision and drainage**. However, simple incision and drainage can often lead to recurrence; therefore, one of two methods can be used.

Word catheter placement is commonly performed in the emergent setting or in the office. This method involves making a small incision (5 mm) to drain and irrigate the abscess. Then a Word catheter with a balloon tip is placed inside the remaining cyst and inflated to fill the space. The balloon is left in place for 4 to 6 weeks, being serially reduced in size, while epithelialization of the cyst and tract occurs (Fig. 13-9).

Marsupialization is usually done for recurrent Bartholin's duct cysts or abscesses. The entire abscess or cyst is incised and the cyst wall is sutured to the vaginal mucosa to prevent reformation of the abscess (Fig. 13-10).

With either treatment, warm sitz baths several times per day are recommended both for pain relief and to decrease healing time. Adjunct antibiotic therapy is only recommended when the drainage is cultured for *Neisseria gonorrhoeae*, which occurs approximately 10% of the time. Concomitant cellulitis or an abscess that seems refractory to simple surgical treatment should also be treated with antibiotics that cover skin flora, primarily *Staphylococcus aureus*.

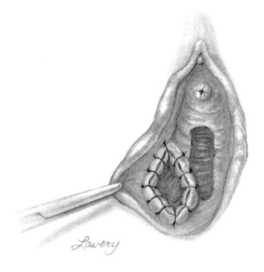

Figure 13-10 • Incision, drainage, and marsupilization of a Bartholin's abscess.

GARTNER'S DUCT CYSTS

Gartner's duct cysts are **remnants of the mesonephric ducts** of the wolffian system. They are found most commonly in the **anterior lateral** aspects of the upper part of the vagina. Most are **asymptomatic**. However, patients may present in adolescence with dyspareunia or difficulty inserting a tampon. These cysts are typically treated by excision. When removal is necessary, an IVP and cystoscopy should be performed preoperatively to locate the position of the bladder and ureters relative to the cyst, and urethral diverticula, ectopic ureters, and vaginal and cervical cancer should be ruled out. Because of the potential for significant bleeding during excision, vasopressin may be used to maintain hemostasis during the procedure.

BENIGN SOLID TUMORS OF THE VULVA AND VAGINA

There are many benign solid tumors of the vulva and the vagina. Some of the most common include lipomas, hemangiomas, and urethral caruncles. **Lipomas** are soft pedunculated or sessile tumors composed of mature fat cells and fibrous strands. These tumors do not require removal unless they become large and symptomatic. **Hemangiomas** are elevated soft red tumors most commonly found in infants. These tumors may grow rapidly and often ulcerate or bleed secondary to trauma. Most subsequently undergo spontaneous involution over several years. **Urethral caruncles** and **urethral prolapse** present as small, red, fleshy tumors found at the distal urethral meatus. These occur almost exclusively in postmenopausal women as a result of vulvovaginal atrophy. This results in formation of an ectropion at the posterior urethral wall. These lesions are usually asymptomatic and no treatment is required. When bloody spotting results, a short course of systemic or topical estrogens is appropriate. Rarely, surgical excision may be needed.

BENIGN CERVICAL LESIONS

CONGENITAL ANOMALIES

Isolated congenital anomalies of the cervix are rare. In case of a uterine didelphys with a double vagina, a **double cervix** (bicollis) may be found, but this does not arise in isolation. However, women who were exposed **in utero to DES** have some abnormality of the cervix approximately 25% of the time. These benign abnormalities include cervical hypoplasia, cervical collars (Fig. 13-11), cervical hoods, cock's comb appearance, and pseudopolyps. These women are also at increased risk of **cervical insufficiency** in pregnancy. Women who have been exposed to DES in utero are also at increased risk of a very rare **clear cell adenocarcinoma** of the cervix and vagina. This cancer is seen in young women under age 20 but only occurs in 0.1% of DES-exposed patients.

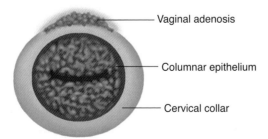

Figure 13-11 • Congenital cervical abnormalities due to in utero DES exposure. Other characteristic DES-associated cervical anomalies include cervical ectropion, cervical ridges, and hypoplastic cervix.
(From Bickley LS, Szilagyi P. *Bates' Guide to Physical Examination and History Taking*, 8th ed. Philadelphia: Lippincott Williams & Wilkins, 2003.)

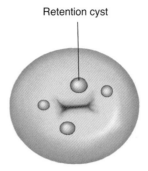

Figure 13-12 • Nabothian cysts of the cervix.
(From Bickley LS, Szilagyi P. *Bates' Guide to Physical Examination and History Taking*, 8th ed. Philadelphia: Lippincott Williams & Wilkins, 2003.)

CERVICAL CYSTS

Most cervical cysts are dilated retention cysts called **nabothian cysts** (Fig. 13-12). These are caused by intermittent blockage of an endocervical gland and usually expand to no more than 1 cm in diameter. Nabothian cysts are more commonly found in menstruating women and are usually asymptomatic. Most often, nabothian cysts are discovered on routine gynecologic examination and require no treatment.

Cervical cysts can also be **mesonephric cysts**. These are remnants of the mesonephric (wolffian) ducts that can become cystic. These cysts differ from nabothian cysts in that they tend to lie deeper in the cervical stroma and on the external surface of the cervix.

Finally, in rare instances, **endometriosis** can implant on or near the cervix. These cysts tend to be red or purple in color and often the patient will have associated symptoms of endometriosis.

CERVICAL POLYPS

True cervical polyps are benign growths that may be pedunculated or broad-based (Fig. 13-13); these can

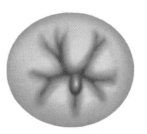

Figure 13-13 • Cervical polyp.
(From Bickley LS, Szilagyi P. *Bates' Guide to Physical Examination and History Taking*, 8th ed. Philadelphia: Lippincott Williams & Wilkins, 2003.)

arise anywhere on the cervix and are often **asymptomatic**. Cervical polyps that do produce symptoms tend to be associated with **intermenstrual or postcoital spotting** rather than pain. Although cervical polyps are not usually considered a premalignant condition, they are generally removed to decrease the likelihood of masking irregular bleeding from another source such as cervical cancer, fibroids, adenomyosis, endometrial polyps, endometrial hyperplasia, and endometrial cancer. Removal of pedunculated cervical polyps is typically quick and easily performed in the office. However, sessile (broad-based) polyps or larger polyps may require removal with electrocautery in the operating room. Hysteroscopy may also be helpful in distinguishing cervical polyps from endometrial polyps.

CERVICAL FIBROIDS

Leiomyomas (myomas or fibroids) are common benign tumors of the uterine corpus but may also arise in the cervix or prolapse into the cervical canal from the endometrial cavity. Leiomyomas can cause symptoms of **intermenstrual bleeding** similar to both uterine fibroids and cervical polyps. Depending on their location and size, these can also cause **dyspareunia** and bladder or rectal pressure. Fibroids of the cervix can cause **problems in pregnancy** and may lead to hemorrhage, poor dilation of the cervix, malpresentation, or obstruction of the birth canal. When evaluating an asymptomatic cervical fibroid, the possibility of cervical cancer should be ruled out, and then the fibroid can be followed with routine gynecologic care. Symptomatic fibroids can be surgically removed but, depending on their location, hysterectomy rather than myomectomy may be required.

CERVICAL STENOSIS

Cervical stenosis can be congenital, a product of **infection**, **atrophy**, **or scarring** (cervical surgical manipulation or radiotherapy). Less frequently, cervical stenosis can result from obstruction with a neoplasm, polyp, or fibroid. Cervical stenosis is typically **asymptomatic** and **does not affect menstruation or fertility**. In these settings, no treatment is indicated. However, if egress from the uterus is completely or partially blocked, oligomenorrhea, amenorrhea, dysmenorrhea, or an enlarged uterus may result. Cervical stenosis can also impede access to the endocervical and endometrial canals for diagnostic and therapeutic procedures. And, it can result in cervical dystocia during labor. When symptoms are present or access to the endocervical or endometrial canals are needed, cervical stenosis can be treated by **gently dilating the cervix**. Prolonged patency can be improved by leaving a catheter in the cervical canal for a few days after the stenosis is relieved. Any obstructive lesions should be removed.

 KEY POINTS

- Labial fusion may be the result of excess androgen exposure or an enzymatic deficiency, most commonly 21-hydroxylase deficiency leading to congenital adrenal hyperplasia and ambiguous external genitalia.
- Patients with imperforate hymen and transverse vaginal septa commonly present with primary amenorrhea at puberty and cyclic abdominal pain. Both can be repaired surgically.
- Vaginal agenesis is seen in MRKH patients who have an absent vagina and partial uterus and tubes. They are genetically female with normal ovarian function and normal secondary sexual characteristics.
- Vulvar itching and lesions can be secondary to a variety of atopic and atrophic skin changes, irritants, and allergens. Lesions can become hypertrophic secondary to chronic irritation and pruritis.

- Diagnosis is made by palpation, colposcopy, and biopsy. Cancer should always be excluded by biopsy.
- Treatment involves hygiene practices, avoidance of irritants, and use of medium- to high-potency topical steroids with a limited role for vaginal estrogens, testosterone, and surgery in the treatment of these disorders.
- A variety of cysts from occlusion of ducts can arise on the vulva, usually from a variety of cysts; and tumors can arise on the vulva and vagina from occlusion of pilosebaceous ducts, sebaceous ducts, and apocrine sweat glands.
- Treatment of benign cystic and solid tumors is only needed if the lesions become symptomatic or infected. This can generally be achieved with incision and drainage or excision.

- Hidradenitis suppurativa is the result of abscess formation from superinfection of apocrine sweat glands and cysts.

- Bartholin's cysts and abscesses are located at 4 o'clock and 8 o'clock on the labia majora. They are usually asymptomatic and resolve on their own.

- When a Bartholin's cyst first appears in a woman over age 40, the cyst wall should be biopsied to rule out the rare possibility of Bartholin's gland carcinoma.

- Large symptomatic Bartholin's cysts and Bartholin's abscesses should be appropriately drained along with placement of a Word catheter or marsupialization. Antibiotics are generally not indicated.

- Congenital anomalies of the cervix are rare and may be associated with abnormalities of the upper genital tract and/or in utero exposure to DES.

- Cervical polyps and fibroids are typically benign and can be removed if symptomatic and to avoid masking bleeding from other sources.

- Cervical stenosis may be congenital or idiopathic or result from scarring from infection or surgical manipulation. When symptomatic, the stenosis can be treated with gentle dilation of the cervical canal.

ANATOMIC ANOMALIES OF THE UTERUS

PATHOGENESIS

All reproductive structures arise from the müllerian system except the ovaries (which arise from the genital ridge) and the lower one-third of the vagina (which arises from the urogenital diaphragm). Specifically, the superior vagina, cervix, uterus, and fallopian tubes are formed by fusion of the **paramesonephric (müllerian) ducts** (see Fig. 13-1). Uterine anomalies arise during embryonic development, generally as a result of incomplete fusion of the ducts, incomplete development of one or both ducts, or degeneration of the ducts (müllerian agenesis). These anomalies (Table 14-1) can vary in scope and severity from the presence of simple septa to bicornuate uterus to complete duplication of the entire female reproductive system (Fig. 14-1). Of the disorders not related to drugs, the most common condition is the **septate uterus** due to malfusion of the paramesonephric ducts. Many anatomic uterine abnormalities may also be associated with **inguinal hernias** and **urinary tract anomalies** (unilateral renal agenesis, pelvic or horseshoe kidneys, or irregularities in the collecting system) (Fig. 14-2).

EPIDEMIOLOGY

Anatomic anomalies of the uterus are extremely rare. Several years ago, the incidence was estimated to be 0.02% of the female population. If estimated today, this percentage would most likely be somewhat higher due to the increased incidence of müllerian anomalies in women who were exposed in utero to **diethylstilbestrol** (DES) from 1940 to 1971 (Fig. 14-3).

CLINICAL MANIFESTATIONS

History

Some uterine anomalies are asymptomatic and may never be discovered, whereas others may not be recognized until the onset of menarche or attempts at childbearing. Some symptoms associated with anomalies of the uterus include dysmenorrhea, dyspareunia, cyclic pelvic pain, infertility, and recurrent miscarriage.

   Uterine septums are positioned vertically and can vary in length and thickness (Fig. 14-1). They are primarily composed of collagen fibers and often lack an adequate blood supply to facilitate placentation and maintain a growing pregnancy. Thus, 25% of women with uterine septums may suffer from recurrent first-trimester **pregnancy loss**. A true **bicornuate uterus** (Fig. 14-1), however, is more commonly complicated by the limited size of the uterine horn (similar to a unicornuate uterus) rather than by blood supply. As such, bicornuate and unicornuate uteri are associated with **second trimester pregnancy loss**, malpresentation, and **preterm labor** and delivery.

Diagnostic Evaluation

The primary investigative tools for uterine abnormalities are pelvic ultrasound, CT, MRI, sonohystogram, hysterosalpingogram, hysteroscopy, and laparoscopy. Keep in mind that uterine septums and bicornuate

■ TABLE 14-1 Classification of Müllerian Anomalies

Class I. Segmented müllerian agenesis or hypoplasia
A. Vaginal
B. Cervical
C. Fundal
D. Tubal
E. Combined
Class II. Unicornuate uterus
A. With a rudimentary horn
1. With a communicating endometrial cavity
2. With a noncommunicating cavity
3. With no cavity
B. Without any rudimentary horn
Class III. Uterus didelphis
Class IV. Bicornuate uterus
A. Complete to the internal os
B. Partial
C. Arcuate
Class V. Septate uterus
A. With a complete septum
B. With an incomplete septum
Class VI. Uterus with internal luminal changes

uteri may appear identical on hysteroscopic evaluation (Fig. 14-4). The two can be better distinguished using MRI or laparoscopy to evaluate the uterine fundus.

Treatment

Many uterine anomalies **require no treatment**. However, when the defect causes significant symptoms such as pain, menstrual irregularities, or infertility, treatment options should be explored. Uterine septa can be excised with operative hysteroscopy once bicornuate uterus has been ruled out. Many women with a bicornuate uterus are able to carry a pregnancy to fruition, although preterm labor and delivery is a significant risk. When a viable pregnancy cannot be achieved in a patient with a bicornuate uterus, viable pregnancies have been achieved with surgical unification procedures. These patients will require delivery via cesarean section to decrease the risk of uterine rupture.

UTERINE LEIOMYOMA

Uterine leiomyomas, also called *fibroids* or *uterine myomas*, are benign **proliferations of smooth muscle cells** of the myometrium. Fibroids typically occur in women of childbearing age and then regress during

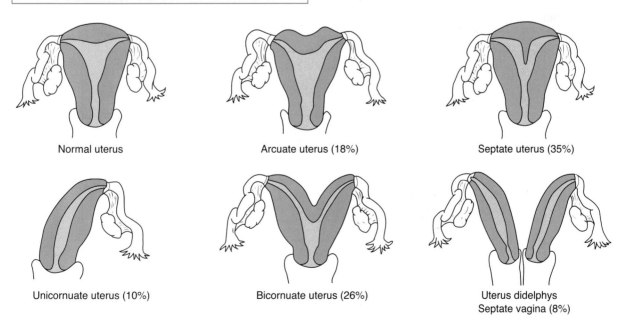

Figure 14-1 • Examples of anatomic anomalies of the uterus. The most common uterine anomalies include arcuate uterus, septate uterus (failure of dissolution of the septum), unicornuate uterus (failure of formation of one müllerian duct), bicornuate uterus (failure of fusion of the mid-müllerian ducts), and uterus didelphys (complete failure of fusion).

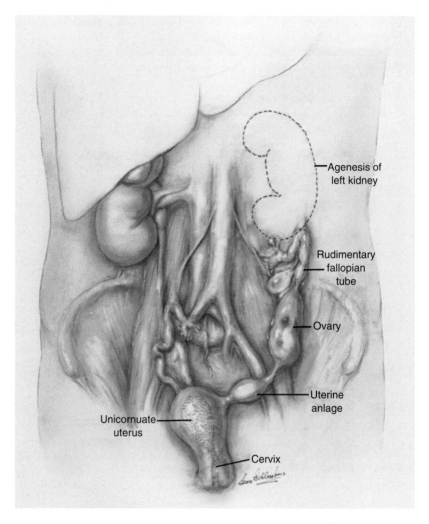

Figure 14-2 • A congenital uterine anomaly (unicornuate uterus) and associated renal anomaly (agenesis of the kidney on the left).
(Image from Rock J, Jones H. *TeLinde's Operative Gynecology,* 10th ed. Philadelphia: Lippincott Williams & Wilkins, 2008.)

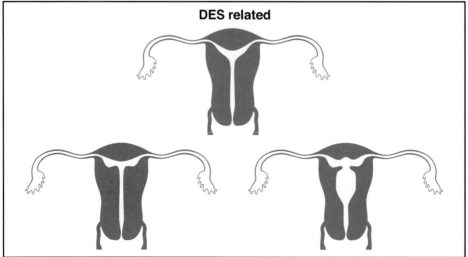

Figure 14-3 • Uterine anomalies associated with in utero DES exposure. Others include hypoplastic uterine cavity, shortened upper uterine segment, and transverse septa. The classic anomaly is a T-shaped uterus.
(From Speroff L, Fritz M. *Clinical Gynecologic Endocrinology and Infertility,* 7th ed. Philadelphia: Lippincott Williams & Wilkins, 2005.)

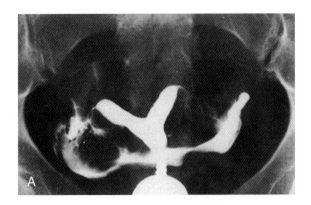

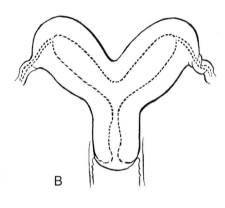
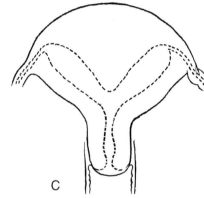

Figure 14-4 • **(A)** A hysterosalpingogram of a double uterus. A bicornuate uterus **(B)** and a septate uterus **(C)** are types of double uteri. Visualization of the fundus is required to determine the type of uterine anomaly.
(Image from Rock J, Jones H. *TeLinde's Operative Gynecology,* 10th ed. Philadelphia: Lippincott Williams & Wilkins, 2008.)

menopause. These benign tumors constitute the **most common indication for surgery** for women in the United States. Approximately one-third of all hysterectomies performed are for uterine fibroids. Most fibroids, however, cause no major symptoms and **require no treatment**. Generally, fibroids only become problematic when their location results in heavy or irregular bleeding or reproductive difficulties. Fibroids may also be identified when they become large enough to cause a mass effect on other pelvic structures resulting in pelvic pain and pressure, urinary frequency, or constipation.

PATHOGENESIS

The cause of uterine leiomyomas is unclear. Fibroids are **monoclonal**, with each tumor resulting from propagation of a single muscle cell. Proposed etiologies include development from smooth muscle cells of the uterus or the uterine arteries, from metaplastic transformation of connective tissue cells, and from persistent embryonic rest cells. Recent studies have identified a small number of genes that mutate in fibroid tissue but not in normal myometrial cells.

Fibroids can vary in size from microscopic to the size of a full-term pregnancy. Fibroids are also **hormonally responsive to estrogen** and progesterone. They can grow quickly and to huge proportions during pregnancy and when exposed to other high levels of endogenous or exogenous estrogens. During menopause, the tumors usually stop growing and may atrophy in response to naturally lower endogenous estrogen levels.

Uterine fibroids are classified by their location in the uterus (Fig. 14-5). The typical classification includes **submucosal** (beneath the endometrium), intramural (in the muscular wall of the uterus), and **subserosal** (beneath the uterine serosa). **Intramural** leiomyomas are the most common type, and submucosal fibroids are commonly associated with heavy or prolonged bleeding. Both submucosal and subserosal fibroids may become pedunculated. A **parasitic** leiomyoma is a pedunculated fibroid that becomes attached to the pelvic viscera or omentum and develops its own blood supply.

Fibroids contain a large quantity of extracellular matrix (fibronectin, collagen, proteoglycan) and are surrounded by a **pseudocapsule** of compressed areolar tissue and smooth muscle cells. This pseudocapsule contains very few blood vessels and lymphatic vessels. This pseudocapsule distinguishes fibroids from adenomyosis, which tends to be more

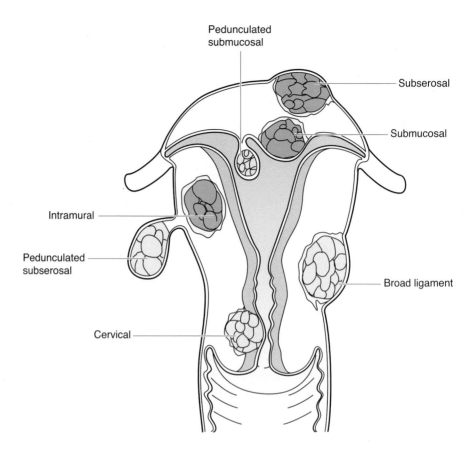

Figure 14-5 • Common locations of uterine fibroids.

diffusely organized in the myometrium (see Chapter 15). As leiomyomas enlarge, they can out-grow their blood supply, infarct, and degenerate, causing pain. Types of **degenerative changes** include hyaline, cystic, red (hemorrhagic), calcific, and sar-comatous. During pregnancy, the growth and de-generation of fibroids can lead to infarction and hemorrhaging (red degeneration) within the tumors in 10% of pregnancies complicated by the presence of fibroids.

It is unclear whether fibroids have any malignant potential. From the available evidence, it is thought that benign leiomyomas and leiomyosarcomas coexist in the same uterus but are independent entities. Leiomyosarcomas are thought to represent separate new neoplasias rather than a degeneration of an exist-ing benign fibroid.

EPIDEMIOLOGY

It is estimated that **30% of all American women** and **50% of African American women** will develop leiomyoma by age 40. African American women are more likely to be younger at the time of diagnosis and have larger fibroids, heavier bleeding, and more se-vere anemia.

RISK FACTORS

Uterine fibroids are more commonly found in African American, nonsmoking, multiparous, peri-menopausal, or hypertensive women. Generally, low-dose oral contraceptive pills are protective against fibroids. The exception to this may be in women who start OCPs between the ages of 13 and 16. The use of hormone replacement in post-menopausal women with fibroids is associated with fibroid growth but typically does not result in clini-cal symptoms.

The incidence of leiomyomas is three to nine times higher in black women in the United States compared to white, Asian, and Hispanic women. There is no known reason for this. The risk of fi-broids is decreased in women who smoke, eat green vegetables or use injectable depot medroxyproges-terone acetate.

CLINICAL MANIFESTATIONS

History

Most women with fibroids (50% to 65%) have **no clinical symptoms**. Of those who do (Table 14-2), **abnormal uterine bleeding** is by far the most common symptom. This is due most commonly to submucosal fibroids impinging on the endometrial cavity (Fig. 14-5). The abnormal bleeding typically presents as increasingly heavy periods of longer duration (**menorrhagia**). Fibroids can also cause spotting after intercourse (postcoital spotting), bleeding between periods (metrorrhagia), or heavy irregular bleeding (menometrorrhagia). Blood loss from fibroids can lead to **chronic iron-deficiency anemia**, dizziness, weakness, and fatigue.

In general, pelvic pain is not usually part of the symptom complex unless vascular compromise is present. This is most common in subserosal pedunculated fibroids. Patients may, however, experience **secondary dysmenorrhea** with menses, particularly when menorrhagia or menometrorrhagia are present. **Pressure-related symptoms** (pelvic pressure, constipation, hydronephrosis, and venous stasis) vary depending on the number and location of leiomyomas. If a fibroid impinges on nearby structures, patients may complain of constipation, urinary frequency, or even urinary retention as the space within the pelvis becomes more crowded.

Uterine myomas are also associated with an increased incidence of infertility but are solely responsible for infertility in only 2% to 10% of cases. Fibroids may distort the endocervical canal, fallopian tubes, or endometrial cavity, thus interfering with conception or implantation and sometimes causing spontaneous abortion. The vast majority of women with fibroids, however, are **able to conceive without any difficulties**. Because fibroids have the potential for excessive growth during pregnancy, they may contribute to intrauterine growth restriction, malpresentation, premature labor, or shoulder dystocia. They may also block the presenting part, necessitating cesarean section.

Physical Examination

Depending on their location and size, uterine leiomyomas can sometimes be palpated on bimanual pelvic examination or on abdominal examination. Bimanual examination often reveals a **nontender irregularly enlarged uterus** with "lumpy-bumpy" or cobblestone protrusions that feel firm or solid on palpation.

DIAGNOSTIC EVALUATION

The differential diagnosis for uterine leiomyoma depends on the patient's symptoms (Table 14-3).

■ **TABLE 14-2** Clinical Symptoms of Uterine Leiomyomas
Bleeding
Longer, heavier periods
Endometrial ulceration
Pressure
Pelvic pressure and bloating
Constipation and rectal pressure
Urinary frequency or retention
Pain
Secondary dysmenorrhea
Acute infarct (especially in pregnancy)
Dyspareunia
Reproductive difficulties
Infertility (failed implantation/spontaneous abortion)
Fetal malpresentation
Intrauterine growth restriction (IUGR)
Premature labor and delivery
Increased cesarean sections

■ **TABLE 14-3** Differential Diagnosis of Uterine Fibroids*
Abnormal bleeding
Adenomyosis
Endometrial polyps
Endometrial hyperplasia
Endometrial cancer
Dysfunctional uterine bleeding (DUB)
Pelvic mass or uterine enlargement
Pregnancy
Adenomyosis
Ovarian cysts
Ovarian neoplasm
Tubo-ovarian abscess
Leiomyosarcoma
*Any of these conditions can coexist with fibroids.

Because most women with leiomyomas are **asymptomatic**, the diagnosis is sometimes made only as an incidental finding.

Pelvic ultrasound is the most common means of diagnosis. Fibroids can be seen as areas of hypoechogenicity among normal myometrial material. Hysterosalpingogram (**HSG**), saline infusion sonogram (**sonohysterogram**), and **hysteroscopy** are additional tools for imaging the location and size of uterine fibroids. In particular, HSG and sonohysterogram can be valuable in identifying submucosal fibroids and in distinguishing fibroids from polyps within the uterine cavity. **MRI** is especially helpful in distinguishing fibroids from adenomyosis (Chapter 15).

TREATMENT

Most cases of uterine fibroids do not require treatment, and **expectant management** is appropriate. However, the diagnosis of leiomyoma must be unequivocal. Other pelvic masses should be ruled out, and the patient with actively growing fibroids should be followed every 6 months to monitor the size and growth.

When leiomyomas result in severe pain, heavy or irregular bleeding, infertility, or pressure symptoms, treatment should be considered. Similarly, when fibroids interfere with examination of the adnexa or when they show evidence of postmenopausal or extremely rapid growth, treatment should be initiated. The choice of treatment depends on the patient's age, pregnancy status, desire for future pregnancies, and size and location of the fibroids.

Medical therapies for leiomyomas, including medroxyprogesterone (Provera), danazol, and gonadotropin-releasing hormone (GnRH) agonists (nafarelin acetate, depot Lupron), have been found to shrink fibroids by **decreasing circulating estrogen levels**. Unfortunately, the tumors usually resume growth after the medications are discontinued. For women nearing menopause, these treatments may be used as a temporizing measure until their own endogenous estrogens decrease naturally. Likewise, **GnRH agonists** may be used to shrink fibroid size, stop bleeding, and increase the hematocrit prior to surgical treatment of uterine fibroids.

Uterine artery embolization (UAE) is being used with greater frequency as a less invasive approach of treating symptomatic fibroids. The procedure is usually preformed by an interventional radiologist who catheterizes the femoral artery under local anesthesia in order to inject an embolizing agent into each uterine artery (Fig. 14-6). The goal is to decrease the blood supply to the fibroid, thereby causing ischemic necrosis, degeneration, and reduction in fibroid size. Because the therapy is not specific to a given fibroid, the blood supply to the

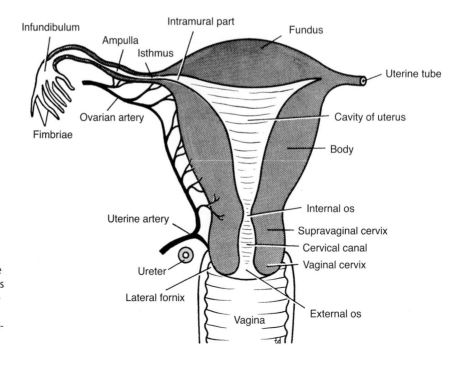

Figure 14-6 • Uterine artery embolization (UAE) for the treatment of uterine fibroids. The uterine artery, shown here, can be catheterized through a femoral approach under fluoroscopy. The catheter is guided to the uterine artery, where polyvinyl alcohol (PVA) microsperes are injected. As a result there is decreased blood flow to the fibroids, causing necrosis and devascularization of the fibroids.

uterus and/or ovaries can be compromised. UAE should not be used in women who are planning to become pregnant after the procedure. Success rates are lower for large and pedunculated fibroids.

One of the newest options for uterine fibroids is the use of **MRI-guided high-intensity ultrasound** (e.g., ExAblate 2000). This uses MRI to locate individual fibroids that are then thermoablated with high-intensity ultrasound waves. The technique is typically reserved for premenopausal women who have completed childbearing and wish to retain their uterus. The procedure can be performed in an outpatient setting but is **expensive and not widely available** at this time.

The indications for surgical intervention for fibroids are listed in Table 14-4. A **myomectomy** is the surgical resection of one or more fibroids from the uterine wall. Myomectomy is usually reserved for patients with symptomatic fibroids who wish to preserve their fertility. Myomectomies can be performed hysteroscopically, laparoscopically, or abdominally. The primary disadvantage of myomectomy is that fibroids **recur in 50% of patients** and adhesions frequently form that may further complicate pain and infertility.

Hysterectomy is the definitive treatment for leiomyomas. Vaginal and laparoscopic hysterectomy can be performed for small myomas and abdominal hysterectomy is generally required for large or multiple myomas. If the ovaries are diseased or if the blood supply has been damaged, then oophorectomy should be performed as well. Otherwise, the ovaries should be preserved in women under age 45 with normal-appearing ovaries. Because of the **potential for hemorrhage**, surgical intervention should be avoided during pregnancy, although myomectomy or hysterectomy may be necessary at some point after delivery.

■ **TABLE 14-4** Indications for Surgical Intervention for Uterine Leiomyomas
Abnormal uterine bleeding, causing anemia
Severe pelvic pain or secondary amenorrhea
Uterine size (>12 weeks) obscuring evaluation of adnexae
Urinary frequency, retention, or hydronephrosis
Growth after menopause
Recurrent miscarriage or infertility
Rapid increase in size

FOLLOW-UP

When hysterectomy is not indicated for a patient with leiomyomas, careful follow-up should take place to monitor the size and location of the tumors. If the size of a fibroid uterus obscures the evaluation of the adnexa, treatment should be recommended. Rapid growth of a tumor in postmenopausal women may be a sign of leiomyosarcoma (extremely rare) or other pelvic neoplasia and should be investigated immediately. **Low-dose oral contraceptives** and hormone replacement therapy at low doses do not appear to pose a risk of recurrence to the patient.

ENDOMETRIAL POLYPS

PATHOGENESIS

Endometrial polyps are benign overgrowths of **endometrial glands and stroma** over a vascular core. These polyps vary in size from millimeters to several centimeters and may be pedunculated or sessile and single or multiple. They are generally within the endometrial cavity but can also prolapse through the endocervical canal.

EPIDEMIOLOGY

The incidence increases with age and they are found most commonly in women **40 to 50 years old**. Women taking **tamoxifen** for breast cancer prevention are at risk of developing endometrial polyps, cysts and cancer.

CLINICAL MANIFESTATIONS

History

Women with endometrial polyps most commonly present with **bleeding between periods** (metrorrhagia) but may also have increasingly heavy menses (menorrhagia) or heavy irregular bleeding (menometrorrhagia).

Diagnostic Evaluation

Ultrasound and sonohysterogram are the best means of evaluation for the presence, size, and number of polyps. As with any other etiology for abnormal bleeding, women 35 or older with abnormal bleeding from endometrial polyps should be evaluated with endometrial biopsy prior to removal.

TREATMENT

Although polyps themselves are benign, they can mask bleeding from another sources such as endometrial hyperplasia without atypia (25%) or endometrial cancer (<1%). For this reason, it is generally recommended that any polyp that is symptomatic or greater than 1 cm in size be removed.

ENDOMETRIAL HYPERPLASIA

PATHOGENESIS

Endometrial hyperplasia is clinically important because it is a **common cause of abnormal uterine bleeding** and because of its link to endometrial cancer. Endometrial proliferation is a normal part of the menstrual cycle that occurs during the follicular (proliferative) estrogen-dominant phase of the cycle. Simple proliferation is an overabundance of histologically normal endometrium.

When the endometrium is exposed to **continuous endogenous or exogenous estrogen stimulation in the absence of progesterone**, simple endometrial proliferation can advance to endometrial hyperplasia. This unopposed estrogen stimulation may be from exogenous or endogenous sources. The most common exogenous source is estrogen hormone replacement without progesterone. In obese women, excess adipose tissue results in increased **peripheral conversion of androgens** (androstenedione and testosterone) to estrogens (estrone and estradiol) by aromatases in the adipocytes. This excess endogenous estrogen stimulation can then stimulate overgrowth of the endometrium resulting in endometrial hyperplasia and even cancer.

Endometrial hyperplasia is the abnormal proliferation of both the **glandular and stromal elements** of the endometrium. In its earliest stages, the stimulation results in changes to the organization of the glands (Fig. 14-7). In its later, more severe forms, the stimulation results in atypical changes in the cells themselves. The changes do not necessarily involve the entire endometrium, but rather may develop **focal patches** among normal endometrium. If left untreated, endometrial hyperplasia can progress to **endometrial carcinoma** (Fig. 14-7) and can also coexist alongside endometrial carcinoma.

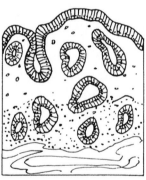

Simple
hyperplasia

Figure 14-7 • Endometrial histology: hyperplasia to carcinoma. Simple hyperplasia without atypia and complex hyperplasia without atypia both represent architectural changes in the endometrium (e.g., crowding of glands) whereas simple or complex hyperplasia with atypia and endometrial carcinoma both demonstrate cytologic (cellular) abnormalities as well as architectural changes.
(From Beckmann C, Ling F. *Obstetrics & Gynecology,* 5th ed. Philadelphia: Lippincott Williams & Wilkins, 2006.)

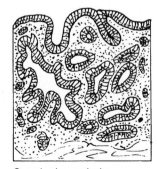

Complex hyperplasia

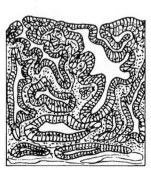

Atypical complex

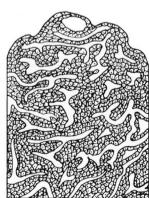

Cancer of the endometrium

■ TABLE 14-5 Classification of Endometrial Hyperplasia and Progression to Endometrial Cancer

Architectural Type	Cytologic Atypia	Progression to Endometrial Cancer (in %)
Simple hyperplasia	Absent	1
Complex hyperplasia	Absent	3
Atypical simple hyperplasia	Present	8
Atypical complex hyperplasia	Present	29

The histologic variations of endometrial hyperplasia and their rates of progression to cancer are outlined in Table 14-5. When only **architectural changes** (changes in the complexity and crowding of the glandular components of the endometrium) are present, the hyperplasia is known as either simple or complex. When **cytologic atypia** (changes in the cellular structure of the endometrial cells) is present, then the hyperplasia is said to be either *atypical* simple or *atypical* complex **hyperplasia**. These cytologic changes include large nuclei with lost polarity, increased nuclear-to-cytoplasmic ratios, prominent nuclei, and irregular clumped chromatin. As noted in Table 14-5, atypical hyperplasia carries a higher risk of **progression to endometrial cancer** and may have **coexistent endometrial cancer** as often as 17% to 52% of the time.

1. **Simple hyperplasia** is the simplest form of hyperplasia. It represents an abnormal proliferation of both the stromal and glandular endometrial elements. Less than 1% of these lesions progress to carcinoma.
2. **Complex hyperplasia** consists of abnormal proliferation of the glandular endometrial elements without proliferation of the stromal elements. In these lesions, the glands are crowded in a back-to-back fashion and are of varying shapes and sizes, but **no cytologic atypia is present**. Approximately 3% of these lesions progress to carcinoma if left untreated.
3. **Atypical simple hyperplasia** involves cellular atypia and mitotic figures in addition to glandular crowding and complexity. These lesions progress to carcinoma in about 8% of cases if untreated.

4. **Atypical complex hyperplasia** is the most severe form of endometrial hyperplasia. It progresses to carcinoma in approximately 29% of untreated cases.

EPIDEMIOLOGY

Endometrial hyperplasia typically occurs in the menopausal or perimenopausal woman, but may also occur in premenopausal women who have prolonged **oligomenorrhea and/or obesity**.

RISK FACTORS

Patients at risk for endometrial hyperplasia, like those at risk for endometrial carcinoma, are at risk due to **unopposed estrogen exposure** (Table 14-6). This includes women with obesity, nulliparity, late menopause, and exogenous estrogen use without progesterone. Chronic anovulation, polycystic ovarian syndrome, and estrogen-producing tumors such as granulosa-theca cell tumors also put women at increased risk for endometrial hyperplasia. Both **hypertension** and **diabetes mellitus** are independent risk factors for endometrial hyperplasia.

CLINICAL MANIFESTATIONS

History

Patients with endometrial hyperplasia typically present with long periods of **oligomenorrhea** or amenorrhea followed by irregular or excessive uterine bleeding. **Uterine bleeding** in a postmenopausal woman should raise high suspicion of endometrial hyperplasia or carcinoma (Chapter 29).

■ TABLE 14-6 Risk Factors for Endometrial Hyperplasia

Chronic anovulation
Obesity
Nulliparity
Late menopause (> age 55)
Exogenous estrogen use without progesterone
Diabetes mellitus
Hypertension
Tamoxifen use

Physical Examination

Occasionally, the uterus will be enlarged from endometrial hyperplasia. This is attributed to both the increase in the mass of the endometrium and to the growth of the myometrium in response to continuous estrogen stimulation. More commonly, the **pelvic exam is unremarkable**. Patients may also have stigmata associated with chronic anovulation such as abdominal **obesity, acanthosis, acne, or hirsutism**.

Diagnostic Evaluation

Pelvic ultrasound may reveal a thickened endometrial stripe that might be suggestive of endometrial hyperplasia. However, **tissue diagnosis is required** for the diagnosis of endometrial hyperplasia. Although dilation and curettage (D&C) was once the gold standard for sampling the endometrium, **endometrial biopsies** enjoy a 90% to 95% accuracy rate without the operative and anesthetic risks. Given this, endometrial biopsies have thus become the **method of choice** for evaluation of abnormal uterine bleeding including that from endometrial hyperplasia. However, when an office biopsy cannot be obtained due to insufficient tissue, patient discomfort, or cervical stenosis, then D&C is required to rule out endometrial hyperplasia and carcinoma, except in women under age 35. D&C is also recommended in patients who have atypical complex hyperplasia on biopsy because approximately 29% of those patients will have a coexistent endometrial carcinoma.

TREATMENT

The treatment of endometrial hyperplasia depends on the histologic variant of the disease and on the age of the patient. Simple, complex, atypical simple, and atypical complex hyperplasia can all be treated medically with **progestin therapy**. Progestins reverse endometrial hyperplasia by activating progesterone receptors, resulting in stromal decidualization, and thinning of the endometrium. Typically, injectable (Depo-Provera) or oral (Provera) **medroxyprogesterone** or other oral progestins such as megestrol (Megace) or norethindrone (Aygestin) are used in doses that will inhibit and eventually reverse the endometrial hyperplasia. **Micronized vaginal progesterone** (Prometrium) and the **levonorgestrel intrauterine system** (Mirena) are alternative dosing modalities. The progestin is usually administered for 3 months and then a repeat endometrial biopsy is performed to evaluate for regression of disease. The progestin therapy may be repeated if residual disease is found on repeat biopsy.

Instead of progestin therapy, patients without cytologic atypia (i.e., those with simple or complex hyperplasia) may be managed with D&C with or without hysteroscopy. These patients should also be reevaluated with endometrial sampling every 3 to 6 months.

Atypical complex hyperplasia is often treated surgically by hysterectomy given the significant (29%) risk of having coexistent endometrial cancer or developing endometrial cancer. Most women with atypical complex hyperplasia are either perimenopausal or postmenopausal. However, in younger patients with atypical complex hyperplasia and chronic anovulation who wish to preserve fertility, endometrial curettage, longer-term progestin management, weight loss, and ovulation induction may assist patients in becoming pregnant.

OVARIAN CYSTS

PATHOGENESIS

In general, ovarian masses can be divided into functional cysts and neoplastic growths. Benign and malignant neoplasms of the ovary are discussed in detail in Chapter 30. **Functional cysts** of the ovaries result from normal physiologic functioning of the ovaries (Chapter 20) and are divided into follicular cysts and corpus luteum cysts.

Follicular cysts are the most common functional cysts. They arise after failure of a follicle to rupture during the follicular maturation phase of the menstrual cycle. Functional cysts may vary in size from 3 to 8 cm and are classically asymptomatic and usually unilateral (Color Plate 9). Large follicular cysts can cause a tender palpable ovarian mass and can lead to ovarian torsion when greater than 4 cm in size. Most follicular cysts resolve spontaneously in 60 to 90 days.

Corpus luteum cysts are common functional cysts that occur during the luteal phase of the menstrual cycle. Most corpus luteum cysts are formed when the corpus luteum fails to regress after 14 days, becomes enlarged (>3 cm) or hemorrhagic (corpus hemorrhagicum). These cysts can cause a delay in menstruation and dull lower quadrant pain. Patients with a ruptured corpus luteum cyst can present with acute pain and signs of hemoperitoneum late in the luteal phase.

Theca lutein cysts are large bilateral cysts filled with clear, straw-colored fluid. These ovarian cysts result from stimulation by abnormally high β-human chorionic gonadotropin (e.g., from a molar pregnancy, choriocarcinoma, or ovulation induction therapy).

EPIDEMIOLOGY

Seventy-five percent of ovarian masses in women of reproductive age are **functional cysts** and 25% are nonfunctional neoplasms. Although functional ovarian cysts can be found in females of any age, they most commonly occur between puberty and menopause. Women who smoke have a twofold increase for functional cysts.

CLINICAL MANIFESTATIONS

History

Patients with functional cysts present with a variety of symptoms depending on the type of cyst. Follicular cysts tend to be **asymptomatic** and only occasionally cause menstrual disturbances such as prolonged intermenstrual intervals or short cycles. Larger follicular cysts can cause aching **pelvic pain**, dyspareunia, and ovarian torsion. Corpus luteum cysts may cause local pelvic pain and either amenorrhea or delayed menses. Acute abdominal pain may result from a **hemorrhagic corpus luteum cyst**, a torsed ovary, or a ruptured follicular cyst.

Physical Examination

The findings on bimanual pelvic examination vary with the type of cyst. Follicular cysts tend to be less than 8 cm and simple or unilocular in structure. Lutein cysts are generally larger than follicular cysts and often feel firmer or more solid on palpation. A ruptured cyst can cause pain on palpation, acute abdominal pain, and rebound tenderness. When an ovarian cyst results in a torsed adnexa, the classic presentation is **waxing and waning pain and nausea**.

Diagnostic Evaluation

After a thorough history and physical, the primary diagnostic tool for the workup of ovarian cyst is the **pelvic ultrasound**. Ultrasonography allows for better characterization of the cyst that can guide the workup and treatment. Because most functional cysts will spontaneously resolve over 60 to 90 days, **serial ultrasounds** may be used to check for cyst resolution. A

CA-125 level is often obtained from patients who are at high risk for ovarian cancer. This should be used solely as a means of evaluating the treatment response to chemotherapy and not as a diagnostic or screening test per the American College of Obstetrics and Gynecology (ACOG) guidelines (see Chapter 30).

The **differential diagnoses** for ovarian cysts include ectopic pregnancy, pelvic inflammatory disease, torsed adnexa, tubo-ovarian abscess, endometriosis, fibroids, and ovarian neoplasms.

Treatment

Treatment of ovarian cysts depends on the age of the patient and the characteristics of the cyst. Table 14-7 outlines the management options using these criteria. In general, a palpable ovary or adnexal mass in a **premenarchal or postmenopausal** patient is suggestive of an ovarian neoplasm rather than a functional cyst and exploratory laparotomy is in order. Likewise, reproductive-age women with cysts larger than 8 cm or that **persist for longer than 60 days** or that are solid or complex on ultrasound probably do not have a functional cyst. These lesions should be closely investigated with diagnostic laparoscopy or laparotomy.

For patients of reproductive age with cysts less than 6 cm in size, **observation** with a **follow-up**

■ **TABLE 14-7** Management of a Cystic Adnexal Mass		
Age	**Size of Cyst (cm)**	**Management**
Premenarchal	>2	Exploratory laparotomy
Reproductive	<6	Observe for 8 to 12 weeks, then repeat ultrasound
	6 to 8	Observe if unilocular; explore if multilocular or solid on ultrasound
	>8	Exploratory laparoscopy/laparotomy for ovarian cystectomy
Postmenopausal	Palpable	Exploratory laparoscopy/laparotomy for ovarian oophorectomy

ultrasound is the appropriate action. Most follicular cysts should resolve spontaneously within 60 to 90 days. During this observation period, patients are often started on **oral contraceptives**. This is not a treatment for existing cysts but rather to suppress ovulation in order to prevent the formation of future cysts. Cysts that do not resolve within 60 to 90 days require evaluation with **cystectomy** and (rarely) oophorectomy via laparoscopy or laparotomy.

KEY POINTS

- Anatomic anomalies of the uterus are extremely rare and result from problems in the fusion of the paramesonephric (müllerian) ducts. Therefore, they are often associated with urinary tract anomalies and inguinal hernias.

- If present, symptoms include amenorrhea, dysmenorrhea, cyclic pelvic pain, infertility, recurrent pregnancy loss, and premature labor.

- Anomalies are diagnosed using physical exam, pelvic ultrasound, CT, MRI, hysterosalpingogram, hysteroscopy, and laparoscopy.

- Both septated uteri and bicornuate uteri can be treated surgically if symptomatic.

- Fibroids are benign, estrogen-sensitive, smooth muscle tumors of unclear etiology found in 20% to 30% of reproductive-age women.

- Fibroid incidence is three to nine times higher in black women compared to white, Asian, and Hispanic women. Risk is also increased in obese, nonsmoking, and perimenopausal women.

- Fibroids may be submucosal, intramural, or subserosal and can grow to great size, especially during pregnancy. They are asymptomatic in 50% to 65% of patients; when symptomatic, they can cause heavy or prolonged bleeding (most common), pressure, pain, and infertility (rare).

- Fibroids are typically diagnosed by pelvic ultrasound. In most cases, no treatment is necessary. However, they can be treated temporarily with Provera, danazol, or GnRH analogs to decrease estrogen and shrink the tumors, or myomectomy to resect the tumors when future fertility is desired.

- Fibroids are treated definitively by hysterectomy in the case of severe pain, when large or multiple, when causing urinary symptoms, or when evidencing postmenopausal or rapid growth.

- Endometrial hyperplasia is classified as simple or complex if only architectural alterations (glandular crowding) exist or as atypical simple or atypical complex if cytologic (cellular) atypia is also present.

- It is caused by prolonged exposure to exogenous or endogenous estrogen in the absence of progesterone. Risk factors include chronic anovulation, obesity, nulliparity, late menopause, and unopposed estrogen use.

- Risk of malignant transformation is 1% in simple hyperplasia, 3% in complex hyperplasia, 8% in atypical simple hyperplasia, and 29% in atypical complex hyperplasia.

- Endometrial hyperplasia is diagnosed by endometrial biopsy or D&C and it is usually treated medically with progestin therapy for 3 months, followed by resampling of the endometrium.

- The risk of atypical complex hyperplasia progressing to endometrial cancer is 29%. Thus, the recommended treatment for atypical complex hyperplasia is hysterectomy.

- Follicular cysts result from unruptured follicles. These are usually asymptomatic unless torsion occurs. Management includes observation for 8 to 12 weeks with or without oral contraceptives, followed by repeat pelvic ultrasound.

- Corpus luteum cysts result from an enlarged and/or hemorrhagic corpus luteum. These may cause a missed period or dull lower quadrant pain. When ruptured, these cysts can cause acute abdominal pain and intra-abdominal hemorrhage. Corpus luteum cysts should resolve spontaneously or may be suppressed with oral contraceptives if recurrent.

- The differential diagnoses for ovarian cysts include ectopic pregnancy, pelvic inflammatory disease, torsed adnexa, tubo-ovarian abscess, endometriosis, fibroids, and ovarian neoplasms.

- Any palpable ovarian or adnexal mass in a premenarchal or postmenopausal patient is suggestive of ovarian neoplasm and should be investigated with exploratory laparoscopy or laparotomy.

- Cysts that do not resolve spontaneously in 60 to 90 days require further evaluation and treatment with cystectomy or oophorectomy (rarely) via laparoscopy or laparotomy.

Endometriosis and Adenomyosis

ENDOMETRIOSIS

PATHOGENESIS

Endometriosis is the presence of endometrial tissue **(glands and stroma)** outside the endometrial cavity. Endometrial tissue can be found anywhere in the body, but the most common sites are the ovary and the pelvic peritoneum. Endometriosis in the ovary appears as a cystic collection known as an **endometrioma**. Other common sites are in the most dependent parts of the pelvis including the uterosacral ligaments, the anterior and posterior cul-de-sacs, and the posterior uterus and broad ligaments (Fig. 15-1). Although not commonly found, endometriosis has been identified in the lung and brain.

There are three main theories about the etiology of endometriosis. The Halban theory proposes that endometrial tissue is transported via the **lymphatic system** to various sites in the pelvis, where it grows ectopically. Meyer proposes that multipotential cells in peritoneal tissue undergo **metaplastic transformation** into functional endometrial tissue. Finally, Sampson suggests that endometrial tissue is transported through the fallopian tubes during **retrograde menstruation**, resulting in intra-abdominal pelvic implants.

Endometrial implants cause symptoms by disrupting normal tissue, forming adhesions and fibrosis, and causing severe inflammation. Interestingly, the **severity of symptoms does not necessarily correlate with the amount of endometriosis**. Women with widely disseminated endometriosis or a large endometrioma may experience little pain, whereas women with minimal disease in the cul-de-sac may suffer severe pain.

EPIDEMIOLOGY

The incidence of endometriosis is estimated to be between 10% and 15%. Because **surgical confirmation** is necessary for the diagnosis of endometriosis, the true prevalence of the disease is unknown. It is found almost exclusively in women of reproductive age, and is the single most common reason for hospitalization of women in this age group. Approximately 20% of women with **chronic pelvic pain** and 30% to 40% of women with **infertility** have endometriosis.

RISK FACTORS

Women with **first-degree relatives** (mother or sisters) with endometriosis are seven times more likely to develop the disorder than women without this risk factor. A relationship has also been demonstrated between endometriosis and some autoimmune disorders (e.g., lupus). For unclear reasons, endometriosis is identified less often in black women.

CLINICAL MANIFESTATIONS

History

The hallmark of endometriosis is **cyclic pelvic pain** beginning 1 or 2 weeks before menses, **peaking 1 to 2 days before the onset of menses**, and subsiding at the onset of flow or shortly thereafter. Women with chronic endometriosis and teenagers with endometriosis may not demonstrate this classic pain pattern. Other symptoms associated with endometriosis are **dysmenorrhea, dyspareunia, abnormal bleeding, and**

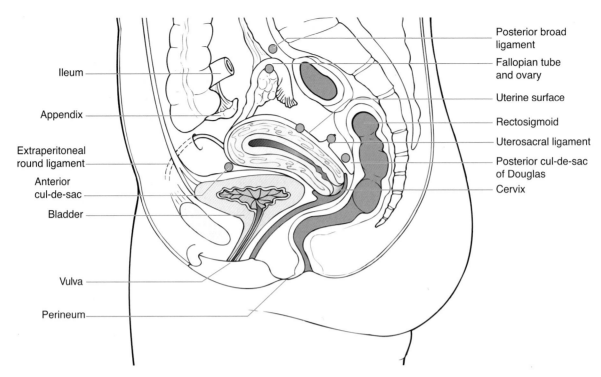

Figure 15-1 • Potential sites for endometriosis. The most common sites (indicated by blue dots) include the ovaries, the uterosacral ligaments, the anterior and posterior cul de sacs, and the posterior uterus and posterior broad ligaments.

infertility. Endometriosis is one of the most common diagnoses in the evaluation of infertility.

Symptoms of endometriosis vary depending on the area involved. Dysmenorrhea usually begins in the third decade, worsens with age, and should be considered in women who develop dysmenorrhea after years of pain-free cycles. Dyspareunia is usually associated with deep penetration that can aggravate endometrial lesions in the cul-de-sac or on the uterosacral ligaments.

Endometriosis is also a cause of **infertility**. Although the exact mechanism is unclear, endometriosis is thought to cause **dense adhesions** which can distort the pelvic architecture, interfere with tubal mobility, and cause tubal obstruction.

Physical Examination

The physical findings associated with early endometriosis may be **subtle or nonexistent**. To maximize the likelihood of physical findings, the physical exam should be performed during early menses when implants are likely to be largest and most tender. When more disseminated disease is present, the clinician may find **uterosacral nodularity** on rectovaginal examination or a **fixed retroverted uterus**. When the ovary is involved, a tender, fixed **adnexal mass** may be palpable on bimanual examination or viewed on pelvic ultrasound (Fig. 15-2).

Diagnostic Evaluation

The only way to definitively diagnose endometriosis is through **direct visualization** with laparoscopy or laparotomy. Endometrial implants may appear as rust-colored to dark brown powder burns or raised, blue-colored mulberry or raspberry lesions. The areas may be surrounded by reactive fibrosis that can lead to dense adhesions in extensive disease. The ovary itself can develop large cystic collections of endometriosis filled with thick, dark, old blood known as endometriomas or **chocolate cysts** (Fig. 15-3). **Peritoneal biopsy** is not necessary but is helpful in histologically confirming the diagnosis of endometriosis.

Once the diagnosis of endometriosis is confirmed, the anatomic location and extent of the disease can be used to properly classify the operative findings. The American Fertility Society's revised classification

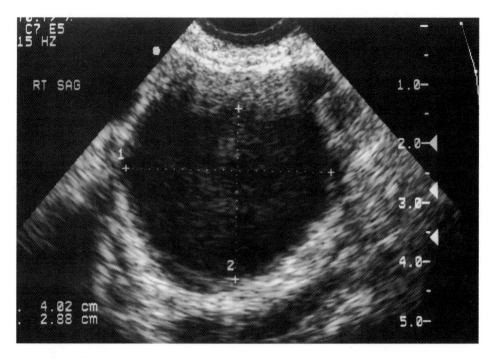

Figure 15-2 • Transvaginal ultrasound of an endometrioma of the ovary. Note the characteristic "ground glass" appearance of the endometrioma on ultrasound.
(From Berek, JS. *Berek & Novak's Gynecology*, 14th ed. Philadelphia: Lippincott Williams & Wilkins, 2006.)

schema is reproduced in Table 15-1. Although not commonly used, this classification method uses a point system to stage endometriosis based on the location, depth, and diameter of lesions and density of adhesions.

DIFFERENTIAL DIAGNOSIS

The differential diagnosis for endometriosis includes other processes that result in recurrent pelvic pain such as pelvic inflammatory disease, recurrent acute

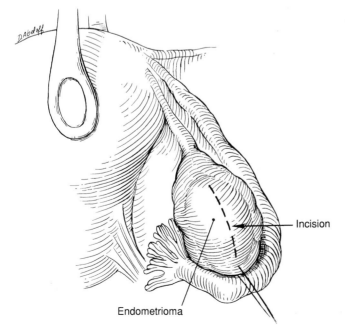

Incision

Endometrioma

Figure 15-3 • Endometrioma.
(From LifeART image copyright © 2006 Lippincott Williams & Wilkins. All rights reserved.)

■ TABLE 15-1 Classification of Endometriosis

Tube	American Society for Reproductive Medicine Revised Classification of Endometriosis		
	Patient's name _____ Date _____ Stage I (minimal) 1 to 5 Stage II (mild) 6 to 15 Laparoscopy _____ Laparotomy _____ Photography _____ Stage III (moderate) 16 to 40 Recommend treatment _____ Stage IV (severe) >40 _____ Total _____ Prognosis _____		

Ovary		Endometriosis	<1 cm	1 to 3 cm	<3 cm
		Superficial	1	2	4
		Deep	2	4	6
	R	Superficial	1	2	4
		Deep	4	16	20
	L	Superficial	1	2	4
		Deep	4	16	20
		Posterior Cul-de-sac Obliteration	Partial		Complete
			4		40

Ovary		Adhesions	<1/3 Enclosure	1/3 to 2/3 Enclosure	>2/3 Enclosure
	R	Filmy	1	2	4
		Dense	4	8	16
	L	Filmy	1	2	4
		Dense	4	8	16
	R	Filmy	1	2	4
		Dense	4*	8*	16
	L	Filmy	1	2	4
Peritoneum		Dense	4*	8*	16

*If the fimbriated end of the fallopian tube is completely enclosed, change the point assignment to 16.
Denote appearance of superficial implant types as red ([R], red, red-pink, flamelike, vesicular blobs, clear vesicles), white ([W], opacifications, peritoneal defects, yellow-brown), or black ([B] black, hemosiderin deposits, blue). Denote percent of total described as R__%, W__%, and B__%. Total should equal 100%.

salpingitis, adenomyosis, fibroids, adhesions, hemorrhagic corpus luteum cysts, ectopic pregnancy, and ovarian neoplasms.

TREATMENT

The treatment choice for patients with endometriosis depends on the extent and location of disease, the severity of symptoms, and the patient's desire for future fertility. **Expectant management** may be used in patients with minimal or nonexistent symptoms and in patients **actively attempting to conceive**. For other patients, both surgical and medical options are available. In the case of severe or chronic endometriosis, a multidisciplinary approach incorporating medical and surgical management as well as pain center involvement and psychiatric support may provide the most comprehensive care.

Medical treatment for endometriosis is aimed at **suppression and atrophy of the endometrial tissue**. Although medical therapies can be quite effective, these are **temporizing measures** rather than permanent treatments because the endometrial implants and symptoms often recur following cessation of treatment. **There is no role for medical management in patients attempting to conceive.** Medical management does not improve conception rates and only serves to delay attempts at conception and/or employment of surgical treatments that have been shown to improve conception rates.

Current medical regimens for the treatment of endometriosis include **NSAIDs**, either continuous or cyclic administration of **oral contraceptives**, and the use of **progestins** (oral and IM medroxyprogesterone, megestrol [Megace]). These treatments induce a state of "**pseudopregnancy**" by suppressing both ovulation and menstruation and by decidualizing the endometrial implants, thereby alleviating the cyclic pelvic pain and dysmenorrhea. This therapy is believed best for patients with mild endometriosis who are not currently seeking to conceive.

Patients can also be placed in a reversible state of **pseudomenopause** with the use of danazol (Danocrine), an androgen derivative, or gonadotropin-releasing hormone (GnRH) agonists such as leuprolide acetate (Lupron) and nafarelin (Synarel). Both classes of drugs suppress follicle-stimulating hormone (FSH) and luteinizing hormone (LH). As a result, the ovaries do not produce estrogen, which would normally stimulate endometrial implants. Subsequently, existing endometrial **implants atrophy**, and new implants are **prevented**.

Side effects associated with OCPs and progestin agents include irritability, depression, breakthrough bleeding, and bloating. The drawback to danazol is that patients may experience some **androgen-related, anabolic side effects** including acne, oily skin, weight gain, edema, hirsutism, and deepening of the voice. GnRH agonists such as Lupron result in **estrogen deficiency**. The side effects of these medications are similar to those seen during menopause including hot flashes, decreased bone density, headaches, and vaginal atrophy and dryness. Moreover, these treatments can be costly and often have limited insurance coverage. Therefore, the use of these medications is generally limited to 6 months.

Fortunately, newer treatment regimens known as **add-back therapy** have been designed for use in conjunction with GnRH agonists. These regimens add a small amount of estrogen to the GnRH agonist to minimize the symptoms caused by estrogen deficiency such as hot flashes and bone density loss. With add-back therapy, the patient receives the benefits of the GnRH agonist (endometriosis suppression and relief of pelvic pain and dysmenorrhea) while the small dose of estrogen minimizes the adverse effects of hypoestrogenation.

Surgical treatment for endometriosis can be classified as either conservative or definitive. **Conservative surgical therapy** typically involves laparoscopy and fulguration of any visible endometrial implants. Endometriomas are best treated using laparoscopic cystectomy with removal of as much of the cyst wall as possible (Fig. 15-4). With conservative therapy, the uterus and ovaries are left in situ to allow for future fertility. For these, the pregnancy rate after conservative surgical treatment depends on the extent of the disease at the time of surgery (Table 15-2). For patients with pain who do not desire immediate pregnancy, pain control can be optimized and recurrences delayed by starting or **restarting medical therapy immediately after surgical treatment.**

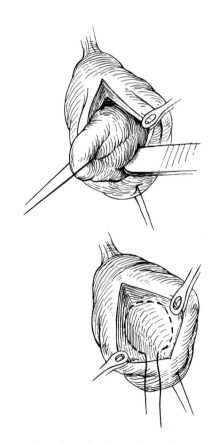

Figure 15-4 • Resection of endometrioma. The cyst wall is removed and the ovarian defect is closed or left to heal spontaneously.
(From LifeART image copyright © 2006 Lippincott Williams & Wilkins. All rights reserved.)

■ **TABLE 15-2** Conception Rates after Ablation of Endometrial Implants		
Extent of Disease	**Stage of Disease**	**Conception Rates (in %)**
Mild	1 & 2	75
Moderate	3	50 to 60
Severe	4	30 to 40

Definitive surgical therapy includes total abdominal hysterectomy and bilateral salpingo-oophorectomy (TAHBSO), lysis of adhesions, and removal of endometriosis lesions. This therapy is reserved for cases in which childbearing is complete and for women with severe disease or symptoms that are refractory to conservative medical or surgical treatment.

ADENOMYOSIS

PATHOGENESIS

Adenomyosis is an **extension of endometrial tissue into the uterine myometrium** (Fig. 15-5). In the past, adenomyosis was referred to as *endometriosis interna*.

This terminology is no longer used because adenomyosis and endometriosis are two distinct and different clinical entities (Table 15-3).

The cause of adenomyosis is not known. The current theory is that high levels of estrogen stimulate **hyperplasia of the basalis layer of the endometrium**. For unknown reasons, the barrier between the endometrium and myometrium is broken and the endometrial cells can then invade the myometrium. Because this disease occurs most frequently in parous women, it is thought that subclinical endomyometritis may be the first insult to the endometrial-myometrial barrier and eventually predisposes the myometrium to subsequent invasion.

Adenomyosis causes the uterus to become diffusely enlarged and globular due to **hypertrophy and hyperplasia** of the myometrium *adjacent to* the ectopic endometrial tissue. The disease is usually most extensive in the **fundus and posterior uterine wall**. Because the endometrial tissue in adenomyosis extends from the basalis layer of the endometrium, it does not undergo the proliferative and secretory changes traditionally seen in normally located endometrium or in endometriosis. Thus, unlike endometriosis, which contains both glandular and stromal endometrial tissue, adenomyosis is **not generally responsive to regulation with OCPs or other hormonal treatments**.

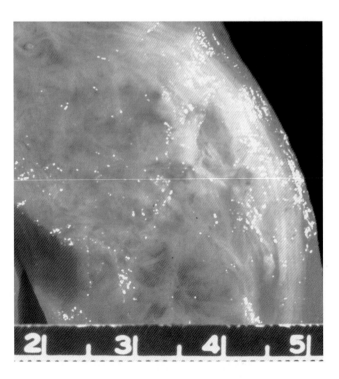

Figure 15-5 • Adenomyosis.
(From Rubin E, Farber JL. *Pathology*, 3rd ed. Philadelphia: Lippincott Williams & Wilkins, 1999.)

■ TABLE 15-3 Terminology of Endometriosis	
Adenomyosis	An extension of endometrial tissue into the uterine myometrium leading to menorrhagia or metromenorrhagia. The uterus becomes soft, globular. The definitive treatment is hysterectomy.
Adenomyoma	A well-circumscribed collection of endometrial tissue within the uterine wall. They may also contain smooth muscle cells and are not encapsulated. Adenomyomas can also extend into the endometrial cavity in the form of a polyp.
Endometriosis	The presence of endometrial cells outside the endometrium. The hallmark of the disorder is cyclic pelvic pain. These estrogen-sensitive lesions can be treated with NSAIDs, OCPs, progestins, GnRH agonists, or surgery.
Endometrioma	A cystic collection of endometrial cells on the ovary; also known as "chocolate cysts."
Leiomyoma	Local proliferations of smooth muscle cells within the uterus, often surrounded by a pseudocapsule. Also known as fibroids, these benign growths may be located on the intramural, subserosal, or submucosal portion of the uterus.

Adenomyosis may also present as a well-circumscribed, isolated region known as an **adenomyoma**. Adenomyomas contain smooth muscle cells as well as endometrial glands and stroma. These nodular growths may be located in the myometrium or extend into the endometrial cavity. Unlike uterine fibroids, which have a characteristic pseudocapsule, individual areas of adenomyosis are not encapsulated. Instead, adenomyosis can infiltrate throughout the myometrium giving the uterus a characteristic boggy feel on palpation.

EPIDEMIOLOGY

The incidence of adenomyosis is 15%. The disease generally develops in parous women in their late 30s or early 40s. It occurs very infrequently in nulliparous women.

RISK FACTORS

Adenomyosis, endometriosis, and uterine fibroids frequently coexist. About 15% to 20% of patients with adenomyosis also have **endometriosis**, and 50% to 60% of patients with adenomyosis also have **uterine fibroids**. Patients with dyspareunia, dyschezia, and menorrhagia or menometrorrhagia have an increased probability of having adenomyosis.

CLINICAL MANIFESTATIONS

History

Thirty percent of patients with adenomyosis are **asymptomatic** or have symptoms minor enough that medical attention is not sought. Symptomatic adenomyosis occurs most often in parous women between age 35 and 50. When symptoms do occur, the most common are **secondary dysmenorrhea** (30%), **menorrhagia** (50%), or both (20%). Patients typically present with increasingly heavy or prolonged menstrual bleeding (menorrhagia). They may also complain of increasingly severe dysmenorrhea that may begin up to 1 week before menses and last until cessation of bleeding. Other patients may only experience pressure on the bladder or rectum due to an enlarged uterus.

Physical Examination

The pelvic examination of a patient with adenomyosis may reveal a **diffusely enlarged globular uterus**. The uterus can be 2 to 3 times normal size but is usually <14 cm. The consistency of the uterus is typically softer and boggier than the firmer, rubbery uterus containing fibroids. The adenomyomatous uterus may be mildly tender just before or during menses but should have normal mobility and no associated adnexal pathology.

DIAGNOSTIC EVALUATION

MRI is the most accurate imaging tool for identifying adenomyosis. However, because the cost of MRI can be prohibitive, pelvic ultrasound is usually the initial imaging modality. MRI is then used if adenomyosis is suggested by **pelvic ultrasound**, most typically to distinguish adenomyosis from uterine fibroids. Ultimately, hysterectomy is the only definitive means of diagnosing adenomyosis.

DIFFERENTIAL DIAGNOSIS

The differential diagnosis for adenomyosis includes disease processes resulting in uterine enlargement, menorrhagia, and/or dysmenorrhea including uterine fibroids, polyps, menstrual disorders, endometrial hyperplasia, endometrial cancer, pregnancy, and adnexal masses.

TREATMENT

Prior to treating adenomyosis, any patient or older age 35 with irregular menses should have an endometrial biopsy and TSH to rule out other causes for irregular menses. The treatment for adenomyosis depends on the severity of the dysmenorrhea and menorrhagia.

Women with minimal symptoms or those near menopause may be managed with analgesics alone. Nonsteroidal anti-inflammatory drugs (**NSAIDs**), oral contraceptive pills (**OCPs**), and menstrual suppression with **progestins** (oral, injectable, or intrauterine) or **continuous OCPs** have also been found to be helpful.

Hysterectomy is the only definitive treatment for adenomyosis. Endometrial biopsy should be performed to rule out concomitant endometrial hyperplasia or carcinoma before a hysterectomy is performed for adenomyosis. Prior to the surgery, it also is particularly important to distinguish adenomyosis from uterine fibroids. If adenomyosis is mistaken for uterine fibroids, a surgeon attempting a myomectomy may find only diffuse adenomyosis and be forced to perform a hysterectomy instead without prior informed consent.

KEY POINTS

- Endometriosis is the presence of endometrial tissue outside the endometrial cavity, most often in the ovary or pelvic peritoneum. It occurs in 10% to 15% of women of reproductive age.

- The hallmark of endometriosis is cyclic pelvic pain which is at its worst 1 to 2 days before menses, and subsides at the onset of flow or shortly thereafter.

- The severity of symptoms of (dysmenorrhea, dyspareunia, abnormal bleeding, and infertility) may not correlate with extent of disease.

- Complications of endometriosis include intra-abdominal inflammation and bleeding that can cause scarring, pain, and adhesion formation, which can lead to infertility and chronic pelvic pain.

- Direct visualization with diagnostic laparoscopy or laparotomy is the only way to definitively diagnose endometriosis.

- Endometriosis can be treated medically (NSAIDs, OCPs, progestins, danazol, GnRH agonists) to reduce pain, but these methods are used mainly as temporizing agents.

- There is no role for the use of medical management in patients trying to conceive or those diagnosed with infertility.

- Endometriosis can be treated surgically with conservative therapy to ablate implants and adhesions, thereby preserving the potential for future fertility. Surgery should be followed immediately by medical therapy.

- Endometriosis can be treated definitively with surgery, including TAHBSO, lysis of adhesions, and removal of endometriosis lesions.

- Adenomyosis is the extension of endometrial tissue into the myometrium, making the uterus diffusely enlarged, boggy, and globular. It occurs in 15% of women, most of whom are parous and in their late 30s or early 40s.

- Patients typically present with increasing secondary dysmenorrhea and/or menorrhagia; 30% of patients are asymptomatic.

- Adenomyosis may be suggested on pelvic U/S. MRI can best distinguish between adenomyosis and fibroids. Patients age 35 and older with irregular menses should also have an endometrial biopsy to rule out hyperplasia and cancer.

- Minimal symptoms may be treated with analgesics, NSAIDs, OCPs, or progestins although adenomyosis is less responsive to hormonal management than endometriosis.

- Hysterectomy is the only definitive means of diagnosing and treating adenomyosis.

Infections of the Lower Female Reproductive Tract

URINARY TRACT INFECTIONS

One of the most common infections of the lower genitourinary tract treated by clinicians is the common **urinary tract infection** (UTI). Women commonly present with symptoms of urethritis (discomfort or pain at the urethral meatus or a burning sensation throughout the urethra with micturition) or cystitis (pain in the midline suprapubic region and/or frequent urination). UTIs are most common in sexually active women, and increased in women with diabetes mellitus and sickle-cell disease. They are diagnosed at a rate of about 1% per year in adult women, although the true rate of occurrence is most likely higher. The rates are higher in women than men secondary to the shorter length of the urethra and its proximity to the vagina and rectum.

DIAGNOSIS

When a woman presents with dysuria and urinary frequency, the diagnosis of UTI should lead the differential. The urine can be sent for urinalysis and sediment. Hematuria, leukocytes, leukocyte esterase, or nitrates in the absence of a vaginal infection are indicative of a UTI. If the sediment has a high bacterial count without the presence of inflammatory cells, this is most likely contamination. To distinguish contamination from true infection, the urinalysis and sediment can be repeated with urine collected via catheterization. Patients are often diagnosed and treated for UTI in the setting of a positive urinalysis with concomitant symptoms of dysuria and urinary frequency once **pyelonephritis** is ruled out with evaluation for fevers and costovertebral angle tenderness (CVAT). The diagnosis can be confirmed with a urine culture. The common organisms that cause UTIs include bacteria that colonize the GI tract such as *E. coli* and *S. saprophyticus*. Other common organisms that cause UTIs are *P. mirabilis*, *K. pneumoniae*, and *Enterococcus*. If the urine culture is negative, the diagnosis should be reconsidered. In patients with symptoms consistent with urethritis, organisms such as *C. trachomatis* and *N. gonorrhoeae* should be considered and screened for using a midstream collection. Another etiology of urethritis is herpes simplex virus (HSV) infection. In patients with symptoms of cystitis, but a negative culture, the diagnosis of interstitial cystitis should be entertained.

TREATMENT

Most uncomplicated UTIs can be treated with oral antibiotics. It is important to both begin treatment on initial diagnosis as well as follow-up culture sensitivities to be certain the pathologic organisms are treated adequately. Initial treatment is often begun with ampicillin, trimethoprim-sulfamethoxazole, macrodantin, or cephalexin. However, the local sensitivities of common organisms should be known. For example, the rates of ampicillin-resistant *E. coli* can range from

5% to 35% in different hospitals. More aggressive treatment of UTIs may use fluoroquinolones such as ciprofloxacin. Patients with symptoms consistent with pyelonephritis are usually admitted and treated in hospital with IV antibiotics. Outpatient management has been studied and is used increasingly in reliable patients without other medical issues.

THE EXTERNAL ANOGENITAL REGION

Various infectious diseases affect the external genitalia. In the female patient, the entire perianal area and mons should be considered in addition to the vulva. The skin overlying these areas is subject to the same infections that can occur anywhere on the epidermis, but the exposure and environment differ and must be considered when discussing these infections. There are also a variety of focal and systemic processes that can cause lesions or symptoms in this region. Anogenital lesions are usually categorized as ulcerative or nonulcerative, and common symptoms include pain and itching.

VULVITIS

The most common cause of vulvitis, and usually of vulvar pruritus, is **candidiasis**. It is also a common cause of vaginitis and is discussed in greater detail later in this chapter. A candidal vulvitis usually presents with vulvar erythema, pruritus, and small satellite lesions. If the vulvitis does not respond to the usual treatment with topical or systemic antifungals, symptoms may be due to other causes such as allergic reaction, chemical or fabric irritants, and vulvar dystrophies. Malignancy should always be ruled out in the setting of chronic vulvar irritation.

ULCERATED LESIONS

Many primary vulvar ulcers are caused by sexually transmitted infections (STIs) (Table 16-1) such as **herpes**, **syphilis**, **chancroid**, and **lymphogranuloma venereum**. However, even with a diagnosis of an infectious process, these lesions can be associated with malignant processes as well.

There are conditions other than infections that can lead to vulvar ulcerations. Crohn disease can have linear "knife cut" vulvar ulcers as its first manifestation, preceding gastrointestinal or other systemic manifestations by months to years. Behçet disease leads to tender and highly destructive vulvar lesions that often cause fenestrations in the labia and extensive scarring.

SYPHILIS

The spirochete *Treponema pallidum* causes the chronic systemic infection of **syphilis**. It is transmitted primarily through sexual contact. The incidence of primary and secondary syphilis in the United States increased through the 1980s until 1990, when the CDC noted a peak of 50,578 reported cases followed by a sharp decline to 8,550 cases reported in 1997 and only 5,979 cases reported in 2000. During this time, there was a concomitant decrease in latent syphilis as well, although at a slower rate of decline. Currently, the incidence is decreasing in both heterosexual men and

■ **TABLE 16-1** Infectious Causes of Ulcerated Lesions				
	Syphilis	**Herpes**	**Chancroid**	**LGV**
Incubation period	7 to 14 days	2 to 10 days	4 to 7 days	3 to 12 days
Primary lesion	Papule	Vesicle	Papule/pustule	Papule/vesicle
Number of lesions	Single	Multiple	1 to 3, occasionally more	Single
Size	5 to 15 mm	1 to 3 mm	2 to 20 mm	2 to 10 mm
Painful	No	Yes	Yes	No
Diagnostic test	Dark-field microscopy RPR/ MHA-TP/FTA-ABS	Viral culture	Gram's stain with "school of fish" appearance	Complement fixation
Treatment	Penicillin	Acyclovir	Ceftriaxone or azithromycin	Doxycycline

women with a decline among the gay population as well, likely secondary to increased safe sexual practices directed at decreasing human immunodeficiency virus (HIV) transmission.

T. pallidum most likely enters the body through minute abrasions in the skin or mucosal surface and replicates locally. Initial lesions therefore commonly occur on the vulva, vagina, cervix, anus, nipples, or lips. The initial lesion that characterizes the primary stage is a painless, red, round, firm ulcer approximately 1 cm in size with raised edges known as a **chancre** (Fig. 16-1). It develops approximately 3 weeks after inoculation and is usually associated with concomitant regional adenopathy. Material expressed from the chancre usually reveals motile spirochetes under dark-field microscopy.

The secondary stage of syphilis occurs as *T. pallidum* disseminates. Between 1 and 3 months after the primary stage resolves, the secondary stage appears as a maculopapular rash and/or moist papules on the skin or mucous membranes. Classically, the rash appears on the palms of the hands or soles of the feet. The dermatologic manifestations of secondary syphilis are why syphilis is known as the "great imitator." There may be other organ system involvement with meningitis, nephritis, or hepatitis. All lesions resolve spontaneously, and this stage can be entirely asymptomatic. After resolution of this stage, the infection enters a latent phase that can last for years.

Tertiary syphilis is quite uncommon today but is characterized by granulomas (gummas) of the skin

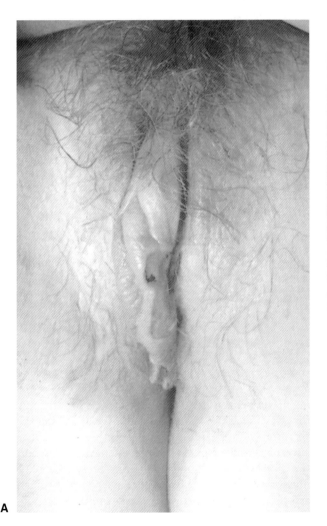

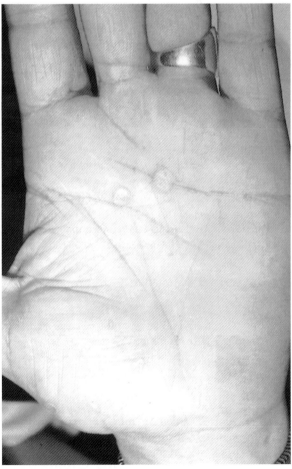

A   B

Figure 16-1 • (A) Slightly indurated primary chancre of 2-days' duration that was neither painful nor tender. It points to the need for a high index of suspicion concerning all genital lesions. Dark-filled microscopy prevents diagnostic error and embarrassment. **(B)** Papulosquamous secondary syphilis involving the palm. *(continued)*

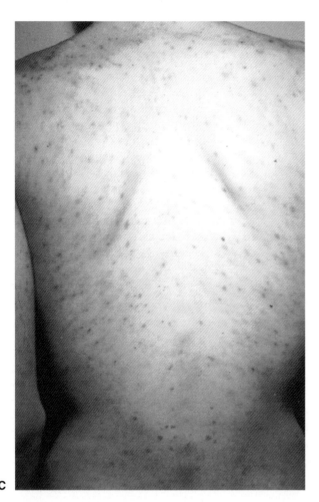

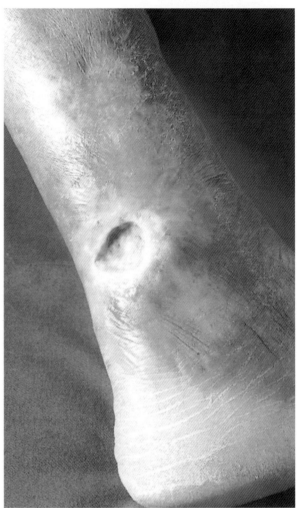

C

D

Figure 16-1 • *(continued)* **(C)** Typical coppery-red papules in secondary syphilis. **(D)** Healing gumma. Delay in diagnosis is suggested by widespread pigmentation and scarring. Response to treatment was slow and the final scarring led to permanent edema of the foot, sometimes called *paradoxical healing*.
(Reproduced with permission from Champion RH. *Textbook of Dermatology*, 5th ed. Oxford: Blackwell Science, 1992:2852.)

and bones; cardiovascular syphilis with aortitis; and neurosyphilis with meningovascular disease, paresis, and tabes dorsalis.

Diagnosis

Screening for *T. pallidum* may be performed with nontreponemal anticardiolipin antibodies. Two types of nontreponemal serologic tests for syphilis are available: the Venereal Disease Research Laboratory (VDRL) test and the Rapid Plasma Reagin (RPR) test. These tests remain positive for 6 to 12 months after treatment of primary syphilis, usually with progres-

sively decreasing titers. In primary syphilis, serologic assays may be negative during early infection, resulting in a lower sensitivity. These tests will become positive several weeks after the initial visit, and should therefore be repeated 1 and 3 months after appearance of the ulcer in the compliant patient in whom the diagnosis cannot be made at first presentation. Of note, the RPR test is now available as a point-of-care assay, a screening tool particularly useful in populations where follow-up is not optimal. A positive result must be confirmed with specific treponemal antibody studies, such as the fluorescent treponemal antibody absorption (FTA-ABS) test and the *Treponema pal-*

lidum particle agglutination assay (TPPA). The microhemagglutination test for antibodies to *Treponema pallidum* (MHA-TP) is no longer available in the United States. False-positive results in confirmatory testing occur less than 1% of the time. Primary, secondary, tertiary, and neurosyphilis can be diagnosed by the presenting signs and symptoms described above. However, patients who are asymptomatic with a positive titer are considered to be in early latent (acquired less than 1 year) or late latent (acquired >1 year) syphilis.

Treatment

Penicillin remains the drug of choice for treatment of syphilis. Primary, secondary, or early latent syphilis can be treated with benzathine penicillin G, 2.4 million units IM one time. For late latent (acquired more than 1 year's duration) or latent of unknown duration syphilis, treatment consists of penicillin G 2.4 million units IM weekly for 3 weeks. Alternative regimens to penicillin, in penicillin-allergic patients, for example, include tetracycline 500 mg orally four times a day or doxycycline 100 mg orally twice a day for 2 weeks, or ceftriaxone 1 g IM or IV daily for 8 to 10 days, or even azithromycin 2 g single oral dose. However, data to support use of alternative regimens in nonpregnant patients is still limited. If compliance is of concern in penicillin-allergic individuals, then desensitization and treatment with penicillin are recommended. Penicillin remains the only recommended treatment in pregnancy, with sufficient evidence demonstrating efficacy for preventing maternal syphilis transmission to the fetus and for treating fetal infection.

Neurosyphilis is a more serious infection and requires aqueous crystalline penicillin G, 3 to 4 million units intravenously every 4 hours for 10 to 14 days. In individuals in whom compliance may be ensured, procaine penicillin 2.4 million units IM once daily plus probenecid 500 mg orally four times a day both for 10 to 14 days is recommended as a treatment alternative for neurosyphilis. Some authorities further recommend following the recommended or alternative neurosyphilis treatment with benzathine penicillin 2.4 million units weekly IM for 3 weeks after completion of either regimen. Patients with a penicillin allergy in whom compliance issues are of concern will therefore require desensitization. Treatment success can be verified by following RPR or VDRL titers at 6, 12, and 24 months. Titers should decrease fourfold by 6 months and become nonreactive by 12 to 24 months after completion of treatment.

The Jarisch-Herxheimer reaction is an acute febrile reaction frequently accompanied by fever, chills, headache, myalgia, malaise, pharyngitis, rash, and other symptoms that usually occur within the first 24 hours (generally within the first 8 hours) after any therapy for syphilis. This reaction was initially recognized in the treatment of neurosyphilis, but can be seen with any syphilitic treatment, most commonly with early syphilis (up to 90% of patients with secondary syphilis). Antipyretics may be used, but they have not been proven to prevent this reaction. The Jarisch-Herxheimer reaction might induce preterm contractions or cause fetal distress in pregnant women, but this should not prevent or delay therapy. This transient inflammatory reaction is not considered a drug reaction, but is related to the treatment of syphilis, and can be seen with the treatment of other spirochetes as well, such as Lyme disease, when injured or dead organisms release endotoxins into the circulation marked by systemic release of cytokines.

GENITAL HERPES

HSV infections are quite common in the perioral and genital regions. Although only about 5% of women report a history of genital herpes infection, as many as 25% to 30% have antibodies on serologic testing. Although some women have the classic severe presentation of genital herpes with painful genital ulcers, many women have a mild initial presentation or are entirely asymptomatic. Because of the asymptomatic nature of many initial presentations it is difficult to get an estimate on the true incidence of disease; however, there has been a steady increase in patient visits to a clinician for herpes over the past two decades, with approximately 200,000 office visits in 2000. Although the majority of genital herpes lesions are caused by HSV-2, up to 30% to 40% of new cases of genital HSV are attributable to HSV-1. Primary infections usually begin with flulike symptoms including malaise, myalgias, nausea, diarrhea, and fever. Vulvar burning and pruritus precede the multiple vesicles that appear next and usually remain intact for 24 to 36 hours before evolving into painful genital ulcers (Fig. 16-2). These ulcers can require a mean of 10 to 22 days to heal. After this initial herpes outbreak, recurrent episodes can occur as frequently as one to six times per year. Because of the possibility of frequent recurrence and the devastating consequences of neonatal herpes, pregnant women should have vaginal examinations around the time of delivery. Those with lesions should be delivered by cesarean delivery.

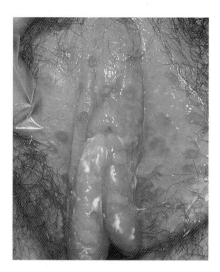

Figure 16-2 • Genital herpes.

Diagnosis

Clinical diagnosis is often made with an examination of the vesicles and ulcers in conjunction with a sexual history. However, this modality has suboptimal sensitivity and specificity. Therefore, clinical diagnosis should be confirmed with laboratory testing. Viral cultures are used as the gold standard for diagnosis; however, sensitivity of culture is low, especially in recurrent or healing lesions. Although DNA PCR assays for HSV are more sensitive than culture, they are not FDA approved and many laboratories may not have this testing capacity. A **Tzanck smear** prepared of the lesions and examined for multinucleated giant cells with a characteristic appearance may reveal typical cytologic changes, but this study is also neither sensitive nor specific. Alternatively, type-specific antibodies for HSV-1 and HSV-2 IgG may be used to determine whether the patient has a primary infection as well as the serotype of the causative organism.

Treatment

Although many palliative treatments have evolved over the years such as sitz baths for comfort and analgesics to reduce the pain, there is no cure for herpes. For a **primary infection**, acyclovir 200 mg five times per day, acyclovir 400 mg three times per day, famiciclovir 250 mg three times per day, or valacyclovir 1 g twice per day orally for 7 to 10 days are recommended therapies in treatment of first clinical outbreak reducing the length of infection and the

length of time a patient has viral shedding. With severe HSV infections, such as those that occur in immunocompromised patients, intravenous acyclovir should be used at a dose of 5 mg/kg every 8 hours. Oral acyclovir 400 mg three times daily or 800 mg twice daily for 5 days may be used for treatment of recurrent lesions. For individuals with frequent recurrences, prophylactic or suppression therapy of 400 mg orally twice daily is recommended. Alternate more costly antiviral medications may also be used, such as valacyclovir, particularly for easier dosing regimens. Additionally, daily treatment with valacyclovir 500 mg daily in the infected partner has been demonstrated to decrease the rate of HSV-2 transmission in discordant, heterosexual couples in which the source partner has a history of genital HSV-2 infection.

CHANCROID

Chancroid is caused by *Haemophilus ducreyi*. Globally, it is a common STI, although the incidence in North America has declined steadily since 1987, with just 78 reported cases in 2000. Reported cases are likely to grossly underestimate true incidence since *H. ducreyi* is difficult to culture. Males are affected more than females by ratios of 3:1 to 25:1. Chancroid is a cofactor for HIV transmission; high rates of HIV infection among patients who have chancroid occur in the United States and other countries. Additionally, approximately 10% of persons who have chancroid that was acquired in the United States are coinfected with *T. pallidum* or HSV.

Chancroid appears as a painful, demarcated, non-indurated ulcer located anywhere in the anogenital region. There is often concomitant painful suppurative inguinal lymphadenopathy. Usually, just a single ulcer is present, but multiple ulcers and occasionally extragenital infections have been known to occur.

Diagnosis

Diagnosis is a challenge because *H. ducreyi* is difficult to culture. A definitive diagnosis of chancroid requires the identification of *H. ducreyi* on special culture media that are not widely available from commercial sources; even when these media are used, sensitivity is <80%. Often, transporting the culture swab in Amies or Stuart transport media or chocolate agar can aid in the culture. Direct Gram's stains have not been a consistent method of diagnosis, and FDA-approved PCR test for *H. ducreyi* are also not available in the United States. The diagnosis is therefore often made clinically by ruling out other sources of infection.

Treatment

Treatment regimens include ceftriaxone 250 mg intramuscularly once, azithromycin 1 g orally once, ciprofloxacin 500 mg orally twice a day for 3 days, or erythromycin 500 mg four times a day for 7 days. As with most other STIs, sexual partners should be treated as well.

LYMPHOGRANULOMA VENEREUM

The *Chlamydia trachomatis* L-serotypes (L1, L2, or L3) cause the systemic disease **lymphogranuloma venereum** (LGV). The primary stage of this illness is often a local lesion that may be either a papule or a shallow ulcer, and is often painless, transient, and can go unnoticed. The secondary stage (inguinal syndrome) is characterized by painful inflammation and enlargement of the inguinal nodes. Systemic manifestations include fever, headaches, malaise, and anorexia. The tertiary stage (anogenital syndrome) of this disease is characterized by proctocolitis, rectal stricture, rectovaginal fistula, and elephantiasis (lymphatic filariasis). Initially, an anal pruritus will develop with a concomitant mucous rectal discharge. Although diagnosis is generally made per clinical suspicion, genital and lymph node specimens may be tested for *C. trachomatis* by culture, direct immunofluorescence, or nucleic acid detection.

Treatment

Treatment of LGV includes doxycycline 100 mg orally twice a day or erythromycin 500 mg orally four times a day for 21 days. With persistent illness, the antibiotic regimen can be repeated. If the external genitalia and rectum are disfigured and scarred, surgical measures may be required.

NONULCERATIVE LESIONS

One of the most common nonulcerative lesions is the condyloma (Fig. 16-3). **Condyloma acuminata** are warty lesions that occur anywhere in the anogenital region and are considered an STI. Other nonulcerative lesions include **molluscum contagiosum**, caused by a pox virus, and lesions caused by *Phthirus pubis*, the crab louse, and *Sarcoptes scabiei*, the itch mite.

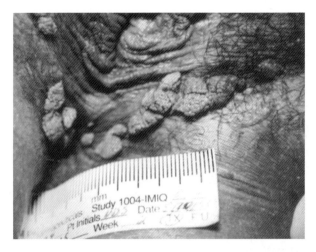

Figure 16-3 • Extensive external condylomata acuminata. These fleshy, exophytic growths are covered with small, papillary surface projections. Some of the lesions are pedunculated; others are sessile.
(Reproduced with permission from Blackwell RE. *Women's Medicine.* Cambridge: Blackwell Science, 1996:317.)

Finally, when considering nonulcerative lesions, folliculitis should always be included in the differential diagnosis because the skin in the pubic region has hair follicles. In rare cases, folliculitis can lead to larger lesions such as boils, carbuncles, and abscesses. The usual source of these infections is skin flora, primarily *Staphylococcus aureus*. Factors contributing to these lesions in the anogenital region include tight undergarments, sanitary pads, poor hygiene, diabetes, and immunosuppression.

HUMAN PAPILLOMAVIRUS

The most clinically evident results of infection with human papillomavirus (HPV) are **condyloma acuminata** or **genital warts**. The annual incidence of genital warts is estimated to be over 1:1,000. However, of more significance in terms of morbidity and mortality, HPV is associated with cervical cancer and other squamous cell malignancies of the female and male reproductive tracts. It is estimated that the incidence of HPV has been increasing in the United States, with an estimated prevalence between 20% and 45%. It is clearly an STI with 60% to 80% of partners being affected.

Although genital warts often occur throughout the lower reproductive tract, patients usually present with anogenital lesions that they have identified or that have become pruritic or caused bleeding. Condyloma acuminata are most commonly caused by serotypes 6 and 11, whereas cervical cancer is more often associated with serotypes 16, 18, and 31. HPV testing is not indicated for patients with genital warts.

Diagnosis

Diagnosis of condyloma acuminata is usually made via clinical examination. The wart has a raised papillomatous or spiked surface. Initially, the lesions are small, 1 to 5 mm diameter lesions, but these can evolve into larger pedunculated lesions and eventually into cauliflower-like growths, particularly in immunocompromised patients. In addition to the vulva, perineal body, and anogenital region, these lesions can also arise in the anal canal, on the walls of the vagina, and on the cervix. When uncertain of diagnosis or for lesions that are unresponsive to therapy, a biopsy of the lesion can be made for definitive diagnosis.

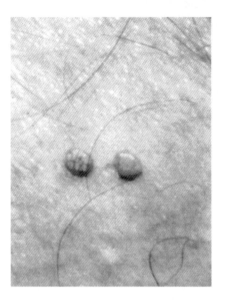

Figure 16-4 • Two typical molluscum lesions, one of which shows a mosaic appearance.

Treatment

Treatment of the lesions includes local excision, cryotherapy, topical trichloroacetic acid, topical 25% podophyllin, and 5-fluorouracil cream (Efudex 5%). The medical treatments are usually repeated weekly by the clinician until all lesions are gone. For motivated patients with uncomplicated condyloma that can be reached, both imiquimod (Aldara) and podofilox (Condylox) can be used. Imiquimod is used three times per week and needs to be washed off after 6 to 10 hours, whereas podofilox is applied twice a day for 3 days and left in place followed by no treatment for 4 days; this therapy regimen may be repeated up to 4 cycles. These patients can self-treat and follow up with clinicians every 3 to 4 weeks until the lesions have resolved. For larger condylomas or those unresponsive to medical treatment, the CO_2 laser may be used to vaporize the lesion. Regardless of treatment modality, a recurrence rate of approximately 20% is seen in all patients.

MOLLUSCUM CONTAGIOSUM

Molluscum contagiosum is caused by a pox virus that is spread via close contact with an infected person or via autoinoculation. The lesion is a small, 1 to 5 mm, domed papule with an umbilicated center (Fig. 16-4). Also known as *water warts*, these lesions contain a waxy material that reveals intracytoplasmic molluscum bodies under microscopic examination when stained with Wright stain or Giemsa stain. Molluscum lesions can occur anywhere on the skin except on the palms of the hands and soles of the feet. These lesions are often asymptomatic and generally resolve on their own. Diagnosis is generally made clinically; however, diagnosis my be confirmed with lesion biopsy for histologic or electron microscopic examination. These can be removed via local excision and/or treatment of the nodule base with trichloroacetic acid or cryotherapy.

PHTHIRUS PUBIS AND *SARCOPTES SCABIEI*

The nonulcerative lesions caused by ***Phthirus pubis***, the crab louse, and ***Sarcoptes scabiei***, the itch mite, are similar. Signs and symptoms of these two infections include pruritis, irritated skin, vesicles, and burrows. The primary difference is that lesions from *P. pubis*, or **pediculosis**, are usually confined to the pubic hair, whereas **scabies** may spread throughout the entire body. Thus, treatment is site specific: pediculosis can be cured with therapy application to specific areas, whereas it is more effective to treat scabies by applying treatment over the entire body. Pediculosis pubis is generally sexually transmitted. Treatment includes permethrin 1% cream rinse applied to affected areas and washed off after 10 minutes or pyrethrins with piperonyl butoxide applied to the affected area and washed off after 10 minutes.

Scabies is commonly sexually transmitted in adults and transmitted by direct contact in children. Treatment for scabies includes permethrin cream (5%) applied to all areas of the body from the neck down and washed off after 8 to 14 hours or ivermectin 200 µg/kg orally, repeated in 2 weeks.

VAGINAL INFECTIONS

Symptoms related to vaginal infections are the leading cause of visits to a gynecologist. The vagina provides a warm, moist environment that can be colonized by various organisms. Imbalance of microflora in the vagina caused by antibiotics, diet, systemic illness; the introduction of a pathogen; or the overgrowth of one variety of organism can lead to symptoms including itching, pain, discharge, burning, and odor. Common organisms that cause symptoms with overgrowth include *Candida* (Fig. 16-5) and *Gardnerella*; the most common pathogenic protozoan is *Trichomonas*. These can each be easily diagnosed and treated quite effectively with antimicrobials. However, any chronic vaginitis with pruritis, pain, bleeding, and/or ulcerated lesions that do not respond to drug therapy should be investigated to rule out malignancy.

BACTERIAL VAGINOSIS

The vagina is commonly colonized with multiple bacteria, predominantly *Lactobacillus* sp. that generally maintain the vaginal pH below 4. **Bacterial vaginosis** (BV) can develop when there is a shift in the pre-

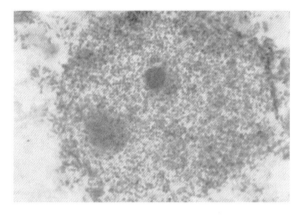

Figure 16-6 • Bacterial vaginosis.

dominant bacterial species in the vagina. Although bacterial vaginosis is likely to be polymicrobial, one of the most common organisms present in culture is *Gardnerella vaginalis*. BV is quite common and is the leading cause of vaginitis, with prevalence rates of 5% of college populations and as high as 60% in STI clinics. Risk factors include new or multiple sexual partners, douching, lack of vaginal lactobacilli, and cigarette smoking. BV is particularly concerning during pregnancy, where it has been associated with preterm birth.

Diagnosis

Many patients with BV may be asymptomatic or have an isolated increase in vaginal discharge. However, symptomatic patients complain of a profuse nonirritating discharge, often with a malodorous fishy amine odor. Diagnosis can be made with three of the following findings: presence of thin, white, homogeneous discharge coating the vaginal walls; an amine odor noted with addition of 10% KOH ("whiff" test); pH of >4.5; or presence of clue cells (vaginal epithelial cells that are diffusely covered with bacteria) on microscopic examination. Gram's stain with examination of bacteria in the vaginal discharge is considered the gold standard diagnostic test for BV.

Performance of vaginal culture for *G. vaginalis*, *Bacteroides*, and other anaerobes is generally not recommended as this is not a specific diagnostic method. Therefore, the clinical diagnosis is usually made from vaginal preps.

Treatment

Treatment of BV is usually with either metronidazole 500 mg orally twice a day for 7 days or clindamycin

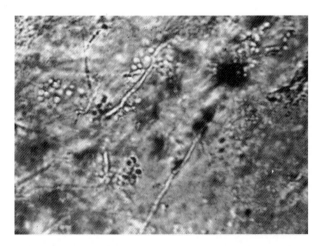

Figure 16-5 • *Candida albicans*, KOH mount of skin scraping. (Reproduced with permission from Crissey JT. *Manual of Medical Mycology.* Boston: Blackwell Science, 1995:90.)

300 mg three times a day for 7 days. Both antibiotics are also available in gel or cream and can be used topically (metronidazole gel 0.75% one applicator intravaginally daily for 5 days or clindamycin cream 2% one applicator intravaginally daily for 7 days). A metronidazole 2 g single dose therapy has been studied. However, it is less than 75% effective in BV when compared to 85% to 90% cure rates for the week-long treatment. Patients should be advised to avoid alcohol consumption during metronidazole treatment due to its antabuse effect.

YEAST INFECTIONS

Candidiasis probably causes 30% of the vaginitis that leads women to be seen by a gynecologist. Many more of these infections are treated by women using over-the-counter (OTC) preparations. Candidiasis is caused by *Candida albicans* in 80% to 90% of all cases, with the remaining cases caused by other candidal species. Predisposing factors for candidal overgrowth include the use of broad-spectrum antibiotics, diabetes mellitus, and decreased cellular immunity as seen in AIDS patients or those on immunosuppressive therapies. Yeast infections are also associated with intercourse and may increase during the late luteal phase of the menstrual cycle.

Diagnosis

Typical symptoms of genital candidiasis include vulvar and vaginal pruritus, burning, dysuria, dyspareunia, and vaginal discharge. On physical examination there is vulvar edema and erythema with a scant vaginal discharge. Only approximately 20% of patients display the characteristic white plaques adherent to the vaginal mucosa or the cottage cheese–like discharge. Diagnosis is usually made by microscopic examination of a 10% KOH preparation of the vaginal discharge which improves visualization of characteristic branching hyphae and spores compared to saline preparation alone. However, the KOH preparation is estimated to have a sensitivity of 25% to 80%. Other diagnostic options include the Gram's stain and culture. Clinically, treatment is often instituted on the basis of clinical signs and symptoms. In recurrent vaginal yeast infection cases (>4 symptomatic episodes in 1 year), vaginal culture should be obtained to identify non-*albicans* species such as *C. glabrata* that may be less responsive to azole therapy.

Treatment

Treatment includes any of the azole agents via topical applications or vaginal suppository, including miconazole as an OTC preparation or terconazole by prescription. Nystatin suppositories may prove to be effective as well. Oral therapy includes fluconazole (Diflucan) 150 mg orally once, which has been shown to be as effective as any of the local treatments. Longer duration of therapy, such as 7 to 14 days of topical regimen or fluconazole oral therapy on day 1, 4, and 7, is recommended for treatment for recurrent cases. First-line maintenance therapy for recurrent cases consists of oral fluconazole weekly for 6 months.

TRICHOMONAS VAGINALIS

Trichomonas vaginalis is a unicellular, anaerobic flagellated protozoan that can cause vaginitis. It inhabits the lower genitourinary tracts of women and men, and there are approximately 3 million cases diagnosed annually in the United States. The disease is sexually transmitted, with 75% of sexual partners possessing positive cultures.

Diagnosis

The signs and symptoms of *T. vaginalis* include a profuse discharge with an unpleasant odor. The discharge may be yellow, gray, or green in coloration and may be frothy in appearance. Vaginal pH is in the 6 to 7 range. Vulvar erythema, edema, and pruritus can also be noted. The characteristic erythematous, punctate epithelial papillae, or "strawberry" appearance of the cervix is apparent in only 10% of cases. Symptoms are usually worse immediately after menses because of the transient increase in vaginal pH at that time.

Diagnosis of *Trichomonas* is made via microscopic examination of wet preps of vaginal swabs. The protozoan is slightly larger than a white blood cell with three to five flagella. Often, active movement of the flagella and propulsion of the organism can be seen (Fig. 16-7). However, microscopy has only 60% to 70% sensitivity. Other more sensitive tests are available, including nucleic acid probe study and immunochromatographic capillary flow dipstick technology. The diagnosis can be confirmed when necessary with culture, which is the most sensitive and specific study.

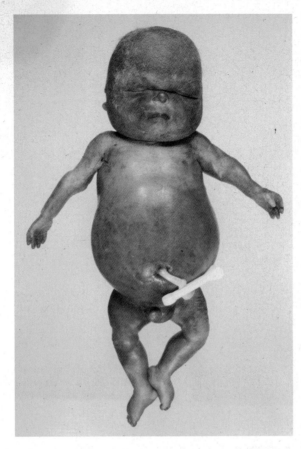

Color Plate 1 • Fetal hydrops caused by the accumulation of fluid in fetal tissues.
(From Sadler TW. *Langman's Medical Embryology*, 10th ed. Philadelphia: Lippincott Williams & Wilkins; 2006.)

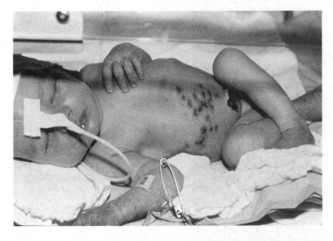

Color Plate 2 • Newborn with disseminated herpes simplex virus infection. Note the healing ulcerations on the abdomen of the infant.
(From Sweet R, Gibbs R. *Atlas of Infectious Diseases of the Female Genital Tract*. Philadelphia: Lippincott Williams & Wilkins; 2005).

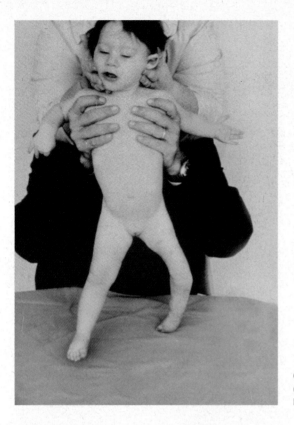

Color Plate 3 • Congenital varicella syndrome.
(From Sweet R, Gibbs R. *Atlas of Infectious Diseases of the Female Genital Tract*.
Philadelphia: Lippincott Williams & Wilkins; 2005).

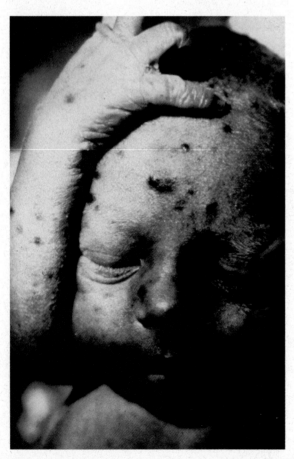

Color Plate 4 • Congenital CMV "blueberry muffin" baby with jaun-
dice and thrombocytopenia purpura.
(From Sweet R, Gibbs R. *Atlas of Infectious Diseases of the Female Genital Tract*.
Philadelphia: Lippincott Williams & Wilkins; 2005).

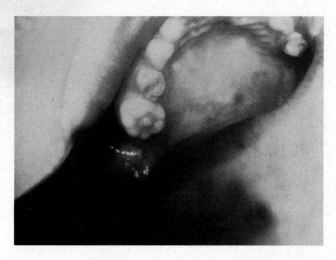

Color Plate 5 • Congenital syphilis—mulberry molar.
(From Sweet R, Gibbs R. *Atlas of Infectious Diseases of the Female Genital Tract*.
Philadelphia: Lippincott Williams & Wilkins; 2005).

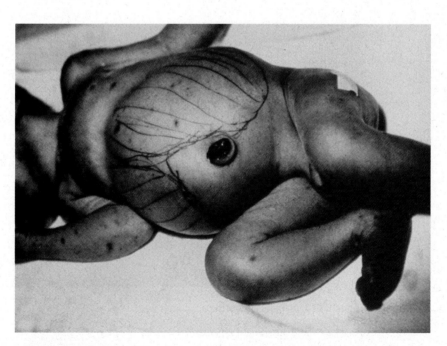

Color Plate 6 • Congenital toxoplasmosis with hepatosplenomegaly, jaundice, and
thrombocytopenia purpura.
(From Sweet R, Gibbs R. *Atlas of Infectious Diseases of the Female Genital Tract*. Philadelphia: Lippincott
Williams & Wilkins; 2005).

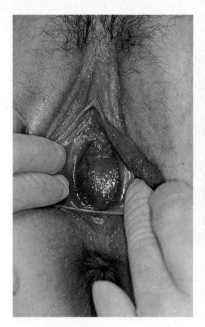
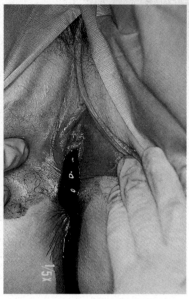

Color Plate 7 • Imperforate hymen.
(From Rock J & Johns H. *TeLinde's Operative Gynecology*, 9th ed. Philadelphia: Lippincott Williams & Wilkins; 2003.)

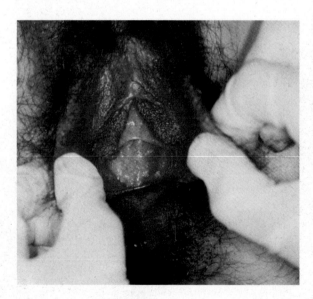

Color Plate 8 • Vaginal agenesis.
(From Emans J, Laufer M, Goldstein DP. *Pediatric and Adolescent Gynecology*, 5th ed. Philadelphia: Lippincott Williams & Wilkins; 2005).

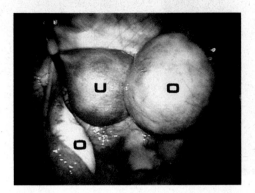

Color Plate 9 • Laparoscopic view of a large ovarian cyst.
(From Emans J, Laufer M, Goldstein DP. *Pediatric and Adolescent Gynecology*, 5th ed. Philadelphia: Lippincott Williams & Wilkins; 2005).

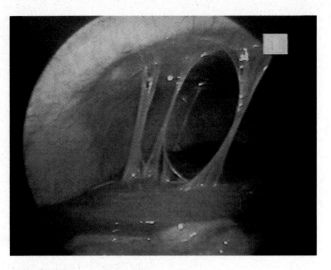

Color Plate 10 • Fitz-Hugh Curtis syndrome.
(From Sweet R, Gibbs R. *Atlas of Infectious Diseases of the Female Genital Tract*. Philadelphia: Lippincott Williams & Wilkins; 2005).

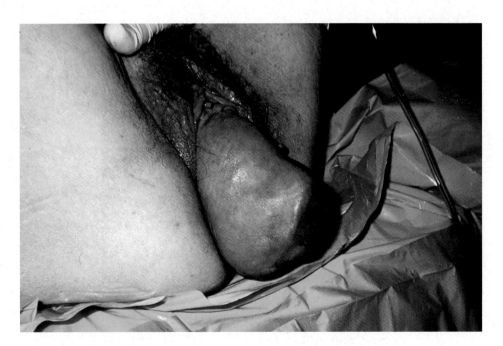

Color Plate 11 • Complete procidentia (prolapse) of the uterus and vagina.
(From Berek, JS. *Berek & Novak's Gynecology*, 14th ed. Philadelphia: Lippincott Williams & Wilkins; 2006.)

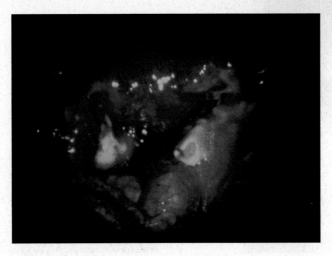

Color Plate 12 • Laparoscopic view of adult pelvic inflammatory disease (PID).
(From Sweet R, Gibbs R. *Atlas of Infectious Diseases of the Female Genital Tract*. Philadelphia: Lippincott Williams & Wilkins; 2005).

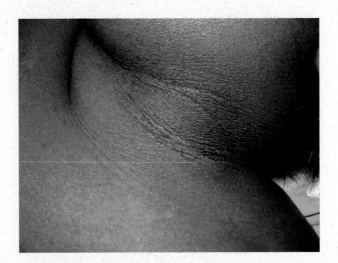

Color Plate 13 • Acanthosis nigricans.
(From Berek, JS. *Berek & Novak's Gynecology*, 14th ed. Philadelphia: Lippincott Williams & Wilkins; 2006.)

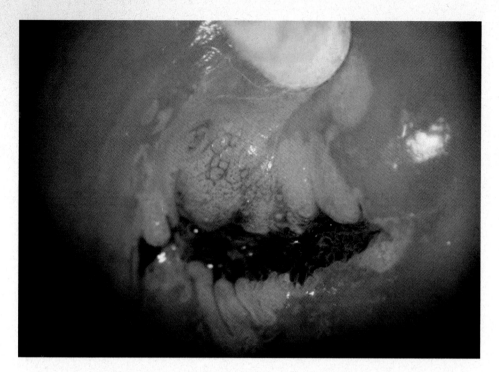

Color Plate 14 • Colposcopic view of cervix with CIN III showing mosaicism and punctations.
(From Berek, JS. *Berek & Novak's Gynecology*, 14th ed. Philadelphia: Lippincott Williams & Wilkins; 2006.)

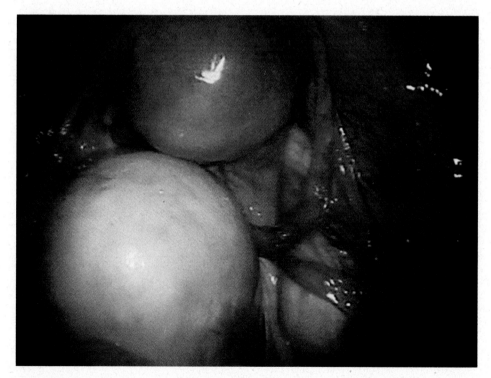

Color Plate 15 • Laparoscopic view of large ovarian mass.
(From Berek, JS. *Berek & Novak's Gynecology*, 14th ed. Philadelphia: Lippincott Williams & Wilkins; 2006.)

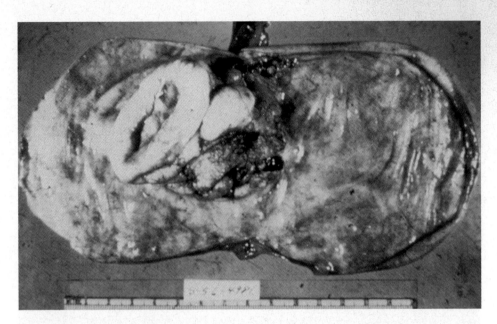

Color Plate 16 • Mature cystic teratoma (dermoid cyst).
(From Berek, JS. *Berek & Novak's Gynecology*, 14th ed. Philadelphia: Lippincott Williams & Wilkins; 2006.)

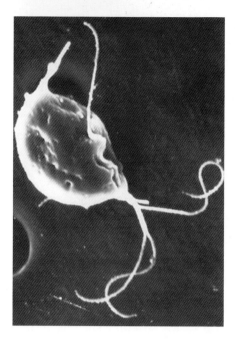

Figure 16-7 • Scanning electron micrograph of *Trichomonas vaginalis*. The undulating membrane and flagella of *Trichomonas* are its characteristic features.
(Reproduced with permission from Cox FEG, ed. *Modern Parasitology: A Textbook of Parasitology*, 2nd ed. Oxford: Blackwell Science, 1993:9.)

Treatment

The mainstay of treatment for *T. vaginalis* infections is metronidazole (Flagyl) 2 g orally or tinidazole 2 g orally in a single dose. As opposed to BV management, this regimen has been found to be as effective as the more traditional 500 mg orally twice a day for 7 days. However, metronidazole resistance may be present in 2% to 5% of vaginal trichomoniasis cases. In cases of metronidazole single-dose treatment failure, metronidazole 500 mg orally twice a day for 7 days or tinidazole 2 g orally in a single dose is recommended. If this treatment is unsuccessful, then tinidazole or metronidazole 2 g orally daily for 5 days, consultation with specialist, and *T. vaginalis* susceptibility through the CDC should be considered. Because of the high rate of concomitant infections in sexual partners, both partners should be treated to prevent reinfection.

INFECTIONS OF THE CERVIX

The organisms that most commonly cause cervicitis and infections of the upper reproductive tract differ from those that most commonly cause infections of the lower reproductive tract. *Neisseria gonorrhoeae* and *Chlamydia trachomatis* are the two most common organisms that cause cervicitis and the only organisms shown to cause mucopurulent cervicitis. Clinically, cervicitis is diagnosed as cervical motion tenderness in the absence of other signs of pelvic inflammatory disease (PID).

Other organisms can cause infections of the cervix including HSV, HPV, *Mycoplasma genitalium*, and BV. HSV causes either herpes lesions or a white plaque that resembles cervical cancer. Infection with HPV leads to condyloma and, depending on the subtype, is also an etiology of cervical cancer. Additionally, frequent douching may also cause cervicitis.

NEISSERIA GONORRHOEAE

Despite a 50% decrease in incidence in the 1990s, **gonococcal** infections remain the second leading reported STIs in the United States, with approximately 360,000 cases reported in 2000. Most cases occur in the 15- to 29-year-old age group. Among sexually active women, 15- to 19-year-olds have two times the incidence of 20- to 24-year-olds. However, the highest overall prevalence is in the 20- to 24-year-old age group because this group includes the highest percentage of sexually active individuals.

Multiple risk factors have been associated with gonococcal infections, including low socioeconomic status, urban residence, nonwhite and non-Asian ethnicity, early age of first sexual activity, illicit drug use, being unmarried, and history of sexually transmitted infections. Condoms, diaphragms, and spermicides decrease the risk of transmission. There are also seasonal variations in the incidence of gonorrhea in the United States with a peak observed in late summer.

Transmission between the sexes is unequal, with male-to-female transmission estimated at 80% to 90% compared to an estimated 20% to 25% female-to-male transmission rate after a single sexual encounter. This difference in transmission is most likely related to the type of epithelium exposed in the different sexes. In males, the external surface of the penis is primarily keratinized epithelium, whereas females receive primary contact with mucosa of the vagina and the nonkeratinized epithelium of the cervix. Further, male ejaculation increases the amount of exposure time in women, which supports the use of condoms as an exceptional prophylactic measure against gonococcal transmission.

Gonococcus can infect the anal canal, the urethra, the oropharynx, and Bartholin glands, in addition to the more commonly reported cervicitis, PID, or tubo-ovarian abscess (TOA). Gonococcal exposure in neonates can cause conjunctivitis. As many as 1% of recognized gonococcal infections may proceed to a disseminated infection. This infection begins with fevers and erythematous macular skin lesions and proceeds to a tenosynovitis and septic arthritis.

Diagnosis

Identification of the causative organism, *N. gonorrhoeae*, a gram-negative diplococcus resembling paired kidney beans, is necessary for definitive diagnosis. Isolation using the modified Thayer-Martin chocolate agar has a sensitivity of 96% in endocervical cultures and provides the option of antimicrobial susceptibility identification. Recently, many hospitals and healthcare facilities have begun using nucleic acid amplification tests (NAAT) for both gonorrhea and *Chlamydia* on urine and cervical specimens. NAAT yield high sensitivity and specificity and provide increased female specimen testing options, including urine.

Treatment

The recommended treatment for uncomplicated gononcoccal infection is ceftriaxone 125 mg intramuscularly once or cefixime 400 mg orally once. Due to increasing resistance, fluoroquinolones are no longer recommended for treatment of gonorrhea infections in the United States. Additionally, because patients infected with *N. gonorrhoeae* frequently are coinfected with *C. trachomatis*, it is recommended that patients diagnosed with gonorrhea infection should also be treated for *Chlamydia* with azithromycin 1 g orally once or amoxicillin 500 mg orally three times a day for 7 days, unless *Chlamydia* coinfection has been ruled out by NAAT.

CHLAMYDIA TRACHOMATIS

Chlamydia trachomatis is a pathogen that causes ocular, respiratory, and reproductive tract infections. In the United States, its transmission is primarily via sexual contact, although vertical transmission from a mother to a newborn is also seen. Interestingly, while there has been a decrease in reported gonococcal infections through the year 2000, reported chlamydial infections have increased to over 700,000. This is most likely secondary to the advent of NAATs for *C. trachomatis* (traditionally difficult to diagnose because they are obligate intracellular organisms and culture poorly) and aggressive screening programs of sexually active women. Prevalence is estimated at 3% to 5% in asymptomatic women, and 5% to 7% of pregnant women have had positive *Chlamydia* tests. Epidemiologically, *C. trachomatis* infections are parallel to those of *N. gonorrhoeae*, with higher rates seen among women age 15 to 29, with earlier age of first coitus, and greater number of sexual partners.

Another reason for the higher prevalence of chlamydial infections is that carriers of both sexes are often entirely asymptomatic. This is particularly unfortunate in women, in whom chronic infections may lead to scarring in the fallopian tubes that may result in infertility or increased risk of ectopic pregnancies. Common sites of infection include the endocervix, urethra, and rectum. Clinical manifestations of symptomatic chlamydial infections are often quite similar to those of *N. gonorrhoeae* and include symptoms of cervicitis, urethritis, and PID. As previously discussed, the L-serotypes of *C. trachomatis* can cause the systemic disease LGV.

Treatment

Treatment of choice for chlamydial infections is azithromycin 1 g orally single dose or doxycycline 100 mg orally twice a day for 7 days. Alternative regimens include erythromycin 500 mg orally four times a day for 7 days. For LGV, the treatment regimen consists of doxycycline 100 mg orally twice a day for 3 weeks.

KEY POINTS

- Syphilis is screened for with the RPR and VDRL tests and confirmed with either the TPPA or FTA-ABS.
- Benzathine penicillin is the drug of choice for treating syphilis. Neurosyphilis requires intravenous penicillin.
- Patients being treated for syphilis may experience the Jarisch-Herxheimer reaction, seen most commonly in treatment of secondary syphilis.
- Thirty to 40% of newly acquired genital herpes infections are caused by HSV-1.
- Primary herpes infection classically appears as multiple vesicles that develop into painful ulcers.
- Treatment of genital herpes is usually palliative, although acyclovir can reduce the length of primary infection and suppressive therapy may decrease the number of recurrences.
- Chancroid manifests as a painful genital ulcer and usually concomitant lymphadenopathy, but can be difficult to diagnose as neither cultures nor Gram's stains have been particularly consistent.
- Treatment of chancroid can include a variety of antibiotics; the simplest are single doses of PO azithromycin or IM ceftriaxone.
- HPV causes condylomata but, more seriously, is associated with cervical cancer.

- Bacterial vaginosis is polymicrobial but usually attributed to *Gardnerella,* and first-line treatment is metronidazole (Flagyl) for a 7-day course.
- Seventy-five percent of sexual partners of those with *Trichomonas* will also be colonized and should be presumptively treated with first-line treatment of metronidazole 2 g orally single dose.
- *N. gonorrhoeae* causes a reported 2 million infections per year with common sequelae including cervicitis, PID, TOA, and Bartholin abscess.
- Treatment for uncomplicated infections is ceftriaxone 125 mg intramuscularly or cefixime 400 mg orally single dose.
- Treatment for *N. gonorrhoeae* should include azithromycin 1 g orally once to treat likely concomitant chlamydial infections.
- Chlamydial infections tend to coincide with gonococcal infections. However, the incidence of gonococcal infections has decreased, whereas the incidence of chlamydial infections has increased.
- Many chlamydial infections are entirely asymptomatic.
- Treatment of *Chlamydia* is a one-time 1 g oral dose of azithromycin.

Upper Female Reproductive Tract and Systemic Infections

THE UPPER FEMALE REPRODUCTIVE TRACT

Women experience more upper reproductive tract, pelvic, and abdominal infections compared to men because of the absence of a mucosal lining or epithelium between these spaces and the external body in the female patient. Although defenses such as ciliary movement creating flow and cervical mucus exist, there is essentially an open tract between the vagina, the pelvis, and abdomen. This can lead to ascending infections of the uterus, fallopian tubes, adnexa, pelvis, and abdomen. This open ascending tract may also lead to the acquisition of toxic shock syndrome (TSS). Further, because the vaginal epithelium is easily abraded during intercourse, transmission of systemic infections such as human immunodeficiency virus (HIV) and hepatitis B and C is more common from men to women than the converse.

ENDOMETRITIS

Pathogenesis

Endometritis is an infection of the uterine endometrium; if the infection invades into the myometrium, it is known as **endomyometritis**. Endometritis and endomyometritis are usually preceded by instrumentation or disruption of the intrauterine cavity. It is seen most commonly after cesarean delivery, but also after vaginal deliveries, dilation and evacuation (D&E) and dilation and curettage (D&C) procedures, and intrauterine device (IUD) placement. Nonpuerperal endometritis is not commonly recognized but is probably coexistent with 70% to 80% of pelvic inflammatory disease (PID). Its etiology is related to ascent of infection from the cervix, which then proceeds to the fallopian tubes to cause acute salpingitis and, eventually, widespread PID. Diagnosis of endomyometritis is made in the clinical settings described above with a bimanual exam revealing uterine tenderness, as well as fever and elevated white blood cell (WBC) count.

Chronic endometritis is often asymptomatic but is clinically significant because it leads to other pelvic infections and, uncommonly, endomyometritis. It is often a polymicrobial infection with a variety of pathogens, including skin and gastrointestinal flora in addition to the usual flora colonizing the lower reproductive tract. It can be suspected in patients with chronic irregular bleeding, discharge, and pelvic pain. The diagnosis can be made in a nonpuerperal patient with endometrial biopsy showing plasma cells.

Treatment

Treatment of severe endomyometritis is usually clindamycin 900 mg intravenously (IV) every 8 hours and gentamicin loaded with 2 mg/kg IV and then maintained with 1.5 mg/kg IV every 8 hours. Single daily intravenous dosing of gentamicin (5 mg/kg every 24 hours) may be substituted for 8-hour dosing. Single antibiotic agent treatment of endometritis may also be considered, including cephalosporins such as cefoxitin 2 g IV every 6 hours. In nonpuerperal infections where *Chlamydia* infection may be the suspected cause, doxycycline should be added to the regimen for a total of 14 days. Treatment course continues until clinical improvement and afebrile status for 24 to 48 hours. Oral antibiotic therapy is not required following successful parenteral treatment. Chronic endometritis, on the other hand, is treated with a 10- to 14-day course of doxycycline 100 mg PO BID.

PELVIC INFLAMMATORY DISEASE

Acute salpingitis, or more generally **pelvic inflammatory disease** (PID), is the most common serious complication of sexually transmitted infections (STIs). As many as 750,000 to 1 million cases are estimated to occur annually in the United States. The annual expense of initial treatment is estimated at $3.5 to $5 billion, which does not account for possible future treatment for the principal sequelae, including infertility and increased ectopic pregnancies. PID is strongly associated with infertility. Specifically, infertility risk increases with the number of PID episodes: 12% with one episode, approximately 20% with two episodes, and 40% with three or more episodes. Additionally, the risk of ectopic pregnancy is increased as much as seven- to tenfold and approximately 20% of women develop chronic pelvic pain during their lifetime. Sequelae, including chronic pelvic pain, dyspareunia, and pelvic adhesions, may also require surgical therapy, contributing to the economic costs and morbidity of this disease.

Among sexually active women, the incidence of this disease is highest in the 15- to 25-year-old age group (at least three times greater than in the 25- to 29-year-old age group). This may be attributed to higher-risk behavior of this age group. It may also be related to decreased immunity to STD agents in younger women, although the pathophysiology is unclear. Finally, the younger age group is less likely to have regular gynecological care or to seek medical attention until bacterial vaginosis or cervicitis has progressed to the more symptomatic PID (Fig. 17-1).

Other risk factors for PID include nonwhite and non-Asian ethnicity, multiple partners, recent history

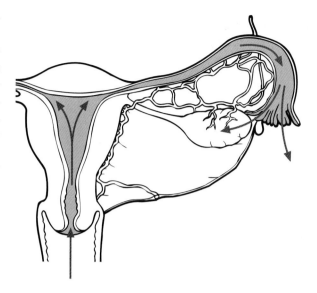

Figure 17-1 • Route of intra-abdominal spread of gonorrhea and other pathogenic bacteria.

of douching, prior history of PID, and cigarette smoking. IUDs are considered a risk factor for PID when insertion occurs in the setting of concurrent *Chlamydia* or gonorrhea infection, where the prevalence of STIs is high, and when aseptic conditions cannot be assured. In contrast, barrier contraceptives have been shown to decrease the incidence of PID, and use of oral contraceptives appears to diminish the severity of PID.

Clinical Manifestations

The principal symptom of acute salpingitis is abdominal or pelvic/adnexal pain. The character of the pain can range (burning, cramping, stabbing) and can be unilateral or bilateral. Pain may also be absent in what has been deemed "silent" PID. Other associated symptoms include increased vaginal discharge, abnormal odor, abnormal bleeding, gastrointestinal disturbances, and urinary tract symptoms. Fever is a less common symptom, seen in only 20% of women with PID.

Diagnosis

Because untreated PID can lead to serious sequelae (e.g., infertility), a low threshold for diagnosis and treatment should be maintained. Minimum criteria for empiric treatment include pelvic or lower abdominal pain, and one or more of the following: cervical motion tenderness, uterine tenderness, or adnexal tenderness. Additional diagnosis criteria include fever (>38.3°C), abnormal cervical or vaginal mucopurulent discharge, abundant WBC on saline microscopy of vaginal secretions, elevated erythrocyte sedimentation rate, elevated C-reactive protein, and cervical *Neisseria gonorrhoeae* or *Chlamydia trachomatis* infection. Cervical cultures are performed to find a causative organism but, due to the disease's polymicrobial nature, should not dictate the treatment regimen. The definitive diagnosis is made via laparoscopy, endometrial biopsy, or pelvic imaging with PID findings. In practice, a more invasive diagnostic laparoscopic surgical procedure is usually performed only when appendicitis cannot be ruled out by clinical examination, although there are several small ongoing trials looking at the effectiveness of laparoscopy under local anesthesia for the diagnosis of PID. Occasionally, PID is complicated by **Fitzhugh-Curtis syndrome** (Color Plate 10). This is a perihepatitis from the ascending infection resulting in right upper quadrant pain and tenderness and liver function test (LFT) elevations.

The principal organisms suspected of causing PID are *N. gonorrhoeae* and *C. trachomatis*; the two organisms combined account for approximately 40% of all PID cases. However, cultures from the upper reproductive tract have shown that most PID is likely to be polymicrobial, including anaerobic organisms such as *Bacteroides* species and facultative bacteria such as *Gardnerella*, *Escherichia coli*, *H. influenzae*, and streptococci.

Treatment

Because of the high rate of ambulatory treatment failures and the seriousness of sequelae, patients are often hospitalized for treatment of PID, particularly those who are teenagers, unable to tolerate POs, pregnant, noncompliant, or who have been refractory to outpatient therapy. PID is usually treated with a broad-spectrum cephalosporin, such as cefoxitin 2 g IV every 6 hours plus doxycycline 100 mg IV or orally every 12 hours because of its polymicrobial nature. The intravenous antibiotic regimen is continued until the patient demonstrates clinical improvement for 24 hours, and doxycycline is continued for a total 14-day course of doxycycline 100 mg orally twice a day. In patients allergic to cephalosporins, IV clindamycin and gentamicin can be used. On an outpatient basis, a single dose of ceftriaxone 250 mg IM or cefoxitin 2 g IM plus 1 g of probenecid orally along with oral doxycycline 100 mg orally twice a day for 14 days with or without metronidazole 500 mg orally twice a day for 14 days is used with close follow-up for resolution of symptoms. PID is rare in pregnant patients; because tetracyclines and fluoroquinolones are avoided in pregnancy, clindamycin and gentamicin is the treatment of choice during pregnancy. Additionally, due to increasing fluoroquinolone-resistant *Neisseria gonorrhoeae* in the United States, fluoroquinolones are no longer recommended by the CDC for treatment of gonorrhea infections or of PID cases in which gonorrhea may be a causative agent.

TUBO-OVARIAN ABSCESS

Persistent PID can lead to the development of tubo-ovarian abscess (TOA) (Fig. 17-2). Most so-called TOAs are actually tubo-ovarian complexes (TOC), the difference being that complexes are not walled off like the true abscess and are thus more responsive to antimicrobial therapy. Estimates of the progression from PID to TOA range from 3% to 16%; thus, any PID not responsive to therapy should be investigated further to rule out TOA. Furthermore, HIV-infected women with PID are at increased risk of development of TOA.

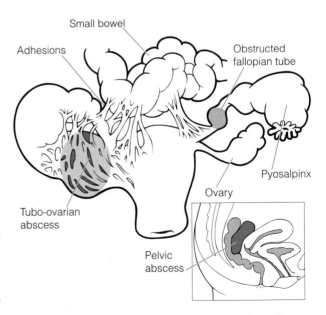

Figure 17-2 • Findings associated with chronic pelvic inflammatory disease, including tubo-ovarian abscess, adhesions, pyosalpinx, and an abscess located in the posterior cul-de-sac.

Diagnosis

The diagnosis of TOA can be made clinically in the setting of PID and the appreciation of an adnexal or posterior cul-de-sac mass or fullness. Most patients will endorse abdominal and/or pelvic pain (90%) and demonstrate fever and leukocytosis (60% to 80%). WBC count is usually elevated with a left shift and the erythrocyte sedimentation rate (ESR) is often elevated as well. Cultures should include endocervical swabs and blood cultures to rule out sepsis. Culdocentesis that reveals gross pus is diagnostic but has been used less as advances in imaging studies have been made. Although most TOA are appreciated by clinical exam, a negative exam does not rule out a TOA. Ultrasound is the imaging study of choice to diagnose TOAs and is able to distinguish between TOAs and TOCs. However, pelvic computed tomography (CT) may be required, particularly in obese patients for whom ultrasound use is limited. Finally, laparoscopy can lead to a definitive diagnosis but is usually only used when the clinical picture is unclear.

Treatment

While treatment of TOAs can be medical or surgical, a trial of medical management with broad-spectrum antibiotics in an inpatient setting is frequently the first step. Unless the abscess is ruptured and causing peritoneal signs or is impenetrable by antibiotics, surgical treatment can often be avoided. The first-line antibiotic choice is often ampicillin (2 g IV every 4 hours), gentamicin (loading dose of 2 mg/kg, followed by 1.5 mg/kg IV every 8 hours or 5 mg/kg IV every 24 hours), plus clindamycin (900 mg every 8 hours) or metronidazole (500 mg PO or IV every 8 hours). In patients allergic to penicillin, ampicillin may be omitted. The course of this disease can be monitored by symptoms, clinical examination, temperature, WBC count, and, if these are equivocal, imaging studies. Typically, a repeat pelvic exam is performed after the patient has been afebrile for 24 to 48 hours to monitor for improvement and eventual resolution of tenderness. If responsive to medical management, the patient can be converted to oral antibiotics to complete a 10- to 14-day course.

For more serious TOAs, either unresponsive to antibiotic therapy or with gross rupture, surgical intervention is necessary. Drainage of TOA using ultrasound guidance or laparoscopy may be considered in patients who do not respond to 48 hours of medical therapy. Unilateral salpingo-oophorectomy is considered as a curative therapy for the unilateral TOA by some authorities. For bilateral TOAs, often a total abdominal hysterectomy and bilateral salpingo-oophorectomy (TAHBSO) may be necessary.

TOXIC SHOCK SYNDROME

Toxic shock syndrome (TSS) reached its peak in the United States in 1980 when the rate was 3:100,000 menstruating women. Since 1984, there have been fewer than 300 cases per year. Initially, TSS was correlated with high-absorbency tampons and menstruation in approximately 50% to 70% of cases over the past two decades. Of note, the proportion of menstrual-related TSS has been decreasing over time. Nonmenstrually related TSS has been associated with vaginal infections, vaginal delivery, cesarean section, postpartum endometritis, miscarriage, and laser treatment of condylomata.

Diagnosis

TSS is caused by colonization or infection with specific strains of *Staphylococcus aureus* that produce an epidermal toxin—toxic shock syndrome toxin-1 (TSST-1). This toxin and other staphylococcal toxins are likely to cause most of the symptoms of TSS. Symptoms include high fever (>38.9°C or 102°F), hypotension, diffuse erythematous macular rash, desquamation of the palms and soles 1 to 2 weeks after the acute illness, and multisystem involvement of three or more organ systems. Gastrointestinal disturbances (abdominal pain, vomiting, and diarrhea), myalgias, mucous membrane hyperemia, increased blood urea nitrogen (BUN) and creatinine, platelet count less than 100,000, and alteration in consciousness can also be seen. Blood cultures are often negative, possibly because the exotoxin is absorbed through the vaginal mucosa.

Treatment

Because of the seriousness of the disease (2% to 8% mortality rate), hospitalization is always indicated. For more severe cases in which patients are hemodynamically unstable, admission to an intensive care unit may be necessary. Of highest priority is supportive treatment of hypotension with IV fluids and pressors if needed. Because this disease is caused by the exotoxin, treatment with IV antibiotics does not often shorten the length of the acute illness. However, it does decrease the risk of recurrence, which has been as high as 30% in women who continued to use high-absorbency tampons. Antibiotic therapy consists of clindamycin plus vancomycin for empiric treatment when specific *S. aureus* isolate sensitivity is unknown, clindamycin plus vancomycin or linezolid in MRSA TSS cases, and clindamycin plus nafcillin or oxacillin in MSSA TSS cases. Treatment duration is generally 10 to 14 days. Currently, there is a lack of controlled studies to support the use of intravenous immune globulin or corticosteroid therapy.

HUMAN IMMUNODEFICIENCY VIRUS

Human immunodeficiency virus (HIV) is the causative agent of acquired immunodeficiency syndrome (AIDS). HIV is transmitted via sexual contact, via parenteral inoculation, and vertically from mothers to infants via a transplacental route, during birth from direct exposure, and via breast milk. As of 2004, there were >123,000 cases of AIDS reported in girls and women in the United States. Although women account for only 18% of AIDS cases in the United States, they are one segment of the population in which the incidence is currently rising. The proportion of AIDS cases among female adults and adolescents (age >13 years) in the United States increased from 7% in 1985 to 27% in 2003. Furthermore, women of color (African American and Latina) have much higher infection rates compared to Caucasian women. More specifically, according to the CDC, African American women accounted for half of all HIV infection in men or women from heterosexual sex between 1999 and 2002. Worldwide, women represent a far more substantial proportion of those affected with HIV. According to the Joint United Nations Program on HIV/AIDS, in 2004, nearly 50% of adults living with HIV worldwide were women. In 2003, there were approximately 38 million patients with HIV, 3 million deaths due to HIV, and 1.1 million deaths directly attributed to HIV in women. There appear to be no differences in disease progression, mortality, or viral decay with use of antiretrovirals between men and women.

Infection with HIV—a retrovirus—leads to decreased cellular immunity because various cells carrying the CD4 antigen become infected, including helper T cells, B cells, monocytes, and macrophages. Initially, the infection is entirely asymptomatic, although the individual is a carrier of the disease; this stage can last from 5 to 7 years. This disease may appear initially with the AIDS-related complex, which includes lymphadenopathy, night sweats, malaise, diarrhea, weight loss, and unusual recurrent infections such as oral candidiasis, varicella zoster, or herpes simplex. As the infection further decreases cellular immunity, full-blown AIDS develops with opportunistic infections such as *Pneumocystis carinii* pneumonia, toxoplasmosis, *Mycobacterium avium intracellulare*, cytomegalovirus, and various malignancies such as Kaposi sarcoma and non-Hodgkin lymphoma.

Diagnosis

The diagnosis of HIV infection is made initially via a screening test. Most commonly, the test is an enzyme-linked immunosorbent assay (ELISA) using HIV antigens, to which patient serum is added. A positive test results when antigen-antibody complexes form. This test does have false-positive results that, in low-risk populations, may occur more often than true positive results. Positive tests are therefore confirmed by a Western blot. Another level of confirmation may be obtained if a viral load is sent and is positive. Viral loads and CD4 cell counts are used to follow the progression of disease.

Treatment

There is no known cure for HIV or AIDS. The approach to this disease is prevention of transmission, prophylaxis of opportunistic infections, and prolonging the lives of infected patients by slowing progression of disease with antiretroviral agents. Great efforts are being directed toward prevention of HIV transmission by encouraging modification of risky behavior. Condoms are recommended for sexually active patients. IV drug users should avoid sharing needles and use clean needles. With improved screening methods, the risk of HIV infection from blood transfusion is currently estimated at less than 1:1,000,000.

Prophylaxis and treatment of the opportunistic infections in HIV-positive patients are discussed in *Blueprints Medicine*. Delaying the progress of the disease is accomplished primarily with nucleoside analogs and protease inhibitors. The nucleoside analogs—zidovudine (AZT), lamivudine (3TC), abacavir, didanosine, and stavudine—act to inhibit reverse transcriptase and interfere with viral replication. Protease inhibitors (lopinavir, atazanavir, indinavir, saquinavir, ritonavir) interfere with the synthesis of viral particles and have been effective in increasing CD4 counts and decreasing viral load. Because the action mechanisms of these two groups differ, a synergistic effect is seen with combination therapy known as highly active antiretroviral therapy (HAART). Other antiretroviral drug classes include nonnucleoside reverse transcriptase inhibitors, and newer drug classes including entry inhibitors and integrase inhibitors.

Beyond this simple review of HIV management, there are issues regarding HIV infection in women that deserve special emphasis. First, obstetric care of the HIV patient demands attention to both the ongoing care of the patient as well as the prevention of vertical transmission to the fetus. Second, the high incidence of invasive cervical cancer in this population requires more aggressive screening than in the general population.

In the United States approximately 7,000 infants are born annually to mothers who are infected with human immunodeficiency virus. With no treatment, approximately 25% of infants born to HIV-infected mothers will become infected with HIV. Increased transmission can be seen with higher viral burden or advanced disease in the mother, rupture of the membranes, and invasive procedures during labor and delivery that increase neonatal exposure to maternal blood. Transmission occurs in utero (1/3) generally late in pregnancy or during labor and delivery (2/3). In 1994, Pediatric AIDS Clinical Trials Group (PACTG) protocol 076 demonstrated that a three-part regimen of **zidovudine** (ZDV) administered during pregnancy and labor and to the newborn could reduce the risk of perinatal transmission by two-thirds in women. Additionally, with the use of HAART to further decrease viral load with potent regimens, the rate of transmission can be further decreased to less than 1% to 2% with an undetectable viral load. Currently, antiretroviral therapy in pregnancy includes a three-drug regimen generally started in the second trimester with a goal for viral suppression by the third trimester, regardless of need for antiretrovirals for maternal health indication.

Cesarean delivery has been shown to lower transmission rates by roughly two-thirds compared to vaginal delivery in patients on no therapy and particularly without onset of labor or rupture of membranes or in the setting of high viral load. However, in women with viral loads of <1,000 copies/mL, there is no additional benefit of cesarean delivery versus vaginal delivery in HIV perinatal transmission. Therefore, cesarean delivery should be considered in HIV-infected pregnant women with viral loads >1,000 copies/mL and without long-standing onset of labor or rupture of membranes. Because of the effective interventions in HIV-positive women to decrease vertical transmission, it is recommended that HIV screening be offered to all pregnant women at their first prenatal visit and again in the third trimester if the woman has specified risk factors for HIV infection. Furthermore, in resource-rich nations where safe bottle feeding alternatives are available, breastfeeding is contraindicated in HIV-infected woman as virus is found in breast milk and is responsible for HIV transmission to the infant. Postnatal HIV transmission from breast milk at 2 years may be as high as 15%. Furthermore, studies are lacking regarding the efficacy of maternal antiretroviral therapy for prevention of transmission of HIV through breast milk and the toxicity of antiretroviral exposure of the infant via breast milk.

The high incidence of invasive cervical cancer in HIV-infected women is an important issue in gynecologic outpatient management. Studies confirm the synergistic association of HIV and human papillomavirus (HPV), the causative agent in squamous cell carcinoma of the cervix. The Centers for Disease Control and Prevention currently recommends routine Pap smears at initial evaluation and 6 months later. Thereafter, yearly evaluations are sufficient if results are negative unless there is documentation of previous HPV infection, squamous intraepithelial lesion, or symptomatic HIV disease, in which case the Pap smear should be repeated at 6-month intervals.

KEY POINTS

- Endomyometritis occurs most commonly after a delivery or instrumentation of the endometrial cavity.
- Diagnosis of endomyometritis is made with uterine tenderness, fever, and elevated WBC count.
- Endomyometritis treatment is with broad-spectrum antibiotics such as intravenous clindamycin and gentamicin; less severe infections are treated with intravenous cephalosporins.
- There may be as many as 1 million cases of PID reported annually.
- Twelve percent of patients with one episode of PID will become infertile.
- Minimal diagnosis criteria for PID consists of pelvic or lower abdominal pain, plus uterine, adnexal, or cervical motion tenderness.
- Because of the seriousness of this disease and its sequelae, patients are often hospitalized and treated with IV antibiotics.
- Chronic or acute PID can lead to TOAs or TOCs.
- Diagnosis of TOA or TOC is most likely when there is an adnexal mass in the setting of PID symptoms. Confirmation is usually achieved with an imaging study such as pelvic ultrasound or CT.

- TOA treatment includes hospitalization and broad-spectrum IV antibiotics. For TOAs not responsive to antibiotics, drainage of TOA is recommended.
- TSS peaked in 1984; currently, there are fewer than 300 cases per year in the United States.
- Symptoms, which include fever, rash, and desquamation of palms and soles, are most likely caused by an *S. aureus* toxin, TSST-1.
- Because of the seriousness of TSS, patients are hospitalized and treated with IV antibiotics and, if necessary, hemodynamic support.
- HIV is transmitted via sexual contact, sharing IV needles, and any activity where infected blood is introduced to a noninfected host.
- HIV infection is screened for with the ELISA test and confirmed with a Western blot.
- There is currently no cure for HIV infection so treatment focuses on antiretroviral agents such as nucleoside analogs and protease inhibitors and treatment of the multiple opportunistic infections.
- Vertical transmission rates during pregnancy have been shown to decrease with antiretroviral treatment and are positively associated with viral load.

18 Pelvic Organ Prolapse

PELVIC ORGAN PROLAPSE

PATHOGENESIS

As shown in Figure 18-1, normal support of the pelvic organs is provided by a complex network of **muscles** (e.g., levator muscles), **fascia** (e.g., urogenital diaphragm, endopelvic fascia), **nerves**, and **ligaments** (e.g., uterosacral and cardinal ligaments). Damage to any one of these structures can potentially result in a weakening or loss of support to the pelvic organs (Fig. 18-2). Damage to the anterior vaginal wall can result in herniation of the bladder (**cystocele**) or urethra (**urethrocele**) into the vaginal lumen. Injuries to the endopelvic fascia of the rectovaginal septum can result in herniation of the rectum (**rectocele**) into the vaginal lumen. And injury or stretching of the cardinal ligaments and other pelvic support structures can result in descensus, or prolapse, of the uterus (**uterine prolapse**). After hysterectomy, some women may experience prolapse of the small intestine (**enterocele**) or vagina secondary to loss of support structures during surgery (**vaginal vault prolapse**).

Pelvic organ prolapse can present with a variety of symptoms including pelvic pressure and pain, urinary incontinence, dyspareunia, and bowel and bladder dysfunction. Pelvic support can be compromised by birth trauma; chronic increases in intra-abdominal pressure from obesity, chronic cough, or heavy lifting; intrinsic weakness; and atrophic changes due to aging or estrogen deficiency.

Pelvic organ prolapse quantitative (POP-Q) refers to an objective, site-specific system for describing, quantifying, and staging pelvic support in women. It provides a standardized means for documenting, comparing, and communicating clinical findings of pelvic organ prolapse that **focuses on the extent of prolapse** and not on which organ part is presumed to be prolapsing within the defect (Fig. 18-3). In order to quantitatively assess the degree of prolapse involved, POP-Q uses six points within the pelvis that are measured in relation to a fixed point of reference: the hymen. POP-Q is not used uniformly by clinicians because it is quite complicated, but it is helpful in the research setting and in comparing patients' exams over time and among different examiners.

Most clinicians utilize the **Baden-Walker Halfway System** for quantifying pelvic organ prolapse. It records the extent of prolapse using a four-point system using the hymen as a fixed point of reference (Fig. 18-4). Zero represents normal anatomic position (i.e., no descensus), 1: descensus halfway to the hymen, 2: descensus to the hymen, 3: descensus halfway past the hymen, and 4: maximum descent. The examination is usually conducted with the patient straining in order to record maximum descent.

EPIDEMIOLOGY

The problem of pelvic relaxation is **increased in postmenopausal** women secondary to decreased endogenous estrogen and increased vaginal deliveries. As a result, tissues become less resilient and the accumulative stresses on the pelvis take effect. Black and Asian women have a much lower rate of uterine prolapse than do white women.

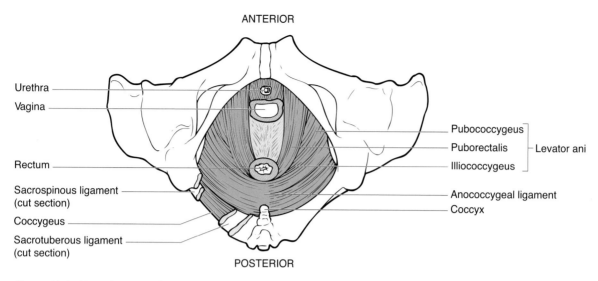

Figure 18-1 • Normal structural support of the pelvic floor as seen from above.

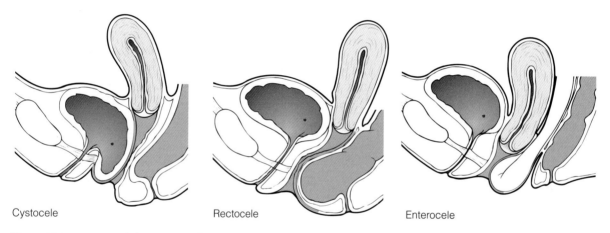

Cystocele

Rectocele

Enterocele

Figure 18-2 • Anatomic defects in pelvic relaxation.

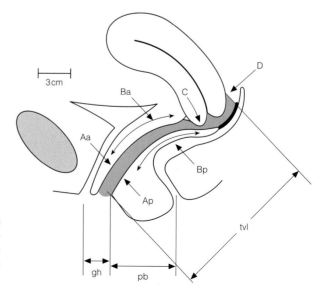

Figure 18-3 • Schematic of the quantified pelvic organ prolapse (POP-Q) system. Six sites (*points Aa, Ba, C, D, Bp, Ap*), genital hiatus (gh), perineal body (pb), and total vaginal length (tvl) are used to quantify the degree of pelvic organ prolapse. The vagina and hymenal ring are shown in blue.

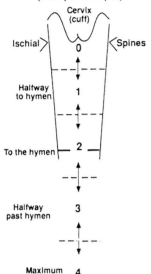

Grading of all sites except perineal
(Example: Prolapse)

Cervix
(cuff)

Ischial — 0 — Spines

Halfway
to hymen — 1

To the hymen — 2

Halfway
past hymen — 3

Maximum
descent — 4

Patient performs Valsalva Maneuver

Grade each site from 0–4
Grade worst site, segment, entire vagina
Grade in doubt? Use the "greater" grade
Grade still in doubt? Examine with patient standing

Figure 18-4 • Baden-Walker halfway system for grading pelvic organ prolapse. In general, grade 1 is given to a defect which descends at least halfway to the hymenal ring. Grade 2 is given to a defect extending to the hymenal ring. Grade 3 is given to a defect extending half-way beyond the hymenal ring. Grade 4 is given if the uterus is completely outside of the vagina.
(Image from Rock J & Jones H. *TeLinde's Operative Gynecology*, 10th ed. Philadelphia: Lippincott Williams & Wilkins, 2008.)

RISK FACTORS

The incidence of pelvic relaxation is increased for those patients who have **chronically increased abdominal pressure** due to chronic cough, chronic constipation, repeated heavy lifting, and large pelvic tumors. Obstructed labor and **traumatic delivery** are also risk factors for pelvic relaxation as are **aging and menopause**.

CLINICAL MANIFESTATIONS

History

The symptoms reported with pelvic relaxation vary depending on the structures involved and the degree of prolapse (Table 18-1). With small degrees of pelvic relaxation, patients are often asymptomatic. With more extensive relaxation, patients often complain of **pelvic pressure**, heaviness in the lower abdomen, or a **vaginal bulge** that may worsen at night or become aggravated by prolonged standing, vigorous activity, or lifting heavy objects. Urinary incontinence, frequency, urgency, and retention are other symptoms that may also be reported by patients with pelvic organ prolapse.

Physical Examination

Pelvic relaxation is best observed by separating the labia and viewing the vagina while the patient strains or coughs. A **split-speculum exam** can also be performed by using a Sims speculum or the lower half of a Grave speculum to provide better visualization of the anterior and posterior vaginal walls individually. Using this method, the speculum is used to retract the posterior vaginal wall and a **cystocele** may cause a downward movement of the anterior vaginal wall when the patient strains (Fig. 18-5). Similarly, **rectoceles and enteroceles** result in an upward bulging of the posterior vaginal wall when the patient strains (Fig. 18-6). This laxity in the rectovaginal wall can

■ TABLE 18-1 Symptoms That May Be Manifested in Pelvic Organ Prolapse	
Pressure Symptoms	**Other Urinary Symptoms**
Pelvic pressure or heaviness	Frequency hesitancy
Backache	Incomplete voiding
Dyspareunia	Recurrent infection
Urinary incontinence	Rectal symptoms
	Constipation
	Painful defecation
	Incomplete defecation
	Splinting*

* Placement of the fingers in the vagina to aid in defecation.

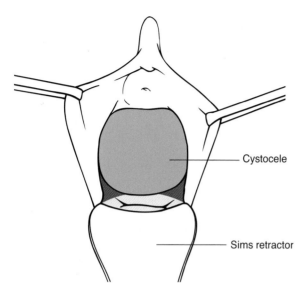

Figure 18-5 • A cystocele (*seen here via split-speculum exam*) is the bulging of the bladder into the anterior vaginal wall. It is usually caused by pelvic floor weakness. It can be repaired with an anterior colporrhaphy.

also be demonstrated on **rectal exam**. A **prolapsed uterus** can also be viewed on split-speculum examination or by bimanual pelvic exam.

The degree of pelvic relaxation is determined by the amount of descent of the structure. In **first-degree** pelvic relaxation, the structure is in the upper two-thirds of the vagina. In **second-degree** pelvic relaxation, the structure descends to the level of the introitus. In **third-degree** pelvic relaxation, the structure protrudes outside of the vagina. In **fourth-degree** pelvic relaxation, the entire structure is outside the vagina (Color Plate 11).

DIAGNOSTIC EVALUATION

The diagnosis of pelvic organ prolapse depends primarily on the history and physical examination. Other tools that may be useful in the diagnosis and preoperative evaluation of cystoceles and urethroceles include urine cultures, cystoscopy, urethroscopy, and urodynamic studies, if indicated. When a rectocele is suspected from a history of chronic constipation and difficulty passing stool, obstructive lesions should be ruled out using anoscopy or sigmoidoscopy. A defecography study (similar to a barium enema) may also help to show a rectocele or enterocele but is not generally essential to diagnosis.

DIFFERENTIAL DIAGNOSIS

Although rare, the differential diagnosis for cystocele and urethrocele includes urethral diverticula, Gartner cysts, Skene gland cysts, and tumors of the urethra and bladder. When a rectocele is suspected, obstructive lesions of the colon and rectum (lipomas, fibromas, sarcomas) should be investigated. Cervical elongation, prolapsed cervical polyp, and prolapsed cervical and endometrial tumors may be mistaken for uterine prolapse as can lower uterine segment fibroids.

TREATMENT

Regardless of the etiology, symptomatic pelvic organ prolapse is essentially a **structural problem** and therefore requires therapies that reinforce the lost support to the pelvis. These structural remedies may include **hormonal therapies** to maximize intrinsic pelvic support or exercises to strengthen the pelvic musculature (**Kegel exercises**). Likewise, mechanical support

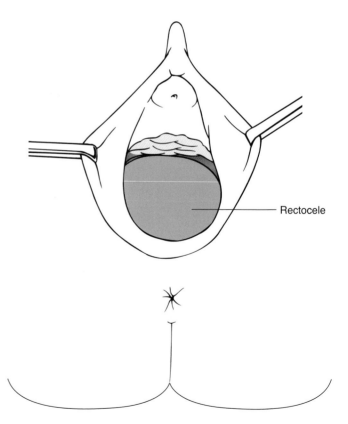

Figure 18-6 • A rectocele is the bulging of the rectum into the posterior vaginal wall. It is usually caused by pelvic floor weakness. It can be repaired with a posterior colporrhaphy.

devices (**pessaries**) may be used or the defect may be **repaired surgically**.

In postmenopausal women, **estrogen replacement** (systemic or vaginal) can be an important supplemental treatment, improving tissue tone and facilitating reversal of atrophic changes in the vaginal mucosa.

In motivated patients with mild symptoms, a first attempt at treatment may involve the use of **Kegel exercises** to strengthen the pelvic musculature. These exercises involve the tightening and releasing of the pubococcygeus muscles repeatedly throughout the day to strengthen the muscles and increase pelvic support.

Vaginal pessaries act as mechanical support devices to replace the lost structural integrity of the pelvis and to diffuse the forces of descent over a wider area. Pessaries are indicated for patients in whom surgery is contraindicated but whose symptoms are severe enough to require treatment. These are used in pregnant and postpartum women as well. These devices are placed in the vagina, positioned like a diaphragm, and serve to hold the pelvic organs in their normal position (Fig. 18-7). The use of vaginal pessaries requires a highly motivated patient and close clinical follow-up to avoid vaginal trauma and ulcerations. Close follow-up also ensures proper placement and hygiene to minimize the risk of leukorrhea and infections.

Symptomatic patients who are not helped by nonoperative approaches may require **surgical correction**. In general, surgical repair for pelvic relaxation produces very good results. As outlined in Table 18-2,

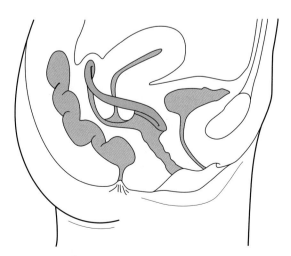

Figure 18-7 • Placement of a vaginal pessary to treat pelvic organ prolapse.

correction of cystoceles and rectoceles can be accomplished by **anterior and posterior colporrhaphy**, respectively. These procedures repair the **fascial defect** through which the herniation occurred (see Figs. 18-8 to 18-10). Enteroceles, which represent the herniation of small bowel into the vaginal canal, can be repaired along with the reinforcement of the rectovaginal fascia and the posterior vaginal wall. With significant uterine prolapse, abdominal or vaginal **hysterectomy** may be indicated. In women who have prolapse of the vaginal vault after hysterectomy the **vaginal vault prolapse** is corrected by suspension of the vaginal apex to fixed points within the pelvis such as the sacrum (abdominal sacral colpopexy) or sacrospinous ligaments (sacrospinous ligament fixation). The degree of success depends on the skill of the surgeon, the degree of pelvic relaxation, and the age, weight, and lifestyle of the patient.

■ **TABLE 18-2** Surgical Treatment of Pelvic Organ Prolapse	
Cystocele	Anterior colporrhaphy: Removal of excess anterior vaginal mucosa and plication (reinforcement) of the endopelvic fascia to resuspend the bladder
Rectocele	Posterior colporrhaphy: Similar to anterior colporrhaphy, except the rectal fascia is plicated posteriorly and excess posterior vaginal wall is removed
Enterocele	Vaginal enterocele repair: The enterocele is repaired along with plication of the rectovaginal fascia and the posterior vagina wall
Uterine prolapse	Vaginal hysterectomy and McCall culdoplasty: Hysterectomy followed by plication of the uterosacral ligaments to decrease the risk of future vault prolapse
Vaginal Vault Prolapse (after hysterectomy)	Sacrospinous ligament suspension: Suturing of the endopelvic fascia of the vaginal apex to the sacrospinous ligament via a vaginal approach
	Abdominal sacral colpopexy: Uses mesh to attach the vaginal apex to the sacrum via an abdominal approach

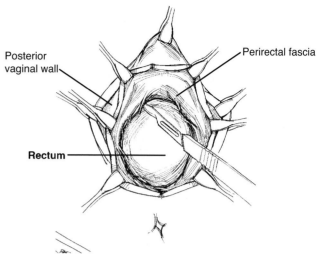

Figure 18-8 • The posterior vaginal wall and rectovaginal fascia are incised and reflected.
(From Bourgeois FJ. *Obstetrics & Gynecology Recall*, 3rd ed. Philadelphia: Lippincott Williams & Wilkins, 2008.)

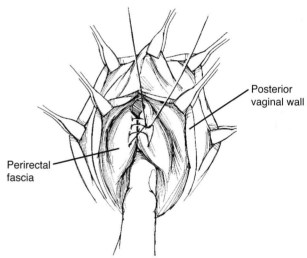

Figure 18-9 • The rectocele is reduced by placating (reinforcing) the perirectal fascia to the midline.
(From Bourgeois FJ. *Obstetrics & Gynecology Recall*, 3rd ed. Philadelphia: Lippincott Williams & Wilkins, 2008.)

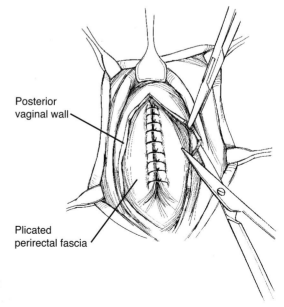

Figure 18-10 • The excess vaginal mucosa is trimmed from the posterior vaginal wall, and the vaginal incision is closed in the midline.
(From Bourgeois FJ. *Obstetrics & Gynecology Recall*, 3rd ed. Philadelphia: Lippincott Williams & Wilkins, 2008.)

KEY POINTS

- Pelvic organ prolapse can result in prolapse of the bladder (cystocele), urethra (urethrocele), rectum (rectocele), small bowel (enterocele), uterus (uterine prolapse) into the vaginal lumen.

- Vaginal vault prolapse occurs most commonly in patients who have undergone hysterectomy. The vagina can then invert into the vaginal canal and potentially outside the body in its most severe form.

- Causes include birth trauma, chronic increases in intra-abdominal pressure, intrinsic weakness, and pelvic change due to aging.

- Pelvic organ prolapse can manifest as pelvic pressure and pain, dyspareunia, bowel and bladder dysfunction, and urinary incontinence.

- Pelvic organ prolapse is diagnosed primarily by history and physical examination, but may also require urine cultures, cystoscopy, urethroscopy, urinary dynamic studies, anoscopy, sigmoidoscopy, and defecography as indicated.

- POP-Q is a system for quantifying the degree of pelvic organ prolapse. It is used more in research while the Baden-Walker Halfway system is used more clinically to quantify pelvic organ prolapse.

- Relaxation of the pelvic organs can be treated non-surgically with Kegel exercises, vaginal pessaries, and/or estrogen replacement.

- Surgical treatment options for pelvic organ prolapse include anterior and posterior colporrhaphy for cystoceles and rectoceles, respectively. These procedures repair the fascial defect and strengthen the existing vaginal wall support.

- Uterine prolapse is most commonly treated with abdominal or vaginal hysterectomy. Vaginal vault prolapse is repaired by resuspending the vaginal vault to a fixed structure in the pelvis.

Urinary Incontinence

URINARY INCONTINENCE

EPIDEMIOLOGY

The involuntary loss of urine is common, affecting an estimated 25 million Americans of all ages. Nearly 50% of all women experience occasional urinary incontinence, and 20% of women over age 75 are affected daily. Urinary incontinence is often a major reason for placing individuals in nursing homes, with some 30% of nursing home residents suffering from urinary incontinence. The incidence of urinary incontinence **increases with age** and with increasing degrees of **pelvic relaxation**.

The four primary types of urinary incontinence are described in Table 19-1. **Stress incontinence** is characterized by urine loss with exertion or straining (coughing, laughing, lifting, exercising) and is typically caused by urethral hypermobility. This differs from **urge incontinence**, also known as *detrusor overactivity*, where urine leakage is due to involuntary and uninhibited bladder contractions. The cause is usually idiopathic but may be due to infection, bladder stones, urinary diverticula, or neurologic disorders such as Alzheimer disease, multiple sclerosis, or stroke. Patients with **mixed incontinence** have components of stress urinary incontinence as well as detrusor overactivity. Finally, **overflow incontinence** may present with incomplete voiding, urinary retention, and overdistension of the bladder due to poor or absent bladder contractions. The causes of overflow incontinence vary widely from the use of certain medications to neurologic disorders and postoperative overdistension.

There are several other conditions which lead to involuntary loss of urine but are not thought of as classic forms of incontinence. Among these is **bypass incontinence**, which is characterized by continuous urine leakage secondary to urinary fistulas. In the United States, almost all cases of total incontinence result from pelvic surgery or pelvic radiation. In many developing nations, total incontinence and urinary fistulas often result from birth trauma and obstructed labor. Similarly, some patients lack the physical or psychological ability to attend to their voiding needs. This type of **functional incontinence** can be seen in nursing home patients and patients with dementia. The mechanisms for voiding and continence may be intact in these patients but they lack the physical or psychological ability to respond to normal voiding cues.

ANATOMY

Understanding the anatomy and physiology of the lower urinary tract and pelvic floor is crucial to understanding the mechanism behind each type of urinary incontinence. The bladder, or detrusor muscle, is a meshwork of smooth muscle layers ending in the trigone area at its base (Fig. 19-1). The **internal sphincter** is at the junction of the bladder and the urethra. This is also known as the UVJ or **urethrovesical junction**. The urethra is also made of smooth muscle. It is suspended by the pubourethral ligaments that originate at the lower pubic bone and extend to the middle third of the urethra to form the **external sphincter**.

Urinary continence at rest is possible because the **intraurethral pressure** exceeds the **intravesical pressure**. Continuous contraction of the **internal sphincter** is one of the primary mechanisms for maintaining continence at rest. The **external sphincter** provides about 50% of urethral resistance and is the second line

■ **TABLE 19-1** Primary Types of Urinary Incontinence	
Stress incontinence	Urine loss with exertion or straining (coughing, laughing, exercising) typically associated with pelvic relaxation and urethral hypermobility
Urge incontinence	Urine leakage due to involuntary and uninhibited bladder contractions known as detrusor overactivity
Mixed incontinence	Urinary leakage with characteristics of both stress urinary incontinence as well as detrusor overactivity
Overflow incontinence	Incontinence due to poor or absent bladder contractions that lead to urinary retention with overdistension of the bladder and overflow incontinence
Other: Bypass incontinence	Continuous urine leakage due to urinary fistula resulting from pelvic surgery or pelvic radiation
Other: Functional incontinence	Urinary incontinence due to a physical or psychological (e.g., dementia) inability to respond to voiding cues. Often seen in nursing home patients and geriatric patients.

of defense against incontinence. When the UVJ is in its proper position, any sudden increase in intra-abdominal pressure is **transmitted equally to the bladder and proximal third of the urethra**. Therefore, as long as the intraurethral pressure exceeds the intravesical pressure, continence is preserved.

In addition to the internal and external sphincters, continence is also maintained via the action of the **submucosal vasculature** of the urethra. When this vasculature complex fills with blood, the intraurethral pressure is increased, thus preventing involuntary loss of urine (Fig. 19-2). The filling mechanism of this system—known as **mucosal coaptation**—is estrogen sensitive, which explains why the estrogen-deficient postmenopausal state can lead to incontinence.

Neurologic control of the bladder and urethra is provided by both the **autonomic** (sympathetic and parasympathetic) and **somatic nervous systems** (Fig. 19-3). The **sympathetic nervous system** provides continence and prevents micturition by contracting the bladder neck and internal sphincter. Sympathetic control of the bladder is achieved via the **hypogastric**

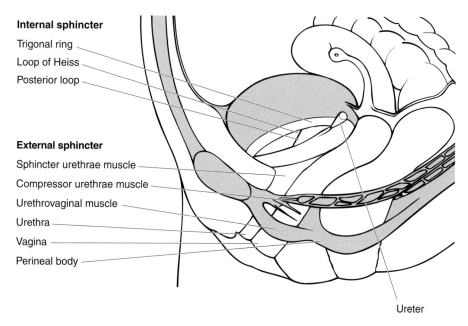

Internal sphincter
Trigonal ring
Loop of Heiss
Posterior loop

External sphincter
Sphincter urethrae muscle
Compressor urethrae muscle
Urethrovaginal muscle
Urethra
Vagina
Perineal body

Ureter

Figure 19-1 • Internal and external bladder sphincters.

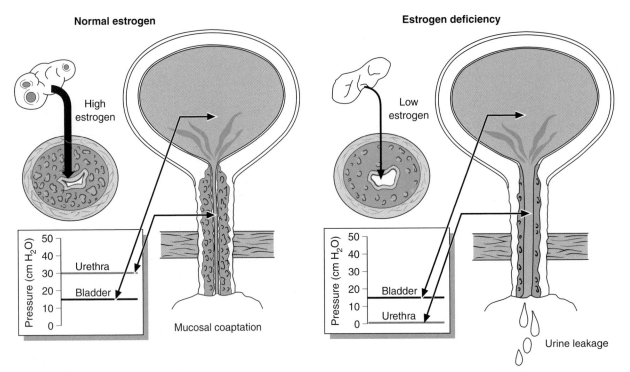

Normal estrogen

High estrogen

Pressure (cm H₂O)

50		
40		
30	Urethra	
20		
10	Bladder	
0		

Mucosal coaptation

Estrogen increases urethral resting pressure, making involuntary urine loss more difficult.

Estrogen deficiency

Low estrogen

Pressure (cm H₂O)

50		
40		
30		
20	Bladder	
10		
0	Urethra	

Urine leakage

Estrogen deficiency decreases urethral resting pressure and facilitates urine leakage.

Figure 19-2 • Urethral mucosal coaptation.

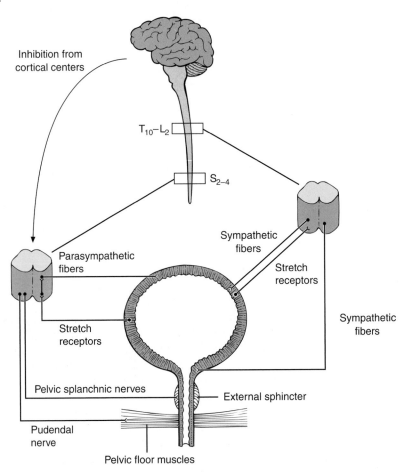

Inhibition from cortical centers

T_{10}–L_2

S_{2-4}

Sympathetic fibers

Parasympathetic fibers

Stretch receptors

Stretch receptors

Sympathetic fibers

Pelvic splanchnic nerves

External sphincter

Pudendal nerve

Pelvic floor muscles

Figure 19-3 • Innervation of the lower urinary tract.

nerve originating from T10 to L2 of the spinal cord. The **parasympathetic nervous system** allows micturition to occur. Parasympathetic control of the bladder is supplied by the **pelvic nerve** derived from S2, S3, and S4 of the spinal cord. Finally, the somatic nervous system aids in voluntary prevention of micturition by innervating the striated muscle of the external sphincter and pelvic floor through the **pudendal nerve**.

During micturition, the bladder releases its contents under voluntary control through a series of coordinated activities resulting in urethral relaxation and bladder contraction. Stretch receptors in the bladder wall send a signal to the central nervous system (CNS) to begin voluntary voiding. This triggers inhibition of the sympathetic sacral and pudendal nerves, thereby causing relaxation of the urethra, external sphincter, and levator ani muscles. This is closely followed by activation of the parasympathetic pelvic nerve, resulting in contraction of the detrusor muscle, and micturition begins.

PHYSICAL EXAMINATION

Care of all patients with urinary incontinence should begin with obtaining a thorough medical and surgical history. The **physical examination** should include both internal and external pelvic examinations. Because the innervation of the lower urinary tract is closely associated with the innervation of the lower extremities and rectum, patients should receive a thorough **neurologic examination**. In particular, deep tendon reflexes, anal reflex, pelvic floor contractions, and the bulbocavernosus reflex (contraction after gentle tapping or squeezing of the clitoris) should be elicited.

DIAGNOSTIC EVALUATION

Fortunately, a variety of diagnostic tests are available for the evaluation of urinary incontinence. The scope of this text precludes an exhaustive compilation of every diagnostic modality. In general, the goal of diagnostic testing is to distinguish between stress urinary incontinence and detrusor overactivity since the treatments for these two conditions are very different. Initial tests typically include the standing stress test, the cotton swab test, cystometrogram, and uroflowmetry. More complex urodynamic studies can be obtained when indicated (considering surgery, patient 65 years old, complicated history, underlying neurologic disease).

A **voiding diary** (Fig. 19-4) can be used to document the specific circumstances of the patient's voiding habits (e.g., intake, amount voided, leak volume, associated activity, urge presence). A **urinalysis and urine culture** should be obtained to rule out infection as a cause of incontinence.

A **standing stress test** is performed by having the patient with a full bladder stand over a towel or sheet with feet placed shoulder distance apart. The patient is asked to cough, and the clinician observes to verify a loss of urine. Alternatively, the clinician can ask the patient to cough while in the lithotomy position. Either method may be used to document stress incontinence. If urine leakage is witnessed by the clinician, the patient is then said to have **stress urinary incontinence**. The stress test has low specificity and sensitivity.

A **postvoid residual** is obtained by catheterization of the bladder after voiding. This specimen can then be used to rule out urinary retention and infection.

The purpose of the **cotton swab test** is to diagnose a hypermobile urethra associated with urinary stress incontinence. The clinician inserts a lubricated cotton swab into the urethra to the angle of the urethrovesical junction (Fig. 19-5). When the patient strains as if urinating, the urethrovesical junction descends and the cotton swab moves upward. The change in cotton swab angle is normally less than 30 degrees (Fig. 19-5A), but will range from 30 to 60 degrees with a hypermobile urethra (Fig. 19-5B).

Urodynamic studies are usually reserved for patients contemplating surgery and for those in whom a clear diagnosis cannot be made on preliminary tests. The three major components of urodynamic studies include evaluation of urethral function, bladder filling (cystometrogram), and bladder emptying (uroflowmetry).

As part of urodynamic testing, a **cystometrogram** measures the response of the bladder, vagina, and rectum to filling the bladder with fluid. To achieve this, pressure sensors are placed in the bladder, vagina, and rectum and are used to determine bladder and sphincter tone as the bladder is filled with fluid in a retrograde fashion. The cystometrogram measures the bladder-filling capacity, the presence or absence of a detrusor reflex in response to filling, and the patient's ability to control or inhibit the strong desire to void. The sensation to void typically occurs after the bladder is instilled with 150 mL of fluid. Normal bladder capacity is 400 to 600 mL.

Urodynamic measurements may also include **uroflowmetry**, which measures the rate of urine flow

Number of pads changed today ___1___
Type of pad used __Maxi pad__

	Urinate in toilet (time and amount)		Accident (time)	Activity during accident	Fluid intake (time, type, amount)
To Bed →	2200	240 cc			1 glass water
	0300	660 cc	0300	Leak on way to bathroom	
	0500	540 cc	0500	Preparing to urinate	
Up For Day →	0700	150 cc			16 oz coffee 1 cup water
	0845	35 cc			
	1145	160 cc			
	1200				16 oz lemonade
	1540	60 cc			
	1800	100 cc			2 glasses wine 2 cups water
	1940	60 cc			16 oz diet coke 1 glass water

Figure 19-4 • Voiding diary (also called bladder chart). This patient's diary demonstrates urinary frequency, nocturia, urge incontinence, and greater consumption of fluid, caffeine, and alcohol in the evening.
(From Berek JS. *Berek & Novak's Gynecology*, 14th ed. Philadelphia: Lippincott Williams & Wilkins, 2006.)

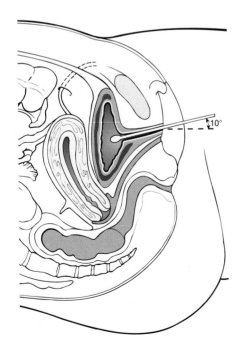

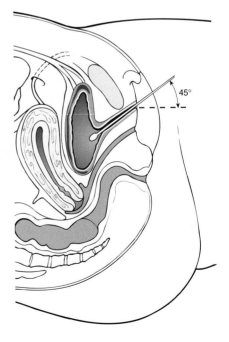

A: During the cotton swab test, a swab is placed in the urethra to the bladder neck. Normal movement of the UVJ with Valsalva (straining) should be less than 30°.

B: When pelvic relaxation results in hypermobility of the bladder neck, there is a large change (30° to 60°) of the UVJ with Valsalva (straining).

Figure 19-5 • **(A,B)** Cotton swab test.

and flow time through the urethra when a patient is asked to spontaneously void while sitting on an uroflow chair. Uroflowmetry is useful in diagnosing outflow obstruction and abnormal bladder reflexes, especially in patients complaining of hesitancy, incomplete bladder emptying, poor stream, and urinary retention.

STRESS INCONTINENCE

PATHOGENESIS

Stress incontinence, also known as genuine stress incontinence or true stress incontinence when witnessed by a clinician, is the involuntary release of urine through the intact urethra in response to a sudden increase in **intra-abdominal pressure** such as coughing, sneezing, or exercise. In most cases, pelvic relaxation results in a **hypermobile urethra**. As a result, increases in intra-abdominal pressure are no longer transmitted equally to the bladder and urethra. Instead, increases in intra-abdominal pressure are transmitted primarily to the bladder. Therefore, as **intravesical pressures exceed intraurethral pressure**, urinary stress incontinence occurs (Fig. 19-6). In a smaller percentage of women, stress urinary incontinence may be due to **weakness in the internal urethral sphincter** known as *intrinsic sphincter deficiency* (ISD).

RISK FACTORS

The risk factors for urinary stress incontinence include factors that affect the normal transmission of intra-abdominal pressure, those that increase intravesical

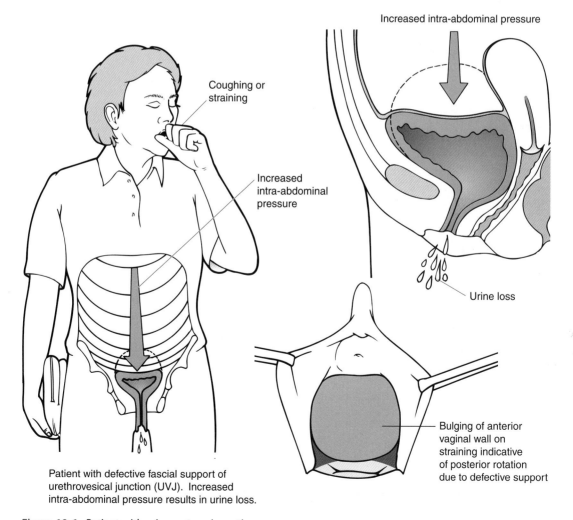

Coughing or straining

Increased intra-abdominal pressure

Patient with defective fascial support of urethrovesical junction (UVJ). Increased intra-abdominal pressure results in urine loss.

Increased intra-abdominal pressure

Urine loss

Bulging of anterior vaginal wall on straining indicative of posterior rotation due to defective support

Figure 19-6 • Patient with urinary stress incontinence.

■ **TABLE 19-2** Risk Factors for Urinary Stress Incontinence

Conditions causing pelvic relaxation
• Vaginal childbirth
• Aging
• Genetic factors
Conditions causing chronic increases in intra-abdominal pressure
• Constipation
• Chronic coughing from lung disease, smoking
• Chronic heavy lifting
• Obesity (does not cause incontinence, but worsens it)
Conditions that weaken the urethral closing mechanism
• Estrogen deficiency
• Scarring
• Denervation
• Medications

pressure, and those that decrease intraurethral pressure (Table 19-2). The three major risk factors for urinary stress incontinence include **pelvic relaxation** (affect transmission), chronically **increased intra-abdominal pressure** (increases intravesical pressure), and **menopause** (decreases intraurethral pressure due to coaptation). Other risk factors are outlined in Table 19-2.

HISTORY

Patients with urinary stress incontinence may present with a sole complaint of involuntary loss of urine with coughing, laughing, sneezing, and straining. With more severe stress incontinence, urine leakage may occur with activities that cause even small increases in intra-abdominal pressure, such as walking or changing positions. If pelvic organ prolapse is also involved, patients may report feeling a bulge, pressure, or pain in the vagina.

DIAGNOSTIC EVALUATION

Table 19-3 lists the criteria for diagnosing urinary stress incontinence.

TREATMENT

The goal of stress incontinence treatment is to maximize pelvic support and to restore the anatomic position of the urethra. This can be accomplished using a number of therapies. However, there are no good medical treatments for stress urinary incontinence due to structurally derived urethral hypermobility. Most nonsurgical treatments have a 30% to 40% success rate.

A variety of **behavior modifications** have been useful in improving mild stress incontinence, including fluid intake regulation, change of medications such as diuretics, biofeedback, and bladder training.

Medical therapies including estrogen and imipramine work to increase urethral sphincter tone and enhance urethral closure. Topical or systemic **estrogen** can be used to increase urethral tone by enhancing mucosal coaptation.

Pelvic diaphragm exercises (**Kegel exercises**) result in an increase in resting and active muscle tone and thereby increase urethral closing pressure in cases of mild incontinence. These can be done with or without biofeedback and/or electrical stimulation.

Pessaries and other intravaginal devices are used to physically elevate and support the urethra, which restores normal anatomic relationships. As a result,

■ **TABLE 19-3** Criteria and Tools for Diagnosing Stress Incontinence

Normal urinalysis
Negative urine culture
Normal neurologic examination
Poor anatomic support (suggesting pelvic relaxation)
Cotton swab test
Urethroscopy
Demonstrable leakage with stress
Stress test
Pad test
Normal cystometrogram or urethrocystometry
Normal residual urine volume
Normal bladder capacity and sensation
No involuntary detrusor contractions

Adapted from DeCherney A, Pernoll M. *Current Obstetric and Gynecologic Diagnosis and Treatment.* Norwalk, CT: Appleton & Lange, 1994:837.

increases in intra-abdominal pressures are transmitted equally to the bladder and urethra and continence is maintained. Incontinence pessaries differ from pessaries for pelvic relaxation in that incontinence pessaries have added features to specifically support the urethra (Fig. 19-7). Because pessaries are non-invasive, they are useful in patients for whom surgery is contraindicated (elderly, ill, or pregnant women). These devices require close medical supervision to avoid infection of the vaginal mucosa or damage to the vaginal tissues. Patients are often given vaginal estrogen to decrease the risk of vaginal trauma and ulceration.

Surgery is the primary method of treating urinary stress incontinence. Most of the procedures aim to **resuspend the hypermobile urethra** to its normal anatomic position (Fig. 19-8). Disadvantages of surgery include the risks of an invasive procedure and the risk of failure with resumption of symptoms over time. Several approaches have been employed with roughly equal success. These include the abdominal retropubic urethropexies (Marshall-Marchetti-Krantz and Burch procedures), and sub-urethral slings (tension-free vaginal tape, transobturator tape, retropubic sling). Patients with **isolated intrinsic sphincter deficiency** without urethral hypermobility benefit from periurethral or transurethral placement of bulking agents to improve sphincter tone (Fig. 19-9).

DETRUSOR OVERACTIVITY

PATHOGENESIS

Detrusor overactivity, also known as **urge incontinence**, is usually caused by involuntary and uninhibited detrusor contractions during the filling phase of bladder function. Under normal circumstances, these contractions should not occur.

Most detrusor overactivity is **idiopathic**. Some conditions known to cause involuntary bladder contractions include urinary tract infections (UTIs), bladder stones, bladder cancer, urethral diverticula, and foreign bodies (Fig. 19-10). Detrusor overactivity, or detrusor hyperreflexia, may also be due to

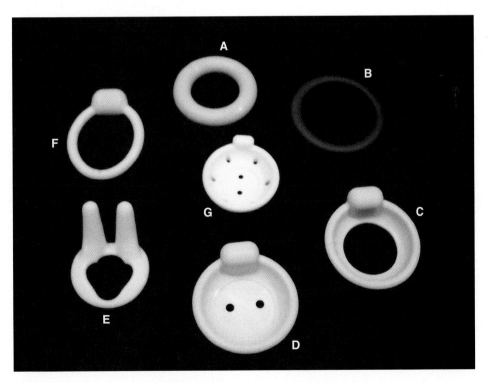

Figure 19-7 • Vaginal incontinence pessaries for treating stress urinary incontinence. Incontinence pessaries differ from more common prolapse pessaries in that most incontinence pessaries have a portion of the device specifically designed to support the bladder neck.
(From Berek JS. *Berek & Novak's Gynecology*, 14th ed. Philadelphia: Lippincott Williams & Wilkins, 2006.)

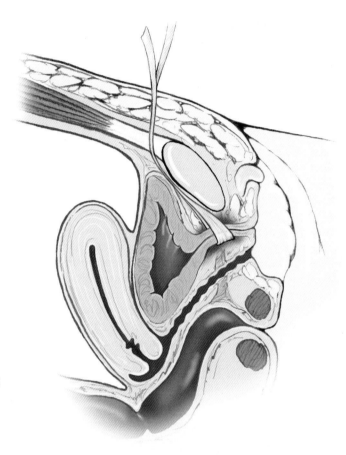

Figure 19-8 • Suburethral sling. The sling is supporting the urethra and bladder neck and the ends are anchored to or above the rectus fascia.
(From Berek JS. *Berek & Novak's Gynecology*, 14th ed. Philadelphia: Lippincott Williams & Wilkins, 2006.)

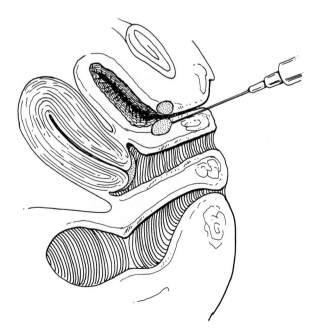

Figure 19-9 • Periurethral injection of collagen around the bladder neck.
(Image from Rock J, Jones H. *TeLinde's Operative Gynecology*, 10th ed. Philadelphia: Lippincott Williams & Wilkins, 2008.)

neurologic disease such as stroke, Alzheimer disease, Parkinson disease, multiple sclerosis, and diabetes mellitus (Table 19-4).

EPIDEMIOLOGY

In the general population, the incidence of detrusor overactivity is 10% to 15%.

CLINICAL MANIFESTATIONS

History

Patients with urge incontinence usually present with a history of involuntary urine loss and urgency whether or not the bladder is full. Many women complain of not being able to reach the bathroom in time or of dribbling or leaking triggered by just seeing a bathroom.

Physical Examination

Detrusor overactivity presents with symptoms that suggest **bladder overactivity**, including urinary

Secondary detrusor overactivity

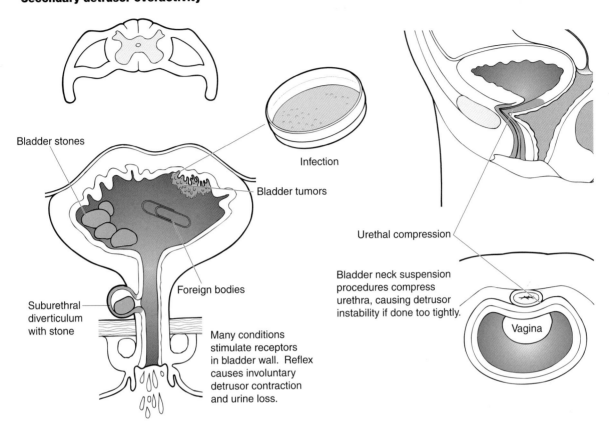

Bladder stones

Infection

Bladder tumors

Urethal compression

Foreign bodies

Bladder neck suspension procedures compress urethra, causing detrusor instability if done too tightly.

Vagina

Suburethral diverticulum with stone

Many conditions stimulate receptors in bladder wall. Reflex causes involuntary detrusor contraction and urine loss.

Figure 19-10 • Causes of detrusor overactivity.

urgency, frequency (more than eight times a day), stress incontinence, and nocturia (more than two times per night). Given the wide differential for detrusor overactivity, patients should also be asked about neurologic symptoms, history of previous anti-incontinence surgery, and hematuria (suggestive of cancer, stones, or infection).

TREATMENT

The treatment of urge incontinence will depend on the etiology of disease. Bladder training, Kegel exercises, biofeedback, hypnosis, and psychotherapy are methods of **behavior modification** that have had moderate success in controlling urge incontinence. Bladder training begins by establishing a regular voiding schedule that is modified to gradually lengthen the intervals between voiding until the patient reestablishes cortical control over the voiding reflex.

Medical therapy for detrusor overactivity is designed to enhance urine storage, relax the bladder, and suppress involuntary bladder contractions. Bladder contractions (micturition) are caused by stimulation of the parasympathetic nervous system through the release of acetylcholine. Continence is maintained in part by the sympathetic nervous system mediated through norepinephrine (Table 19-5). It is therefore not surprising that drugs to treat the frequent unexpected bladder contractions seen in detrusor overactivity are often anticholinergic (suppressing micturition) or alpha-adrenergic (supporting continence).

The most frequently used and most effective medications for urge incontinence are **anticholinergics** (e.g., Pro-Banthine, oxybutynin). Similarly, **smooth muscle relaxants** (e.g., Detrol, tolterodine) can be used to increase bladder capacity, decrease frequency of bladder contractions, and to improve the symptoms of urgency. The tricyclic antidepressant imipramine (Tofranil) is useful in patients with mixed incontinence (DI and SUI) because it has **anticholinergic** and **alpha-adrenergic** activity. As a result,

■ TABLE 19-4 Common Causes of Detrusor Overactivity

Nonneurologic causes
UTIs
Urethral obstruction
Urethral compression (previous surgery)
Bladder stones
Bladder cancer
Suburethral diverticula
Foreign bodies
Neurologic causes
Cerebrovascular accident
Alzheimer disease
Parkinsonism
Multiple sclerosis
Diabetes
Peripheral neuropathies
Autonomic neuropathies
Cauda equine lesions

■ TABLE 19-5 Neurologic Control of Continence and Micturition and Resultant Classifications of Drug Therapies

Continence	
Norepinephrine	Adrenergic medications to increase bladder storage
Sympathetic	
Micturition	
Acetylcholine	Anticholinergic medications to block bladder contractions
Parasympathetic	

it increases bladder storage, improves bladder compliance, and increases bladder outlet resistance (Table 19-6). These medications used alone or in concert are effective in 50% to 80% of patients.

There are no effective surgical procedures to treat detrusor overactivity.

OVERFLOW INCONTINENCE

PATHOGENESIS

Overflow incontinence in women is usually due to **detrusor insufficiency** (bladder hypotonia) or **detrusor areflexia** (bladder acontractility). As a result, bladder contractions are weak or nonexistent, causing incomplete voiding, urinary retention, and overdistension of

■ TABLE 19-6 Medications Used to Treat Detrusor Overactivity

Generic Name	Trade Name	Drug Class	Indication	Mechanism of Action
Propantheline bromide	Pro-Banthine	Anticholinergic	Detrusor overactivity	Decreases bladder contractions
Oxybutynin chloride	Ditropan, Ditropan XL	Anticholinergic and smooth muscle relaxant	Detrusor overactivity	Decreases frequency of bladder contractions, increases bladder capacity
Tolterodine	Detrol, Detrol LA	Bladder-specific anticholinergic and smooth muscle relaxant	Overactive bladder, detrusor overactivity	Decreases frequency of bladder contractions, increases bladder capacity
Flavoxate hydrochloride	Urispas	Smooth muscle relaxant	Detrusor overactivity	Relaxes detrusor muscle
Imipramine hydrochloride	Tofranil	Tricyclic antidepressant	Mixed incontinence (DI and SUI)	Increases bladder storage and compliance, increases bladder outlet resistance

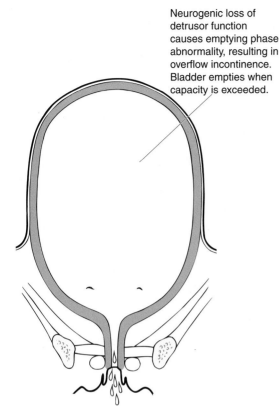

Neurogenic loss of detrusor function causes emptying phase abnormality, resulting in overflow incontinence. Bladder empties when capacity is exceeded.

Figure 19-11 • Overdistended bladder with overflow incontinence.

■ **TABLE 19-7** Causes of Overflow Incontinence
Neurogenic causes
Lower motor neuron disease
Spinal cord injuries
Diabetes mellitus (autonomic neuropathy)
Multiple sclerosis
Obstructive causes
Postsurgical urethral obstruction (rare)
Post-operative overdistention
Pelvic masses
Fecal impaction
Pharmacologic causes
Anticholinergic drugs
Alpha-adrenergic agonists
Epidural and spinal anesthesia
Other causes
Cystitis and urethritis
Psychogenic (psychosis or severe depression)
Idiopathic

the bladder (Fig. 19-11). The causes of overflow incontinence due to detrusor insufficiency vary widely from fecal compaction, to use of certain medications, to neurologic diseases including lower motor neuron disease, autonomic neuropathy (diabetes), spinal cord injuries, and multiple sclerosis (Table 19-7).

Outflow obstruction, typically due to surgical procedures that result in urethral kinking, stenosis, or obstruction, can also cause bladder overdistension and overflow incontinence, but it is rarely seen in women. **Postoperative overdistension** of the bladder due to unrecognized urinary retention and the use of epidural anesthesia are common causes of overflow incontinence.

CLINICAL MANIFESTATIONS

Patients with overflow incontinence may present with a wide variety of symptoms including frequent or **constant urinary dribbling**, along with the symptoms of stress incontinence and urge incontinence.

Outflow obstruction (rare) involves a history of urinary retention, straining to void, poor stream, and incomplete emptying.

TREATMENT

Treatment strategy in overflow incontinence is geared toward relieving urinary retention, increasing bladder contractility, and decreasing urethral closing pressure.

Medical management of overflow incontinence includes the use of various agents to reduce urethral closing pressure (prazosin, terazosin, phenoxybenzamine) and **striated muscle relaxants** (diazepam, dantrolene) to reduce bladder outlet resistance. **Cholinergic agents** (bethanechol) are used to increase bladder contractility (Table 19-6). Intermittent **self-catheterization** may also be used in overflow incontinence to avoid chronic urinary retention and infection.

Patients with overflow incontinence due to **urinary obstruction** benefit from surgical correction of the obstruction. Postoperative overdistension of the bladder is typically temporary and may be managed by continuous bladder drainage for 24 to 48 hours.

OTHER INCONTINENCE: BYPASS INCONTINENCE

PATHOGENESIS

Bypass incontinence (continuous urine flow) is typically the result of a **urinary fistula** formed between the bladder and the vagina (vesicovaginal fistula), as shown in Figure 19-12, or between the urethra and the vagina (urethrovaginal fistula) or the ureter and the vagina (ureterovaginal fistula).

In developing countries, the most common cause of urinary fistulas is **obstetric trauma** from an obstructed labor, prolonged second stage, or operative deliveries (e.g., forceps, vacuum extraction). However, in the United States, genitourinary fistulas are most often caused by **pelvic radiation** or **pelvic surgery**. Ectopic ureters and urethral diverticula may also produce total incontinence.

EPIDEMIOLOGY

Pelvic radiation and **pelvic surgery** account for over 95% of total urinary incontinence cases in the United States. In particular, simple **abdominal hysterectomy** and **vaginal hysterectomy** alone account for over 50% of vesicovaginal fistulas. Urethrovaginal fistulas may also occur as complications of surgery for urethral di-

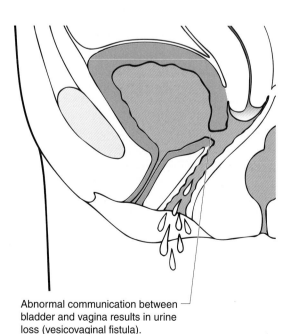

Abnormal communication between bladder and vagina results in urine loss (vesicovaginal fistula).

Figure 19-12 • Vesicovaginal fistula.

verticula, anterior vaginal wall prolapse, or stress urinary incontinence. Ureterovaginal fistulas, as seen after 1% to 2% of **radical hysterectomies**, are usually due to devascularization rather than direct injury. Obstetric injuries associated with **operative vaginal deliveries** (forceps, vacuum) were once the leading cause of urinary fistulas but are now rare causes of total urinary incontinence in the United States, Canada, and western Europe.

RISK FACTORS

The incidence of fistula formation after surgery is higher if the patient has a history of preoperative radiation, endometriosis, pelvic inflammatory disease (PID), or previous pelvic surgery.

HISTORY

Patients with a urinary fistula usually present with a history of painless and continuous loss of urine, usually after pelvic surgery or pelvic radiation. Fistulas due to surgery become clinically apparent in 5 to 14 postoperative days.

DIAGNOSTIC EVALUATION

Methylene blue dye instilled **into the bladder** in a retrograde fashion will leak onto a tampon if a vesicovaginal fistula is present. To diagnose a ureterovaginal fistula, **indigo carmine** is given intravenously. As the compound is filtered through the kidneys and passes through the ureters, it will stain the tampon. If a ureterovaginal fistula is present, the methylene blue test will be negative and the indigo carmine test will be positive. **Cystourethroscopy** and the **voiding cystourethrogram** (VCUG) can then be used to identify the number and location of the fistulas. Intravenous pyelogram (IVP) and retrograde pyelogram may also be used to localize urinary fistulas as well.

TREATMENT

Surgery is the primary treatment for urinary fistulas. Most **obstetric fistulas** can be repaired immediately; however, it is typical to wait 3 to 6 months before attempting to repair **postsurgical fistulas**. This waiting period allows inflammation to decrease and vascularity and pliability of the area to increase. **Antibiotics** for urinary infection and **estrogen** for postmenopausal women are also used during this period. **Steroids** have been used to decrease inflammation, although their use is still controversial.

OTHER INCONTINENCE: FUNCTIONAL INCONTINENCE

Functional incontinence is attributed to factors outside the lower urinary tract. These might include physical or mental impairments which prevent the patient from being able to response normally to cues to void. These are particularly common in nursing home residents and in geriatric patients in general. Factors such as physical immobility, dementia, delirium, medications, and systemic illness can all contribute to functional incontinence. Once an etiologic agent is identified, treatment should be aimed at addressing the root cause.

 KEY POINTS

- Under normal circumstances, urinary incontinence is avoided due to the complex system of muscles, ligaments, sphincters, and nerves that keep the intraurethral pressure greater than the intravesical pressure.

- Diagnostic evaluation includes a thorough history and physical, urine culture and analysis, standing stress test, cotton-swab test, and use of a voiding diary. Simple urodynamics (cystometrogram, uroflowmetry) can be used as indicated.

- The incidence of urinary incontinence increases with age and with increasing degrees of pelvic relaxation. The four primary types are stress incontinence, detrusor overactivity, mixed incontinence, and overflow incontinence.

- Stress urinary incontinence is characterized by leaking with physical activity such as coughing, sneezing, lifting, or exercising. It is most commonly due to urethral hypermobility and occasionally from intrinsic sphincter weakness.

- Risk factors for stress urinary incontinence include pelvic relaxation, chronically increased intra-abdominal pressure (e.g., obesity, chronic cough), and estrogen deficiency in menopause.

- Stress incontinence can be treated with pelvic exercises, medication to enhance urethral sphincter closure (estrogen, imipramine), or surgery to stabilize the hypermobile urethra.

- Detrusor overactivity results from involuntary and uninhibited bladder contractions. Symptoms include urinary urgency, frequency, and nocturia. Most cases of detrusor overactivity are idiopathic. Other cases are caused by UTI, bladder stones, cancer, diverticula, and neurologic disorders (stroke, multiple sclerosis, Alzheimer disease).

- The goal of medical treatment is to relax the bladder, suppress involuntary bladder contractions, and enhance urine storage. This can be achieved with bladder training, behavior modification, and medication (especially anticholinergics).

- When neurologic etiologies exist, treatment of the disorder may result in improved detrusor stability. There are no effective surgical procedures for the treatment of detrusor overactivity.

- Overflow incontinence is most commonly due to decreased detrusor contractions due to medications or neurologic disease; obstruction and postoperative overdistension occur less frequently in women.

- The primary symptom is urinary retention with continuous dribbling and it is usually treated with self-catheterization and/or medications to increase bladder contractility (cholinergic agents) and lower urethral resistance (*alpha-adrenergic agents*).

- *Bypass incontinence* is painless, continuous urine leakage usually due to vesicovaginal, urethrovaginal, or ureterovaginal fistulas. Bypass incontinence is treated surgically with repair of the urinary fistula.

- The most common causes of urinary fistulas in the United States are pelvic radiation and pelvic surgery. In developing countries, total incontinence is attributable to obstetric trauma, often leading to urinary fistula.

- *Functional incontinence* is urinary loss due to the physical and/or mental inability to attend to voiding cues. Causes include physical impairment, dementia and delirium, and medications.

- Functional incontinence occurs most commonly in nursing homes and in geriatric and psychiatric patients.

Puberty, the Menstrual Cycle, and Menopause

PUBERTY

Puberty describes the series of events in which a child matures into a young adult. It encompasses as series of neuroendocrine and physiologic changes, which result in the ability to ovulate and menstruate (Fig. 20-1). These changes include the development of secondary sex characteristics, the growth spurt, and achievement of fertility. Before any perceived phenotypic change, **adrenarche** occurs with regeneration of the zona reticularis in the adrenal cortex and production of androgens. **Gonadarche** follows with pulsatile gonadotropin-releasing hormone (GnRH) secretion stimulating the anterior pituitary to produce luteinizing hormone (LH) and follicle-stimulating hormone (FSH). These in turn trigger the ovary to produce estrogens. Subsequently physical changes are triggered, including breast development (**thelarche**), development of pubic and axillary hair (**pubarche**), the growth spurt (peak height velocity), and onset of menstruation (**menarche**). These stages usually occur in that order (Fig. 20-2). Concerned parents can be reassured by knowing that, on average, the length of time from breast bud development to menstruation is typically 2.5 years.

ADRENARCHE AND GONADARCHE

Adrenarche occurs between ages 6 and 8 when the adrenal gland begins regeneration of the zona reticularis. This inner layer of the adrenal cortex is responsible for the **secretion of sex steroid hormones**. As a result of the regeneration, the adrenal gland produces increased quantities of the androgens

dehydroepiandrosterone sulfate (DHEAS), dehydroepiandrosterone (DHEA), and androstenedione. Production of these androgenic steroid hormones increases from age 6 to 8 up until age 13 to 15.

Gonadarche begins around age 8, when pulsatile GnRH secretion from the hypothalamus is increased. This leads to subsequent pulsatile secretion of LH and FSH from the anterior pituitary. Initially, these increases occur mostly during sleep and fail to lead to any phenotypic changes. As a girl enters early puberty, the LH and FSH pulsatility lasts throughout the day, eventually leading to stimulation of the ovary and subsequent estrogen release. This, in turn, triggers the characteristic physical changes associated with puberty. The positive feedback of estradiol also results in the initiation of the LH surge and the ability to ovulate.

THELARCHE

The first stage of **thelarche**, the development of breast buds, usually occurs around age 10. Thelarche is usually the **first phenotypic sign of puberty** and occurs in response to the increase in levels of circulating estrogen. Concomitantly, there is estrogenation of the vaginal mucosa and growth of the vagina and uterus. Further development of the breast will continue throughout puberty and adolescence, as described by Marshall and Tanner (Table 20-1 and Fig. 20-3).

PUBARCHE

The onset of **growth of pubic hair** (Fig. 20-3) usually occurs around age 11 and is often accompanied by growth of **axillary hair**. Pubarche usually follows

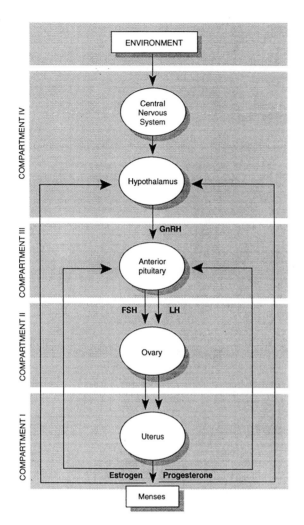

COMPARTMENT IV

COMPARTMENT III

COMPARTMENT II

COMPARTMENT I

ENVIRONMENT

Central Nervous System

Hypothalamus

GnRH

Anterior pituitary

FSH   LH

Ovary

Uterus

Estrogen   Progesterone

Menses

Figure 20-1 • Basic principles of menstrual function. The hypothalamic-pituitary-ovarian axis can be segmented into distinct compartments; each is necessary for normal menstrual function. (From Bourgeois FJ. *Obstetrics & Gynecology Recall*, 3rd ed. Philadelphia: Lippincott Williams & Wilkins, 2008.)

thelarche, but a normal variant in order is seen with pubarche preceding thelarche, particularly in African American girls. The growth of pubic and axillary hair is likely secondary to the increase in **circulating androgens**.

PEAK GROWTH VELOCITY

The growth spurt is characterized by an acceleration in growth rate around age 9 to 10, leading to a peak growth velocity around age 12 of about 9 cm per year. The increased rate of growth is likely secondary to increasing levels of **estrogen**, which result in increased levels of **growth hormone and somatomedin-C**.

MENARCHE

The average age at onset of menstruation is between 12 and 13 or **2.5 years after the development of breast buds**. The adolescent menstrual cycle is usually irregular for the first 1 to 2 years after menarche, reflecting anovulatory cycles. On average, it takes about 2 years after menarche before regular ovulatory cycles are achieved. Failure to achieve a regular menstrual cycle after this point may represent a reproductive disorder. Menarche is often delayed in gymnasts, distance runners, and ballet dancers. Some theories propose that this is due to an **insufficient percentage of body fat** that may result in hypothalamic anovulation and amenorrhea. Others postulate that the **exercise and stress** on the body may inhibit ovulation through positive effects on norepinephrine and GnRH, thus interfering with menarche.

THE MENSTRUAL CYCLE

The hypothalamus, pituitary, ovaries, and uterus are all involved in maintaining the menstrual cycle (Fig. 20-1). The menstrual cycle is divided into two 14-day phases, **the follicular and luteal phases**, which describe changes in the ovary over the length of the cycle, and the **proliferative and secretory phases**, which describe concurrent changes in the endometrium over the same period of time (Fig. 20-4).

During the **follicular phase** the release of **follicle-stimulating hormone** (FSH) from the pituitary gland results in development of a primary ovarian follicle. The ovarian **follicle produces estrogen**, which causes the uterine lining to proliferate. At midcycle—approximately day 14 there is an LH spike in response to a preceding estrogen surge, which stimulates ovulation, the release of the ovum from the follicle (Fig. 20-4). After ovulation the **luteal phase** begins. The remnants of the follicle left behind in the ovary develop into the corpus luteum. This corpus luteum is responsible for the **secretion of progesterone**, which maintains the endometrial lining in preparation to receive a fertilized ovum. If fertilization does not occur, the corpus luteum degenerates and progesterone levels fall. Without progesterone, the endometrial lining is sloughed off, which is known as *menstruation* (Fig. 20-4).

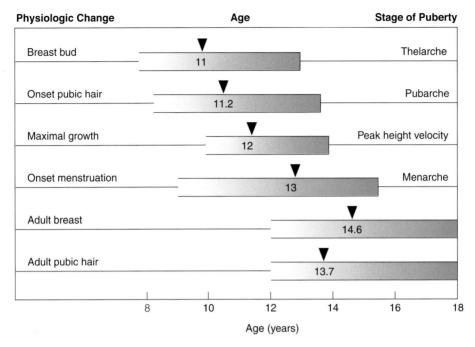

Figure 20-2 • Average age and age range for onset of the major physical changes associated with puberty.

FOLLICULAR PHASE

The withdrawal of estrogen and progesterone during the luteal phase of the prior cycle causes a gradual increase in FSH. In turn, FSH stimulates growth of approximately 5 to 15 **primordial ovarian follicles**, initiating the **follicular phase**. Of these primordial follicles, one becomes the **dominant follicle** and develops and matures until ovulation. The developing dominant follicle destined to ovulate produces estrogen that enhances follicular maturation and increases the production of FSH and LH receptors in an autocrine fashion.

The estrogens are produced in a two-cell process with the **theca interna cells** producing **androstene-dione** in response to LH stimulation and the **granulosa cells** converting this **androstenedione to estradiol** when stimulated by FSH. LH also rises and stimulates the synthesis of androgens, which are converted to estrogen. As rising estrogen levels negatively feed back on pituitary FSH secretion, the dominant follicle is protected from the decrease in FSH by its increased number of FSH receptors (Fig. 20-5).

OVULATION

Toward the end of the follicular phase, estrogen levels eventually surge to reach a critical level that triggers the anterior pituitary to release an LH spike. Ovulation occurs as the increase in LH levels causes

■ **TABLE 20-1** The Tanner Stages of Breast Development	
Stage 1	Preadolescent: Elevation of papilla only
Stage 2	Breast bud stage: Elevation of breast and papilla, areolar enlargement
Stage 3	Further enlargement of breast and areola without separation of contours
Stage 4	Projection of areola and papilla to form a secondary mound
Stage 5	Mature stage: Projection of papilla only as areola recesses to breast contour
Adapted from Speroff L, Glass RH, Kase NG. *Clinical Gynecologic Endocrinology and Infertility*, 5th ed. Baltimore: Williams & Wilkins; 1994:377.	

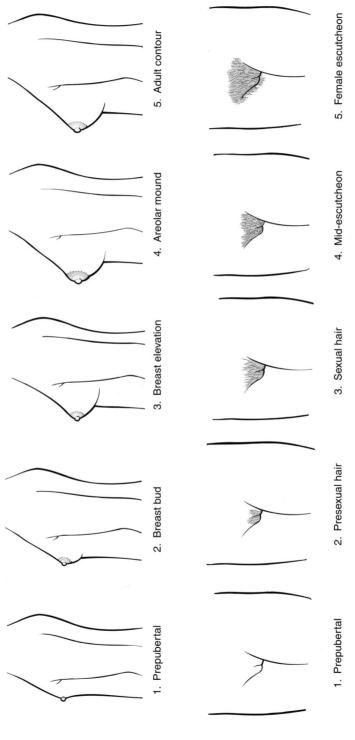

Figure 20-3 • Tanner stages of thelarche (breast development) and of pubarche (onset of pubic hair growth).

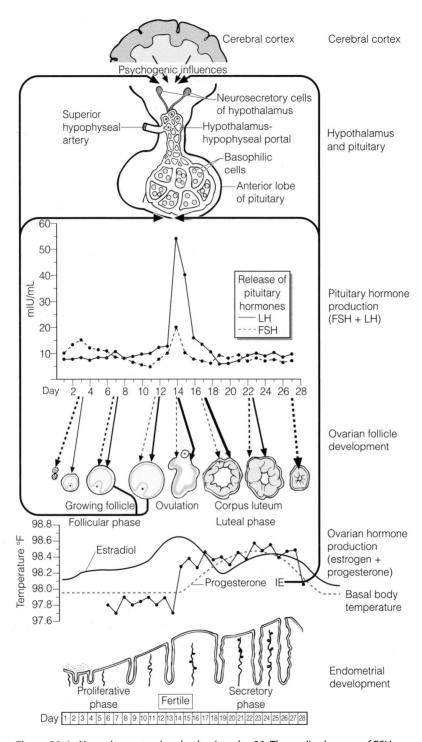

Figure 20-4 • Normal menstrual cycle, day 1 to day 28. The cyclic changes of FSH and LH and the resultant changes in the ovarian histology (follicular and luteal phases) in estrogen and progesterone levels, in basal body temperature, and the endometrial histology (proliferative and secretory phases) are shown. Note how the LH surge near day 14 of a 28-day cycle triggers ovulation and a rise in basal body temperature, signifying the time of maximum fertility during the cycle.

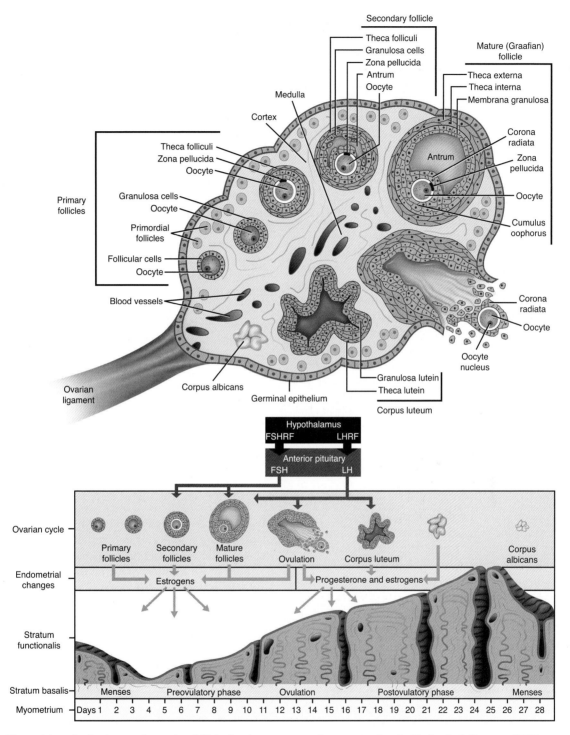

Figure 20-5 • Cyclic changes in ovarian follicle development over the menstrual cycle. Under the influence of FSH, the primordial follicle matures into the preantral follicle and then into the graafian follicle. During the last few days of the growing period, the estrogen produced by the follicular and theca cells stimulate the formation of LH in the pituitary. The LH surge triggers ovulation and the oocyte is discharged from the ovary together. During the luteal phase of the cycle, the follicular cells remaining inside the collapsed follicle differentiate into luteal cells. The corpus luteum is formed by hypertrophy and accumulation of lipid in the granulose and theca interna cells. The remaining cavity of the follicle is filled with fibrin. If pregnancy does not occur, the corpus luteum then degenerates into the corpus albicans and menstruation begins.

(From Eroschenko VP. *Di Fiore's Atlas of Histology, with Functional Correlations*, 9th ed. Baltimore: Lippincott Williams & Wilkins, 2000.)

the follicle to rupture and release the mature ovum (Fig. 20-5). The ovum usually passes into the adjoining fallopian tube and is swept down to the uterus by the cilia lining the tube. This process takes 3 to 4 days. **Fertilization of the ovum must occur within 24 hours of ovulation** or it degenerates.

LUTEAL PHASE

After ovulation, the luteal phase ensues. The **granulosa and theca interna cells** lining the wall of the follicle form the corpus luteum under stimulation by LH. The corpus luteum synthesizes estrogen and significant quantities of progesterone, which cause the endometrium to become more glandular and secretory in preparation for implantation of a fertilized ovum (Fig. 20-5). If fertilization occurs, the developing **trophoblast synthesizes human chorionic gonadotropin (hCG)**—a glycoprotein very similar to LH—that maintains the corpus luteum so that it can continue production of estrogen and progesterone to support the endometrium until **the placenta develops its own synthetic function (at 8 to 10 weeks' gestation)**. If fertilization, with its concomitant rise in hCG, does not occur, the corpus luteum degenerates, progesterone levels fall, the endometrium is not maintained, and menstruation occurs.

MENSTRUATION

The endometrium of the uterus undergoes cyclical changes during the menstrual cycle (Fig. 20-4). During the follicular phase, the endometrium is in the **proliferative phase**, growing in response to estrogen. During the luteal phase, the endometrium enters the **secretory phase** as it matures and is prepared to support implantation. If the ovum is not fertilized, the corpus luteum degenerates after approximately 14 days, leading to a fall in estrogen and progesterone levels. The withdrawal of progesterone causes the endometrium to slough, initiating the **menstrual phase**. At the same time, FSH levels begin to slowly rise in the absence of negative feedback and the follicular phase starts again.

MENOPAUSE AND POSTMENOPAUSE

Menopause is defined by **12 months of amenorrhea after the final menstrual period**. At this point, nearly all the oocytes have undergone atresia, although a few remain and can be found on histologic examination. It is characterized by complete, or near complete, ovarian follicular depletion and absence of ovarian estrogen secretion.

The **average age** at menopause in the United States is **51 years**. Five percent of women will have **late menopause** (occurring after age 55) and another 5% of women have **early menopause** (occurring between ages 40 and 45). Early menopause is more common in women with a history of cigarette smoking, short cycles, nulliparity, type 1 diabetes, and family history of early menopause. **Premature ovarian failure** (PMOF) is the onset of spontaneous menopause before the age of 40.

Various physiologic and hormonal changes occur during this period, including a decrease in estrogen, increase in FSH, and classic symptoms such as hot flashes, night sweats, mood swings, and vaginal dryness. Ten percent of women will begin having these symptoms during perimenopause and 50% will experience an increase in symptoms during menopause. For most women, symptoms may last during the **first year or two of menopause** before gradually decreasing and stopping. Rarely do symptoms extend beyond the first 5 years of menopause. When this occurs, it's important to look for other causes for the symptoms.

ETIOLOGY

Menopause is generally heralded by menstrual irregularity as the number of oocytes capable of responding to FSH and LH decreases and **anovulation** becomes more frequent. During this period, LH and FSH levels gradually rise because of decreased negative feedback from **diminished estrogen production**. The fall in estradiol levels leads to hot flashes, mood changes, insomnia, depression, osteoporosis, and vaginal atrophy (Fig. 20-6). Premature menopause resulting from premature ovarian failure is usually idiopathic or autoimmune. If it occurs before age 30, chromosomal studies can be ordered to rule out a genetic basis (e.g., mosaicism).

DIAGNOSIS

The diagnosis of menopause can usually be made by history and physical examination and confirmed by testing FSH levels. Patients classically present between ages 48 and 52 (average age is 51) complaining of

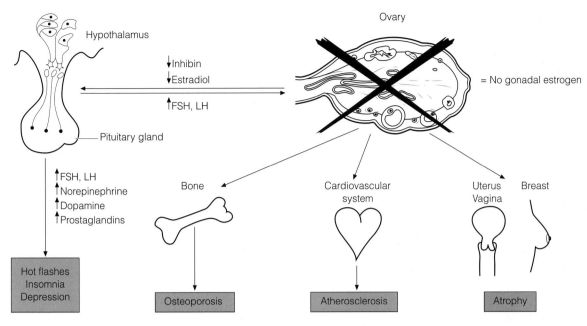

Figure 20-6 • Changes in both the ovary and the hypothalamus contribute to the physiologic changes of menopause.

amenorrhea, and vasomotor instability, sweats, mood changes, depression, dyspareunia, and dysuria. These symptoms generally **disappear within 12 months**, although a substantial proportion of women can remain symptomatic for years.

On physical examination there may be a decrease in breast size and change in texture. Vaginal, urethral, and cervical **atrophy** may all be seen, which are consistent with **decreased estrogen levels**. If there is any question about the diagnosis, an **elevated FSH** is diagnostic of menopause. During the perimenopausal period, the FSH level may be increased or decreased. Therefore, as a diagnostic test, FSH is best reserved for patients with a combination of amenorrhea or oligomenorrhea and menopausal symptoms.

PATHOGENESIS

Although menopause is a naturally occurring event, there are two important long-term consequences of the estrogen decrease (Fig. 20-6). From a cardiovascular standpoint, the protective benefits of estrogen on the lipid profile (increased high-density lipoprotein [HDL], decreased low-density lipoprotein [LDL]) and on the vascular endothelium (prevents atherogenesis, increases vasodilatation, inhibits platelet adherence) are lost, and women are at **increased risk for coronary artery disease**. With menopause, **bone resorption accelerates** because estrogen plays an impor-

tant role in regulating osteoclast activity. The increased bone resorption leads to osteopenia and finally osteoporosis (particularly in thin, fair, and Caucasian women).

HORMONE REPLACEMENT THERAPY AND ESTROGEN REPLACEMENT THERAPY

Hormone replacement therapy (HRT) refers to the use of a **combination of estrogen and progesterone** to treat menopausal related symptoms in women who still have their uterus in situ. Menopausal symptoms are due to decreased estrogen levels. The estrogen component on HRT supplies the patient with an exogenous source of estrogen and thereby treats the symptoms of menopause. However, **unopposed estrogen exposure**, whether endogenous or exogenous but can result in endometrial hyperplasia and/or endometrial cancer. Therefore, when estrogens are being used to treat menopausal symptoms in women who still have a uterus in situ, **progestins must be used to decrease the risk of endometrial hyperplasia and cancer**. In menopausal patients who have undergone a hysterectomy, there is no risk of endometrial hyperplasia or endometrial cancer from unopposed estrogen exposure. Thus, these women can use **estrogen replacement therapy (ERT)** for the treatment of their menopausal symptoms. This therapy utilizes estrogen only and does not require complementary progesterone use.

The risks and benefits of HRT and ERT have been the center of numerous studies over the past few decades. Initial studies suggested that, in addition to treating the symptoms of menopause and preventing osteoporosis, HRT may also be cardioprotective (reduce the risk of strokes and heart attacks). During this era, women were started on HRT during menopause and left on it indefinitely. However, more recent studies have shown that, not only are HRT and ERT *not* cardioprotective, they actually carry significant increased cardiovascular risks. As a result, the current recommendation is that HRT and ERT be used **only for the treatment of menopausal symptoms** and that the use be limited to a **short period of time** (6 to 12 months) and be at the **smallest dose** which controls the patient's symptoms. Symptomatic relief involves reduction of vasomotor flushing, mood and sleep improvement, prevention of urogenital and vaginal atrophy, and improvement in skin and muscle tone.

The other major value of HRT is the **prevention and treatment of osteoporosis**. This is a particularly important preventative measure since 15% of women over age 50 will be diagnosed with osteoporosis and 50% with osteopenia. In fact, a woman can lose 20% of her original bone density in the first 5 to 7 years after menopause. By reducing the incidence and severity of osteoporosis, HRT subsequently reduces the incidence of hip and vertebral fractures, pain, loss of height, and immobility.

Treatment must be considered carefully, however, and each patient's symptoms, risk factors, and relative risks and benefits should be individually evaluated. **Contraindications to hormone replacement therapy** include chronic liver impairment, pregnancy, known estrogen-dependent neoplasm (breast, ovary,

uterus), history of thromboembolic disease (DVT, PE, CVA), and undiagnosed vaginal bleeding.

Additional Therapeutic Regimens

Alternative regimens for postmenopausal women who are unable or unwilling to take hormone replacement therapy or who have completed short-term HRT or ERT, should be targeted toward the individual's symptoms and treatment goals (Table 20-2). **Vasomotor flushes** can be managed with clonidine (Catapres), selective serotonin reuptake inhibitors (SSRIs) such as paroxetine (Paxil) and serotonin and norepinephrine reuptake inhibitors (SNRIs) such as venlafaxine (Effexor). Other causes for hot flashes such as thyroid disease, autoimmune disorders, tumors, and selective estrogen receptor modulator (SERMs) (tamoxifen/raloxifene) use should also be ruled out when indicated. **Vaginal atrophy** can be managed locally with lubricants and moisturizers. Vaginal estrogen can have excellent local effects on vaginal and urethral atrophy, with only minimal systemic absorption.

The **prevention and treatment for osteoporosis** has been refined over the past few years and includes calcium and vitamin D supplementation, bisphosphonates (etidronate, alendronate, risedronate), calcitonin, raloxifene, and tamoxifen (SERMs), and weight-bearing exercise such as walking, hiking, and stair climbing. Reduction in smoking and in caffeine and alcohol intake has also been shown to lower the rate of bone loss. A bone-density measurement may be determined to follow bone mass in postmenopausal women. It is recommended that all postmenopausal women receive a bone-density measurement at age 65. Women who are at higher risk of osteoporosis (thin, Caucasian, Asian, smoker, family history) or those using medications that predispose to bone loss

■ **TABLE 20-2** Treatment Options to Address the Various Symptoms of Menopause	
Menopausal Symptom	**Treatment Option**
Cardiovascular changes	Blood pressure and lipid control medications, smoking cessation, weight loss, exercise
Osteoporosis risk	HRT, calcium, calcitonin, bisphosphonates, raloxifene, weight-bearing exercise
Hot flashes	HRT, clonidine, SSRIs, black cohosh, evening primrose, dong quai
Vaginal dryness/dyspareunia	HRT, vaginal estrogen, water-based lubricant, isoflavones, chasteberry, ginseng
Mood disturbances	HRT, SSRIs, St. John's wort, black cohosh
HRT, hormone replacement therapy; SSRIs, selective serotonin reuptake inhibitors.	

(levothyroxine, steroids, heparin) should be scanned earlier, perhaps at the time of menopause or by age 60.

With respect to **cardiovascular risks**, improvement in lifestyle and diet are key factors, as well as optimal blood pressure control to decrease morbidity and mortality.

The Women's Health Initiative (WHI) was a major 15-year research program to address the most common causes of death, disability and poor quality of life in postmenopausal women—cardiovascular disease, cancer, and osteoporosis.

 KEY POINTS

- The typical order of the events puberty is thelarche (breast development), pubarche (pubic hair development), peak height velocity, and menarche (onset of menstruation).

- During the normal menstrual cycle, the ovary goes through a follicular and luteal phase at the same time that the endometrium goes through the proliferative and secretory phases.

- Ovulation occurs in response to the LH surge signaling the mature follicle to break open and release the mature oocyte. Fertilization of the ovum must occur within 24 hours of ovulation.

- Menstruation occurs as the result of decreasing progestin levels resulting in the sloughing of the endometrium.

- Menopause marks the termination of the reproductive phase of a woman's life. It is characterized by the cessation of menses and the onset of an estrogen-deficient state.

- The average age of menopause is 51. Menopausal patients present with amenorrhea, hot flashes, vaginal

atrophy, and mood and sleep changes, all consistent with decreased levels of estrogen.

- Menopause can be diagnosed with after 12 months of amenorrhea and the presence of menopausal symptoms which may include hot flashes, night sweats, mood and sleep disturbances, and vaginal dryness. It can be confirmed by elevated levels of FSH.

- Women who wish to use HRT and still have a uterus in place should use both estrogen and progesterone therapy to avoid endometrial hyperplasia and endometrial cancer from unopposed estrogen exposure.

- Two major advantages of HRT are the prevention of bone loss and osteoporosis and the relief of symptoms associated with menopause.

- When used, HRT and ERT should be reserved for the treatment symptoms and be used only for the short term (6 to 12 months) at the lowest amount needed to treat symptoms.

- If HRT is completed, not tolerated, or not desired, alternative therapies are available to address each of the symptoms and side effects of menopause.

Amenorrhea

Amenorrhea—the absence of menses—is classified as either primary or secondary. **Primary** amenorrhea is the absence of menses in women who have not undergone menarche by age 16 or have not had menstruation by 4 years after thelarche (the onset of breast development). **Secondary** amenorrhea is the absence of menses for three menstrual cycles or a total of 6 months in women who have previously had normal menstruation. The pathophysiology underlying these two processes differs greatly, as do the differential diagnoses.

PRIMARY AMENORRHEA

If menses has not occurred by age 16, the diagnosis of primary amenorrhea is made. In the United States, the prevalence of primary amenorrhea is 1% to 2%. The causes of primary amenorrhea include congenital abnormalities, hormonal aberrations, chromosomal abnormalities, hypothalamic-pituitary disorders, and the variety of causes of secondary amenorrhea that may present before menarche. These causes are divided into three categories: outflow tract obstruction, end-organ disorders, and central regulatory disorders (Table 21-1).

OUTFLOW TRACT ANOMALIES

Imperforate Hymen

The hymen sometimes fails to canalize during fetal development and remains as a solid membrane across the vaginal introitus. If the hymen is imperforate, it will not allow egress of menstrual blood or menses.

Thus, despite having begun to menstruate, patients appear to have primary amenorrhea. After a time, patients present with pelvic or abdominal pain from the accumulation and subsequent dilation of the vaginal vault and uterus by menses. On physical examination these patients have a bulging membrane just inside the vagina, often with purple-red discoloration behind it consistent with hematocolpos. The treatment of imperforate hymen is surgical; usually a cruciate incision is made and the hymen is sewn open to allow the egress of menses.

Transverse Vaginal Septum

A transverse vaginal septum may result from failure of the müllerian-derived upper vagina to fuse with the urogenital sinus–derived lower vagina. Commonly found at the level of the midvagina, it is usually patent. However, in some cases it may be imperforate and cause primary amenorrhea. Diagnosis is made on careful examination of the female genital tract. The diagnosis is commonly mistaken as imperforate hymen, and can be differentiated by the presence of a hymeneal ring below the septum. Surgical correction involves resection of the septum.

Vaginal Agenesis

Patients with **Mayer-Rokitansky-Kuster-Hauser (MRKH)** syndrome have müllerian agenesis or dysgenesis. They may have complete vaginal agenesis and absence of a uterus or partial vaginal agenesis with a rudimentary uterus and distal vagina. This differs from **vaginal atresia** where the müllerian system is developed, but the distal vagina is composed of fibrosed

■ **TABLE 21-1** Etiologies of Primary Amenorrhea

Outflow tract abnormalities
Imperforate hymen
Transverse vaginal septum
Vaginal agenesis
Vaginal atresia
Testicular feminization
Uterine agenesis with vaginal dysgenesis
MRKH syndrome
End-organ disorders
Ovarian agenesis
Gonadal agenesis 46,XX
Swyer syndrome/gonadal agenesis 46,XY
Ovarian failure
Enzymatic defects leading to decreased steroid biosynthesis
Savage syndrome—ovary fails to respond to FSH and LH
Turner syndrome
Central disorders
Hypothalamic
Local tumor compression
Trauma
Tuberculosis
Sarcoidosis
Irradiation
Kallmann syndrome—congenital absence of GnRH
Pituitary
Damage from surgery or radiation therapy
Hemosiderosis deposition of iron in pituitary

tissue. Diagnosis is made with physical examination that reveals no patent vagina, chromosomes that are 46,XX, and ovaries visualized on ultrasound. With partial vaginal agenesis or vaginal atresia, a rectal examination may reveal a pelvic mass consistent with a uterus. The uterus can be visualized with ultrasound (US), computed tomography (CT), or magnetic resonance imaging (MRI). Creation of a neovagina can be achieved either by serial dilation of the perineal body by the patient over an extended period of time or by reconstructive surgery. In true vaginal atresia, the neovagina created may be connected with the upper genital tract.

Testicular Feminization

Testicular feminization or androgen insensitivity results from a dysfunction or absence of the testosterone receptor that leads to a phenotypical female with 46,XY chromosomes. This syndrome occurs in 1 in 50,000 women. Because these patients have testes, **müllerian inhibiting factor** (MIF) was secreted early in development, and these patients therefore have an absence of all müllerian-derived structures. Of note, the testes may be undescended or have migrated down to the labia majora. The diminished testosterone sensitivity commonly leads to an absence of pubic and axillary hair. Usually estrogen is produced, and these patients develop breasts but present with primary amenorrhea because they have no uterus. Patients commonly have a vagina that ends as a blind pouch. For those patients with the absence of or a foreshortened vagina, therapy involves creating a neovagina for sexual function; however, these patients are unable to reproduce.

END-ORGAN DISORDERS

Ovarian Failure

Primary ovarian failure results in low levels of estradiol but elevated levels of gonadotropins termed **hypergonadotropic hypogonadism**. There are a variety of causes of primary ovarian failure (Table 21-2). **Savage syndrome** is characterized by failure of the ovaries to respond to follicle-stimulating hormone (FSH) and luteinizing hormone (LH) secondary to a receptor defect. In **Turner syndrome** (45,XO), the ovaries undergo such rapid atresia that by puberty there are usually no primordial oocytes. Defects in the enzymes involved in steroid biosynthesis, particularly 17-α-hydroxylase, can result in amenorrhea and absence of breast development because of lack of estradiol.

Gonadal Agenesis with 46,XY Chromosomes

If there is a defect in the enzymes that are involved in testicular steroid production—**17-α-hydroxylase** or **17,20 desmolase**—these patients will not produce

■ **TABLE 21-2** Causes of Primary Gonadal Failure (Hypergonadotropic Hypogonadism)

Idiopathic premature ovarian failure
Steroidogenic enzyme defects (primary amenorrhea)
Cholesterol side-chain cleavage
3β-ol-dehydrogenase
17-hydroxylase
17-desmolase
17-ketoreductase
Testicular regression syndrome
True hermaphroditism
Gonadal dysgenesis
Pure gonadal dysgenesis (Swyer syndrome) (46,XX and 46,XY)
Turner syndrome (45,XO)
Turner variants
Ovarian resistance syndrome (Savage syndrome)
Autoimmune oophoritis
Postinfection (e.g., mumps)
Postoophorectomy (also wedge resections)
Post irradiation
Post chemotherapy

Adapted from DeCherney A, Pernoll M. *Current Obstetric and Gynecologic Diagnosis and Treatment.* Norwalk: Appleton & Lange, 1994:1009.

CENTRAL DISORDERS

Hypothalamic Disorders

The pituitary will not release FSH and LH if the hypothalamus is unable to produce gonadotropin-releasing hormone (GnRH), transport it to the pituitary, or release it in a pulsatile fashion. Anovulation and amenorrhea result from this hypogonadotropic hypogonadism. **Kallmann syndrome** involves a congenital absence of GnRH and is commonly associated with anosmia. GnRH transport may be disrupted with compression or destruction of the pituitary stalk or arcuate nucleus. This can result from tumor mass effect, trauma, sarcoidosis, tuberculosis, irradiation, or Hand-Schuller-Christian disease. There may be defects in GnRH pulsatility in cases of anorexia nervosa, extreme stress, athletics, hyperprolactinemia, hypothyroidism, rapid or severe weight loss, and constitutionally delayed puberty.

Pituitary Disorders

Primary defects of the pituitary are a rare cause of primary amenorrhea. Pituitary dysfunction is usually secondary to hypothalamic dysfunction. It may be caused by tumors, infiltration of the pituitary gland, or infarcts of the pituitary. Surgery or irradiation of pituitary tumors may lead to decreases in or absence of LH and FSH. Hemosiderosis can result in iron deposition in the pituitary, leading to destruction of the gonadotrophs that produce FSH and LH.

DIAGNOSIS

A patient who presents with primary amenorrhea can be worked up based on the phenotypic picture (Table 21-3, Fig. 21-1). Lack of a uterus is seen in males because of the release of MIF by the testes and in females with müllerian agenesis. Breast development is dependent on estradiol secretion by the ovaries. Patients who have neither a uterus nor breasts are generally 46,XY males with steroid synthesis defects or varying degrees of gonadal dysgenesis, in which adequate MIF is produced by gonadal tissue but androgen synthesis is insufficient.

If breasts are present but no uterus, the etiologies can include congenital absence of the uterus (müllerian agenesis) in the female or testicular feminization in the male. In the latter case, estradiol from direct testicular secretion as well as peripheral

testosterone. However, MIF will still be produced; hence, there will be no female internal reproductive organs. These patients will otherwise be phenotypically female, usually without breast development. Patients with an absence of or defect in the testosterone receptor develop testicular feminization syndrome.

While testicular feminization results from peripheral effects of diminished or absent sensitivity of testosterone receptors, another situation in which the patient is genetically male but phenotypically female is gonadal agenesis. The congenital absence of the testes in a genotypical male, **Swyer syndrome**, results in a phenotypical picture similar to that of ovarian agenesis. Because the testes never develop, MIF is not released and these patients have both internal and external female genitalia. However, without estrogen they will not develop breasts.

■ TABLE 21-3 Diagnosis of Etiology of Primary Amenorrhea

	Uterus Absent	**Uterus Present**
Breasts Absent	Gonadal agenesis in 46,XY	Gonadal failure/agenesis in 46,XX
	Enzyme deficiencies in testosterone synthesis	Disruption of hypothalamic-pituitary axis
Breasts Present	Testicular feminization	Hypothalamic, pituitary, or ovarian pathogenesis similar to that of secondary amenorrhea
	Müllerian agenesis or MRKH	Congenital abnormalities of the genital tract

conversion of testosterone and androstenedione leads to breast development.

For patients who have a uterus but the absence of breast development, the differential includes hypergonadotropic hypogonadism, as seen in gonadal dysgenesis in both sexes, and with defects in steroid pathways in 46,XX patients and hypogonadotropic hypogonadism, which is seen in central nervous system (CNS), hypothalamic, and pituitary dysfunction. A serum FSH level differentiates between these two, with elevation seen in hypergonadotropic hypogonadism.

The workup for amenorrhea in phenotypic females with the absence of either a uterus or breasts should include a karyotype analysis, followed by testosterone and FSH assays. Further biochemical and hormonal assays may be performed to elucidate specific enzyme defects. Patients with both a uterus and breast development should be evaluated to determine whether there is a patent outflow tract from

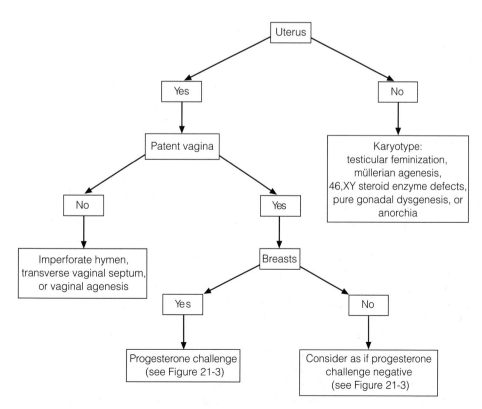

Figure 21-1 • Diagnostic flowchart for patients with primary amenorrhea.

the uterus. If the vagina, cervix, and uterus are continuous, these can be evaluated as if the patient were presenting with secondary amenorrhea.

TREATMENT

Patients with congenital abnormalities may be treated surgically with plastic procedures to allow egress of menses in those with a functional uterus or to create a functional vagina. Patients with an absent uterus and breasts can be treated with estrogen replacement to effect breast development and prevent osteoporosis. Patients who have breast development but an absent uterus may not require medical intervention.

Patients with a uterus but without breast development and with hypergonadotropic hypogonadism often have irreversible ovarian failure and will require estrogen replacement therapy. Patients with hypogonadotropic hypogonadism require further workup as patients with secondary amenorrhea.

SECONDARY AMENORRHEA

Secondary amenorrhea is the absence of menses for more than 6 months or for the equivalent of three menstrual cycles in a woman who previously had menstrual cycles. **The most common cause of secondary amenorrhea is pregnancy**. Other causes can be categorized as anatomic abnormalities, ovarian dysfunction, prolactinoma and hyperprolactinemia, and CNS or hypothalamic disorders.

ANATOMIC ABNORMALITIES

The common anatomic causes of secondary amenorrhea are Asherman syndrome and cervical stenosis. **Asherman syndrome** is the presence of intrauterine synechiae or adhesions, usually secondary to intrauterine surgery or infection. The potential etiologies of Asherman syndrome include dilation and curettage (D&C), myomectomy, cesarean delivery, or endometritis. **Cervical stenosis** can manifest as secondary amenorrhea and dysmenorrhea. It is usually caused by scarring of the cervical os secondary to surgical or obstetric trauma.

OVARIAN FAILURE

Ovarian failure may result from ovarian torsion, surgery, infection, radiation, or chemotherapy. **Premature ovarian failure** (POF) is often idiopathic.

Any time menopause occurs without another etiology before age 40, it is considered POF. Before age 35, chromosomal analysis is usually performed to diagnose a genetic basis for POF. Patients with either idiopathic POF or a known cause of early ovarian failure are generally treated with supplemental estrogen to decrease the risk of cardiovascular disease and osteoporosis.

POLYCYSTIC OVARIAN DISEASE

Stein-Leventhal syndrome, also known as *polycystic ovarian syndrome* (PCOS), was described in 1935 and included the constellation of anovulation, oligomenorrhea or amenorrhea, hirsutism, obesity, and enlarged polycystic ovaries. This syndrome is now understood to represent one end of the spectrum of patients with polycystic ovarian disease (PCOD), who have anovulation in common but can have any or all of the other findings. It is not entirely clear what precipitates the disease, but once it begins, a self-perpetuating cycle occurs.

Chronic anovulation leads to elevated levels of estrogen and androgen. The increased androgen released from the ovaries and the adrenal cortex is converted peripherally in the adipose tissue into estrone. Further, the elevated androgens lead to a decrease in the production of sex hormone binding globulin (SHBG), resulting in even higher levels of free estrogens and androgens. This hyperestrogenic state leads to an increased LH:FSH ratio, atypical follicular development, anovulation, and increased androgen production. Once again, the androgens are peripherally converted to estrogens, leading to a cyclical propagation of the disease. Many patients with PCOD who are hyperandrogenic and obese also develop insulin resistance and hyperinsulinemia. Not surprisingly, the incidence of type 2 diabetes mellitus is increased in these patients.

Treatment of these patients depends on the particular symptoms and the desires of the patient. For patients desiring fertility, ovulation induction (OI) using clomiphene citrate (Clomid) is begun. Patients with PCOD are particularly resistant to OI and there is evidence that the probability of ovulation can be increased by weight loss or the concomitant use of corticosteroids. In patients with hyperinsulinemia and insulin resistance, metformin has been shown to increase spontaneous ovulation. For patients who are not currently interested in fertility, either cyclic progestins or Depo-Provera should be used to decrease the risk of endometrial hyperplasia and cancer secondary to the unopposed estrogen. In addition, obese patients should be strongly urged to lose weight because this will decrease the risk of cardiovascular disease and diabetes and can actually break the cycle of anovulation. Obviously, such patients should undergo a screen for type 2 diabetes mellitus.

HYPERPROLACTINEMIA-ASSOCIATED AMENORRHEA

Excess prolactin leads to amenorrhea and galactorrhea. Menstrual irregularities often result from abnormal gonadotropin (FSH and LH) secretion due to alterations in dopamine levels typically seen in hyperprolactinemia. The etiologies and consequences of excess prolactin are numerous. Prolactin release is inhibited by dopamine and stimulated by serotonin and thyrotropin-releasing hormone (TRH). Because of the constant suppression of prolactin release by hypothalamic release of dopamine, any disturbance in this process by a hypothalamic or pituitary lesion can lead to disinhibition of prolactin secretion.

Hyperprolactinemia has several possible etiologies (Table 21-4). Primary hypothyroidism that leads to elevated thyroid-stimulating hormone (TSH) and TRH can cause hyperprolactinemia. Medications that increase prolactin levels (by a hypothalamic-pituitary effect) include dopamine antagonists (Haldol, Reglan, phenothiazines), tricyclic antidepressants, estrogen, monoamine oxidase (MAO) inhibitors, and opiates. A prolactin-secreting pituitary adenoma leads to elevated prolactin levels. The empty sella syndrome, in which the subarachnoid membrane herniates into the sella turcica, causing it to enlarge and flatten, is another cause of hyperprolactinemia. Other conditions associated with high prolactin include pregnancy and breastfeeding. Any patient with an elevated prolactin level should have an imaging study to rule out prolactinoma.

DISRUPTION OF THE HYPOTHALAMIC-PITUITARY AXIS

As in the hypothalamic and pituitary causes of primary amenorrhea, disruption in the secretion and transport of GnRH, absence of pulsatility of GnRH, or acquired pituitary lesions will all cause hypogonadotropic hypogonadism (Table 21-5). Common causes of hypothalamic dysfunction include stress, exercise, anorexia nervosa, and weight loss.

TABLE 21-4 Differential Diagnosis of Galactorrhea-Hyperprolactinemia

Pituitary tumors secreting prolactin

Macroadenomas (>10 mm)

Microadenomas (<10 mm)

Hypothyroidism

Idiopathic hyperprolactinemia

Drug-induced hyperprolactinemia

Dopamine antagonists

  Phenothiazines

  Thioxanthenes

  Butyrophenone

  Diphenylbutylpiperidine

  Dibenzoxazepine

  Dihydroindolone

  Procainamide derivatives

Catecholamine-depleting agents

False transmitters (α-methyldopa)

Interruption of normal hypothalamic-pituitary relationship

Pituitary stalk section

Peripheral neural stimulation

Chest wall stimulation

  Surgery (e.g., mastectomy)

  Burns

  Herpes zoster

  Bronchogenic tumors

  Bronchiectasis/chronic bronchitis

Nipple stimulation

Stimulation of nipples

Chronic nipple irritation

Spinal cord lesion

Tabes dorsalis

Syringomyelia

CNS disease

Encephalitis

Craniopharyngioma

Pineal and hypothalamic tumors

Hypothalamic tumors

Pseudotumor cerebri

■ **TABLE 21-5** Differential Diagnosis of Hypoestrogenic Amenorrhea (Hypogonadotropic Hypogonadism)
Hypothalamic dysfunction
Kallmann syndrome
Tumors of hypothalamus (craniopharyngioma)
Constitutional delay of puberty
Severe hypothalamic dysfunction
Anorexia nervosa
Severe weight loss
Severe stress
Exercise
Pituitary disorder
Sheehan syndrome
Panhypopituitarism
Isolated gonadotropin deficiency
Hemosiderosis (primarily from thalassemia major)

Adapted from DeCherney A, Pernoll M. *Current Obstetric and Gynecologic Diagnosis and Treatment.* Norwalk: Appleton & Lange, 1994:1013.

Diagnosis

The approach to secondary amenorrhea always begins with a **β-hCG** (beta human chorionic gonadotropin) assay to **rule out pregnancy** often before a formal history is taken. If this is negative, the standard history should include focused questions toward hypothyroidism (e.g., lethargy, weight gain, cold intolerance) and hyperprolactinemia (e.g., nipple discharge, usually bilateral), and hyperandrogenism (e.g., recent changes in hirsutism, acne, or virilism; see Chapter 23). **TSH** and **prolactin** levels should then be checked to rule out hypothyroidism and hyperprolactinemia, both of which can cause amenorrhea. If both are elevated, the hypothyroidism should be treated and the prolactin level can be checked after thyroid studies have normalized to verify resolution.

If the prolactin level is elevated and TSH is normal, a workup for the other causes of prolactinemia should ensue (Fig. 21-2). In the diagnostic evaluation of the patient, a careful history should be taken, including a complete list of medications and clear documentation of the onset of symptoms. A thorough physical examination should include visual fields, cranial nerves, breast examination, and an attempt to express milk from the nipple. An MRI can rule out a hypothalamic or pituitary lesion.

If the prolactin level is normal, a **progesterone challenge test** (10 mg orally for 7 to 10 days to mimic progesterone withdrawal) can be performed to assess the adequacy of endogenous estrogen production and the outflow tract. Withdrawal bleeding occurring after the progesterone challenge indicates the presence of estrogen and an adequate outflow tract. In this case, amenorrhea is usually secondary to anovulation, which can be caused by a variety of endocrine disorders that alter pituitary/gonadal feedback such

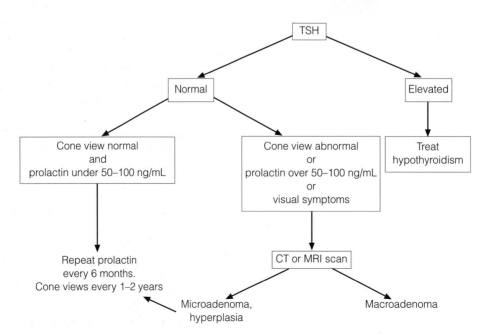

Figure 21-2 • Diagnostic flowchart for patients with amenorrhea-galactorrhea-hyperprolactinemia.

as polycystic ovaries, tumors of the ovary and adrenals, Cushing syndrome, thyroid disorders, and adult-onset adrenal hyperplasia (Table 21-6).

Absence of withdrawal bleeding in response to progesterone alone must then be evaluated with estrogen and progesterone administration. If there is still no menstrual bleeding, an outflow tract disorder such as Asherman syndrome or cervical stenosis is suspected. If menstrual bleeding does occur in response to estrogen and progesterone administration, this suggests an intact and functional uterus without adequate endogenous estrogen stimulation. Measurement of FSH and LH will help differentiate between a hypothalamic/pituitary disorder (low/normal FSH and LH levels) and ovarian failure (high FSH and LH levels) (Fig. 21-3).

Treatment

Patients with hypothyroidism are treated with thyroid hormone replacement. Those with pituitary macroadenomas are treated with surgical resection.

■ **TABLE 21-6** Differential Diagnosis of Eugonadotropic Eugonadism (Progesterone Challenge Positive)

Mild hypothalamic dysfunction
Emotional stress
Psychologic disorder
Weight loss
Obesity
Exercise-induced
Idiopathic
Hirsutism-virilism
Polycystic ovary syndrome
Ovarian tumor
Adrenal tumor
Cushing syndrome
Congenital and adult-onset adrenal hyperplasia
Systemic disease
Hypothyroidism
Hyperthyroidism
Addison disease
Chronic renal failure
Many others seen in other chronic diseases

Adapted from DeCherney A, Pernoll M. *Current Obstetric and Gynecologic Diagnosis and Treatment.* Norwalk: Appleton & Lange, 1994:1013.

Some patients with macroadenomas and most with microadenomas are treated with bromocriptine, a dopamine agonist that often causes tumor regression and the resumption of ovulation. Other hyperprolactinemic patients can also be treated with bromocriptine in order to resume ovulation. Further, this treatment should be followed with serial prolactin levels and cone view radiographs to diagnose development of a macroadenoma.

Patients who respond to a progesterone challenge should be withdrawn with progesterone on a regular basis to prevent endometrial hyperplasia. Oral contraceptive pills (OCPs) are useful in this case and may be beneficial in the management of hirsutism. However, if the patient is a smoker over age 35, progesterone alone is indicated due to the increased risk of cerebrovascular accidents and venous thromboembolism with estrogen usage in these patients.

For patients who are hypoestrogenic, consideration should be given to estrogen and progesterone replacement for the effects these have on bone density and genital atrophy. OCPs are often used for women under age 35 or nonsmokers over age 35. For other patients, a regimen of 0.625 mg of conjugated estrogen cycled with 5 to 10 mg of medroxyprogesterone acetate is suitable. These patients should also receive 1.2 g of elemental calcium supplementation per day.

Ovulation Induction

Ovulation induction with bromocriptine can be used in patients with hyperprolactinemia. If the cause of hyperprolactinemia is medication related, discontinue or decrease the medication if possible. Patients who respond to the progesterone challenge have evidence of estrogenation. Any specific cause of this amenorrheic state should be corrected. If menses do not resume, ovulation induction may be performed with clomiphene citrate (Clomid), which acts as an antiestrogen to stimulate gonadotropin release. Patients with elevated androgens may need combined therapy with Clomid and corticosteroids.

Patients who do not respond to progesterone alone are presumed to have low estrogen levels; however, these patients will occasionally respond to Clomid as well. For patients who do not respond to Clomid, human menopausal gonadotropin (hMG) or recombinant GnRH can be used to stimulate ovulation. Careful monitoring with ultrasound and estradiol levels should be done in the case of gonadotropin ovulation induction because of the risk of ovarian hyperstimulation.

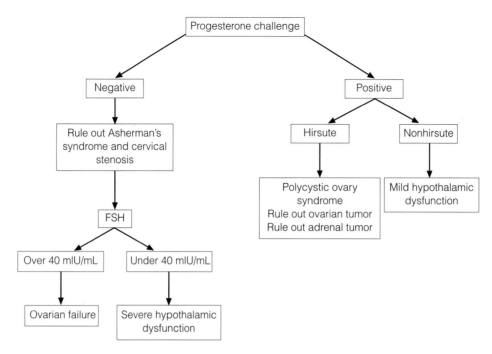

Figure 21-3 • Diagnostic flowchart for patients with secondary amenorrhea.

 KEY POINTS

- Primary amenorrhea is the absence of menarche by age 16 or 4 years after thelarche.

- Primary amenorrhea can be caused by congenital abnormalities of the genital tract, chromosomal abnormalities, enzyme or hormonal deficiencies, gonadal agenesis, ovarian failure, or disruption of the hypothalamic-pituitary axis.

- The workup of primary amenorrhea is usually organized into four categories based on the presence or absence of a uterus and the presence or absence of breast development.

- In the absence of both uterus and breasts, karyotype usually reveals 46,XY.

- In the absence of a uterus and presence of breasts, karyotype will differentiate between müllerian agenesis and testicular feminization.

- In the absence of breasts and presence of a uterus, FSH will differentiate between hypergonadotropic and hypogonadotropic hypogonadism. Karyotype may be necessary to rule out gonadal agenesis in a 46,XY.

- Patients with both a uterus and breasts should be evaluated as if presenting with secondary amenorrhea.

- Anatomic abnormalities including Asherman syndrome and cervical stenosis may lead to secondary amenorrhea. These patients fail to respond to estrogen and progesterone withdrawal.

- Hyperprolactinemia is a common cause of secondary amenorrhea.

- Patients with normal prolactin levels may be given a progesterone challenge to investigate whether or not the endometrium is estrogenized.

- With progesterone challenge failure, the differential diagnosis becomes hypergonadotropic or hypogonadotropic hypogonadism that can be differentiated by an FSH measurement.

- For patients not seeking current fertility, it is important to treat the specific cause of amenorrhea and to consider hormone replacement in the hypoestrogenic patient.

- For patients who desire fertility, ovulation induction can usually be achieved. Patients with hyperprolactinemia require bromocriptine, whereas patients with other forms of hypogonadism may respond to clomiphene and gonadotropins.

22

Abnormalities of the Menstrual Cycle

DYSMENORRHEA

Dysmenorrhea is defined as **pain and cramping** during menstruation that **interferes with normal activities** and requires over-the-counter or prescription medication. Mild pain during menses is normal. Discomfort during menstruation ranges from mild discomfort to severe pain that causes some patients to be bedridden. Fifty percent of menstruating women suffer from dysmenorrhea and 10% of these are incapacitated for 1 to 3 days each month.

Dysmenorrhea is classified as primary or secondary. **Primary dysmenorrhea** is idiopathic menstrual pain without identifiable pathology; **secondary dysmenorrhea** is painful menses due to underlying pathology (endometriosis, fibroids, adenomyosis, PID, cervical stenosis).

PRIMARY DYSMENORRHEA

Primary dysmenorrhea usually occurs before age 20. Because primary dysmenorrhea is almost always associated with ovulatory cycles, it is usually diagnosed in late teens rather than at menarche when cycles are often anovulatory. Although there is no obvious organic cause, primary dysmenorrhea is thought to result from **increased levels of endometrial prostaglandin production** derived from the arachidonic acid pathway. Additionally, there may be a psychological component involved for some patients that depends on attitudes toward menstruation learned from mothers, sisters, and friends.

Diagnosis

The diagnosis of primary dysmenorrhea is made on the basis of history and the **absence of organic causes**. The most common misdiagnosis of primary dysmenorrhea is endometriosis. Often, the pain of dysmenorrhea occurs with ovulatory cycles on the first or second day of menstruation, whereas pain from endometriosis may begin 1 to 2 weeks before menstruation, worsens 1 to 2 days before menstruation, and is relieved at or right after the onset of menstrual flow (Chapter 15). Associated symptoms include nausea, vomiting, and headache. On physical examination there are no obvious abnormalities except a generalized tenderness throughout the pelvis.

Treatment

The first-line medical treatment for primary dysmenorrhea is **nonsteroidal anti-inflammatory drugs** (NSAIDs). The most commonly used agents include aspirin, ibuprofen, ketoprofen, and naproxen. These are all available without prescription; however, patients may need prescription-strength dosages to obtain adequate symptom relief. Because antiprostaglandins work by blocking prostaglandin synthesis and metabolism, these medications should be taken with the onset of menses, continued for 1 to 3 days and then taken as needed. **COX-2 inhibitors** such as Celebrex (celecoxib) are another class of NSAIDs that have been shown to be effective in the treatment of primary dysmenorrhea. However, potential side effects have limited their use in the United States.

Oral contraceptive pills (OCPs) are the second line of treatment for women who do not get adequate pain relief from antiprostaglandin agents and NSAIDs alone or who cannot tolerate them. More than 90% of women with primary dysmenorrhea find adequate pain relief with the use of oral contraceptives given in a continuous (preferred) or cyclic fashion. The same is true for other estrogen/progestin combination contraceptives such as the Ortho Evra patch and NuvaRing. The mechanism of relief is either secondary to the **cessation of ovulation** or due to the **decrease in endometrial proliferation** leading to **decreased prostaglandin production**. Most patients who have been cycled for 1 year on OCPs experience a reduction of symptoms even if the OCPs are discontinued.

Nonmedical options for the treatment of primary dysmenorrhea include the use of heating pads to the lower abdomen, exercise, massage, acupuncture, and hypnosis. Most recently, the use of transcutaneous electrical nerve stimulation (TENS) has been shown to relieve or decrease pain in women suffering from primary dysmenorrhea.

Surgical therapies including cervical dilation, uterosacral ligament ligation, and presacral neurectomy have been used in the past but **have little use in** current management of true primary dysmenorrhea. Often, primary dysmenorrhea will decrease throughout a patient's 20s and early 30s. In addition, a pregnancy carried to viability will usually decrease the symptoms of primary dysmenorrhea. Very rarely, a patient with true primary dysmenorrhea may require hysterectomy to relieve her pain. Prior to this a thorough evaluation, possibly including questioning about childhood molestation or sexual assault, pelvic ultrasound, MRI, and laparoscopy should be performed to look for secondary causes of dysmenorrhea.

SECONDARY DYSMENORRHEA

Secondary dysmenorrhea implies that the symptoms are secondary to an identifiable cause (Fig. 22-1) such as endometriosis and adenomyosis (Chapter 15), uterine fibroids (Chapter 14), cervical stenosis, or pelvic adhesions. Because the first three causes are discussed in other chapters, refer to those particular chapters for detailed management.

Cervical Stenosis

Cervical stenosis causes dysmenorrhea by obstructing blood flow during menstruation. The stenosis can be

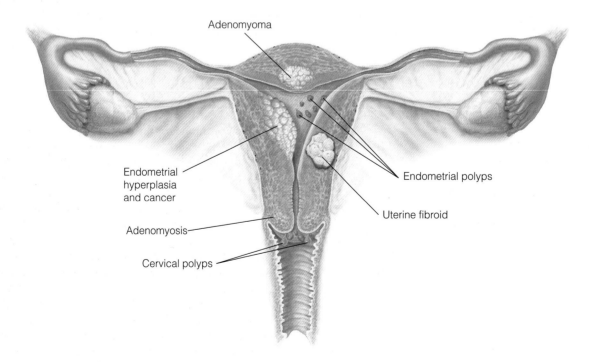

Adenomyoma

Endometrial hyperplasia and cancer

Adenomyosis

Cervical polyps

Endometrial polyps

Uterine fibroid

Figure 22-1 • Common causes of abnormal vaginal bleeding.
(From Anatomical Chart Co.)

congenital or secondary to scarring from infection, trauma, or surgery. Patients often complain of scant menses associated with severe cramping pain that is relieved with increased menstrual flow. On physical examination there may be obvious scarring of the external os; often the clinician is unable to pass a uterine sound through the cervical canal.

Treatment

Dilation of the cervix is the treatment for cervical stenosis. Either a surgical dilation can be performed or laminaria tents can be used. Surgical dilation is usually performed in the operating room, but can be attempted in the office with a paracervical block. Progressively larger dilators are placed through the cervical canal until it becomes patent. Ultrasound guidance can be helpful in avoiding creation of a false passage or uterine perforation.

Laminaria may be placed in the cervix in the office setting. Made from seaweed, these dilate over a 24-hour period by absorbing water from the surrounding tissue. Slow dilation of the cervix results from expansion of the laminaria. Dilation will provide relief; however, symptoms often recur, requiring multiple dilations. Pregnancy with vaginal delivery often leads to a permanent cure.

PELVIC ADHESIONS

Patients with a history of **pelvic infections** including cervicitis, pelvic inflammatory disease (see Color Plate 12), or tubo-ovarian abscess may have symptoms of dysmenorrhea secondary to adhesion formation. Patients with other local **inflammatory diseases** (appendicitis, endometriosis, or Crohn's disease) or **prior pelvic surgery** (especially myomectomy) may also have adhesions leading to dysmenorrhea. If a patient has a history of any of these problems and reports pain associated with movement or activity, pelvic adhesions should be suspected. In some patients, pelvic adhesions can be so extensive as to "cement" the uterus into a fixed position, which may be noted on pelvic examination. Adhesions are **not visible using traditional imaging modalities** such as pelvic ultrasound, MRI, or CT.

Treatment

These patients will occasionally respond to the antiprostaglandins prescribed for primary dysmenorrhea. When suspicions are high and the pain necessitates treatment, pelvic adhesions can be both **diagnosed and treated via laparoscopy**. Occasionally, the adhesions may be so dense as to necessitate laparotomy for safe lysis. However, the patient should be aware that surgery can lead to further adhesions and further problems with dysmenorrhea and/or chronic pelvic pain.

PREMENSTRUAL SYNDROME AND PREMENSTRUAL DYSPHORIC DISORDER

Premenstrual syndrome (PMS) and its more severe variant, premenstrual dysphoric disorder (PMDD) are characterized by is a constellation of physical and/or behavioral changes that occur in the second half of the menstrual cycle. These changes might include headache, weight gain, bloating, breast tenderness, mood fluctuation, restlessness, irritability, anxiety, depression, fatigue, and a feeling of being out of control. These symptoms must occur in the 2 weeks prior to menstruation and there must be at least a 7-day symptom-free interval in the first half of the menstrual cycle. Symptoms must occur in at least two consecutive cycles for the diagnosis to be made.

Some 75% of women suffer from some recurrent PMS symptoms; of these, 30% report significant problems and 5% of women are incapacitated or severely distressed by PMDD at some point during their cycle. The highest incidence occurs among women in their late 20s to early 30s.

Pathogenesis

The exact etiology of PMS and PMDD is unknown but is likely **multifactorial** and includes both physiologic and psychological causes. Past hypotheses have included abnormalities in estrogen-progesterone balance, disturbance in the renin-angiotensin-aldosterone pathway, excess prostaglandin and prolactin production, and psychogenic factors. Recent studies also suggest that PMS and PMDD may be due to the interaction between the **neurotransmitter serotonin** and cyclic changes in the **ovarian steroids**. The serum concentrations of estrogen and progesterone are no different in patients with PMS/PMDD and those without. However, studies have suggested that although women with PMS and PMDD have normal levels of estrogen and progesterone, they may have **an abnormal response to normal hormonal changes**.

Treatment

Effective treatments for PMS and PMDD have been identified after systematic reviews. The **selective serotonin reuptake inhibitors** (SSRIs) have demonstrated clear efficacy in treating both the physical and mood symptoms of these disorders. **Prozac** (fluoxetine) has been approved by the U.S. FDA for the treatment of PMDD. Other drugs in this category, including Celexa (citalopram), Paxil (paroxetine), and Zoloft (sertraline), have also been shown to be effective.

The serotonin and norepinephrine reuptake inhibitor (SNRI) **Effexor** (venlafaxine) and the benzodiazepine **Xanax** (alprazolam) have also shown efficacy in treating these disorders. In small trials, both Lupron (leuprolide acetate) and Danocrine (danazol) have shown efficacy in treating PMS and PMDD. Their side effects, however, prevent widespread use of these options.

A number of additional medications may have possible efficacy in the treatment of PMS and PMDD. Several older studies showed oral contraceptives to have no greater efficacy than placebo in managing PMS and PMDD. A new OCP, **Yaz**, which is formulated with low-dose estrogen and uses **drospirenone** (a spironolactone with antimineralocorticoid and antiandrogenic activity) as its progestin, has been found to be effective in the treatment of PMS and has been approved for that use. Spironolactone itself has not consistently shown to be effective. There is some suggestion that **exercise** and **relaxation** techniques may improve the symptoms of PMS and PMDD.

Several studies have looked at **vitamin supplementation** as a treatment for PMS and PMDD. There appears to be some role for the use of calcium (600 mg BID), vitamin D (800 mg per day), vitamin B6 ($\leq$100 mg/day), magnesium (200 to 360 mg/day), and chasteberry extract (one tablet/day) in the treatment of these disorders. Several studies also showed that complex **carbohydrate-rich beverage** consumption improved both the psychological symptoms and appetite cravings. This is thought to work by modulating tryptophan the serotonin synthesis.

Other supplements such as evening primrose oil, essential fatty acids, and ginkgo biloba extract have not been found to be effective nor has the use of progesterone and progestins.

ABNORMAL UTERINE BLEEDING

The normal menstrual cycle consists of cyclic bleeding approximately **every 28 days** (normal range, 21 to 35 days), lasting **3 to 5 days** with about **30 to 50 mL** of blood loss per cycle. Abnormal uterine bleeding refers to any departure from the norm in the menstrual cycle. It can involve **too much bleeding** (heavy periods, frequent menses, or bleeding between periods) or **too little bleeding** (light periods, infrequent periods, or complete absence of periods). The most common causes of abnormal uterine bleeding are covered briefly in this chapter and in more detail in other chapters of this text (Fig. 22-1).

Dysfunctional uterine bleeding (DUB) describes idiopathic heavy and/or irregular bleeding that **cannot be attributed to another cause.** Amenorrhea—complete absence of periods for at least 6 consecutive months—is discussed in Chapter 21.

PATTERNS OF ABNORMAL UTERINE BLEEDING

The typical patterns of abnormal uterine bleeding are summarized in Table 22-1.

MENORRHAGIA

Patients with menorrhagia have regularly timed menstrual cycles but the flow is either excessive in its duration (>7 days) or its volume (>80 mL/cycle). Patients with menorrhagia occasionally describe the blood as **flooding** or **gushing**, and may have blood clots along with their excessive flow. Most gynecologists use a history of greater than 24 menstrual pads in a day or soaking through a pad every hour as indicative of menorrhagia. Menorrhagia is most commonly caused by **uterine fibroids**, **adenomyosis**, **endometrial polyps**, and less commonly by endometrial hyperplasia or cancer or cervical polyps or cancer (Fig. 22-1). Teenagers with menorrhagia should be evaluated for **primary bleeding disorders** such as von Willebrand disease, idiopathic thrombocytopenic purpura (ITP), platelet dysfunction, and thrombocytopenia from malignancy.

HYPOMENORRHEA

Patients with hypomenorrhea have **regularly timed menses** but an unusually **light amount of flow**. This is commonly caused by hypogonadotropic hypogonadism in anorexics and athletes. Atrophic endometrium can also occur in the case of Asherman's syndrome (**intrauterine adhesions** or synechiae), congenital malformations, infection, and intrauterine

TABLE 22-1 Patterns of Uterine Bleeding

Bleeding Pattern	Definition	Timing of Cycle	Flow Amount
Normal menses	Regular bleeding, average Q 28 days (range, 21 to 35), lasting 3 to 5 days, bleeding on average 30 to 50 mL/cycle	Regular	Normal
Menorrhagia (hypermenorrhea)	Heavy (>80 mL/cycle) or prolonged (>7 days) menstrual flow occurring at regular intervals	Regular	Heavy
Hypomenorrhea	Regularly timed menses but light flow	Regular	Light
Metrorrhagia (intermenstrual bleeding)	Any bleeding between normal menses, usually lighter than normal menstrual bleeding	Irregular	Normal-light
Menometrorrhagia	Excessive or prolonged bleeding at irregular intervals	Irregular	Heavy
Oligomenorrhea	Irregular cycles >35 days apart	Irregular	Varies
Polymenorrhea	Frequent regular cycles but <21 days apart	Regular	Normal
Amenorrhea, secondary	No menses for 6 or more consecutive months	N/A	N/A
Amenorrhea, primary	No menses by age 14 in the absence of secondary sexual characteristics *or* No menses by age 16 in the presence of secondary sexual characteristics	N/A	N/A
Dysfunctional uterine bleeding (DUB)	Idiopathic heavy and/or irregular bleeding with no identifiable causes	Regular or irregular	Varies

trauma. Patients on **OCPs, Depo-Provera, and the progestin-containing IUDs** also have atrophic endometrium and often have light menses as do women who have undergone endometrial ablation. Outlet obstruction secondary to cervical stenosis or congenital abnormalities can also result in hypomenorrhea.

METRORRHAGIA AND MENOMETRORRHAGIA

Metrorrhagia is characterized by bleeding that occurs between regular menstrual periods. This bleeding is usually less than or equal to menses. Primary causes include cervical lesions (polyps, eversion, carcinoma) and endometrial polyps and carcinoma. **Menometrorrhagia** is excessive (greater than 80 mL) or prolonged bleeding at irregular intervals. The usual causes include uterine fibroids, adenomyosis, endometrial polyps, hyperplasia, and cancer (Fig. 22-1). Thyroid disorders can result in increased or decreased flow or no change in menstrual flow.

OLIGOMENORRHEA

Patients with periods **greater than 35 days apart** are described as having oligomenorrhea. The causes are similar to those for amenorrhea with disruption of the hypothalamic-pituitary-gonadal axis or systemic diseases such as hyperprolactinemia and thyroid disorders (Chapter 21). The most common causes of oligomenorrhea are **polycystic ovarian syndrome (PCOS), chronic anovulation, and pregnancy. Thyroid disease** should also be considered. When a patient has no period for 6 consecutive months, secondary amenorrhea is diagnosed.

POLYMENORRHEA

Polymenorrhea, or **frequent periods**, describes regular periods that occur less than 21 days apart. Polymenorrhea can be confused with metrorrhagia (intermenstrual bleeding). However, if all of the bleeding episodes are similar in amount and fewer than 21 days apart, polymenorrhea should be considered. This is usually caused by **anovulation**.

Evaluation

The workup for abnormal uterine bleeding includes a careful **history and physical** followed by diagnostic tests to determine the underlying etiology. The history should include timing of bleeding, quantity of bleeding, menstrual history with menarche and recent periods, and associated symptoms. It should also include a family history of bleeding disorders, particularly if menorrhagia appears at menarche.

On physical examination, **rectal, urethral, vaginal, and cervical causes of bleeding should be ruled out**. Care should be taken to look for sequelae of polycystic ovarian syndrome (hirsutism, acne, truncal obesity, acanthosis nigricans), thyroid disease (thyromegaly, skin changes, diaphoresis, increased pulse), and signs of bleeding disorder (bruising, petechiae). The bimanual examination may reveal uterine or adnexal masses consistent with fibroids, adenomyosis, pregnancy, or cancer. A **Pap smear** is used to screen for cervical dysplasia and cancer and **cervical cultures** should be taken to rule out infection.

Laboratory evaluation should be tailored to the type of menstrual irregularity. For light or skipped cycles, evaluation would include a **pregnancy test, TSH, PRL, and an FSH** if menopause or premature ovarian failure (PMOF) is suspected. The spectrum of hormonal tests that can be performed are discussed with the workup of amenorrhea or polycystic ovarian syndrome, and PMOF are discussed elsewhere in the text.

For heavy, frequent, or prolonged cycles, appropriate laboratory tests would include a **pregnancy test, TSH, and CBC**. A primary bleeding disorder evaluation should be done when menorrhagia presents at menarche, in teenagers or in women with symptoms suggestive of a systemic or hematologic etiology such as easy bruising (>5 cm), frequent nosebleeds, or bleeding gums, and excessive bleeding after surgery, dental extraction, or childbirth. Evaluation for these women might include a complete blood count **(CBC) including platelet count, PT/PTT, factor VIII, and von Willebrand factor antigen and activity**.

Importantly, any woman age 35 or older with abnormal uterine bleeding (excessive or insufficient) should undergo an **endometrial biopsy** to rule out endometrial hyperplasia and cancer even if other testing reveals a potential explanation for the abnormal bleeding. **Obese patients with prolonged oligomenorrhea**

should also undergo endometrial biopsy even if they are under the age of 35. These women are at increased risk of endometrial hyperplasia and cancer due to the peripheral conversion of androgens into estrogens in their adipose cells.

A **pelvic ultrasound** can be used to identify endometrial polyps, fibroids, hyperplasia, cancers, and adnexal masses. If intrauterine pathology is suspected on pelvic ultrasound, a **sonohysterogram** or hysterosalpingogram can be performed to show intrauterine defects. **MRI** is expensive but useful in distinguishing adenomyosis from uterine fibroids. **Hysteroscopy** allows direct visualization of the intrauterine cavity. A dilation and curettage (D&C) provides tissue for diagnosis.

Treatment

The treatment of abnormal uterine bleeding **depends on the specific underlying etiology**. The most common causes and treatments are detailed in Table 22-2. Symptomatic fibroids and polyps can be treated by removal (Chapter 14). Adenomyosis is occasionally responsive to hormonal regulation with estrogens and/or progestins or endometrial ablation but often requires hysterectomy (Chapter 15). Endometrial hyperplasia is most commonly managed with progestin therapy and occasionally with D&C or hysterectomy (Chapter 14). Anovulation is treated with menstrual regulation with estrogens and/or progestins and weight loss (Chapter 21). Treatment for PMOF and menopause is directed toward relief of specific symptoms (Chapter 20).

DYSFUNCTIONAL UTERINE BLEEDING

If **no pathologic cause** of abnormal uterine bleeding is identified, the diagnosis of dysfunctional uterine bleeding (DUB) is made. DUB is a **diagnosis of exclusion**. Most patients with DUB are **anovulatory**. In these instances, the ovary produces estrogen but no corpus luteum is formed, and thus no progesterone is produced. Subsequently, there is continuous estrogenic stimulation of the endometrium without the usual progesterone-induced bleeding. Instead, in DUB, the endometrium continues to proliferate until it outgrows its blood supply, breaks down, and sloughs off in an irregular fashion. DUB is most likely to occur with anovulatory cycles and thus is most common during times in a woman's life when she is

■ **TABLE 22-2** Common Causes and Treatments for Abnormal Uterine Bleeding

Bleeding Disorder	Bleeding Amount	Typical Treatment
Neoplasms		
Uterine fibroids	Heavy	Myomectomy vs. hysterectomy
Adenomyosis	Heavy	Hormonal management vs. hysterectomy
Cervical polyps	Light	Polypectomy in office
Endometrial polyps	Heavy	Hysteroscopy, polypectomy ± D&C
Endometrial hyperplasia	Varies	Progestin therapy vs. hysterectomy
Endometrial cancer	Heavy	Hysterectomy, BSO, radiation
Pregnancy problems		
Pregnancy	Varies	Expectant management vs. delivery
Miscarriage	Heavy	Expectant management vs. D&C
Ectopic pregnancy	Varies	Methotrexate vs. surgical removal
Hormonal problems		
Hypothyroidism	Varies	Thyroid hormone replacement
Hyperprolactinemia	None	Dopamine agonists
Anovulation	Varies	Cyclic OCPs or progestins

most likely to be anovulatory such as adolescence, perimenopause, lactation, and pregnancy. Pathologic anovulation occurs in **hypothyroidism, hyperprolactinemia, hyperandrogenism, and PMOF**.

DIAGNOSIS

The diagnosis of DUB is made by history, physical, lab tests, and imaging to **rule out other causes of abnormal bleeding** as described in the prior section. In **adolescence**, the risk of structural causes of abnormal bleeding is small. However, any congenital anomalies and bleeding disorders should be eliminated. In the **reproductive years**, there is an increased risk of structural and hormonal etiologies for abnormal bleeding. During **perimenopause**, the risk of DUB increases, but so does the risk of other causes of abnormal bleeding including hyperplasia, polyps, and cancer. A careful workup of abnormal uterine bleeding must therefore be performed before the diagnosis of DUB is given. Importantly, **any woman over age 35 with abnormal uterine bleeding should undergo an endometrial biopsy to rule out endometrial hyperplasia and cancer.** The same is true for obese women under age 35 who have had extended periods of oligomenorrhea.

Because DUB is commonly associated with anovulation, efforts should be made to determine whether a patient is ovulating. A basal body temperature can be graphed daily to determine whether ovulation is occurring. This can also be accomplished with ovulation prediction kits, which are at-home tests for detecting the LH surge from urine samples. A midluteal, day 21 to 23 serum progesterone level may also indicate if a patient is ovulating.

TREATMENT

Once the diagnosis of DUB is made, treatment depends on the cause, the age of the patient, desire for fertility, and the acute versus chronic nature of the bleeding.

In the case of **acute hemorrhage**, therapy to stop the bleeding should be initiated immediately. Intravenous estrogen (25 mg conjugated estrogen every 4 hours up to 24 hours) provides a quick response but also carries an increased risk of thromboembolic events (DVT, PE). For patients with excessive blood loss who are hemodynamically stable, high-dose oral estrogens can control the bleeding within 24 to 48 hours. A typical dosing might be 2.5 mg every 4 hours for 14 to 21 days followed by medroxyprogesterone acetate 10 mg per day for 7 to 10 days. Instead of this sequential hormone therapy, an OCP taper can be used for endometrial stabilization. A typical taper would use a monophasic pill containing 35 mcg ethinyl estradiol given three times a day for 3 days, then two times a day for 2 days, and then daily for the remainder of the pack.

For chronic DUB, nonhormonal therapy with **NSAIDs** (e.g., 800 mg ibuprofen TID × 5 days) has been shown to decrease menstrual blood loss by 20% to 50%. This is typically reserved for ovulatory women with DUB. This therapy may be used alone or in conjunction with estrogen and progesterone therapy.

Menstrual regulation using hormonal therapy is the primary treatment for anovulatory DUB. This can include use of combination **estrogen and progesterone** in the form of oral contraceptive pills, Ortho Evra patch, or NuvaRing. These may be dosed in a continuous (preferred) or cyclic fashion depending on the patient's desire.

In patients in whom the use of estrogen is contraindicated (women with hypertension, thrombophilias, history of DVT or PE and those 35 and older who smoke), or those who prefer an alternative to estrogen/progestin combination, similar cycle control can be achieved **progestin-only dosing**. Options include cyclic progestin administration (10 mg medroxyprogesterone acetate per day for 10 consecutive days each month), or progesterone in the form of Depo Provera, levonorgestrel-releasing IUS (Mirena), or Implanon. These latter three are likely to result in light menses or amenorrhea over time. The Mirena IUS is particularly helpful in anovulatory and ovulatory patients with menorrhagia who are at increased risk for developing endometrial hyperplasia or cancer (obese, diabetic, hypertension, smoker, positive family history, chronic anovulation due to polycystic ovary syndrome).

Surgical intervention may be required for patients with DUB who do not respond to medical therapy. **D&C** may be both diagnostic and therapeutic but the result can be temporary. In women who have completed childbearing, **endometrial ablation** can also be used to treat DUB by destroying the majority of the endometrium down to its basalis layer. A variety of ablation modalities are available including laser, roller ball, hydrothermal balloon, cryo-, bipolar mesh, microwave, or hydrothermal (circulating hot water). Each of these carries an 85% to 97% success rate over 5 years. Success for the procedure is measured as more controllable amounts of bleeding and patient satisfaction. About 15% to 20% of patients will be amenorrheic after ablation and 10% to 25% will subsequently require hysterectomy.

Hysterectomy is the definitive surgery for DUB but should be reserved for those cases refractory to all other treatments or for women for whom childbearing is complete. Hysterectomy may be performed laparoscopically, vaginally, or abdominally. The patient's personal risk factors and age may be used to determine if the ovaries and/or cervix is left in situ or removed.

POSTMENOPAUSAL BLEEDING

Menopause is marked by 12 months of amenorrhea after the final menstrual period. Postmenopausal bleeding, then, is any vaginal bleeding that occurs more than 12 months after the last menstrual period. **Any postmenopausal bleeding is abnormal** and should be investigated given the increased risk of reproductive cancers in women in this age group. The most common cause of postmenopausal bleeding, however, is **endometrial and/or vaginal atrophy**, not cancer (Table 22-3). Endometrial cancer in responsible for only 10% to 15% of all postmenopausal bleeding.

ETIOLOGIES

Bleeding in postmenopausal women can be due to nongynecologic etiologies, lower and upper genital tract sources, reproductive tumors, or exogenous hormonal stimulation. **Nongynecologic causes** include rectal bleeding from hemorrhoids, anal fissures, rectal prolapse, and lower gastrointestinal (GI) tumors. Urethral caruncles are another source of bleeding in the postmenopausal woman. These disorders can be identified by history and physical, anoscopy, occult blood stool screening, barium enema, or colonoscopy.

■ **TABLE 22-3** Causes of Postmenopausal Bleeding

Etiology	Percentage
Vaginal/endometrial atrophy	30
Exogenous estrogens	30
Endometrial cancer	15
Endometrial polyps	10
Endometrial hyperplasia	5
Other	10

Vaginal atrophy due to the lack of endogenous estrogen is the most common source of **lower genital tract** postmenopausal bleeding. The thin vaginal mucosa is easily traumatized and therefore likely to bleed. Other causes of lower genital tract bleeding are benign and malignant lesions of the vulva, vagina, or cervix.

Pathologic causes of postmenopausal bleeding from the **upper genital tract** include endometrial atrophy, endometrial polyps, endometrial hyperplasia, and endometrial cancer. Estrogen-secreting ovarian tumors can cause stimulation of the endometrium that presents as postmenopausal bleeding. Each of these disorders can be identified with a combination of Pap smear, endometrial biopsy, and pelvic ultrasound.

The use of **exogenous hormones** is the most common cause of postmenopausal uterine bleeding. Despite the occurrence of bleeding with the use of hormone replacement therapy, thorough evaluation of the postmenopausal patient with endometrial biopsy is still required to rule out endometrial hyperplasia and cancer.

DIAGNOSIS

A careful history is important. Physical examination should include a careful inspection of the external anogenital region, vulva, vagina, and cervix. A **Pap smear** should be performed as well as a digital rectal examination and occult blood screening. Laboratory tests might include a **CBC, TSH, prolactin, and FSH levels**. If an ovarian mass is identified, tumor markers (LDH, hCG, AFP, CEA, inhibin, and estradiol) should also be considered. **Endometrial biopsy** should be performed to rule out endometrial cancer even if there is an identifiable source of postmenopausal bleeding.

A **pelvic ultrasound, sonohysterogram, and MRI** can be useful in evaluation of the endometrial stripe and uterine cavity. In the postmenopausal woman, the endometrial stripe should be thin and ≤3 mm. **Hysteroscopy**—either in the office or operating room—can further elucidate intrauterine abnormalities such as endometrial polyps and fibroids. **D&C** is both diagnostic and therapeutic for some lesions of the uterus and cervix.

TREATMENT

Treatment of postmenopausal bleeding should be directed at **treating the causal agent**. Lesions of the vulva and vagina should be biopsied and treated accordingly. Lacerations of the vaginal mucosa should be repaired. Vaginal atrophy can be treated with vaginal estrogen. Commonly, vaginal estrogen preparations in the form of creams, pill, and rings are very effective. Systemic treatment can also be obtained with hormone replacement therapy (HRT) if the uterus is in situ or with estrogen replacement therapy (ERT) if the uterus has been removed.

Endometrial polyps may be removed by hysteroscopic resection or D&C. Endometrial hyperplasia (Chapter 14) can be treated with progestin therapy or hysterectomy, and endometrial cancer is usually treated by TAHBSO performed in conjunction with possible lymph node dissection, radiation, or chemotherapy therapy (less common).

 KEY POINTS

- Primary dysmenorrhea is severe pain with menses that cannot be attributed to any identifiable cause. It is thought to be due to increased levels of prostaglandins.
- Most primary dysmenorrhea is managed with NSAIDs and/or combination estrogen and progesterone in pill, patch, or ring form. TENS units, heating pads, exercise, massage, acupuncture, and hypnosis may also help. There is little role for surgery in the management of primary dysmenorrhea.
- Secondary dysmenorrhea is painful menses due to an identifiable cause such as adenomyosis, endometriosis, fibroids, cervical stenosis, or pelvic adhesions. The treatment should be tailored to the cause.
- PMS and PMDD represent a multifactorial disease with physiologic and psychological components including headache, weight gain, bloating, breast fluctuation, irritability, fatigue, and a feeling of being out of control.
- In order to make the diagnosis, symptoms must be in the second half of the menstrual cycle with at least a 7-day symptom-free interval during the first half of the menstrual cycle. Symptoms must occur in at least two consecutive cycles.

KEY POINTS *(continued)*

- Although the cause is unknown, it is thought to be to an interaction between serotonin and the ovarian hormones. A variety of treatments offer relief including SSRIs (Prozac, Zoloft), Xanax, Yaz OCPs, as do diet modification, exercise, and vitamin supplementation (calcium, vitamin D, vitamin B6, and magnesium).

- The normal menstrual cycle occurs, on average, every 28 days (range, 21 to 35 days) and lasts 3 to 5 days with 30 to 50 mL of blood loss per cycle.

- Menorrhagia is regular bleeding that is heavy or prolonged. Metrorrhagia is bleeding between periods and menometrorrhagia is heavy or prolonged irregular bleeding. The most common causes of heavy or prolonged bleeding include polyps, fibroids, adenomyosis, cancer, and pregnancy complications.

- The most common causes of oligomenorrhea (periods greater than 35 days apart) include chronic ovulation, PCOS, and pregnancy.

- The initial evaluation of abnormal uterine bleeding should include a history and physical, laboratory tests (pregnancy test, TSH, prolactin, FSH), endometrial biopsy (for women 35 and older), and pelvic ultrasound. Treatment should be directed at the cause of the abnormal bleeding.

- DUB is a diagnosis of exclusion when no other source for abnormal bleeding can be identified. It is thought to be secondary to anovulation, and is therefore more prevalent in adolescents and perimenopausal woman.

- Most women with DUB can achieve menstrual regularity using a daily monophasic birth control pill or cyclic progestins when estrogens are contraindicated.

- In cases of acute hemorrhage, IV estrogens and high-dose oral estrogens can be used to stop acute bleeding. DUB that is not responsive to medical therapy may require surgical treatment with D&C, endometrial ablation, or, rarely, hysterectomy.

- The most common cause of postmenopausal bleeding is vaginal/endometrial atrophy. Other causes of postmenopausal bleeding include cancer of the upper and lower genital tract, endometrial polyps, exogenous hormonal stimulation, and bleeding from nongynecologic sources.

- Postmenopausal bleeding should always be investigated to rule out endometrial hyperplasia and cancer. The evaluation of postmenopausal bleeding should include a thorough history and physical, CBC, TSH, PRL, and FSH as well as an endometrial biopsy and pelvic ultrasound.

Hirsutism and Virilism

Adults have two types of hair: vellus and terminal. Vellus hair is nonpigmented, soft, and covers the entire body. Terminal hair is, on the other hand, pigmented, thick, and covers the scalp, axilla, and pubic area. Androgens are responsible for the conversion of vellus to terminal hair at puberty, resulting in pubic and axillary hair. An abnormal increase in terminal hair is due to androgen excess or increased **5α-reductase** activity; this enzyme converts testosterone to the more potent dihydrotestosterone (DHT). DHT is believed to be the main stimulant of terminal hair development.

Hirsutism refers to the increase in terminal hair on the face, chest, back, lower abdomen, and inner thighs in a woman. Often, the pubic hair is characterized by the development of a male escutcheon, which is diamond shaped as opposed to the triangular female escutcheon. **Virilization** refers to the development of male features, such as deepening of the voice, frontal balding, increased muscle mass, clitoromegaly, breast atrophy, and male body habitus.

The evaluation of hirsutism and virilism in the female patient is complex and requires the understanding of pituitary, adrenal, and ovarian function with detailed attention to the pathways of glucocorticoid, mineralocorticoid, androgen, and estrogen synthesis.

NORMAL ANDROGEN SYNTHESIS

The adrenal gland is divided into two components: the adrenal cortex, which is responsible for glucocorticoid, mineralocorticoid, and androgen synthesis, and the adrenal medulla, which is involved in catecholamine synthesis. The adrenal cortex is composed of three layers.

An outer **zona glomerulosa** layer produces aldosterone and is regulated primarily by the renin-angiotensin system. Because this zone lacks **17α-hydroxylase**, cortisol and androgens are not synthesized. In contrast, the inner layers, the **zona fasciculata** and the **zona reticularis**, produce both cortisol and androgens but not aldosterone because they lack the enzyme **aldosterone synthase**. These two inner zones are highly regulated by adrenocorticotropic hormone (ACTH).

ACTH regulates the conversion of cholesterol to pregnenolone by hydroxylation and side-chain cleavage. Pregnenolone is then converted to progesterone and eventually to aldosterone or cortisol or shunted over to the production of sex steroids (Fig. 23-1).

In the adrenal glands, androgens are synthesized from the precursor **17α-hydroxypregnenolone**, which is converted to **dehydroepiandrosterone** (DHEA) and its sulfate (DHEAS), androstenedione, and finally to testosterone. DHEA and DHEAS are the most common adrenal androgens, whereas only small amounts of the others are secreted.

In the ovaries, the theca cells are stimulated by luteinizing hormone (LH) to produce androstenedione and testosterone. Both androstenedione and testosterone are then aromatized to estrone and estradiol, respectively, by the granulosa cells in response to follicle-stimulating hormone (FSH). Elevations in the ratio of LH to FSH may therefore lead to elevated levels of androgens.

PATHOLOGIC PRODUCTION OF ANDROGENS

Elevation of androgens can be due primarily to adrenal or ovarian disorders. Because synthesis of steroid

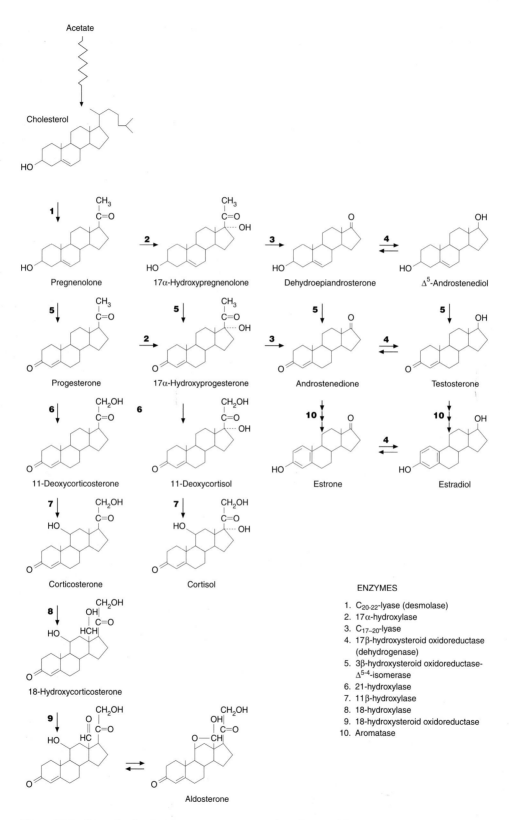

Figure 23-1 • Biosynthesis of androgens, estrogens, and corticosteroids.
(Reproduced with permission from Mishell DR, Davajan V, Lobo RA. *Infertility, Contraception, and Reproductive Endocrinology*, 3rd ed. Cambridge: Blackwell Science, 1991.)

hormones in the adrenal cortex is stimulated by ACTH at a nondifferentiated step, elevated ACTH levels increase all the steroid hormones, including the androgens. If enzymatic defects are present, the precursor proximal to the defect accumulates and is shunted to another pathway. Thus, enzymatic blockade of either cortisol or aldosterone synthesis can lead to increased androgen production. Because DHEAS is derived almost entirely from the adrenal glands, its elevation is used as a marker for adrenal androgen production.

In the ovary, any increase in LH or in the LH:FSH ratio appears to lead to excess androgen production. Further, tumors of both the adrenal gland and the ovary can lead to excess androgens. Regardless of the source, elevated androgens lead to hirsutism and possibly virilism.

ADRENAL DISORDERS

The adrenal disorders leading to virilization in a woman are divided into two categories: nonneoplastic and neoplastic etiologies. Androgen-producing adrenal tumors may be either adenomas or carcinomas. Adrenal adenomas typically cause glucocorticoid excess and virilizing symptoms are rare. Carcinomas, on the other hand, can be more rapidly progressive and lead to marked elevations in glucocorticoid, mineralocorticoid, and androgen steroids.

CUSHING SYNDROME

Cushing syndrome is characterized by excess production of cortisol. Because the intermediates in production are androgens, there will be a concomitant hyperandrogenic state. Cushing syndrome may be caused by pituitary adenomas, ectopic sources of ACTH, and tumors of the adrenal gland. **Cushing syndrome** is caused by pituitary adenomas that hypersecrete ACTH. Paraneoplastic syndromes, such as nonpituitary ACTH-secreting tumors, also lead to increased ACTH levels. Adrenal gland tumors usually result in decreased levels of ACTH secondary to the negative feedback from the increased levels of adrenal steroid hormones. All three of these situations lead to the glucocorticoid excess characteristic of Cushing syndrome, as well as hirsutism, acne, and menstrual irregularities related to adrenal androgen production.

When Cushing syndrome is suspected, it can be diagnosed with the overnight dexamethasone sup-

pression test. Essentially, if there is normal negative feedback from exogenous steroid hormone, then the adrenal gland should decrease production in response to the dexamethasone. A plasma cortisol level is drawn the next morning and if it is <5 µg/dL the patient does not have Cushing syndrome. A cortisol level >10 µg/dL is diagnostic, whereas a value between 5 and 10 is indeterminate. The diagnosis can be confirmed by collecting a 24-hour urine specimen and checking free cortisol levels.

CONGENITAL ADRENAL HYPERPLASIA

Congenital adrenal hyperplasia (CAH) refers to a constellation of enzyme deficiencies involved in steroidogenesis. The most common disorder is **21α-hydroxylase** deficiency. As seen in Figure 23-1, an enzymatic block at this step will lead to the accumulation of **17α-hydroxyprogesterone** (17-OHP), which is then shunted to the androgen pathway. Patients with CAH do not synthesize cortisol or mineralocorticoids and thus present with salt wasting and adrenal insufficiency at birth. Female infants will have ambiguous genitalia due to androgen excess. In milder or adult-onset forms, the degree of deficiency can vary, and often the only presenting sign is mild virilization and menstrual irregularities.

The other types of CAH that can be associated with virilization include **11β-hydroxylase** and **3β-hydroxysteroid dehydrogenase** (3β-HSD) deficiencies. Patients with 11β-hydroxylase deficiency present with similar symptoms of androgen excess as accumulated precursors are shunted to androstenedione and testosterone production pathways. Patients with 3β-HSD deficiency actually accumulate DHEA because they are unable to convert pregnenolone to progesterone or DHEA down the androgen synthesis pathway. DHEA and its sulfate, DHEAS, both have mild androgenic effects. Importantly, because this defect is also present in gonadal steroidogenesis, males have feminization and females have hirsutism and virilization. All patients have impaired cortisol synthesis and varying degrees of either mineralocorticoid excess or deficiency, depending on the location of the enzymatic block.

When CAH is suspected, a 17-OHP level should be checked because 21α-hydroxylase deficiency is the most common etiology. If 17-OHP is elevated (>200 ng/dL), the diagnosis can be confirmed with an ACTH stimulation test in which Cortrosyn (ACTH) is given IV and a 17-OHP level is checked after 1 hour. A marked increase in 17-OHP is consistent with CAH, with lower elevated values being seen in late-onset CAH and heterozygote carriers for the 21α-hydroxylase deficiency.

FUNCTIONAL OVARIAN DISORDERS

The ovarian disorders leading to virilization are divided into nonneoplastic and neoplastic etiologies. Polycystic ovaries, theca lutein cysts, stromal hyperplasia, and stromal hyperthecosis all involve nonneoplastic lesions. Neoplastic lesions vary and often cause rapid onset of virilization.

NONNEOPLASTIC OVARIAN DISORDERS

Polycystic Ovarian Syndrome

Polycystic ovarian syndrome (PCOS), previously known as the Stein-Leventhal syndrome and also known as polycystic ovarian disease (PCOD), is a common disorder affecting up to 4% of reproductive age women. Patients present with a constellation of symptoms including hirsutism, virilization, anovulation, amenorrhea, and obesity. There is also an increased incidence of hyperinsulinemia, diminished insulin sensitivity, and type 2 diabetes mellitus in this population. The cause of androgen excess appears to be related to excess LH stimulation leading to cystic changes in the ovaries and increased ovarian androgen secretion. Typically, the LH:FSH ratio is greater than 3:1. What actually causes the elevation in LH levels is not clear, although it appears that any number of factors may be involved in this cycle including obesity, insulin resistance, and excessive adrenal androgen production.

Theca Lutein Cysts

The **theca cells** of the ovary are stimulated by LH to produce androstenedione and testosterone. These androgens are normally shunted to the **granulosa cells** for aromatization to estrone and estradiol. Theca lutein cysts produce an excess amount of androgens that are secreted into the circulation. These cysts may be present in either normal or molar pregnancy. The ovaries are enlarged, and patients present with hirsutism and, occasionally, virilization. Diagnosis is made by ovarian biopsy.

Stromal Hyperplasia and Hyperthecosis

Stromal hyperplasia is common between age 50 and 70 and can cause hirsutism. The ovaries are uniformly enlarged. **Stromal hyperthecosis** is characterized by foci of utilization within the hyperplastic stroma. It is more likely than simple hyperplasia to result in virilization as the utilized cells continue to produce ovarian androgens. The ovaries typically appear enlarged and fleshy, with the more florid cases seen in younger patients.

NEOPLASTIC OVARIAN DISORDERS

Functional Ovarian Tumors

Functional ovarian tumors that can produce varying amounts of androgen include the sex-cord mesenchymal tumors, Sertoli-Leydig cell tumors (arrhenoblastoma), granulosa-theca cell tumors, hilar (Leydig) cell tumors, and germ cell tumors (gonadoblastomas). Sertoli-Leydig cell tumors usually occur in young women and account for less than 1% of all ovarian neoplasms. Hilar cell tumors are even rarer than Sertoli-Leydig cell tumors and are usually seen in postmenopausal women. These tumors may secrete androgens, leading to hirsutism and virilism.

In pregnancy, there may be a luteoma—a benign tumor that grows in response to human chorionic gonadotropin. This tumor can result in high levels of testosterone and androstenedione and virilization in 25% of patients. There will also be virilization of 65% of female fetuses. These findings should resolve in the postpartum period.

Nonfunctional Ovarian Tumors

Androgen excess can also occur in the case of nonfunctional ovarian tumors (e.g., a cystadenoma or Krukenberg's tumor). Although these tumors do not secrete androgens themselves, they do stimulate proliferation in the adjacent ovarian stroma, which in turn may lead to increased androgen production.

DRUGS AND EXOGENOUS HORMONES

A variety of drugs can affect the circulating levels of sex hormone binding globulin (SHBG). SHBG is one of the major proteins that bind circulating testosterone, leaving a small proportion of free testosterone to interact at the cellular level. Androgens and corticosteroids decrease SHBG, leaving a greater percentage of free testosterone circulating. Patients who use anabolic steroids often present with hirsutism and virilization. In addition, drugs such as minoxidil, phenytoin, diazoxide, and cyclosporin will cause hirsutism without using androgenic pathways.

IDIOPATHIC HIRSUTISM

Hirsutism is considered idiopathic in the absence of adrenal or ovarian pathology, an exogenous source of androgens, or use of the above-listed drugs. Patients may actually have occult androgen production, but many will have normal circulating androgen levels. There may be an increase in peripheral androgen production due to elevated 5α-reductase activity at the level of the skin and hair follicles.

Clinical Manifestations

A detailed history including time of onset, progression, and symptoms of virilization/hirsutism should be obtained, as well as a pubertal, menstrual, and reproductive history. Because various medications can affect androgen levels by affecting SHBG or intrinsic androgenic activity, a detailed drug history should be obtained. A family history is also important in order to look for genetic disorders such as CAH.

Physical Examination

On physical examination, the hair pattern should be noted, with attention to facial, chest, back, abdominal, and inner thigh hair, as well as the presence of frontal balding. The body habitus and presence or absence of female contours should be described. Breast examination may reveal atrophic changes, and a careful pelvic examination should include inspection of the escutcheon (pattern of pubic hair), clitoris (for clitoromegaly), and palpation for ovarian masses. Cushingoid features should be ruled out and inspection for acanthosis nigricans (velvety, thickened hyperpigmentation) in the axilla and nape of neck should be performed because this dermatologic finding is often associated with polycystic ovaries.

Diagnostic Evaluation

Laboratory evaluation should include free testosterone, 17-OHP, and DHEAS, the latter of which is normally exclusive to the adrenal gland. An elevation in free testosterone confirms androgen excess and a concomitant elevation in DHEAS suggests an adrenal source. An elevated 17-OHP is suggestive of CAH. If an adrenal source is suspected, an abdominal computed tomography (CT) should be performed to rule out an adrenal tumor, as well as further tests to diagnose Cushing syndrome or CAH.

If the DHEAS is normal or minimally elevated, an ovarian source should be considered and a pelvic ultrasound or CT should be performed to rule out an ovarian neoplasm. An elevation in the LH:FSH ratio greater than 3 is suggestive of PCOS. However, most obstetrician-gynecologists do not diagnose PCOS with the LH:FSH ratio any longer. Rather, the absence of another etiology for either secondary amenorrhea or oligomenorrhea or hirsutism plus two out three of the Rotterdam criteria for PCOS: secondary amenorrhea or oligomenorrhea, evidence of hyperandrogenism, or evidence for polycystic ovaries as assessed by ultrasound.

Rapid onset of virilization and testosterone levels >200 ng/dL may indicate an ovarian neoplasm. At times the source of androgen excess is not readily evident and further diagnostic tests such as abdominal magnetic resonance imaging (MRI) and selective venous sampling need to be done for localization. In the hirsute woman with normal free testosterone, an assay for 5α-reductase activity is performed to determine whether increased peripheral enzymatic activity is responsible for the development of hirsutism.

Treatment

Adrenal nonneoplastic androgen suppression can be achieved with glucocorticoid administration, such as prednisone 5 mg qhs. Finasteride inhibits the 5α-reductase enzyme, thus diminishing peripheral conversion of testosterone to DHT. Antiandrogens such as spironolactone have been helpful as well, but are temporizing at best. In the case of ovarian or adrenal tumors, the underlying disorder should be treated. Often surgical intervention is required.

In general, ovarian nonneoplastic androgen production can be suppressed with oral contraceptives that will suppress LH and FSH as well as increase SHBG. Progesterone therapy alone may help patients with contraindications to estrogen use. Progesterone decreases levels of LH and thus androgen production;

further, the catabolism of testosterone is increased, resulting in decreased levels. Gonadotropin-releasing hormone (GnRH) agonists can also be used to suppress LH and FSH. However, this leads to a hypoestrogenic state and requires concomitant estrogen replacement.

Patients using exogenous androgens or other drugs leading to increased androgens or hair growth should be advised to discontinue use. For patients with idiopathic hirsutism or contraindications to hormonal use, waxing, depilatories, and electrolysis will often provide cosmetic improvement.

KEY POINTS

- Hirsutism is excess hair growth with a male pattern on the face, back, chest, abdomen, and inner thighs, usually in response to excess androgens.

- Virilism is a constellation of symptoms including hirsutism, deepening of the voice, frontal balding, clitoromegaly, and increased musculature.

- Primary causes of hirsutism and virilization include PCOS, ovarian tumors, adrenal tumors, CAH, and Cushing syndrome.

- Diagnosis is made by history and physical, serum assays for testosterone, DHEAS, and 17-OHP, and imaging studies.

- Management involves primary treatment for the underlying cause; hormonal therapy with OCPs, GnRH, or progestins; and cosmetic treatment of hirsutism.

Contraception and Sterilization

Approximately 90% of women of childbearing age use some form of contraception. Despite this, nearly 50% of pregnancies in the United States are unintentional. Of these, 43% result in live births, 13% in miscarriages, and 44% end in elective abortion. In weighing the risks and benefits of contraception methods, couples must keep in mind that no contraceptive or sterilization method is 100% effective. Table 24-1 outlines relative failure rates or the number of women likely to become pregnant within the first year of using a particular method. **Theoretical efficacy rate** refers to the efficacy of contraception when used exactly as instructed. **Actual efficacy rate** refers to efficacy when used in real life, assuming variations in the consistency of usage.

NATURAL METHODS

The methods of contraception described in this section—periodic abstinence, coitus interruptus, and lactational amenorrhea—are **physiology-based methods** that use neither chemical nor mechanical barriers to contraception. Many couples, for deeply held religious or philosophic reasons, prefer these methods to other forms of contraception. However, these are the least effective methods of contraception and should not be used if pregnancy prevention is a high priority.

PERIODIC ABSTINENCE

Method of Action

Periodic abstinence (the rhythm or calendar method) is a physiologic form of contraception that emphasizes **fertility awareness and abstinence** shortly before and after the estimated ovulation period. This method requires instruction on the physiology of menstruation and conception and on methods of determining ovulation. **Ovulation assessment methods** may include the use of ovulation prediction kits, basal body temperature measurements (Fig. 24-1), menstrual cycle tracking, cervical mucous evaluation, and documentation of any premenstrual or ovulatory symptoms.

Effectiveness

The average effectiveness of periodic abstinence is relatively low (55% to 80%) compared to other forms of pregnancy prevention.

Advantages/Disadvantages

Periodic abstinence uses neither chemical nor mechanical barriers to conception and is therefore the method of choice for many couples for philosophical and/or religious reasons. However, this method requires a highly motivated couple willing to learn reproductive physiology, predict ovulation, and abstain from intercourse. Periodic abstinence is relatively unreliable compared to the more traditional methods of contraception. This low reliability may require prolonged periods of abstinence and regular menstrual cycles, making it less desirable for some couples.

COITUS INTERRUPTUS

Method of Action

Coitus interruptus, or withdrawal of the penis from the vagina before ejaculation, is one of the oldest methods

■ **TABLE 24-1** Failure Rates for Various Contraceptive Methods During the First Year of Use in the United States

Method	Percent of Women Who Become Pregnant	
	Theoretical Failure Rate (%)	Actual Failure Rate (%)
No method	85.0	85.0
Periodic abstinence		
Calendar	9.0	25.0
Ovulation method	3.0	25.0
Symptothermal	2.0	25.0
Postovulation	1.0	25.0
Withdrawal	4.0	27.0
Lactational amenorrhea	2.0	15.0 to 55.0
Condom		
Male condom	2.0	15.0
Female condom	5.0	21.0
Diaphragm with spermicide	6.0	16.0
Cervical cap with spermicide		
Parous women	26.0	32.0
Nulliparous women	9.0	16.0
Spermicide alone	18.0	29.0
Intrauterine devices		
Copper-T IUD (ParaGard)	0.6	0.8
Levonorgestrel IUS (Mirena)	0.1	0.1
Combination estrogen and progesterone		
Combination pill	0.1	3.0
Transdermal patch (Ortho Evra)	0.3	0.8
Vaginal ring (NuvaRing)	0.3	0.8
Progesterone-only methods		
Progestin-only pill (POPs)	0.5	8.0
Depo-Provera	0.3	0.3
Subdermal implant (Implanon)	0.4	0.4
Surgical sterilization		
Female sterilization	0.5	0.5
Male sterilization	0.1	0.15

of contraception. With this method, the majority of semen is deposited outside of the female reproductive tract with the intent of preventing fertilization.

Effectiveness

The failure rate for coitus interruptus is quite high (27%) compared to other forms of contraception. Failure can be attributed to the deposition of semen

(pre-ejaculate) into the vagina before orgasm or the deposition of semen near the introitus after intracrural intercourse.

Advantages/Disadvantages

The primary disadvantage of coitus interruptus is its high failure rate and the need for sufficient self-control to withdraw the penis before ejaculation.

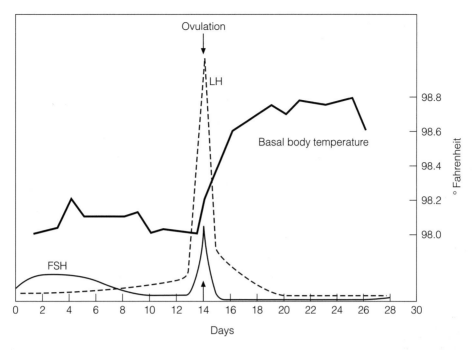

Figure 24-1 • The relationship between ovulation and basal body temperature.

LACTATIONAL AMENORRHEA

Method of Action

Continuation of nursing has long been a widespread method of contraception for many couples. After delivery, the restoration of ovulation is delayed because of a nursing-induced hypothalamic **suppression of ovulation**. Specifically, there is a **prolactin-induced** inhibition of pulsatile GnRH from the hypothalamus resulting in suppression of ovulation.

Effectiveness

The duration of ovulatory suppression during nursing is highly variable. In fact, 50% of lactating mothers will begin to ovulate between 6 and 12 months after delivery, even while breastfeeding. Importantly, return of ovulation occurs *before* the return of menstruation. As a result, 15% to 55% of mothers using lactation for contraception subsequently become pregnant.

The effectiveness of lactational amenorrhea as a method of contraception can be enhanced by following certain principles. First, breastfeeding should be the only form of nutrition for the infant. Second, this method of contraception should be used only as long as the woman is experiencing amenorrhea and, even then, it should only be used for a **maximum of 6 months** after delivery. Following these guidelines, lactational amenorrhea as a method of contraception can have a much lower failure rate. In practice, however, most mothers are not able to meet these stringent requirements.

Advantages/Disadvantages

Lactational amenorrhea has no effect on nursing and has no monetary cost. However, while the theoretical failure rates are reasonable, the failure rates for actual practice are so high as to make this an unacceptable and unreliable sole means of contraception.

BARRIER METHODS AND SPERMICIDES

These contraceptive methods work by preventing sperm from entering the endometrial cavity, fallopian tubes, and peritoneal cavity. Figure 24-2 shows the various barrier method contraceptives and spermicides.

MALE CONDOMS

Method of Action

Condoms are latex sheaths placed over the erect penis before ejaculation. They prevent the ejaculate

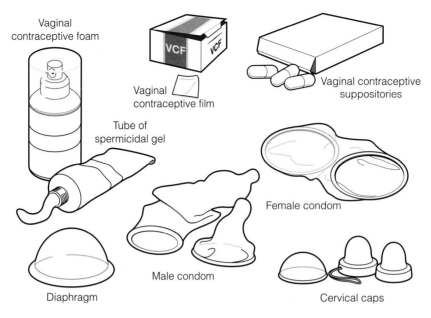

Figure 24-2 • Barrier methods and spermicides.

from being released into the reproductive tract of the woman.

Effectiveness

When properly used, the condom can be 98% effective in preventing conception. The actual efficacy rate in the population is 85% to 90%. To maximize effectiveness and decrease the risk of condom breakage, it is important to leave a well at the tip of the condom to collect the ejaculate and to avoid leakage of semen as the penis is withdrawn. Efficacy is also increased by use of spermicide-containing condoms or by using a spermicide along with condoms.

Side Effects

Some individuals may experience a hypersensitivity to the latex, lubricant, or spermicide in condoms.

Advantages/Disadvantages

Condoms are widely available for a moderate cost and carry the added benefit of preventing the transmission of many **sexually transmitted infections** (STIs). Condoms are the only method of contraception that offers protection against human immunodeficiency virus (HIV). Drawbacks of the condom include coital interruption and possible decreased sensation or hypersensitivity.

FEMALE CONDOMS

Method of Action

The female condom (FC; formerly the Reality Vaginal Pouch) is a pouch made of polyurethane that has a flexible ring at each end. One ring fits into the depth of the vagina, and the other stays outside the vagina near the introitus (Fig. 24-3).

Effectiveness

Initial studies show that the failure rate of the female condom is 20% to 25%, somewhat higher than that of the male condom. However, these were short-term studies and may not reflect the failure rate with long-term usage.

Advantages/Disadvantages

Female condoms protect against many STIs while also placing the control of contraception with the female partner. Major drawbacks include cost and overall bulkiness. The acceptability rating is somewhat higher for the male partner (75% to 80%) than for the female partner (65% to 70%).

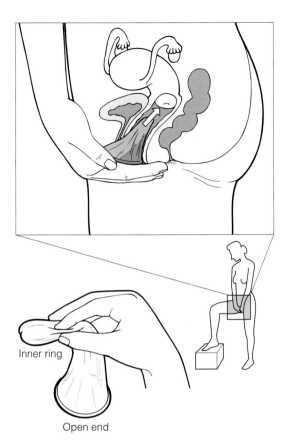

Figure 24-3 • Placement of the female condom.

DIAPHRAGM

Method of Action

The vaginal diaphragm is a dome-shaped latex rubber sheet stretched over a thin coiled rim. Spermicidal jelly is placed on the rim and on either side of the diaphragm, and it is placed into the vagina so that it covers the cervix (Fig. 24-4). The diaphragm and spermicide should be placed in the vagina before intercourse and left in place for **6 to 8 hours** after intercourse. If further intercourse is to take place within 6 to 8 hours after the first episode of intercourse, additional spermicide should be placed in the vagina without removing the diaphragm.

Effectiveness

The theoretical effectiveness of the diaphragm approaches 94%. The actual effectiveness rate of the diaphragm with spermicide is 80% to 85%.

Side Effects

Possible side effects include bladder irritation, which can lead to UTIs. If the diaphragm is left in place too long, colonization by *Staphylococcus aureus* may lead to the development of **toxic shock syndrome** (TSS). Some women also experience a hypersensitivity to the rubber, latex, or spermicide.

Advantages/Disadvantages

The diaphragm must be fitted and prescribed by a clinician, making its initial cost significantly higher than over-the-counter methods of contraception. The diaphragm should be replaced every 2 years or when the patient gains or loses more than 20% of her body weight. It should also be checked after each pregnancy. Women who are not comfortable with inserting the diaphragm or who cannot be properly fitted due to pelvic relaxation defects are poor candidates for the diaphragm, as are women who are at high risk of HIV.

CERVICAL CAP

Method of Action

The cervical cap (FemCap, Lea's Shield) is a small, soft, silicone cap that fits directly over the cervix (Fig. 24-5). It is held in place by suction and acts as a

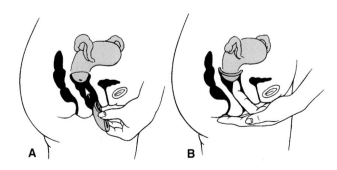

Figure 24-4 • **(A)** Insertion of the vaginal diaphragm. **(B)** Checking to ensure the diaphragm covers the cervix. (From Beckmann C, Ling F. *Obstetrics & Gynecology*, 5th ed. Philadelphia: Lippincott Williams & Wilkins, 2006.)

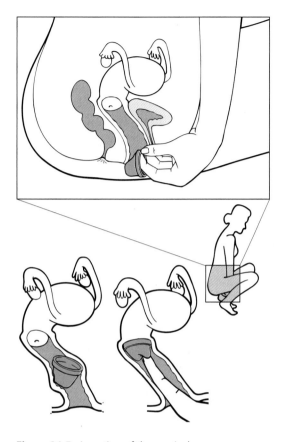

Figure 24-5 • Insertion of the cervical cap.

barrier to sperm. The cap must be **fitted by a clinician** and must be **used with a spermicidal jelly**. Because of the variability in cervix size, proper fit and usage of the cap are essential to its effectiveness. Although it is widely used in Britain and Europe, the cervical cap is not widely available in the United States.

Effectiveness

The actual efficacy rate of the cervical cap is 68% to 84% (16% to 32% failure rate) depending on the woman's parity. There is an increased risk of failure in parous women. **Dislodgment** is the most common cause of failure.

Advantages/Disadvantages

One advantage of the cervical cap is that it can be inserted up to 6 hours prior to intercourse and can be left in place for 1 to 2 days. However, a foul discharge often develops after the first day. The cap must be refitted after a pregnancy or in the event of large weight change. Also, many women have a difficult time mastering the placement and removal techniques for the cervical cap; as a result, the continuation rate is low (30% to 50%).

SPERMICIDES

Method of Action

Spermicidal agents come in varying forms including vaginal creams, gels, films, suppositories, and foams (Fig. 24-2). The most widely used spermicides are **nonoxynol-9** and **octoxynol-9**. Other agents such as menfegol and benzalkonium chloride are used around the world but are not available in the United States. Nonoxynol-9 and octoxynol-9 both disrupt the cell membranes of spermatozoa and also act as a mechanical barrier to the cervical canal. In general, spermicides should be placed in the vagina at least 30 minutes before intercourse to allow for dispersion throughout the vagina. Spermicides may be used alone but are far more effective when used in conjunction with condoms, cervical caps, diaphragms, or other contraceptive methods.

Effectiveness

When properly and consistently used with condoms, spermicides can have an effectiveness rate as high as 95%. However, in actual usage, the efficacy of spermicides when used alone is only 70% to 75%. This effectiveness is further reduced by failure to wait long enough for the spermicide to disperse in the vagina prior to intercourse.

Side Effects

Spermicides can irritate the vaginal mucosa and external genitalia.

Advantages/Disadvantages

Spermicidal agents are widely available in a variety of forms and are relatively inexpensive. Some formulations can also be messy to use.

In addition to providing contraception, it was initially thought that spermicides might provide some protection against sexually transmitted infections (STIs). However, it now appears that these agents *do not* confer any protection against STIs. They may, in fact, make the user **more susceptible to STIs** including HIV by causing vaginal irritation. For this reason,

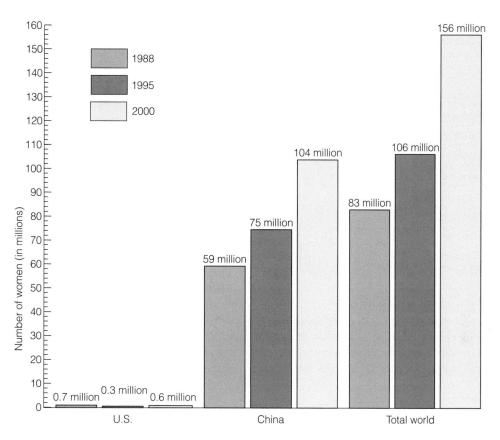

Figure 24-6 • Use of the IUD in the United States, China, and the rest of the world.

spermicides should not be used by women with HIV or at high risk of contracting HIV. This is of special significance in developing nations where contraception and STI prevention are paramount. For the general public, it is strongly recommended that **consistent condom use** be employed whenever protection against STIs is desired.

INTRAUTERINE DEVICES

Intrauterine devices (IUDs) have been used to prevent pregnancy since the 1800s. In the 1960s and 1970s,

IUDs became extremely popular in the United States. However, legal ramifications stemming from pelvic infections associated with one particular IUD—the Dalkon shield—resulted in consumer fear and limited availability of all IUDs. Currently, only two IUDs are available in the United States (Fig. 24-7): the **intrauterine Copper-T IUD** (TCu-380A or ParaGard) and the **levonorgestrel intrauterine system** (LNG-20 or Mirena). Despite previous fears, there are nearly 100 million IUD users globally, making the IUD the **most widely used method of reversible contraception in the world** (Fig. 24-6).

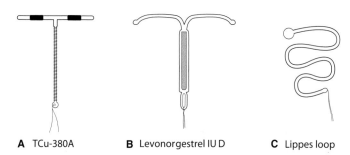

A TCu-380A   **B** Levonorgestrel IUD   **C** Lippes loop

Figure 24-7 • Intrauterine devices. **(A)** ParaGard Copper T (TCu-380A). **(B)** Mirena (Levonorgestrel IUS). **(C)** Lippes loop (used throughout the world but not available in the United States).
(From Speroff L, Fritz M. *Clinical Gynecologic Endocrinology and Infertility*, 7th ed. Philadelphia: Lippincott Williams & Wilkins, 2005.)

■ **TABLE 24-2** Contraindications for IUD Use

Absolute contraindications
Known or suspected pregnancy
Undiagnosed abnormal vaginal bleeding
Acute cervical, uterine, or salpingeal infection
Copper allergy or Wilson disease (for ParaGard only)
Current breast cancer (for Mirena only)
Relative contraindications
Prior ectopic pregnancy
History of STIs in past 3 months
Uterine anomaly or fibroid distorting the cavity
Current menorrhagia or dysmenorrhea (for ParaGard only)

IUD (Mirena) has also been used off label to treat menorrhagia and dysmenorrhea and in post-menopausal women receiving estrogen therapy. Absolute and relative contraindications for IUD use are outlined in Table 24-2.

METHOD OF ACTION

Intrauterine devices are introduced into the endometrial cavity using a cervical cannula (Fig. 24-8). IUDs have two monofilament strings that extend through the cervix where they can be checked to detect expulsion or migration. The strings also facilitate removal of the device by the clinician.

The mechanism of action for IUDs is not completely understood, but they act mainly by killing sperm (spermicidal) and preventing fertilization. Specifically, the primary method of action is to elicit a **sterile inflammatory response** resulting in sperm being engulfed, immobilized, and destroyed by inflammatory cells. The IUD is also thought to **reduce tubal motility** that in turn inhibits sperm and blasto-

The IUD is especially indicated for women in whom oral contraceptives are contraindicated, those who are at low risk for STIs, and in monogamous women of any age. The levonorgestrel-containing

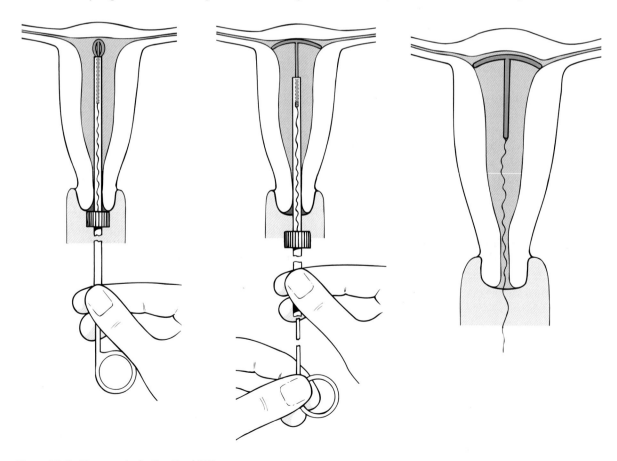

Figure 24-8 • Placement of a ParaGard IUD.

cyst transport. IUDs do not affect ovulation, nor do they act as abortifacients. Their presumed mechanisms of action are augmented by the addition of levonorgestrel in the Mirena IUD and copper in the ParaGard IUD. Progesterone in the Mirena **thickens the cervical mucus** and **atrophies the endometrium** to prevent implantation. Copper in the ParaGard is thought to hamper sperm motility and capitation so sperm rarely reach the fallopian tube and are unable to fertilize the ovum.

EFFECTIVENESS

The efficacy for IUDs rivals that of permanent sterilization with prolonged use. The failure rate is 0.8% for the ParaGard and 0.1% for the Mirena IUD. The cumulative 10-year failure rate for the ParaGard is 2.1% to 2.8% and the cumulative 5-year failure rate for the Mirena is 0.7%. During the first year of use, however, the failure rate is near 3%. This is believed to be due to unrecognized expulsions.

SIDE EFFECTS

Although extremely safe, uncommon side effects and complications of IUDs can be potentially severe and dangerous. These include pain and bleeding, pregnancy, expulsion, perforation, and infection.

Placement of IUDs in women with cervical infections can lead to **insertion-related PID**. This increased risk is now believed to be due to contamination of the endometrial cavity at the time of insertion. Otherwise, pelvic infection is rarely seen beyond the first 20 days after insertion. Antibiotic prophylaxis is not needed for IUD insertion nor is it indicated for bacterial endocarditis prophylaxis. Instead, emphasis should be placed on appropriate patient selection and screening women for gonorrhea and *Chlamydia* prior to insertion of the IUD. Moreover, studies now show that women using the Mirena IUD have a decreased risk of PID due to the protection of progesterone-induced cervical mucus thickening. Given these findings, Mirena IUDs are being used more liberally in younger women, women who have not completed childbearing, and nulliparous women.

The pregnancy rate with IUD use is very low; however, when pregnancy does occur, the **spontaneous abortion** rate is increased to 40% to 50% for women who become pregnant with an IUD in place. Given this, if intrauterine pregnancy occurs while an IUD is in place, the device should be removed by **gentle traction on the string**. The risk of life-threatening spontaneous septic abortion has only been seen with the Dalkon shield, which is no longer available. The IUD is not associated with any increased risk of congenital abnormalities.

ADVANTAGES/DISADVANTAGES

The IUD must be prescribed, inserted, and removed by a clinician. However, once in place, it is highly effective, cost-effective, long-lasting, and rapidly reversible. The user must do little other than a monthly string check to ensure the device has not been expelled. This improves coital spontaneity and decreases fear of pregnancy. In the United States, the **ParaGard IUD has been approved for use for 10 years** but has been shown to maintain its effectiveness for 12 years. The **Mirena IUD has been approved for use for 5 years** but is effective for at least 7 years. One IUD can be removed and another one can be inserted on the same visit. Also, an IUD may be inserted **immediately after induced or spontaneous first trimester abortions** without increased risk of infection or perforation. The ParaGard IUD can be inserted immediately postpartum (within 10 minutes of placental delivery) with an increased risk of expulsion but no increased risk of infection or perforation. Both the Mirena and ParaGard IUDs can be used safely at **6 weeks postpartum** and are safe in breastfeeding women.

In general, because IUDs are so effective at preventing pregnancy that the risk of **ectopic pregnancy is reduced** in IUD users compared to that of noncontraceptive users. In the rare event that a woman does become pregnant with an IUD in place, however, **the risk of ectopic pregnancy may be as high as 30% to 50%** of those patients. Although controversial, the IUD is an acceptable form of contraception for women with a **prior history of ectopic pregnancy**.

The Mirena IUD has been found to **decrease menorrhagia** (90% less blood loss) and **dysmenorrhea**. It is also as effective as oral progestins in treating endometriosis, endometrial hyperplasia, and cancer. It also protects the user from PID. As a result, this decreases the number of surgeries needed for pain and bleeding (hysterectomies, D&Cs, endometrial ablations). Some 20% of women will experience amenorrhea while using a Mirena IUD for 1 year and 60% will experience amenorrhea after using the Mirena for

5 years. FDA approval is currently being sought for use of the Mirena IUD for the treatment of menorrhagia.

HORMONAL CONTRACEPTIVE METHODS

Hormonal contraceptives are the most commonly used reversible means of preventing pregnancy in the United States and consist of combined (estrogen and progesterone) and progesterone-only methods. Currently, combined hormonal methods are available in oral, transdermal, and vaginal forms, whereas progesterone-only methods are available in oral, injectable, implantable, and intrauterine forms. At this time, there are several hormonal contraceptives in various stages of the FDA approval process in the United States including new formulations for oral use, new subdermal implants and vaginal delivery systems, self-injectables, and male hormonal methods.

COMBINED ESTROGEN AND PROGESTIN METHODS

Oral Contraceptive Pills (OCPs)

Method of Action

Oral contraceptive pills (OCPs) are composed of progesterone alone or a combination of progesterone and estrogen. (The progesterone-alone pill is described later in the progesterone-only section.) Over 150 million women worldwide—including one-third

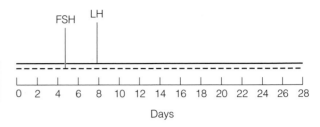

Figure 24-10 • Serum levels of FSH and LH while taking monophasic oral contraceptive pills.

of sexually active women in the United States—use oral contraceptives.

Oral contraceptives place the body in a **pseudopregnancy** state by interfering with the pulsatile release of follicle-stimulating hormone (FSH) and luteinizing hormone (LH) from the anterior pituitary. This pseudo-pregnancy state **suppresses ovulation** and prevents pregnancy from occurring. Figure 24-9 illustrates the serum levels of FSH and LH during the normal menstrual cycle, and Figure 24-10 shows FSH and LH levels during a cycle on the combination pill. Because the FSH and LH surges do not occur, follicle growth, recruitment, and ovulation do not occur. The bleeding that takes place during the hormone-free interval is actually a bleed due to the withdrawal of hormone rather than a menstrual period induced by endogenous hormone fluctuation.

Secondary mechanisms of action for OCPs include thickening the **cervical mucus** to render it less penetrable by sperm and changing the **endometrium** to make it unsuitable for implantation.

Monophasic (Fixed-Dose) Combination Pills

Monophasic combination pills contain a **fixed dose of estrogen and a fixed dose of progestin in each tablet**. Nearly 30 combinations of estrogen and progestins are available in the United States. In general, the selection of a particular pill for each patient depends on the individual side effects and risk factors for each patient.

The combination pill containing both estrogen and progestin is taken for the first 21 days out of a 28-day monthly cycle. During the last 7 days of the cycle, a placebo pill or no pill is taken. Bleeding should begin within 3 to 5 days of completion of the 21 days of hormones. Newer formulations are now available that give 24 days of hormone (rather than the traditional 21 days) and a 4-day hormone-free interval. So-called 24/4 regimens (i.e., Yaz and Loestrin 24 Fe) result in a shorter 3- to 4-day menstrual cycle for most users.

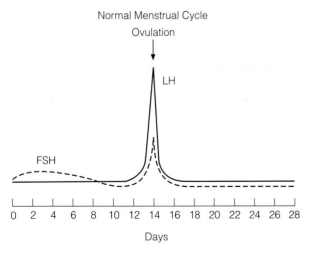

Figure 24-9 • Serum levels of FSH and LH during a normal menstrual cycle.

Women with menstrual-related disorders (such as endometriosis, menorrhagia, anemia, dysmenorrhea, menstrual irregularity, menstrual migraines, PMS, PCOS, or ovarian cysts) may benefit from extending the number of consecutive days of hormonal pills taken from 21 days to 1, 2, or 3 months, thus increasing the length of continuous hormonal suppression and decreasing the number of withdrawal bleeds. These extended or long-cycle regimens provide continued suppression of ovulation and decreased menstrual-related symptoms (such as pain, heavy bleeding, anemia, headaches) for their users.

Seasonale and **Seasonique** contains **84 consecutive hormonal pills** followed by 7 placebo pills, or 7 low-estrogen pills, respectively. These dosing regimens were designed to decrease the number of withdrawal bleeds to four per year, again, with the goal of minimizing menstrual-related symptoms. Most recently, a **365-day OCP regimen** known as Lybrel was approved by the FDA. **Lybrel** provides a combination estrogen and progestin pill each day, 365 days of the year. There is more breakthrough bleeding in this regimen but no formal monthly withdrawal bleed.

Multiphasic (Dose Varying) Combination Pills

Multiphasic oral contraceptives differ from monophasic pills only in that they **vary the dosage of estrogen and/or progestin** in the active hormone pills in an

■ **TABLE 24-4** Complications Associated with Oral Contraceptives

Cardiovascular*
Deep vein thrombosis (DVT)
Pulmonary embolism (PE)
Cerebrovascular accident (CVA)**
Myocardial infarction (MI)**
Hypertension
Other
Cholelithiasis
Cholecystitis
Benign liver adenomas (rare)
Cervical adenocarcinoma (rare)
Retinal thrombosis (rare)

*These complications occur mainly in smokers.
**Most MIs and CVAs occur in users of high-dose estrogen products.

effort to mimic the menstrual cycle. The advantage of the multiphasic dosing is that it may provide a lower level of estrogen and progestin overall but is still highly effective at preventing pregnancy.

Effectiveness

OCPs are remarkably effective in preventing pregnancy. In fact, the theoretical failure rate for the first year of use is less than 1%. However, the failure rate with actual real-life usage is closer to 8%. Nausea, breakthrough bleeding, and the necessity of taking the pill every day are often cited as reasons for discontinuing the pill.

Several medications are thought to interact with oral contraceptives and reduce the effectiveness of the pill. Conversely, oral contraceptives can also reduce the efficacy of many medications (Table 24-3).

Side Effects

Table 24-4 lists some of the cardiovascular, neoplastic, and biliary complications associated with oral contraceptive use.

Oral contraceptives with estrogen doses greater than 50 mg can increase coagulability, leading to higher rates of myocardial infarction, stroke, thromboembolism, and pulmonary embolism, particularly in women who smoke. Even at lower doses of estrogen (35 mcg or less), women over 35 who smoke

■ **TABLE 24-3** Interactions of Oral Contraceptives with Other Medications

Medications That Reduce the Efficacy of Oral Contraceptives	Medications Whose Efficacies are Changed by Oral Contraceptives
Barbiturates	Chlordiazepoxide (Librium)
Carbamazepine (Tegretol)	Diazepam (Valium)
Griseofulvin	Hypoglycemics
Phenytoin (Dilantin)	Methyldopa
Rifampin	Phenothiazides
St. John's wort	Theophylline
Topiramate (Topamax)	Tricyclic antidepressants

more than one pack of cigarettes per day are still at increased risk of **heart attack, stroke, DVT, and PE** if they use OCPs. The progestins in oral contraceptives have been found to raise low-density lipoproteins while lowering high-density lipoproteins in pill users smoking more than 1 pack per day. For these reasons, oral contraceptives are **contraindicated in women over age 35 who smoke 15 or more cigarettes a day**. The advent of new progestins and lower estrogen doses has led to pill formulations that are essentially neutral in terms of cardiovascular effect. However, combination oral contraceptive use is still contraindicated in women over age 35 who smoke. These women often benefit from progesterone-only IUDs or permanent female or male sterilization.

Neoplastic complications of oral contraceptive use are rare. The effect of long-term oral contraceptive use on breast cancer has been studied extensively over the past decade with no conclusive findings. There is, however, an **increased incidence of gallbladder disease and benign hepatic tumors** associated with oral contraceptive use.

Table 24-5 outlines both the absolute and relative contraindications to oral contraceptive use.

■ **TABLE 24-6** Noncontraceptive Health Benefits of Oral Contraceptives
Decrease risk of serious diseases
Ovarian cancer
Endometrial cancer
Ectopic pregnancy (combination pills only)
Severe anemia
Pelvic inflammatory disease
Salpingitis
Improve quality-of-life problems
Iron-deficiency anemia
Dysmenorrhea
Functional ovarian cysts
Benign breast disease
Osteoporosis (increased bone density)
Rheumatoid arthritis
Treat/manage many disorders
Dysfunctional uterine bleeding
Control of bleeding in bleeding disorders and anovulation
Dysmenorrhea
Endometriosis
Acne/hirsutism
Premenstrual syndrome

■ **TABLE 24-5** Contraindications to Combination Estrogen-Progesterone Contraceptives	
Absolute Contraindications	**Relative Contraindications**
Thromboembolism	Uterine fibroids
Pulmonary embolism	Lactation
Coronary artery disease	Diabetes mellitus
Cerebrovascular accident	Sickle-cell disease or sickle C disease
Smokers over the age of 35	Hepatic disease
Breast/endometrial cancer	Hypertension
Unexplained vaginal bleeding	Lupus (SLE)
Abnormal liver function	Age 40+ and high risk for vascular disease
Known or suspected pregnancy	Migraine headaches
Severe hypercholesterolemia	Seizure disorders
Severe hypertriglyceridemia	Elective surgery

Advantages/Disadvantages

The major advantages of OCPs include their **extremely high efficacy** rates and the **noncontraceptive health benefits** primarily attributable to decreased pregnancy, decreased menstrual flow, and decreased ovulation. These benefits include a reduced incidence of ovarian cancer, endometrial cancer, ectopic pregnancy, pelvic inflammatory disease (PID), and benign breast disease (Table 24-6). By taking OCPs, nearly 50,000 women avoid hospitalizations; of these, 10,000 avoid hospitalization for life-threatening illnesses.

Disadvantages include cardiovascular complications, increased gallbladder disease, increased incidence of benign hepatic tumors, and the need to take a medication every day. Because they contain estrogen, combination OCPs are not suitable for many women. Many women also complain of nausea, headaches, breakthrough bleeding, and weight gain associated with OCP use. Most of these symptoms are generally mild and transient.

Transdermal Estrogen and Progestin Hormonal Contraception—Ortho Evra

Mechanism of Action

The contraceptive patch (Fig. 24-11) with the brand name **Ortho Evra** releases progestin and **ethinyl estradiol. The patch releases 150 mg per day of the progestin, norelgestromin, and 20 μg per day of ethinyl estradiol**. Although it is difficult to compare the estrogen levels in Ortho Evra users to those in women taking standard OCPs, limited data suggests that the overall average estrogen concentration is higher in Ortho Evra users. Therefore, these patients should be made aware of the possible **increased risk of thromboembolism**, specifically **DVT and PE** in Ortho Evra users. There does not appear to be an increased risk of heart attack and stroke in these patients.

Women apply one patch each week for 3 weeks followed by 1 week patch-free during which they will have a withdrawal bleed. This hormone-free period can be skipped to allow for continuous 3-month dosing. Again, just like combined OCPs, the primary mechanism of action is suppression of ovulation by decreasing endogenous FSH and LH levels (Figs. 24-9 and 24-10).

Effectiveness

The patch has been shown to have a 1% pregnancy rate in actual use—similar to other combination hormonal methods. Ortho Evra has been found to have a **decreased effectiveness in markedly overweight women (greater than 198 pounds or 90 kg)**.

Advantages/Disadvantages

The same primary side effects and noncontraceptive health benefits of OCPs apply to the patch as well. The patch can cause skin irritation in some users. The patch has the added benefit of being self-administered only once a week.

Vaginal Estrogen and Progestin Hormonal Contraception-NuvaRing

Method of Action

The hormone-releasing vaginal ring (Fig. 24-11) with the brand name of **NuvaRing** releases a daily dose of 15 mcg of ethinyl estradiol and 120 mcg of etonogestrel (the active form of desogestrel). The ring is **placed in the vagina for 3 weeks** (it is likely effective for 4 weeks), and is removed for 1 week to allow for a withdrawal bleed. Again, this hormone-free period can be skipped to allow for continuous dosing, typically for 3 months.

Effectiveness

Clinical studies are ongoing, but the vaginal ring is **highly effective** (0.8% failure rate in actual use), similar to other forms of combined hormonal contraception.

Advantages/Disadvantages

Because one size of vaginal ring fits all women, the vaginal ring need does not need to be fitted by a

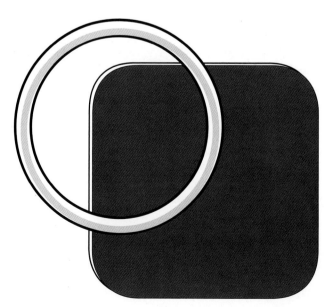

Figure 24-11 • Vaginal contraceptive ring (NuvaRing) and transdermal contraceptive patch (Ortho Evra). Both contain a combination of estrogen and progesterone, which are released over time; 1 week and 3 weeks, respectively.
(From Speroff L, Fritz M. *Clinical Gynecologic Endocrinology and Infertility*, 7th ed. Philadelphia: Lippincott Williams & Wilkins, 2005.)

clinician. Women place the ring in the vagina themselves for 3 continuous weeks and then remove it for 1 week. Because the ring is left in place continuously it provides a low, steady release of hormone with lower total hormone exposure compared to other combination hormone methods. And, while douching with the NuvaRing in place is discouraged, the use of antifungal agents and spermicides is permitted.

The disadvantages of the vaginal ring include a woman's (or partner's) concern with having a foreign body in the vagina and the potential for expulsion. Studies have shown that women do not feel the ring inside once placed in the vagina and **the ring does not need to be removed for intercourse.** If it is removed for intercourse, it should be rinsed in cool water and replaced within 3 hours. Reasons for discontinuation include discomfort, headache, vaginal discharge, and recurrent vaginitis.

PROGESTERONE-ONLY CONTRACEPTION

Progesterone-only contraception consists of oral, injectable, implantable, and intrauterine options (the Mirena IUS is discussed earlier in the IUD section). These all function primarily using the same mechanisms: thickening the cervical mucus, inhibiting sperm motility, and thinning the endometrial lining so that it is not suitable for implantation.

Progestin-Only Oral Contraception Pills (The Minipill)

Method of Action

Progestin-only pills (POPs; Micronor, Nor-QD) deliver a **small daily dose of progestin** (0.35 mg norethindrone) without any estrogen. POPs have lower progestin doses than combination pills, thus the nickname *minipills*. POPs also differ from traditional pills in that **they are taken every day of the cycle** with no hormone-free days. POPs are believed to **thicken the cervical mucus** making it less permeable to sperm. This effect, however, decreases after 22 hours so the minipill must be **taken at the same time each day.** Other mechanisms of action include endometrial atrophy and ovulation suppression (50% of cycles).

Effectiveness

Progestin-only pills are generally **not as effective** (failure rate of 8%) as combination hormone regimens.

This failure rate increases if punctual dosing is not achieved.

Side Effects

Side effects of the progesterone-only OCP include irregular ovulatory cycles, breakthrough bleeding, increased formation of follicular cysts, and acne. POPs can also cause breast tenderness and irritability.

Advantages/Disadvantages

Because they contain no estrogen, progestin-only pills are ideal for nursing mothers and **women for whom estrogens are contraindicated** including women over 35 who smoke and women with hypertension, CAD, CVD, lupus, migraines, and those with a personal history of thromboembolism. The disadvantages **include irregular menses** ranging from amenorrhea to irregular spotting. Also, POPs must be taken at the same time each day. A delay of more than 3 hours is akin to a missed pill.

Injectable Progesterone-Only Contraception—Depo-Provera

Method of Action

Although it was only approved for contraceptive use in the United States in 1992, Depo-Provera (**medroxyprogesterone acetate; DMPA**) has been used in other countries since the mid-1960s. Depo-Provera is injected intramuscularly every 3 months in a vehicle that allows the slow release of progestin over a 3-month period. Depo-Provera acts by suppressing ovulation, thickening the cervical mucus, and making the endometrium unsuitable for implantation. After an injection, ovulation does not occur for 14 weeks; therefore, patients have a 2-week grace period in their every 12-week dosing.

Effectiveness

With a first-year failure rate of only 0.3% when used correctly, Depo-Provera is one of the most effective contraceptive methods available. A newer low-dose DMPA is also available although not widely used yet. This formulation carries the benefit of lower progestin levels but the same efficacy rates.

Side Effects

The primary side effects experienced by Depo-Provera users include **irregular menstrual bleeding,** depression, weight gain, hair loss, and headache. Over 70% of patients experience spotting and irregular menses during the first year of use. Irregular bleeding is the primary reason for discontinuing Depo-Provera. It is anticipated that **50% of DMPA users will have amenorrhea after 1 year** of use and 80% after 5 years of DMPA use. However, the possibility of amenorrhea makes Depo-Provera a good option for women with bleeding disorders, women on anticoagulation, women in the military, and women who are mentally or physically disabled.

Women using DMPA for more than 2 years may experience a **reversible decrease in bone mineralization** similar to that seen in lactating women. The effect of Depo-Provera use on bone mineralization is summarized in Table 24-7. Thus, calcium, vitamin D, weight-bearing exercise, and smoking cessation should be encouraged in all women using Depo-Provera. Subcutaneously administered Depo-Provera regimens that do not result in decreased bone density are now available but not in wide use in the United States.

Advantages/Disadvantages

The primary advantages of Depo-Provera are that it is **highly effective**, acts independent of intercourse, and only requires injections every 3 months. Like other progestins, Depo-Provera **reduces the risk of endometrial cancer and PID** and also the amount of menstrual bleeding. It is also useful in the treatment of menorrhagia, dysmenorrhea, endometriosis, menstrual-related anemia, and endometrial hyperplasia. DMPA is especially useful in women who desire effective contraception but may have **concomitant medical conditions** that prevent the use of estrogen-containing contraceptives such as women with migraines, seizure disorders, lupus, hypertension, coronary artery disease, and who smoke.

Irregular bleeding, weight gain, and mood changes are the major disadvantages. Although not contraindicated, Depo-Provera should be used with caution in patients with a history of depression, mood disorders, PMS, and PMDD. Similarly, Depo-Provera use is not contraindicated in obese women but weight monitoring should be employed when using the medicine in women who may be at increased risk for weight gain.

After discontinuation of Depo-Provera injections, some women may experience a significant **delay in the return of regular ovulation** (6 to 18 months; average is 10 months). This is independent of the number of injections but may be directly related to the weight of the patient. Within 18 months, however, fertility rates return to normal levels.

Implantable Progesterone-Only Contraception—Implanon

Method of Action

Implanon is a **single-rod**, **progestin implant** that provides **3 years** of uninterrupted contraceptive coverage. The progestin used in Implanon is **etonogestrel**, the same progestin as used in the NuvaRing. The device provides slow release of 68 mg of etonogestrel over 3 years. It is the size of a matchstick and is placed in the subdermal skin of a woman's upper arm. When appropriate timing of placement is utilized, Implanon is affective 24 hours after placement and has quick return to fertility once the device is removed by a clinician.

Jadelle is a two-rod implantable subdermal device also approved by the FDA. It uses **levonorgestrel** to provide 5 years of contraceptive coverage. At this time, Jadelle has not yet been marketed in the United States but has been used in most other countries.

Effectiveness

Implanon is **highly effective** with only a 0.4% failure rate.

Side Effects

Irregular and unpredictable light bleeding is the major side effect of Implanon. In the majority of cases (75%), the bleeding is lighter than a normal

■ **TABLE 24-7** The Effects of Depo-Provera Use on Bone Mineralization
Bone density is decreased in women using Depo-Provera
The decrease in bone density is most rapid in the first year of use
The decrease in bone density increases with length of use
The decrease in bone density is reversible and occurs over 6 mo to 2 years
There is no role for the use of bone density screening (DEXA) in DMPA users
There is no role for the use of bisphosphonates, estrogens, SERMS in DMPA users
Women on Depo-Provera should be encouraged to take calcium and vitamin D, to stop smoking, and to do regular weight-bearing exercise

menstrual bleed and requires only a panty liner or less for protection. However, irregular bleeding was the reason for 20% of discontinuations.

Advantages/Disadvantages

The major advantage of Implanon is that it is implantable and provides 3 uninterrupted years of contraceptive coverage. There is **no maintenance** associated with the device and thus **no interruption of sexual spontaneity**. The disadvantages include the need for a provider to insert and remove the device and the **unpredictable bleeding profile**.

EMERGENCY CONTRACEPTION

The emergency contraception pill (ECP) can **prevent pregnancy** after unprotected intercourse or in the case of contraceptive failure (condom break, diaphragm dislodgment, IUD expulsion, missed pill, late Depo-Provera injection). It is used only if a woman is not already pregnant from a previous act of intercourse. ECP use is not indicated in women with a known or suspected pregnancy. However, there is no known evidence of harm to the patient, her pregnancy, or to the fetus if ECPs are unintentionally taken during pregnancy.

Emergency contraception works by preventing pregnancy, not by disrupting an implanted pregnancy. In fact, ECP is thought to account for a 40% **decline in therapeutic abortions** in the past 10 years while also **decreasing the number of teen pregnancies**. It is available in two forms: emergency contraceptive pills (also called the *postcoital* or the *morning-after pill*) and an emergently inserted Copper T IUD (ParaGard). Although **mifepristone** (RU 486) has been approved in the United States for the termination of pregnancy up to 49 days' gestation, its use has not been approved for emergency contraception use in the United States.

EMERGENCY CONTRACEPTIVE PILLS

Methods of Action

Emergency contraceptive pills use high doses of both estrogen and progestins or progesterone alone (Plan B, Norlevo, Vikela) to prevent pregnancy after unprotected intercourse has taken place. Several differing regimens exist including those using high doses of regularly prescribed OCPs and some using prepackaged regimens.

The most common prepackaged formulation is **Plan B (progestin only)**. All regimens are usually **taken in two doses, 12 hours apart**. However, studies now show that Plan B is equally effective if taken in a single dose rather than splitting the dose into two with minimal increased side effects. Regardless of the regimen, **the first dose must be taken within 72 hours of unprotected vaginal intercourse**. An antiemetic is often prescribed at the same time to prevent nausea (more common in estrogen-containing regimens).

The **mechanism of action** for emergency contraceptive pills depends on the point during the cycle when the pills are taken. Emergency contraception is used to prevent pregnancy by inhibiting ovulation, interfering with fertilization and tubal transport, preventing implantation, or causing regression of the corpus luteum.

Effectiveness

When taken within 72 hours of intercourse, emergency contraceptive pills have a failure rate of 0.2% to 3%. The sooner an ECP is taken after unprotected intercourse, the more effective it is. The risk of pregnancy is reduced by 75% to 90% in women who have had unprotected intercourse during the second or third week of their menstrual cycles, when they are most likely ovulating. Of all the oral EC regimens, the progesterone-only formulations (Plan B) are the most effective and have fewer side effects. Thus, **Plan B should be used as a first choice** when it is available rather than using a combination method.

Side Effects

The primary side effects of emergency contraception include **nausea (50%)**, **vomiting (20%)**, headaches, dizziness, and breast tenderness. Most of these symptoms are thought to be secondary to the high doses of estrogen in the combined regimens. The side effects of the progesterone-only formulations are less severe than symptoms experienced with estrogen and progesterone-containing methods.

While there are relative and absolute contraindications for use of oral contraceptives in women with certain medical conditions (history of stroke, heart attack, DVT, PE), these contraindications do not apply to women using emergency contraceptives. However, repeated use of ECP is not recommended in this high-risk group.

Advantages/Disadvantages

Emergency contraceptive pills are extremely effective in preventing pregnancy and are safe for the user. In 2006, the FDA approved over-the-counter dispensing of Plan B emergency contraception without a prescription for men and women age 18 and older.

The major disadvantages include the short window of time when they can be used (within 72 hours of intercourse). Additionally, these cannot be used as long-term contraception.

EMERGENCY IUD INSERTION

Method of Action

The Copper T IUD (Fig. 24-7A) can be inserted in the uterine cavity within 120 hours (or 5 to 8 days) of unprotected intercourse as a form of emergency contraception. The IUD functions primarily by eliciting a **sterile inflammatory response** within the uterus, making the environment unsuitable for implantation.

Effectiveness

Emergency IUD insertion reduces the risk of pregnancy by 99.8%; therefore, only 1 in 1,000 become pregnant after emergency IUD insertion, **making it the most effective form of emergency contraception.**

Side Effects

The side effects are the same as those discussed in the IUD section. This is not an acceptable form of emergency contraception in women who are not candidates for IUDs including those with multiple sexual partners and victims of rape.

Advantages/Disadvantages

Emergency IUD insertion is extremely effective, even more effective than the oral regimens. It differs from emergency contraceptive pills in that it **can be used long term (10 years)**, whereas the ECPs have a one-time-only use. Disadvantages are that the IUD must be placed by a provider and that it has potential (rare) complications such as infection and perforation that are described in the IUD section above. The ParaGard IUD is also associated with heavier menses and dysmenorrhea.

SURGICAL STERILIZATION

The rate of surgical sterilization as a method of contraception has increased dramatically over the past 3 decades. Approximately 30% of reproductive-age couples in the United States and Great Britain choose female sterilization for contraceptive purposes. A similar number of men seek vasectomies each year. The rate of sterilization is higher in women who are married, divorced, over age 30, or African American.

Before performing any sterilization procedure, careful counseling should be provided and informed consent obtained. The patient should understand the **permanent and largely irreversible nature** of the procedure, operative risks, chance of failure, and possible side effects. Sterilization is ideal in stable monogamous relationships where no additional children are desired. It is also indicated in women in whom pregnancy would be life threatening such as those with major cardiac issues.

TUBAL STERILIZATION

Method of Action

Tubal sterilization prevents pregnancy by surgically occluding both fallopian tubes to prevent the ovum and sperm from uniting. When tubal ligation is performed outside the postpartum period, it is either done via laparoscopic (**laparoscopic tubal ligation [LTL]**) or hysteroscopic (Essure, Adiana) approach.

Laparoscopically, there are a number of methods by which tubal occlusion can be accomplished including bipolar cautery (Fig. 24-12), Silastic banding with Falope (Fig. 24-13) or Yoon rings, clipping with Hulka clips or Filshie clips (Fig. 24-14), and ligation sutures. Tubal ligation can also be performed immediately postpartum (**postpartum sterilization [PPS]**) through a small subumbilical incision using epidural or spinal anesthesia. The most commonly used method, the modified Pomeroy tubal ligation, is illustrated in Figure 24-15.

Most recently, a new procedure using a **hysteroscopic transcervical nonincisional approach (Essure)** was introduced in the United States and abroad. In this method, flexible form-fitting microinserts are introduced into the interstitial (uterine) portions of the fallopian tubes. An outer spring coil molds to the shape of the fallopian tube to anchor the microinsert. **Over about 12 weeks, sterilization is accomplished as**

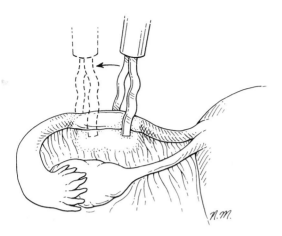

Figure 24-12 • Tubal occlusion with the bipolar cautery. A 3 cm portion of the isthmic tube is desiccated with bipolar forceps. (From Rock J, Jones H. *TeLinde's Operative Gynecology*, 10th ed. Philadelphia: Lippincott Williams & Wilkins, 2008.)

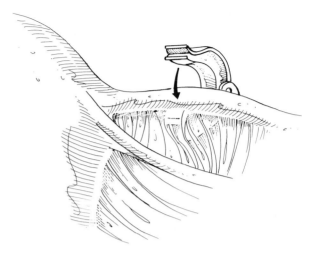

Figure 24-14 • Tubal occlusion with the Filshie clip. The clip is applied to the mid-isthmic portion of the tube about 2 cm from the cornua. The lower jaw of the clip should be visible through the mesosalpinx to ensure inclusion of the entire circumference of the tube. (From Rock J, Jones H. *TeLinde's Operative Gynecology*, 10th ed. Philadelphia: Lippincott Williams & Wilkins, 2008.)

in-growth of tissue around the coils result in tissue barrier occlusion in the fallopian tubes.

The advantages include the lack of general anesthesia and the lack of a surgical incision. As a result, when Essure can be performed, very little recuperative time is needed. Essure can often be performed in the office setting, making it a preferable option to surgical sterilization for obese women, women with prior abdominal surgeries, or those at risk from anesthesia use.

Because the tubal blockage is accomplished over time, a **backup method of birth control** is recommended for 3 months after the procedure until such time that a **hysterosalpingogram** (HSG) can confirm

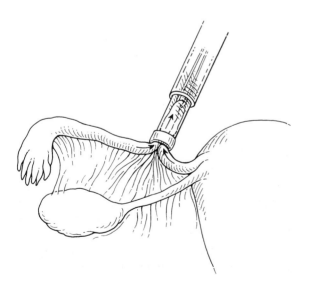

Figure 24-13 • Tubal occlusion with the silicone band (Falope ring). The isthmic portion of the tube is retracted into the applicator barrel using grasping tongs. During this retraction process the ring is rolled forward to occlude the portion of tube. The intervening "knuckle" of tube becomes ischemic and necroses. (From Rock J, Jones H. *TeLinde's Operative Gynecology*, 10th ed. Philadelphia: Lippincott Williams & Wilkins, 2008.)

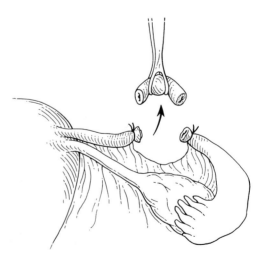

Figure 24-15 • The Parkland (modified Pomeroy) method of postpartum tubal ligation. A 2 to 3 cm segment of the tube is doubly ligated and the intervening segment is removed. This technique is typically performed during the immediate postpartum period through a small subumbilical incision. (From Rock J, Jones H. *TeLinde's Operative Gynecology*, 10th ed. Philadelphia: Lippincott Williams & Wilkins, 2008.)

complete tubal occlusion. Some patients are reassured by this confirmatory test while others are burdened by the additional step to achieving permanent sterilization. Prior to the procedure, patients should understand that tubal occlusion by this method is **essentially irreversible**.

Effectiveness

Tubal ligation has a failure rate of 0.5% but varies by method, patient age, and surgeon's experience. The highest success rates are achieved with postpartum sterilization and Essure tubal occlusion. When the laparoscopic approach is undertaken, the Falope ring has been found to be most effective in women under age 28. Electrocautery and Falope rings are equally effective in women over age 30. More recently, titanium Filshie clips have been used for tubal ligation, but long-term efficacy rates are not yet available. It appears that Essure may offer the lowest rates of all of these methods although long-term data are not available yet.

Side Effects

There are no side effects associated with tubal sterilization. Some women report pain and menstrual disturbances. This phenomenon was once described as **posttubal ligation syndrome** but has largely been discounted by the literature. In most of these women, symptoms are due to discontinuation of hormone-containing contraceptives. As a result, patients may experience heavier baseline menses and dysmenorrhea.

Advantage/Disadvantages

Tubal ligation offers the advantage of permanent effective contraception without continual expense, effort, or motivation. The **mortality rate** of bilateral tubal ligation is 4 in 100,000 women. The major risks are those associated with surgery including the risk of infection, hemorrhage, conversion to laparotomy, viscus injury, vascular damage, and anesthesia complications.

Tubal ligation results in a **very low risk of pregnancy**. However, when pregnancy does occur, there is an **increased risk of ectopic pregnancy** (1 in 15,000). However, nearly 1,000 maternal lives are saved due to sterilization during the period from the time of sterilization to the end of the woman's re-

■ TABLE 24-8 Success Rates of Tubal Occlusion Reversal, by Method

Method of Tubal Sterilization	Success Rates for Reversal (%)
Clips	84
Bands	72
Pomeroy	50
Electrocauterization	41

productive life. Patients may also benefit from a **reduction in the risk of ovarian cancer**. The reason for this is unclear but it's speculated that tubal ligation may limit the migration of carcinogens from the lower genital tract into the peritoneal cavity.

Of women who undergo permanent sterilization, **regret is highest in women who were under age 30** when the procedure was performed. However, it is estimated that only 1% of women seek reversal of tubal sterilization. The success of reversal varies from 41% to 84% depending on the method used (Table 24-8). The success rate of reanastomosis is highest when clips are used since they destroy a much smaller segment of the tube. When pregnancy is desired after tubal ligation, in vitro fertilization (IVF) offers a greater likelihood of pregnancy than tubal microplasty. However, when multiple future pregnancies are desired, tubuloplasty may be a more economical alternative than multiple IVF cycles.

VASECTOMY

Method of Action

Vasectomy is a simple and safe option for permanent sterilization involving **ligation of the vas deferens**. This procedure may be performed in a provider's office under local anesthesia through a small incision in the upper outer aspect of each scrotum (Fig. 24-16). In 1985, the **no-scalpel vasectomy** technique was introduced. With this procedure both vas are ligated through a single small midline incision that reduces the already low rate of complications associated with vasectomy. Unlike female tubal ligations, **vasectomy is not immediately effective**. Because sperm can remain viable in the proximal collecting system after vasectomy, patients should use **another form of contraception** until azoospermia is confirmed by semen analysis, usually in 6 to 8 weeks.

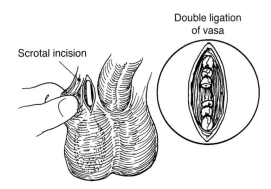

Figure 24-16 • Sterilization by vasectomy. Typically performed in an office setting under local anesthesia.
(From Beckmann C, Ling F. *Obstetrics & Gynecology*, 5th ed. Philadelphia: Lippincott Williams & Wilkins, 2006.)

Effectiveness

The failure rate for vasectomy in actual practice is 0.15%. In fact, vasectomy is **safer, simpler, and more effective than female sterilization**. When pregnancies occur after vasectomy, many are due to having inter-course too soon after vasectomy rather than from re-canalization of the vas deferens.

Side Effects

Complications after vasectomy are rare and usually involve slight bleeding, skin infection, and reactions to the sutures or local anesthesia. Fifty percent of patients form **antisperm antibodies** after the procedure. However, there are no long-term side effects of vasectomy.

Advantages/Disadvantages

Vasectomy is a permanent, highly effective form of contraception with few, if any, side effects. Vasectomy is generally safer and less expensive than tubal ligation and can be performed as an outpatient under local anesthesia. Vasectomy offers permanent sterilization. The success rate of vasal reanastomosis is 60% to 70%. Pregnancy rates after vasectomy reversal range from 18% to 60%.

 KEY POINTS

- Natural family planning methods and coitus interruptus are the least effective methods of contraception and should not be used if pregnancy prevention is a high priority.

- Lactational amenorrhea provides a prolactin-induced suppression of GnRH and subsequent suppression of ovulation. It should only be used for a maximum of 6 months after delivery in an amenorrheic woman and breastfeeding should be the only source of nutrition for the infant.

- Condoms, diaphragms, and cervical caps act as mechanical barriers between sperm and egg. Their efficacy rate is 75% to 85% with practical use.

- Male and female condoms carry the added benefit of prophylaxis against STIs.

- Efficacy of spermicides is 70% to 80%, but variability in user technique can significantly lower efficacy. Spermicides DO NOT protect against STIs and may, in fact, make the vaginal mucosa more susceptible to infections such as HIV.

- IUDs provide long-term, highly effective, cost-effective contraception. There are currently two IUDs on the U.S. market: ParaGard (copper containing;

10 years of use) and Mirena (progestin containing; 5 years of use).

- The primary mechanism of action for IUDs is a sterile spermicidal inflammatory response. Other mechanisms include inhibition of implantation and alteration in tubal motility. Potentially serious side effects include insertion-related PID, uterine perforation, and spontaneous abortion.

- Hormonal contraceptives have extremely low failure rates and are available in oral, injectable, transdermal, implantable, vaginal, and intrauterine forms.

- Combined hormonal contraception methods (OCPs, Ortho Evra, NuvaRing) prevent pregnancy by suppressing ovulation, altering cervical mucus, and causing atrophic changes in the endometrium.

- Serious complications from combined hormonal contraception use occur mainly in smokers over age 35, including pulmonary embolism, stroke, deep venous thrombosis (DVT), and heart attack.

- Benefits of combined hormonal contraception include protection from ovarian and endometrial cancer, anemia, PID, osteoporosis, dysmenorrhea, acne, hirsutism, and benign breast disease.

- Progesterone-only contraception (progestin-only OCPs, Depo-Provera, Implanon, and the Mirena IUD) use progestins to suppress ovulation, thicken the cervical mucus, and make the endometrium unsuitable for implantation.
- Primary side effects of Depo-Provera include irregular bleeding, reversible bone demineralization, and a significant delay in return of fertility after discontinuation. It should be used with caution in women with depression and obesity.
- Implanon is a single-rod, subdermal implant of etonogestrel that is placed in the upper arm of the patient. It provides 3 years of contraception without impacting the patient's bone density, weight, or mood.
- Emergency contraceptive pills contain high doses of estrogen and progestin or progesterone alone and must be taken within 72 hours of intercourse to prevent pregnancy. These pills act to suppress ovulation and to prevent fertilization and implantation. They do not cause abortions.
- When available, a single dose of progesterone-only ECP (Plan B), should be used preferentially given its increased effectiveness and lower rate of side effects.
- Emergency IUD insertion (Copper T only) must be performed within 120 days of unprotected intercourse; it can then be used as long-term contraception.
- Both vasectomy and tubal occlusion are highly effective forms of permanent sterilization. Vasectomies are safer, simpler, and more effective than female sterilization.
- Patients requesting sterilization should be counseled of the permanent and largely irreversible nature of the procedures. The risk of regret is highest among women under 30 regardless of their parity.
- The most effective tubal ligations are those done immediately postpartum or those utilizing the Essure tubal occlusion system.
- When interval laparoscopic approach is undertaken, Falope rings have the highest efficacy in women under 28. Electrocautery and Falope rings have equal efficacy in women 28 and over.
- Essure offers a hysteroscopic transcervical approach to tubal ligation. It does not require a surgical incision or general anesthesia but it does require use of a backup method for 3 months and an HSG to confirm complete tubal occlusion.
- Reversal rates for tubal occlusion vary from 41% to 84% depending on the method used for sterilization. These procedures are costly and are associated with a higher rate of ectopic pregnancy.

In the United States nearly 50% of all pregnancies are unintended and 44% end in elective abortion. As such, the availability of safe and effective means of elective pregnancy termination is an important means of fertility control and an integral part of obstetrics and gynecologic care. Of the over 1.3 million abortions performed annually in the United States; one-third are performed on women under age 20, one-third on women aged 20 to 24, and the remaining one-third on women over age 25. Over 80% of all abortions are performed on unmarried women, 60% have one or more children, and 55% are Caucasian.

The abortion procedures used legally in the United States are both safe and effective. Importantly, the maternal morbidity from induced abortion has decreased significantly, from an estimated 39% in 1972 prior to the legalization of abortion in the United States to 1 per 100,000 in 2004. This is in comparison to a maternal morbidity of 7.7 per 100,000 for completed pregnancy and delivery. In general, maternal morbidity is lowest if legal abortion is performed before 8 weeks' gestation (Fig. 25-1). The major causes of abortion mortality are complications of **general anesthesia**, followed distantly by hemorrhage, infection, and thromboembolism.

There are many surgical and medical procedures by which pregnancy termination can be achieved (Fig. 25-2). Over 85% of induced abortions are done in the first trimester of pregnancy and 97% are accomplished using a surgical evacuation of the uterus (D&C). Evacuation of the uterus is an **important technique** in the field of obstetrics and gynecology. Not only is it used for elective termination of pregnancy, but it is an integral part of managing spontaneous abortion, missed abortion, intrauterine fetal demise, retained products of conception, and gestational trophoblastic neoplasia.

The options for first trimester abortion include **suction curettage** (97%), manual vacuum aspiration, and **medical abortion** (3%) using either mifepristone or methotrexate. Second trimester options include **surgical evacuation** of the uterus and medical **induction of labor**. In general, the technique used for termination is determined by the duration of the pregnancy. Table 25-1 outlines the various options available during the first and second trimesters. Nearly **95% of all induced abortions are performed before 16 weeks' gestation**, 4% are performed between 16 and 20 weeks' gestation, and fewer than 1.5% are performed after 21 weeks' gestation. Laws vary from state to state, but generally speaking, terminations are performed up until the fetus has reached what is considered to be the **stage of viability at about 24 weeks'** gestation. After week 24, abortions are only performed when necessary for the preservation of maternal life. In 2000, 87% of counties in the United States had **no access** to an abortion provider.

All Rh-negative women should receive RhoGAM at the time of termination. **Gestational age** should be confirmed by last menstrual period, bimanual examination, and ultrasound evaluation. Two to 4 weeks after completion of termination of pregnancy, routine follow-up should include an assessment of the **emotional and physical status** of the patient. Clinical, laboratory, or imaging studies should be used as needed to confirm completion of the abortion and any complications should be treated. Women should be counseled on reliable forms of **contraception**. This may also be an opportune time to obtain a **cervical cytology** if the Pap smear is not up-to-date.

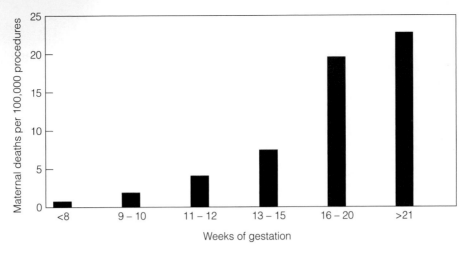

Figure 25-1 • The effect of gestational age on maternal mortality for legal abortions.

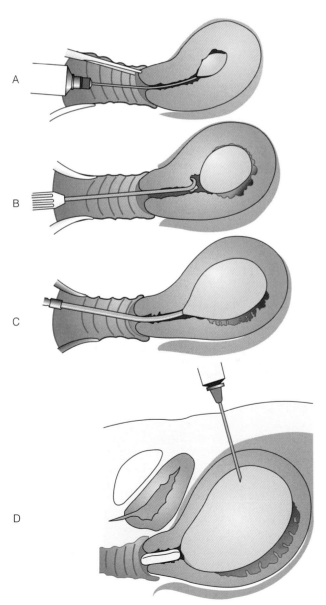

A

B

C

D

Figure 25-2 • Various techniques used for termination of pregnancy. **(A)** Manual extraction. **(B)** Suction curettage (D&C). **(C)** Dilation and evacuation (D&E). **(D)** Induction of labor by intra-amniotic instillation.
(From Pillitteri A. *Maternal and Child Nursing*, 4th ed. Philadelphia: Lippincott Williams & Wilkins; 2003.)

■ **TABLE 25-1** Termination of Pregnancy Options, by Gestational Age
First trimester terminations
Evacuation of the uterus
Suction curettage (D&C)
Manual vacuum aspiration
Medical abortion*
Mifepristone plus misoprostol
Methotrexate plus misoprostol
Second trimester terminations
Surgical evacuation of the uterus (D&E)
Medical induction of labor
High-dose oxytocin
Intra-amniotic installation agents
Prostaglandins
*Only used up to 49 days after LMP.

FIRST TRIMESTER OPTIONS

Ninety percent of all abortions are performed **before 12 weeks' gestation**. Suction curettage (D&C), manual vacuum extraction, and medical abortions are all methods of inducing abortion in the first trimester.

Ninety percent of all abortions in the United States are achieved using suction curettage (D&C). However, this number may change since FDA approval (September 2000) of the use of mifepristone (RU 486) for pregnancy termination in the United States. The maternal mortality for suction curettage is 1 in 100,000 patients. In general, the risk of complications after suction curettage is small and directly proportional to the gestational age.

SUCTION CURETTAGE/MANUAL VACUUM ASPIRATION

Method of Action

Suction curettage is both a safe and effective means of terminating a pregnancy between 7 and 13 weeks of gestation. This procedure is used for 97% of all induced abortions. D&C typically involves **mechanical dilation of the cervix** and removal of the products of conception using a **suction cannula** (Fig. 25-3). A **sharp curettage** may then be performed to ensure the uterus is completely evacuated. This is generally performed using a **paracervical or uterosacral block** with a local anesthetic often in conjunction with **IV conscious sedation**. Less commonly, general anesthesia is used. **Antibiotic prophylaxis** (doxycycline, ofloxacin, or ceftriaxone) on

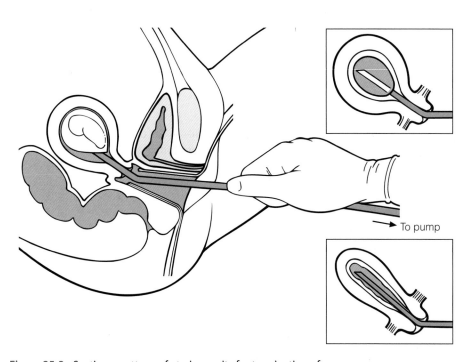

Figure 25-3 • Suction curettage of uterine cavity for termination of pregnancy.

the day of procedure is recommended to avoid the risk of postabortion endometritis. Maternal complications are rare with suction curettage and the **maternal mortality rate is 1 in 100,000.**

For early pregnancies up to 7 weeks' gestation, **manual vacuum aspiration** can be performed. This technique involves insertion of a 3- to 6-mm cannula (Karman) into the undilated cervical os. The uterine contents are then manually extracted using a 50- or 60-mL self-locking vacuum syringe instead of a suction machine. Evacuation is achieved by moving the cannula in and out of the uterus while also rotating the unit along the long axis to ensure clearance of all aspects of the uterine wall. Sharp curettage is not performed in this procedure.

Effectiveness

When performed by a trained physician, the success rate for suction curettage is 98% to 99%. If the gestational age is less than 6 weeks, it is possible to fail to remove the small fetus with the suction curette. In these early pregnancies, an effort should be made to identify villi after the procedure by floating the evacuated tissue in saline. If no villi are identified, or the menses have not returned within 6 weeks or the patient has persistent vaginal bleeding, then serial β-hCG levels should be taken to rule out ectopic pregnancy, gestational trophoblastic disease, or an ongoing pregnancy.

Side Effects

First trimester termination using suction curettage (D&C) is **the safest of all surgical termination methods.** Complications of suction curettage are rare and include infection (1% to 5%), excessive bleeding (2%), uterine perforation (1%), and incomplete abortion (1%). Some data suggest that women who have three or more cervical dilation procedures (for termination, hysteroscopy, D&Cs, etc.) may be at higher risk for cervical insufficiency and uterine scarring (Asherman's syndrome). The maternal mortality rate for suction D&C is **1 in 100,000.**

MEDICAL ABORTION

Mifepristone (RU 486)

Mifepristone was approved for use in termination of pregnancies by the FDA in September 2000. Since

that time, over 460,000 medical terminations have been achieved using mifepristone in the United States.

Mifepristone (RU 486) is a synthetic **progesterone receptor antagonist** that binds to progesterone receptors in the uterus, thus blocking the stimulatory effects of progesterone on endometrial growth. Mifepristone thereby disrupts the pregnancy by making the **endometrial lining unsuitable** to sustain the pregnancy. This leads to detachment of the embryo.

Mifepristone can be used **up to 49 days from the last menstrual period** (LMP). While it can be used alone, the success rate of completed pregnancy is greatly improved when used in combination with a prostaglandin analog. Both the manufacturer and the FDA recommend a single 600-mg dose of mifepristone. However, more recent data support using a lower dose with equal effectiveness. The **typical protocol** used for termination involves a single oral dose (200 to 600 mg) of RU 486 followed by an oral (400 to 800 mcg) or vaginal (800 mcg) dose of **misoprostol** (Cytotec) 36 to 48 hours later. Of note, the FDA has only approved the 400-mcg oral dose of misoprostol for medical termination.

Approximately 2 weeks after the procedure, the success of completion should be confirmed with ultrasound or a **serum β-hCG level.** Rh-negative patients should receive RhoGAM.

Methotrexate

Methotrexate is a chemotherapeutic agent and **dihydrofolate reductase inhibitor** that works by interfering with DNA synthesis, thereby **preventing placental villi proliferation.** Because methotrexate has been approved for use for a variety of medical conditions including ectopic pregnancy, it has been used by clinicians on an **off-label** basis as an abortifacient. Like mifepristone, methotrexate is also **used with a prostaglandin analog.** Methotrexate is administered intramuscularly or orally within 49 days of the LMP, followed by misoprostol (Cytotec) 6 to 7 days later. Two weeks after the procedure, the success of completion should be confirmed with **ultrasound** or a **serum β-hCG level.** Rh-negative patients should receive RhoGAM.

Effectiveness

When used alone, the efficacy rate of mifepristone is approximately 65% to 85%. However, when given with misoprostol, the **success rate is approximately**

92% to 98%. The efficacy rate of methotrexate with misoprostol for induced abortion is **94% to 96%**. The regimen is also therapeutic for ectopic pregnancy in 90% to 95% of cases. The efficacy rates of both mifepristone and methotrexate **decline significantly for pregnancies greater than 7 weeks' gestation**. Failed medical abortions require suction D&C.

Side Effects

The most common side effects of medical abortion are **abdominal pain and cramps**. Other side effects include nausea, vomiting, diarrhea, and **excessive or prolonged uterine bleeding**. Vaginal bleeding averages 10 to 17 days. However, with methotrexate in particular, 15% to 20% of women may have to wait 4 weeks for abortion to occur. The rate of endometritis for medical abortion is lower than after surgical abortion.

Advantages/Disadvantages

Medical abortion offers the advantages of being a **highly effective noninvasive means of termination** that can be achieved on an **outpatient basis**. In a medical abortion a miscarriage is induced and the woman must go through the experience of miscarriage, which generally involves substantial uterine cramping and bleeding. Medical abortion requires at least three total visits to a health provider: two for the treatment and then a 2-week follow-up visit. The contraindications of medical abortion are shown in Table 25-2.

■ **TABLE 25-2** Contraindications of Medical Abortion
Pregnancy greater than 49 days
Pregnancy with an IUD in place
Obstruction of the cervical canal
Ectopic pregnancy
Gestational trophoblastic disease
Bleeding disorder, chronic adrenal failure, or severe asthma
Allergy to mifepristone or misoprostol
Inability to sign the consent agreement because of lack of competence
Minor without parental consent or court order

SECOND TRIMESTER OPTIONS

Second trimester abortions are elective terminations performed between weeks 14 and 24. **Congenital abnormalities are the primary reason for second trimester abortions**. Other indications include severe hyperemesis, previable preterm premature rupture of membranes (PPROM), life-threatening maternal condition, and undesired pregnancy.

Options for second trimester termination of pregnancy include **dilation and evacuation (D&E) and induction of labor** using systemic or intrauterine installation agents (Table 25-1). When a second trimester termination is necessary, **dilation and evacuation is the most common and safest method** of second trimester termination of pregnancy. D&E has a lower maternal mortality and comparable morbidity to second trimester induction of labor.

DILATION AND EXTRACTION/EVACUATION

Method of Action

D&E is the general term to describe cervical dilation and extraction of uterine contents after 14 weeks of gestation. This method of termination is very similar to first trimester suction curettage except that **wider cervical dilation** is required. A combination of **extraction forceps, suction, and sharp curettage** that may be needed to assist in complete evacuation of the uterus, especially after 16 weeks' gestation. This is generally performed using **IV conscious sedation** in combination with a **paracervical block**. Spinal, epidural, and general anesthesias are only rarely used.

Typically, D&E involves the gradual dilation of the cervix to accommodate the larger volume of uterine contents. Cervical preparation can be achieved with careful manual dilation, multiple osmotic dilators, or prostaglandin agents. Osmotic dilators are generally preferred given that manual dilation for second trimester terminations may result in increased cervical laceration and hemorrhage and prostaglandin agents such as misoprostol can take some time to provide sufficient cervical dilatation.

Osmotic dilators can be synthetic (Lamicel, Dilapan) or natural (seaweed-based laminaria). These dilators are placed into the cervix the day before the procedure and gradually dilate and soften the cervix as they absorb the cervical moisture (Fig. 25-4). These

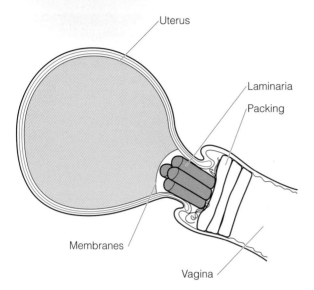

Figure 25-4 • Osmotic dilation of the cervix. Multiple laminaria are placed inside the cervix through both the internal and external os. They slowly expand by absorbing moisture from the vagina, thereby dilating the cervix.

osmotic dilators slowly expand over 12 to 18 hours to dilate the cervix prior to D&E. **Once dilated, a large suction cannula (12 to 14 mm) can be introduced into** the uterus to extract the fetal tissue and placenta. At more advanced gestational ages greater than 16 weeks, **forceps** designed to extract uterine contents (e.g., Sopher forceps) are often needed in addition to suction curettage to remove fetal parts. Upon completion of the procedure, the clinician should verify extraction of the major fetal parts. **Ultrasound** can be used to guide the extraction and to rule out retained products of conception.

Effectiveness

When performed by a highly experienced clinician, the success rate for second trimester extraction procedures is 98% to 99%.

Side Effects

Complications from D&E are uncommon but may include **cervical laceration, hemorrhage, uterine perforation, infection, and retained tissues.** These can be lessened by visual inspection of the fetal parts to ensure complete evacuation of the products of conception. For pregnancies at 16 weeks' gestational age and less, D&E has been found to be safer than induc-

tion of labor. The **maternal mortality rate for D&E is 4 in 100,000.**

Advantages/Disadvantages

As a method of second trimester abortion, D&E offers the advantage of being performed on an **outpatient basis** without the need to undergo induction of labor and delivery. Also, there is no risk of delivering a live-born fetus with extraction procedures. Complications from D&E occur at lower rates than those for intra-amniotic instillation or intravaginal prostaglandin abortions. Some patients may feel the **decreased amount of time** for this procedure is advantageous over an induction of labor; however, other patients may feel that the **delivery of a nonintact fetus** is unacceptable. Perceptions of advantages and disadvantages of these procedures depend greatly on patient preference.

INDUCTION OF LABOR

Method of Action

Termination of a second trimester pregnancy can also be achieved with induction of labor. Although the greater majority of second trimester terminations are achieved with D&E, the percentage of terminations with induction of labor **increases as gestational age increases.**

In the past, installation of intrauterine abortifacient agents such as hypertonic saline, prostaglandin $F_2\alpha$, or hyperosmolar urea was a common method of inducing labor for second trimester terminations. These methods have largely been abandoned for safer methods (D&E or induction of labor).

Termination through induction of labor is typically done using **cervical ripening agents, amniotomy,** and **high-dose IV oxytocin** infusion. Vaginal or oral prostaglandins (prostaglandin E2, misoprostol) can be used to induce labor in second trimester termination. Prostaglandins usually result in higher rates of fever and gastrointestinal side effects. Fetacidal agents (intra-amniotic saline or digoxin, intracardiac potassium chloride) are used in conjunction with prostaglandins to circumvent the possibility of live birth.

Effectiveness

Depending on the regimen used, the success rate for second trimester abortions using induction of labor is **80% to 100%.**

Side Effects

General complications of induction of labor for termination of pregnancy include retained placenta, uterine rupture, hemorrhage, and infection (Table 25-3). Oral and vaginal prostaglandins have a higher incidence of **live births** and significant gastrointestinal side effects (**nausea, vomiting, diarrhea**), whereas instillation agents have a higher rate of **retained placenta** (13% to 46%). The maternal mortality rate for second trimester terminations using oxytocin, vaginal prostaglandins, or instillation agents is **8 in 100,000**, similar to that of term delivery (7 in 100,000).

TABLE 25-3 Complications Associated with Second Trimester Abortion by Induction of Labor

Complications	Side Effects
Retained placenta	Nausea
Incomplete abortion	Vomiting
Hemorrhage	Diarrhea
Infection	Fever
Cervical laceration	Chills

Advantages/Disadvantages

Induction of labor is a **longer process** than a D&E. It requires an **inpatient admission** and can potentially become a **multiday process**. However, induction of labor allows for the potential **delivery of an intact fetus**. This may be emotionally important for some patients and also facilitates more comprehensive **postmortem evaluation** of the fetus, particularly when fetal anomalies are involved and fetopsy is requested.

KEY POINTS

- First trimester abortion options include suction curettage, manual vacuum extraction (Karman), and medical abortion up until week 7.
- Ninety percent of all abortions in the United States are achieved using suction curettage.
- Suction curettage can be performed anytime during the first trimester but is most effective between 7 and 13 weeks' gestation.
- Complications are rare but can include infection, bleeding, and perforation of the uterus.
- Mifepristone (RU 486) is an abortifacient that blocks progesterone stimulation of the endometrial lining, thus causing detachment of the embryo.
- Methotrexate is a chemotherapeutic agent that blocks dihydrofolate inhibitor that interrupts placental proliferation.
- Both mifepristone and methotrexate are used in combination with a prostaglandin and have high efficacy rates (92% to 90%) for medical termination when used within 49 days of the LMP.
- During the second trimester, abortion may be achieved via D&E or induction of labor. D&E has lower maternal mortality and comparable morbidity to induction of labor for second trimester abortions.
- D&E is similar to suction curettage (D&C) but requires wider cervical dilation and the use of special forceps to assist with extraction of fetal parts.
- Complications of D&E include cervical laceration, hemorrhage, infection, uterine perforation, and retained tissue.
- Induction of labor techniques most commonly include cervical ripening and amniotomy followed by induction of labor with high-dose oxytocin.
- Oral and vaginal prostaglandins can be used to induce terminations in the second trimester but they have a higher rate of live birth and gastrointestinal side effects.
- Complications from induction of labor include retained placenta, hemorrhage, infection, and cervical laceration.
- Maternal morbidity is 4 in 100,000 for D&E and 8 in 100,000 for induction of labor compared to 7.7 in 100,000 for continued pregnancy and delivery.

Infertility and Assisted Reproductive Technologies

INTRODUCTION

Infertility is a complex medical disorder that requires the **evaluation and treatment of a couple** rather than an individual. *Infertility* is defined as failure of a couple to conceive after 12 months of unprotected sexual intercourse. If the female partner is 35 years of age or older, evaluation should be initiated after 6 months of unprotected intercourse. In the United States, 1.2 million women (2% of reproductive-age women) had sought medical care to help them become pregnant in 2002 and 10% of women had received infertility services during their lifetime.

Fecundability, or the ability to achieve pregnancy in one menstrual cycle, is a more accurate measurement to evaluate fertility potential. The **fecundity rate** in a normal couple who had unprotected intercourse is approximately **20% to 25% for the first 3 months**, and then 15% during the next 9 months. This means that 80% to 90% of couples are able to spontaneously conceive within 12 months (Table 26-1) and that the fecundability of the cohort decreases over time. For the remaining 10% to 20% of couples who are incapable of conceiving on their own within that time frame, the factors contributing to infertility vary widely.

Of those couples who undergo evaluation for infertility, approximately 45% to 55% is attributed to **female factors** and 35% attributed to **male factors** (Fig. 26-1). After evaluation, 10% of couples will have **no identifiable cause** for their infertility. In as many as 10% to 20% of infertility cases, **both male and female factors** are detected (Table 26-2). Once the cause of infertility is identified, therapy is aimed at correcting reversible conditions or overcoming irreversible conditions. The overview of infertility evaluation is shown in Figure 26-2.

Over the past three decades, multiple different therapies have become available to help the infertile couple conceive. Strictly defined, **assisted reproductive technologies** (ART) involve all therapies in which both sperm and the eggs are handled for the purpose of increasing the rate of conception. In 2005, 134,260 assisted reproductive cycles were performed, resulting in 38,910 live births (deliveries of one or more living infants) and 52,041 infants.

FEMALE FACTOR INFERTILITY

The World Health Organization (WHO) task force on Diagnosis and Treatment of Infertility performed a study of 8,500 infertile couples and found that the most common identifiable female factors were **ovulatory disorders** (32%), **fallopian tube abnormalities** including pelvic adhesions (34%), and **endometriosis** (15%). Other factors include uterine and cervical factors, luteal phase defect, and genetic disorders (Table 26-3 and Fig. 26-3).

TABLE 26-1 Average Conception Rates for All Couples	
Percent of Couples	**Length of Time Before Conception (months)**
20	Conceive within 1
60	Conceive within 6
75	Conceive within 9
80	Conceive within 12
90	Conceive within 18

OVULATORY DISORDERS

Disruption in the **hypothalamic-pituitary-gonadal axis** (Fig. 20-1) can result in menstrual disorders and infertility through impairment of folliculogenesis, ovulation, and endometrial maturation (Table 26-4). The WHO has classified ovulatory disorders into four groups: WHO group 1, hypogonadotropic hypogonadal anovulation (hypothalamic amenorrhea);

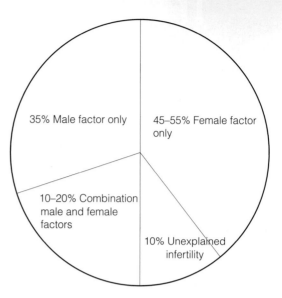

Figure 26-1 • Contribution of male and female factors to infertility.

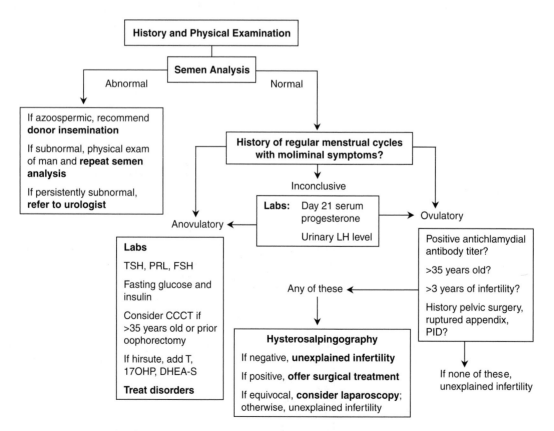

Figure 26-2 • Algorithm for evaluation and treatment of the infertile couple.
(From Curtis M. *Glass' Office Gynecology*, 6th ed. Philadelphia: Lippincott Williams & Wilkins, 2005.)

TABLE 26-2 Contribution of Various Male and Female Factors to the Incidence of Infertility

Etiology	Incidence (%)
Male factor	35
No identifiable cause	25
Idiopathic abnormal sperm	15
Varicocele	10
Miscellaneous factors	
Female factor	45 to 55
Ovulatory factors	32
Peritoneal/tubal factors	34
Endometriosis	15
Uterine and cervical factors	10
Combined male and female factors	10 to 20
Unexplained infertility	10

TABLE 26-3 Causes of Female Factor Infertility

Ovarian
PCOS
Advanced maternal age
Premature ovarian failure
Hypothalamic amenorrhea
Hyperprolactinemia
Tubal factors
PID/salpingitis
Tubal ligation
Endometriosis
Pelvic adhesions
Uterine factors
Congenital malformations
Submucosal fibroids
Uterine polyps
Intrauterine synechiae (Asherman's syndrome)
Cervical factors
Müllerian duct abnormality
Cervical stenosis
Cervicitis or chronic inflammation
DES exposure in utero

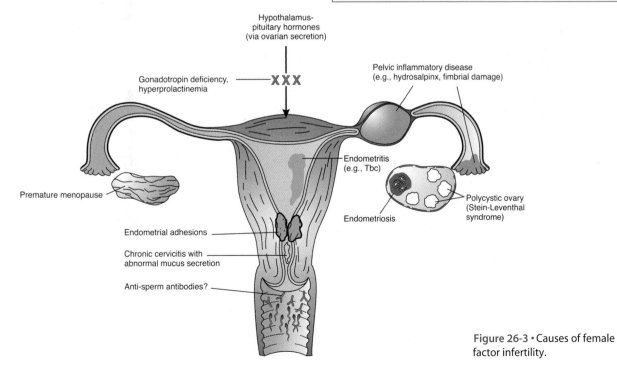

Figure 26-3 • Causes of female factor infertility.

WHO group 2, normogonadotropic normoestrogenic anovulation (polycystic ovarian syndrome [PCOS]); WHO group 3, hypergonadotropic hypoestrogenic anovulation (premature ovarian failure, advanced maternal age); and WHO group 4, hyperprolactinemic anovulation. The most common ovulatory disorders that lead to infertility are **PCOS and advanced maternal age**.

Oocyte aging in an important factor affecting female fertility. During fetal life, the ovary contains the greatest number of germ cells, approximately 6 to 7 million in midgestation. The germ cell population then begins an **exponential decline** through gene-mediated apoptosis, numbering 1 to 2 million at birth and 300,000 at the onset of puberty (Fig. 26-4). The number of viable follicles continues to decline throughout the reproductive years and the rate of loss **accelerates after the mid-30s**. At the time of menopause, the ovary contains fewer than 1,000 follicles. Other factors that result in decreased ovarian reserve and premature ovarian failure include tobacco smoking, radiation and chemotherapy, and autoimmune disease.

The age-related decrease in fecundability is due to both the **decline of quantity and quality of the oocytes**. It is generally accepted that oocyte age is the single most important factor affecting the probability of success with ART. The live birth rates for nulliparous women undergoing ART using fresh nondonor eggs exponentially declines after 35 years of age. However, if donor eggs were utilized, the live birth rate is determined by the age of the donor (Fig. 26-5). The age-related decrease in fertility may be due to the corresponding increase in the rate of aneuploidy.

PCOS is the most common cause of oligo-ovulation and anovulation among all women and among women with infertility. Since it was first described by Stein and Leventhal in 1935, the diagnostic criteria of this syndrome have been avidly debated. In general, most clinicians use the minimal criteria set forth by the NIH. These criteria to diagnose PCOS are menstrual irregularity due to **oligo-ovulation or anovulation**, clinical or biochemical evidence of **hyperandrogenism** (hirsutism, acne, male pattern balding, or elevated serum androgen concentrations), and exclusion of other causes of hyperandrogenism and menstrual irregularity.

The prevalence of reproductive-age women with PCOS based on the NIH 1990 criteria is **6.5% to 8%**. Risk factors include obesity, insulin resistance, diabetes, infertility, premature adrenarche, and a positive family history of PCOS among first-degree relatives.

Currently PCOS is thought to be a complex disorder with a **multifactorial etiology** where multiple genetic variants and environmental factors interact, resulting in the development of this disorder. Suspected genetic variants include genes which are responsible for the regulation of gonadotropin, androgen, or insulin secretion and action (Fig. 26-6). These genetic polymorphisms interplay with diet and obesity. The end result is **hyperinsulinemia** which contributes to **hyperandrogenism** by stimulating androgen biosynthesis in the ovary and decreasing the circulating level of sex hormone binding globulin. Hyperandrogenism then leads to disruption of the HPGA manifest by infrequent or absent menses due to **chronic anovulation**.

TUBAL FACTORS

Tubal disease and pelvic adhesions (Color Plate 12) result in infertility by preventing the transport of the oocyte and sperm through the fallopian tube (Fig. 26-7). The primary cause of tubal factor infertility is **pelvic inflammatory disease**. In countries where infection by gonorrhea and *Chlamydia* is increasing and

---

■ **TABLE 26-4** Causes of Ovulatory Factor Infertility
Central
Pituitary insufficiency (trauma, tumor, congenital)
Hypothalamic insufficiency
Hyperprolactinemia (drug, tumor, empty sella)
Luteal phase defects
Peripheral defects
Gonadal dysgenesis
Premature ovarian failure
Ovarian tumor
Ovarian resistance
Metabolic disease
PCOS (chronic hyperandrogenemic anovulation)
Thyroid disease
Liver disease
Obesity
Androgen excess (adrenal, neoplastic)

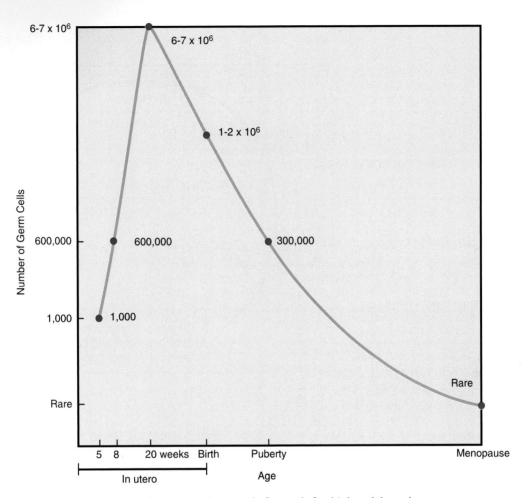

Figure 26-4 • The number of oocytes in the ovary before and after birth and through menopause.
(From Berek JS. *Berek & Novak's Gynecology*, 14th ed. Philadelphia: Lippincott Williams & Wilkins, 2006.)

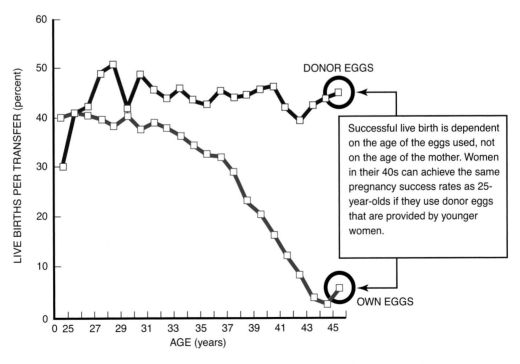

Successful live birth is dependent on the age of the eggs used, not on the age of the mother. Women in their 40s can achieve the same pregnancy success rates as 25-year-olds if they use donor eggs that are provided by younger women.

Figure 26-5 • Live births per embryo transfer comparing use of a patient's own versus donor oocytes.
(From Berek JS. *Berek & Novak's Gynecology*, 14th ed. Philadelphia: Lippincott Williams & Wilkins, 2006.)

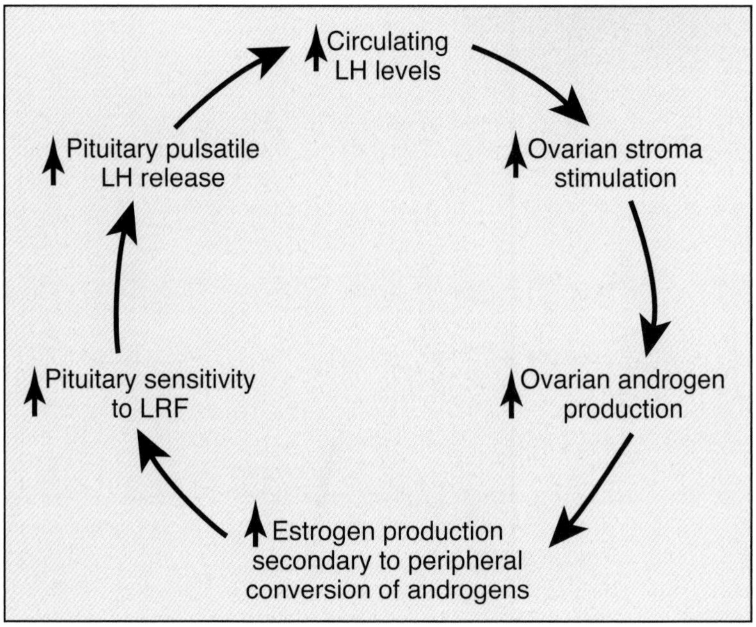

Figure 26-6 • A proposed mechanism for polycystic ovarian syndrome. (LH, luteinizing hormone; LRH, luteinizing releasing hormone). (From Beckmann C, Ling F. *Obstetrics & Gynecology*, 5th ed. Philadelphia: Lippincott Williams & Wilkins, 2006.)

treatment is limited, tubal factor infertility is on the rise. Other conditions which can interfere with normal tubal transport include severe **endometriosis**, history of **ectopic pregnancy**, and pelvic adhesions from **previous surgery** or **nongynecologic infection** such as appendicitis or diverticulitis.

ENDOMETRIOSIS

Although the true prevalence of endometriosis is unknown, it is believed that approximately **15% of infertile women** have endometriosis. Endometriosis is the presence of endometrial cells outside the uterine cavity (Chapter 15). It can invade local tissues and cause severe **inflammation and adhesions** (Color Plate 12).

Although the presence of endometriosis has been associated with an increased risk of infertility, the exact mechanism is not understood. Endometriosis can interfere with tubal mobility, cause tubal obstruction, or result in tubal or ovarian adhesions that contribute to infertility by holding the fallopian tube away from the ovary or by trapping the released oocyte. However, infertility has also been diagnosed in women with minimal endometriosis and minimal to no adhesive disease. It is thought that endometriosis may stimulate the production of **inflammatory mediators** which impair ovulation, fertilization, or implantation.

UTERINE AND CERVICAL FACTORS

Uterine and cervical factors account for less than **10% of female factor infertility** cases (Table 26-2). Varying **uterine conditions** can contribute to infertility including submucosal fibroids, polyps, intrauterine synechiae, and congenital malformations (especially uterine septums) (Table 26-3). Similarly, **endometrial abnormalities** such as hyperplasia, out-of-phase endometrium, and carcinoma can cause infertility. These factors may distort the uterine cavity, prevent implantation, or affect endometrial development.

Risk factors for uterine factor infertility include conditions that predispose to **intrauterine adhesions** such as history of pelvic inflammatory disease, infection after pregnancy loss, and multiple curettages of the uterus. Diethylstilbestrol (DES) exposure in utero also increases uterine factor infertility (Table 26-3 and Fig. 14-3).

Cervical problems can contribute to infertility through structural abnormalities of the cervix, cervicitis, and abnormal cervical mucous production. **Cervical stenosis** may be iatrogenic and may result from scarring after conization, multiple (four or more) mechanical dilations (e.g., cervical dilation for miscarriage, termination of pregnancy, or hysteroscopy), extensive laser, or cauterization of the cervix. These procedures may result in stenosis as well as destruction of the endocervical epithelium, leading to **inadequate mucous production**.

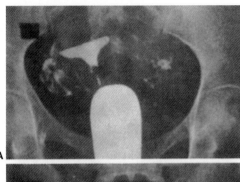
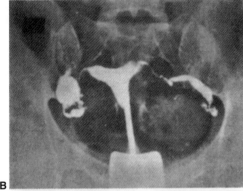
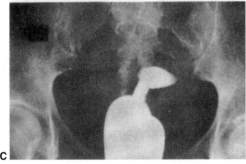

Figure 26-7 • Hysterosalpingograms showing **(A)** normal uterine cavity and patent tubes, **(B)** bilateral hydrosalpinx, and **(C)** bilateral tubal occlusion.
(From Beckmann C, Ling F. *Obstetrics & Gynecology*, 5th ed. Philadelphia: Lippincott Williams & Wilkins, 2006.)

OTHER FACTORS

Luteal phase defect is a controversial and poorly understood disorder. The defect may possibly begin with disruption of the HPGA (Fig. 20-1), resulting in inadequate production of progesterone by the corpus luteum and subsequent delay in endometrial maturation. This results in impaired implantation following fertilization.

In couples in which no other cause of infertility can be determined, infertility may be due to **genetic abnormalities** (trisomies, mosaics, translocations, etc). The most common aneuploidy associated with female infertility is 45X (Turner syndrome).

Clinical Manifestations

History

The evaluation should begin with a thorough **medical history** including a **menstrual history** (Fig. 26-2). The physician should guide the interview systematically while looking for symptoms related to ovarian, tubal, uterine, and cervical factors which can lead to infertility.

Patients with **ovulatory dysfunction** may report amenorrhea, oligomenorrhea, or menorrhagia. Additional questioning should elicit symptoms related to PCOS, thyroid dysfunction, hyperprolactinemia, and ovarian failure. Patients with PCOS may report hirsutism, irregular menses, and/or weight changes. A detailed social history might reveal reasons for centrally mediated ovulatory dysfunction including eating disorders, extreme exercise, or unusual stress.

Women with **endometriosis** often give a history of cyclic pelvic pain, dysmenorrhea, and/or dyspareunia. Pelvic adhesions may be asymptomatic or may be associated with varying degrees of pelvic pain, especially with movement or lifting.

The clinical presentation of **uterine factor** infertility varies with the etiology. For many of these factors, infertility may be the only symptom. Among the most common causes, endometritis may present with pelvic pain and fever; submucosal fibroids and polyps may present with menorrhagia. Uterine anomalies such as uterine septum may present with a history of recurrent pregnancy loss. **Cervical factor** infertility may present with a history of prior cryotherapy, conization, cervical dilations, or in utero DES exposure.

Physical Examination

A physical examination should be performed to look for signs which may point toward a disorder associated with infertility. Careful evaluation may uncover **signs of PCOS** such as acne, hirsutism, acanthosis nigricans (Color Plate 13), achrochordons, and central obesity (BMI >27). Similar care should be taken in evaluating for **thyroid dysfunction** (goiter, changes in hair/nails, tachycardia). The exam should also look for breast development as a sign of past estrogen secretion.

When performing a **pelvic exam**, premature ovarian failure might present with signs of estrogen deficiency such as vaginal atrophy. Visualization of the cervix may demonstrate **cervical stenosis**, signs of infection, or malformations. The findings associated with **endometriosis** or pelvic adhesions include a fixed or retroverted uterus, uterosacral nodularity, or tender fixed adnexa. With **pelvic adhesions**, the pain can sometimes be reproduced on abdominal or pelvic exam. Uterine size should be evaluated and the physician should look for **leiomyoma** and any signs of current or prior pelvic infection. Endometriomas and other **ovarian pathology** may be palpated during the pelvic exam.

Diagnostic Evaluation

The primary tests for the evaluation of ovulatory factor infertility involve looking for **evidence of ovulation** by tracking the menstrual cycle, measuring the basal body temperature (Fig. 24-1), monitoring the cervical mucus, and measuring the **mid-luteal progesterone** (days 21 to 23). Over-the-counter ovulation prediction kits have made predicting the presence and timing of ovulation much easier.

A **clomiphene citrate challenge test** (CCCT) can be used to assess for decreased ovarian reserve-the oocyte-related decline in fertility. The test involves administration of 100 mg of clomiphene citrate (Clomid) on days 5 through day 9 of the menstrual cycle. An FSH level is measured on days 3 and 10. Even small elevations in FSH levels correlate with decreased fecundity. This is especially useful in women over 30 years of age, those with prior ovarian surgery or only one ovary, those with a history of prior chemotherapy or radiation exposure, and in women who have had a poor response to ovulation induction.

A **progestin challenge test** may be used to demonstrate the endometrium's ability to respond with bleeding after progesterone is withdrawn from the system. This involves administration of a progestin over 5 to 10 days to build up the endometrium. When the progestin is stopped, the patient should experience a withdrawal bleed within 1 week. If this fails to produce bleeding, a **combined estrogen and progesterone challenge** can be performed.

Endocrine evaluation may include measurement of FSH, LH, prolactin, thyroid function tests (TFTs), and thyroid antibodies. If Cushing syndrome is suspected, serum testosterone, dehydroepiandrosterone sulfate (DHEAS), 17-hydroxyprogesterone, 24-hour urine cortisol levels, and an overnight dexamethasone suppression test are helpful. When intracranial lesions are suspected, **MRI or CT imaging** of the head should be done.

Endometriosis or pelvic adhesions may be strongly suspected based on the patient's history, but direct visualization with **laparoscopy or laparotomy** is necessary to confirm the diagnosis. Ovarian

endometriomas (cystic collections of endometrial cells on the ovaries) can be diagnosed on **pelvic ultrasound** (Fig. 15-2).

Tubal patency can be demonstrated with a **hysterosalpingogram** (HSG) performed during the follicular phase or tubal lavage (chromopertubation) performed during laparoscopy. HSG is one of the primary investigative tools for evaluation of **anatomic abnormalities** of the female reproductive tract. This involves installation of a contrast dye transcervically to evaluate for filling defects in the cavity and to test for **tubal patency** (Fig. 26-7).

The **pelvic ultrasound** is also useful in evaluating the uterus for structural defects such as fibroids, polyps, adenomyosis, hyperplasia, and cancer. A **saline sonohysterogram** can complement the pelvic ultrasound by allowing better visualization of the uterine cavity. This is accomplished by transcervical infusion of saline into the cavity while ultrasound examination of the uterus is performed.

Hysteroscopy may be used to directly visualize the cavity of the uterus. **MRI** can also be useful in better delineation of adenomyosis and uterine anomalies.

A **Pap smear** and **cervical cultures** for gonorrhea and *Chlamydia* should be performed in all women undergoing an infertility evaluation. Cervical mucous studies and a postcoital test may be used to evaluate the quality of the cervical mucous. This assesses both sperm quality and sperm–mucous interaction 2 to 8 hours after coitus. The **postcoital test** is generally not performed because pregnancy rates were not affected by testing in couples undergoing infertility evaluation and therapy.

Treatment

The **underlying etiology** of infertility should be **identified and corrected**. For uncorrectable cases, ovulation induction with fertility drugs, **intrauterine insemination** (IUI) with sperm, or **in vitro fertilization** (IVF) with placement of the embryo into the uterus can be used.

Regular ovulation can be restored in 90% of infertility cases that are due to endocrine factors by treating the underlying disorder. The most common etiology of ovulatory infertility is **PCOS**. For these patients, weight loss, metformin, and ovulation induction with Clomid or letrozole (Femara) have been effective in establishing ovulation and producing viable pregnancies. In PCOS patients, even small amounts of weight loss can result in lowered fasting insulin levels, testosterone, and androstenedione.

Metformin (Glucophage) is an oral biguanide typically used for the treatment of non-insulin-dependent diabetes mellitus. This insulin sensitizer results in inhibition of gluconeogenesis and **increased peripheral glucose uptake**. PCOS patients using metformin experience a decrease in fasting insulin levels and testosterone levels. These improvements can help promote the reestablishment of **spontaneous ovulation** in PCOS patients.

If spontaneous ovulation cannot be established, ovulation inducing medications can be utilized to stimulate ovulation (Table 26-5). Of these the most frequently used are **Clomid and letrozole** (Femara). If theses treatments are unsuccessful, ovulation induction and pregnancy can be attempted with a combination of Clomid, letrozole, or human gonadotropins with IUI or IVF.

For patients with **hypothalamic-pituitary failure (WHO Group 1)**, ovulation can usually be achieved with pulsatile GnRH therapy or human gonadotropins (Table 26-5). Of note, there is **no treatment** for WHO Group 3 patients with **ovarian failure** because these patients lack viable oocytes. Patients with this diagnosis should be offered the options of egg donation, gestational surrogacy, or adoption.

Symptomatic relief of **endometriosis** can be achieved medically or surgically. However, **there is no role for medical management in the treatment of infertility caused by endometriosis**. Medical treatments such as Danazol, Lupron, oral medroxyprogesterone (Provera), or continuous oral contraceptives can temporarily relieve symptoms but do not increase fertility rates.

For patients with endometriosis fertility rates can be improved by surgical ligation of periadnexal adhesions during laparoscopy or laparotomy with excision, coagulation, vaporization, or **fulguration of endometrial implants**. Pregnancy rates after surgical treatment depend on the extent of the disease, with increased conception rates for severe endometriosis. Conflicting data exists regarding conception rates following surgical therapy for mild endometriosis. However, the consensus is that surgical adhesion lysis and ablation of endometrial implants does increase fertility.

Microsurgical **tuboplasty with tubal reanastomosis** or neosalpingostomy has proven to be effective for treating tubal occlusion due to prior infection or from prior tubal ligation. However, because it is more effective, most couples undergo **IVF rather than attempt tuboplasty**. The advantage of tuboplasty is that it allows for more than one future pregnancy without the cost and difficulty of multiple IVF cycles. When tubal occlusion, tubal damage, or hydrosalpinx results from prior salpingitis, reproductive endocrinologists will often remove the damaged tube and opt for **IVF** to treat the resulting infertility.

Operative hysteroscopy is used to treat **uterine factors** such as uterine synechiae, septae, polyps, or

■ **TABLE 26-5** Medications Used in the Treatment of Infertility and in Assisted Reproductive Technologies

Commercial Name	Generic Name	Mechanism
Clomid Serophene	Clomiphene citrate	Antiestrogen, stimulates follicular development for ovulation induction
Glucophage	Metformin	Insulin sensitizer, decreases insulin, testosterone, BMI; promotes ovulation
Repronex Menopur Pergonal Humegon	Human menopausal gonadotropins (menotropins)	Purified FSH/LH, stimulates follicular development during ovulation induction
Follistim Puregon Gonal-F Fertinex	Follistatins (recombinant FSH)	Gonadotropins containing FSH that stimulates follicular development during ovulation induction
Novarel Pregnyl Profasi	Human chorionic gonadotropin	Similar structure to LH, triggers ovulation after gonadotropin follicle stimulation
Lutrepulse Factrel	Pulsatile GnRH/ gonadorelin	GnRH agonist, stimulates release of FSH/LH from pituitary
Femara	Letrozole	Aromatase inhibitor, reduces androgen conversion to estrogen, stimulates follicular development for ovulatory induction

Intrauterine

Cervical-vaginal

Cervical cap

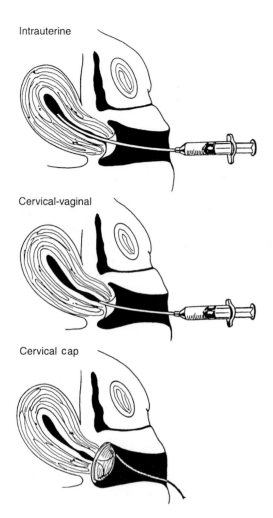

Figure 26-8 • Techniques of artificial insemination.
(From Beckmann C, Ling F. *Obstetrics & Gynecology*, 5th ed. Philadelphia: Lippincott Williams & Wilkins, 2006.)

submucosal fibroids. Following surgical ligation of synechiae or septae, estrogen therapy or intrauterine devices are often used to **prevent recurrence** of adhesions. Fertility is restored in 50% of these cases. Most surgeons reserve myomectomy for treatment after recurrent pregnancy loss or when symptomatic fibroids have been identified.

Treatment of cervical factor infertility varies with the cause. Cervical stenosis can often be treated with **surgical or mechanical dilation** of the endocervical canal. Both cervical stenosis and abnormal cervical mucus can be treated by **bypassing the cervix with IUI** (Fig. 26-8). IUI appears to be the most effective treatment for cervical factor infertility. In cases that are refractory to other treatments, patients should be offered IVF.

MALE FACTOR INFERTILITY

PATHOGENESIS

There are multiple causes of male factor infertility (Table 26-6) including endocrine disorders, anatomic defects, problems with abnormal sperm production and motility, as well as sexual dysfunction.

EPIDEMIOLOGY

Thirty five percent of infertility is due to **purely male factors** (Fig. 26-1). Of couples undergoing infertility

■ TABLE 26-6 Common Etiologies of Male Factor Infertility
Abnormal semen
Cryptorchidism (congenital)
Mumps orchitis
Antisperm antibodies
Endocrine disorders
Hypogonadotropic hypogonadism
Thyroid disease
Environmental exposures
Radiation
Heat
Chemicals
Genetic
Klinefelter's syndrome
Immobile cilia syndrome
Cystic fibrosis
Sexual dysfunction
Erectile dysfunction
Ejaculation failure
Retrograde ejaculation
Structural factors
Varicocele
Testicular torsion
Vasectomy
Unexplained
No identifiable cause
Idiopathic abnormal semen

evaluation, 10% to 20% are affected by a combination of male and female factors.

RISK FACTORS

Men with **occupational or environmental exposure** to chemicals, radiation, or excessive heat are at increased risk for infertility, as are those with a history of varicocele, mumps, hernia repair, pituitary tumor, anabolic steroid use, testicular injury, and impotence. **Certain medications** have also been found to depress semen quantity and quality, cause erectile dysfunction, or result in ejaculation failure (Table 26-7).

CLINICAL MANIFESTATIONS

History

The physician should ask about previous pregnancies fathered by the patient, environmental exposures, medications, and any history of sexually transmitted infections (STIs), mumps orchitis, hernia repair, and surgery or trauma to the genitals.

Physical Examination

The physical examination should include a search for signs of testosterone deficiency and varicocele, identification of the urethral meatus, and measurement of testicular size.

DIAGNOSTIC EVALUATION

A **semen analysis** is the primary investigative tool for male factor infertility. Sperm count, volume, motility, morphology, pH, and white blood cell count are analyzed (Table 26-8). In the case of an abnormal semen analysis, an endocrine evaluation should include thyroid function tests, serum testosterone, prolactin, and follicle-stimulating hormone (FSH) (may identify parenchymal damage to testes).

The **postcoital test** is rarely performed but can be used to examine the interaction between sperm and the cervical mucus. An abnormal postcoital test, sperm agglutination, and reduced sperm motility are suspicious for the presence of **antisperm antibodies**. Several tests are presently available to detect such antibodies.

TREATMENT

In general, the probability of conception can be enhanced by **improvements in coital practice**. This includes having intercourse every other day near ovulation. Men should avoid the use of tight underwear, saunas and hot tubs, and unnecessary environmental exposures such as radiation, excess heat, and certain medications (Table 26-7).

Treatment of male factor infertility **depends upon the etiology**. Hypothalamic-pituitary failure can be treated with injections of human menopausal gonadotropins (hMGs) and varicoceles can be repaired by ligation.

Assisted reproductive techniques can be used to overcome an abnormal semen analysis when treating the underlying disorder is not effective. Low semen volume, low sperm density, and low sperm motility are most often treated by **washed sperm for IUI** (Fig. 26-8).

■ **TABLE 26-7** Drugs That Decrease Semen Quality and Quantity

Medications		**Exogenous Exposures**
Cimetidine	Metoclopramide	Anabolic steroids
Sulfasalazine	Chemotherapeutic agents	Marijuana
Spironolactone	Beta blockers	Alcohol abuse
Antidepressants	Nitrofurans	Heroin/cocaine abuse

■ **TABLE 26-8** Semen Analysis Normal Parameters

Volume	>2.0 mL
pH	7.2 to 7.8
Concentration	>20 million/mL
Morphology	>30% normal forms
Motility	>50% with forward progression
WBC	<1 million/mL

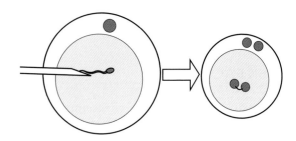

Figure 26-9 • Intracytoplasmic sperm injection (ICSI). A spermatid or spermatozoon is collected by ejaculation or aspiration from the epididymus or testis. One sperm is injected directly into each harvested egg. The embryos are then transferred back into the uterine cavity (IVF) or fallobian tube (GIFT).

Intracytoplasmic sperm injection (ICSI) is another option for patients with low sperm density or impaired motility and has revolutionized the treatment of male factor infertility (Fig. 26-9). This method involves retrieving sperm from the male, preparing it, individually injecting a single sperm directly into an egg, and then placing the fertilized egg into the uterus cavity (IVF). The sperm can be retrieved from the male by ejaculation, or by direct aspiration from the testis (testicular sperm extraction [TSE]) or epididymis (microsurgical epididymal sperm aspiration [MESA]).

In refractory cases of male factor infertility, artificial insemination with **donor sperm is highly effective.**

UNEXPLAINED INFERTILITY

For those couples who complete an initial assessment, **10% find no cause for their infertility** (Fig. 26-1). When the initial infertility evaluation reveals no cause for infertility, the problem often involves abnormalities in sperm transport, the presence of antisperm antibodies, or problems with penetration and fertilization of the egg. When problems in sperm transport, motility, or functional capacity are identified, **IVF and ICSI** may be used for treatment. If this fails, the use of **donor sperm** may result in pregnancy.

When no cause for infertility is identified after in-depth testing, studies show that most therapies have **no higher success rates than no treatment at all.** Although some patients with unexplained infertility may undergo three to six cycles of gonadotropin stimulation with IUI before trying IVF, many opt for no treatment. The eventual pregnancy rate for couples with unexplained infertility who receive no treatment approaches **60% over 3 to 5 years**. Other options include use of donor sperm, surrogacy, adoption, or acceptance of childlessness.

ASSISTED REPRODUCTIVE TECHNOLOGIES

Since their inception, the treatment of infertility with assisted reproductive technologies has progressed rapidly and now includes not only fertility drugs that stimulate multiple follicular development but also technologies that combine **ovulation induction** agents with **IUI, IVF, or ICSI.** Oocytes may also be obtained via natural, nonstimulated cycles but the number of eggs per cycle is increased by ovulation induction.

OVULATION INDUCTION

Clomiphene citrate (Clomid) is an **antiestrogen** that **competitively binds to estrogen receptors** in the hypothalamus. This results in increased pulsatile GnRH. Subsequently, **FSH and LH production is increased** leading to follicular growth and ovulation (Table 26-5). Clomid is generally administered orally starting on day 3 or 5 of the follicular phase of the menstrual cycle for approximately 5 days.

Letrozole is an **aromatase inhibitor** that **decreases the conversion of androgens into estrogens** (Table 26-5). Lower estrogen levels reduce the negative feedback effect on the hypothalamus and pituitary which leads to an increase of FSH and follicular development.

Absent or infrequent ovulation is the major indication for Clomid and letrozole use in women with PCOS or mild hypothalamic amenorrhea. Specific causes of anovulation should be ruled out first and patients should have normal TSH, FSH, and prolactin levels. Although Clomid is used as a first-line therapy in couples with unexplained infertility, it has no use in patients with premature ovarian failure.

The other major category of ovulation induction agents is **human menopausal gonadotropins** (hMGs).

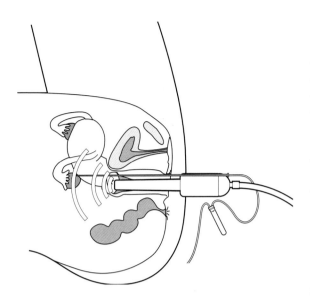

Figure 26-10 • Transvaginal ultrasound-guided needle aspiration of oocytes. Following ovulation induction, multiple eggs are removed from the ovaries by placing a vaginal probe into the vagina. A fine needle is guided toward the ovary while the physician visualizes the follicles on ultrasound. Fluid around the follicles is then collected through a needle connected to a test tube.

These are best used when the pituitary gland fails to secrete sufficient FSH and LH to stimulate follicular maturation and ovulation, and when Clomid is also incapable of stimulating ovulation. Patients with mild to severe hypothalamic dysfunction fall into this category and often require hMGs for ovulation induction.

The hMGs (Table 26-5) often come in combined preparations of FSH and LH or of FSH alone. They are administered via intramuscular injection during the follicular phase of the menstrual cycle. The patient's response to ovulation induction should be **monitored closely** through **serial estrogen levels and pelvic ultrasounds** to measure the number of follicles, size of follicles, and total estrogen production level.

Each means of **ovulation induction** can potentially produce multiple follicular development. Once ovulation occurs, **fertilization** may be attempted by intercourse or IUI. Conversely, after ovulation induction, the **oocyte retrieval** may be accomplished with **transvaginal aspiration** (Fig. 26-10). The oocytes are then fertilized via **ICSI** (Fig. 26-9) or **in vitro fertilization** is allowed to occur (Fig. 26-11). Selected **embryos are then transferred** into the uterus under ultrasound guidance. Progesterone is often used to promote **endometrial receptivity** beginning after embryo transfer and lasting through the first trimester. Any remaining embryos are saved using **cryopreservation** techniques for future cycles, embryo donation, or research.

Effectiveness

Clomiphene citrate is successful in **inducing ovulation in 80% of correctly selected patients** and **36% will become pregnant**. If pregnancy does not occur after 3 to 6 cycles of Clomid, more aggressive therapies are needed. Gonadotropins have an **80% to 90% ovulation success rate** and a **10% to 40% pregnancy success rate** per cycle depending on the diagnosis (recall fecundity is only 20% to 25% in the

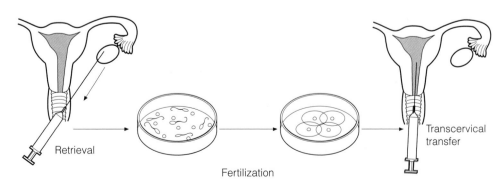

Figure 26-11 • In vitro fertilization (IVF). **(A)** After ovulation induction, oocytes are harvested transvaginally. **(B)** The egg and sperm are placed together in the laboratory and fertilization takes place. **(C)** The fertilized embryos are transferred into the uterine cavity through the cervix.

general population). Gonadotropins carry a much higher risk of **ovarian hyperstimulation** (1% to 3%) and **multiple gestation pregnancy** (20%).

Side Effects and Complications

The potential side effects of Clomid are related to its **antiestrogen effects**: hot flashes, abdominal distension and bloating, emotional lability, depression, and visual changes. These side effects are mostly mild and disappear after discontinuation of the medication.

Multiple gestation pregnancy is a major side effect of OI and assisted reproductive technologies. Multiple gestation pregnancies occur in 8% of Clomid-induced pregnancies and 20% of pregnancies from gonadotropins.

The other major complication of OI with gonadotropins is ovarian **hyperstimulation syndrome** (OHSS). This is a potentially life-threatening condition caused by overstimulation of the ovaries occurring in 1% to 3% of patients undergoing ovulation induction. This completely iatrogenic disorder can range from ovarian enlargement and minimal symptoms to significant ovarian enlargement, torsion, or rupture. This may be complicated by ascites, pleural effusions, hemoconcentration, hypercoagulability, electrolyte disturbances, renal failure, and even death.

ADVANCED REPRODUCTIVE TECHNOLOGIES (IVF, ICSI, PGD)

Method of Action

Assisted reproductive technologies have advanced the treatment of infertility by allowing physicians to successfully **bypass the normal mechanisms of gamete transportation and fertilization**. In conjunction with OI, multiple oocytes may be harvested from the ovary using ultrasound (Fig. 26-10).

During IVF, the oocytes are allowed to mature briefly in vitro before washed sperm are added. **Fertilization** is verified 14 to 18 hours later by the presence of two pronuclei. In the case of IVF, the conceptuses are then **placed into the uterus** through the cervix using a catheter (Fig. 26-11), making IVF a relatively noninvasive procedure.

ICSI has revolutionized the treatment of male factor infertility by allowing a single spermatid or **spermatozoon to be directly injected into the cytoplasm of a harvested oocyte** (Fig. 26-9). The result-

ing embryos can then be placed back into the uterus for implantation.

Preimplantation genetic diagnosis (PGD) refers to the evaluation of the embryo for genetic abnormalities prior to transfer during an IVF cycle. PGD involves removing 1 or 2 cells from a 6- to 8-cell embryo and then screening for common **chromosomal abnormalities** or **genetic mutations** such as sickle cell anemia, Tay-Sachs disease, cystic fibrosis, Down syndrome, hemophilia A, and fragile X syndrome. This technique is usually performed when a patient has a known inherited genetic disease, is a carrier of a chromosomal translocation that has resulted in recurrent miscarriages, has an affected child, or is of advanced maternal age (increased risk of aneuploidy). PGD is used in approximately 5% of ART cycles nationwide.

Effectiveness

The success rate of these advanced reproductive technologies varies from center to center. On average, with IVF, **delivery** is achieved in **28% of retrievals using fresh nondonor embryos and 54% using fresh donor embryos**. Success rates vary by maternal age; diagnosis; and the number and quality of eggs, sperm, and embryos. The most favorable rates are seen in **women under 35**, those **without hydrosalpinges**, those with **adequate ovarian reserve**, and in couples where there is **no male infertility** factor. Keep in mind that the normal fecundity rate in a couple with normal fertility is approximately 20% to 25% per month.

Again, **multiple gestation pregnancies** are a major complication of ART. The Society for Assisted Reproductive Technologies reports that in 2005 the rate of multiple gestations at delivery was **32% for IVF** (29.6% twins, 2.4% triplets and higher-order multiples). The rate of multiple gestations is important because these pregnancies carry much higher rates of **maternal complications** (preeclampsia, gestational diabetes, placenta previa, premature delivery, postpartum hemorrhage) and **fetal complications** (IUGR, respiratory distress syndrome, intraventricular hemorrhage, neonatal sepsis, low birth weight, stillbirth).

The rate of multiple gestation pregnancies in ART can be reduced by **close ultrasound surveillance** and **estradiol monitoring** during ovulation induction and by **limiting the number of embryos**, oocytes, or zygotes transferred during ART.

KEY POINTS

- Female factor infertility is purely responsible for 45% to 55% of all infertility cases. These can be divided into ovulatory, tubal, uterine, and cervical factors.

- Female factor infertility may be due to ovulatory factors that interrupt the hypothalamic-pituitary-ovarian axis such as polycystic ovarian syndrome, premature ovarian failure, hyperprolactinemia, and thyroid diseases. The most common causes of ovulatory factor infertility are PCOS and advanced maternal age.

- Ovulatory factors are diagnosed by confirming ovulation through menstrual history, basal body temperature measurements, mucous analysis, ovulation detection kits, midluteal progesterone level, followed by endocrine evaluation (TSH, prolactin, FSH, LH, CCCT).

- Ovulatory factors are best addressed by treating the cause of the ovulatory dysfunction. PCOS-related infertility can be treated with weight loss, metformin, and ovulation induction with Clomid or letrozole. When refractory to treatment, ovulation induction with human gonadotropins can be used along with along with IUI or IVF.

- The most common causes of tubal factor infertility are endometriosis and pelvic adhesions. These factors are diagnosed by history and laparoscopy or laparotomy and treated surgically to improve fertility rates. Tubal occlusion may be repaired with microsurgical tuboplasty, but most couples opt for IVF.

- Female infertility may be due to uterine factors such at uterine synechiae, polyps, submucosal fibroids, congenital malformations, or endometritis. Uterine factors are diagnosed by pelvic ultrasound, hysterosalpingogram, saline sonohysterogram, hysteroscopy, and laparoscopy. Uterine factors are treated according to the cause of the infertility. Synechiae, fibroids, and polyps can be resected; endometritis is treated with antibiotics.

- Female infertility may also be due to cervical factors such as cervical stenosis from surgical or mechanical dilation. These factors are diagnosed by exam and treated with surgical or mechanical dilation of the endocervical canal or IUI to bypass the cervix.

- Male factor infertility is purely responsible for 35% of all infertility cases.

- It may be idiopathic or due to improper coital practices; sexual dysfunction; endocrine disorders; or abnormalities in spermatogenesis, sperm volume, density, or mobility.

- Male factor infertility is diagnosed by semen analysis and endocrine evaluation if indicated. The treatment of male factor infertility depends on the causal agent and includes improved coital practices, repair of anatomic defects, ICSI, and use of donor sperm.

- Ten percent of couples find no explanation for infertility after their initial assessment. When this occurs, further assessment may be done to search for problems with sperm transport, ability to penetrate and fertilize the egg, and antisperm antibodies. IVF/ICSI can be used to treat these patients.

- Most therapies for unexplained infertility have not been shown to have higher success rates than no treatment. Couples with unexplained infertility who choose no treatment will conceive up to 60% of the time over 3 to 5 years.

- Clomiphene citrate is an antiestrogen that binds to estrogen receptors in the hypothalamus to cause increased FSH and LH production, thereby promoting follicular maturation and ovulation.

- Clomiphene citrate is best used for ovulation induction in women with chronic anovulation or mild hypothalamic insufficiency after specific causes of hypothalamic dysfunction have been ruled out.

- Human menopausal gonadotropins are forms of FSH or FSH and LH that directly stimulate follicular maturation in patients for whom Clomid has failed, or those with hypothalamic or pituitary failure or unexplained infertility.

- The primary complications of fertility drugs include ovarian hyperstimulation and multiple gestation pregnancy.

- IVF and ICSI may be used to bypass the normal mechanisms of gamete transport and fertilization with deliveries in about 30% of cases.

Neoplastic Disease of the Vulva and Vagina

Benign lesions of the vulva and vagina are discussed in Chapter 13. This chapter discusses preinvasive neoplasia of the vulva and vagina and invasive cancers of the vulva and vagina (Table 27-1). It is important to distinguish between benign disease and neoplastic disease so that appropriate treatment and follow-up can be offered to patients.

PREINVASIVE NEOPLASTIC DISEASE OF THE VULVA

Preinvasive neoplastic disease of the vulva is divided into two categories: squamous (**vulvar intraepithelial neoplasia**) and nonsquamous intraepithelial neoplasias (**Paget disease, melanoma in situ**). Histologically, vulvar intraepithelial neoplasia, Paget disease, and melanoma of the vulva can all be quite similar. Therefore, immunohistochemical staining is often used to assist in the diagnosis of vulvar lesions.

VULVAR INTRAEPITHELIAL NEOPLASIA (VIN)

Pathogenesis

Just as the incidence of cervical dysplasia has been rising in younger women, so has the incidence of vulvar intraepithelial neoplasia (VIN). VIN is defined as **cellular atypia contained within the epithelium**. It is characterized by a loss of epithelial cell maturation, cellular crowding, nuclear hyperchromatosis, and abnormal mitosis. Lesions are designated as VIN I (mild dysplasia), II (moderate dysplasia), or III (severe dysplasia), based upon the depth of epithelial involve-

ment. Twenty percent of patients with VIN will have a coexistent invasive carcinoma, which has penetrated the basement membrane.

The concomitant rise in VIN and cervical intraepithelial neoplasia (CIN) is not surprising because both cervical and vulvar neoplastic disease are correlated with **human papillomavirus (HPV) infection**; 80% to 90% of VIN lesions will have DNA fragments from HPV and 60% of women with VIN have cervical neoplasia as well.

Other risk factors for VIN include **cigarette smoking** and an **immunocompromised state**. This disease has **two distinct forms** which differ by the age of the patient. Younger, premenopausal women are more likely to have more aggressive multifocal lesions (Fig. 27-1) that rapidly become invasive and are associated with HPV. Older, postmenopausal women have another form which is more likely to involve unifocal lesions that are slow to become invasive and are not typically associated with HPV.

Epidemiology

In the past, VIN was thought of as a disorder primarily affecting postmenopausal women. However, in the past few decades, the incidence of VIN has nearly doubled. Today, the majority of cases occur in **premenopausal women (75%)** and the median age is 40. Interestingly, despite the increased incidence in VIN, the incidence of vulvar cancer has stayed relatively stable over the same period of time. Risk factors for VIN include infection with **HPV types 16 and 18**, **cigarette smoking**, immunodeficiency, and immunosuppression. The incidence of HPV-associated VIN decreases as age increases. There is no racial predisposition to VIN.

■ **TABLE 27-1** Classification of Neoplastic Diseases of the Vulva and Vagina		
	Vulvar Disease	**Vaginal Disease**
Premalignant	VIN	VAIN
Malignant	Squamous cell (85%)	Squamous cell (90%) Adenocarcinomas (6%)

Diagnosis

As many as 50% of patients with VIN are **asymptomatic**. This highlights the need for a **thorough inspection** of the vulva for masses, ulcerations, and color changes at the annual exam. When symptoms are present, the most common are **vulvar pruritus** or vulvar irritation. Patients may also experience a **palpable abnormality, perineal or perianal burning, or dysuria**. Often, these women have been seen several times and diagnosed with candidiasis but will have no relief of symptoms with antifungal treatments or topical steroids. Any time a pruritic area of the vulva does not respond to topical antifungal creams—particularly in the postmenopausal woman—further workup with **biopsy should be performed** (see Fig. 13-6).

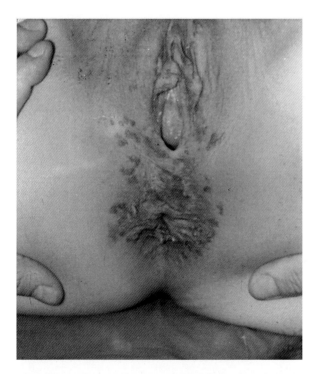

Figure 27-1 • Severe vulvar intraepithelial neoplasia (VIN III). (From Rock J, Jones H. *TeLinde's Operative Gynecology*, 10th ed. Philadelphia: Lippincott Williams & Wilkins, 2008.)

On **physical examination** there may be a variety of lesions that are discrete and often multifocal. Lesions may appear white, red, or pigmented and may be raised or flat. If there are no obvious lesions, **colposcopic-directed biopsy** may be performed to reach a pathologic diagnosis. Extensive colposcopy of the entire vulvar region will often reveal multiple suspicious lesions that can be biopsied in order to make a pathologic diagnosis (Fig. 27-1). VIN appears as distinct acetowhite lesions with or without punctations. Associated vascular abnormalities are more commonly associated with invasive disease.

Treatment

Unlike cervical intraepithelial neoplasia, VIN encompasses a mixed group of lesions with varying potential for **progression to invasive vulvar cancer**. Although spontaneous regression can be seen in women under 40, the risk of progression of untreated disease may be as high as **100% for women over 40**. The options for treatment include wide local excision, laser vaporization, and superficial skinning vulvectomy with and without split-thickness skin grafting.

If all of the biopsies taken reveal VIN without any evidence of invasion, then **wide local excision** can be used for distinct, unifocal disease. The goal is to have a **disease-free margin of at least 5 to 10 mm**. When multifocal disease is diagnosed a simple vulvectomy or skinning vulvectomy may be used. **Split-thickness skin grafts** are often used to replace the excised lesions. More recently, **laser vaporization** has been used to eradicate multi-focal lesions; this results in less scar tissue and decreased healing time, but it provides no pathologic specimen and should therefore only be used when previous biopsies show no invasive disease.

In younger patients, conservative treatment with topical **5-fluorouracil** (5-FU) and imiquimod (Aldara) has been attempted in order to preserve vulvar anatomy. Effectiveness varies from 40% to 75%. These therapies require thorough evaluation to rule out invasive disease prior to use.

Follow-Up

These therapies can be curative for VIN, but close follow-up is required since at least **one-third of women will have a recurrence of disease**. Recurrence is more common with multifocal lesions, moderate and severe dysplasia, and in patients with positive margins. Patients should have follow-up colposcopy of the entire genital tract every 6 months for 2 years and then annually.

PAGET DISEASE OF THE VULVA

Aside from VIN, the two other noninvasive neoplasias of the vulva, Paget disease and noninvasive melanoma, are extremely rare. Paget disease is covered here since melanoma is much more likely to present as invasive disease.

Extramammary Paget disease is an intraepithelial neoplasia of the skin overlying the vulva. About 20% of patients with Paget disease will have **coexistent adenocarcinoma** underlying the outward changes. When this occurs, metastasis is common. When adenocarcinoma is not present, Paget disease can be treated locally without concern for metastases.

Diagnosis

The lesions of Paget disease are consistent with **chronic inflammatory changes**—hyperemic, sharply demarcated, and thickened with areas of excoriation and induration. Commonly, there is a long-standing **pruritus** that accompanies **velvety red lesions** of the skin that eventually become eczematous and scar into **white plaques**. These lesions may be focal on the labia, perineum, or perianal region or may encompass the entire region. The disease is most common in **patients over age 60**, but the symptoms of **vulvar pruritus and vulvodynia** can precede the diagnosis by years. Absolute diagnosis is made with vulvar biopsy (see Fig. 13-6).

Treatment

In the absence of invasion, **wide local excision** of this intraepithelial lesion can be curative. Because microscopic Paget disease often extends beyond the obvious gross lesions, wide margins should be taken and excised segments checked in pathology for clean margins. It is also important to rule out underlying adenocarcinoma during pathologic evaluation. Finally, even with clean margins, Paget disease has a **high recurrence rate** and may require multiple local excisions. Without nodal metastases, the disease is commonly cured with local excision; however, the disease is **almost invariably fatal if it spreads to lymph nodes**.

CANCER OF THE VULVA

Pathogenesis

Cancers of the vulva may arise from the skin, glandular tissue, subcutaneous tissue, or the mucosa of the lower vagina. The most common type of vulvar cancer is **squamous cell carcinoma** (SCC), which makes up 90% of cases. The other types of vulvar cancers include malignant melanoma (5%), basal cell carcinoma (2%), and soft tissue sarcomas (1%). Although lesions can appear anywhere on the vulva, most are on the **labia majora**. These lesions range in appearance from cauliflower-like masses to hard indurated ulcers (Fig. 27-2). Spread of disease is

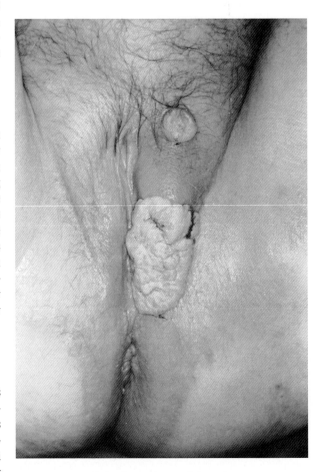

Figure 27-2 • Multifocal carcinoma of the vulva. (From Rock J, Jones H. *TeLinde's Operative Gynecology*, 10th ed. Philadelphia: Lippincott Williams & Wilkins, 2008.)

primarily via the **lymphatics** to the superficial inguinal lymph nodes with a smaller degree of spread via **direct extension** to vagina, urethra, and anus. It is rare for patients without metastases to the inguinal nodes to have spread to the intra-abdominal pelvic nodes.

Epidemiology

Vulvar cancer accounts for only **5% of gynecologic malignancies**, with over 3,800 new cases diagnosed and 800 deaths in the United States each year. Although the rate of noninvasive neoplasia of the vulva has increased dramatically over time, the rate of vulvar carcinoma has **remained relatively stable**. This is thought to be due to the disproportionate increase in VIN in younger women. These women are more likely to undergo early detection and treatment resulting in cancer prevention.

Risk factors for vulvar cancer include menopausal status, cigarette smoking, VIN, CIN, HPV, immunosuppression and history of cervical cancer. The average age of diagnosis is 65. Young women are more likely to have associated HPV infections and VIN.

Diagnosis

Annual examination of the vulva by a healthcare provider is an important component in the diagnosis of vulvar cancer. Patients with vulvar cancer often present with long histories of **vulvar pruritus**, **pain, and bleeding**. Focal lesions tend to be merely inflamed and erythematous in early cancers and heaped up or ulcerated as the lesions progress. They may also present with a **vulvar mass** that may be fleshy, nodular, or warty (Fig. 27-2).

The most common location is the labia majora. Ninety percent of lesions are **unifocal**. Final diagnosis is made by pathologic examination of a biopsy specimen which should be taken even if the patient is asymptomatic. Twenty percent of patients will have a secondary neoplasia (usually cervical). The presence of bleeding, discharge, or a clear mass is strongly suggestive of invasive carcinoma.

Staging

Vulvar carcinoma is **surgically staged** using the International Federation of Gynecology and Obstetrics (FIGO) staging criteria based on tumor size and invasiveness, nodal involvement, and distant metastases (Table 27-2). Staging is the most important prognostic factor for vulvar cancer. The most common surgical approach is **radical local excision** with **inguinofemoral lymph node dissection**. Patients with superficial (<1 mm invasion) and unilateral disease can forego unilateral lymph node dissection. Patients with deeper disease (>1 mm invasion), bilateral disease, or disease which crosses the midline may require ipsilateral bilateral lymph node dissection depending on the location of the lesion.

And given its method of spread, **inguinal lymph node dissection** is required to definitely stage vulvar cancer. Staging may be approximated by a thorough examination for palpable lymph nodes, although 25% of those with positive nodes will have no palpable nodes on physical examination. The use of **sentinel node biopsy** is under investigation as a means of preventing some of the complications associated with complete inguinal node dissection. Metastasis to the intra-abdominal pelvic lymph nodes is very unlikely if the inguinal nodes are disease-free.

■ TABLE 27-2 Staging of Vulvar Cancer

Ia Lesions 2 cm or less in size confined to the vulva or perineum and with stromal invasion no greater than 1.0 mm (no nodal metastasis)

Ib Lesions 2 cm or less in size confined to the vulva or perineum and with stromal invasion greater than 1.0 mm (no nodal metastasis)

II Tumor confined to the vulva and/or perineum—more than 2 cm in greatest dimension (no nodal metastasis)

III Tumor any size with
(a) adjacent spread to the lower urethra and/or distal vagina and/or anus;
(b) unilateral regional lymph node metastasis

IVa Tumor invades any of the following: upper urethra, bladder, mucosa, bone bilateral regional node metastasis

IVb Any distant metastasis including pelvic lymph nodes

Treatment

Prior to definitive treatment, women with vulvar cancer should have a **complete pelvic examination** including palpation of the inguinal nodes, cervical cytology and colposcopy of the cervical vagina, vulva, and perianal area.

For a primary occurrence of squamous cell carcinoma of the vulva carcinoma, **wide radical local excision** with **inguinal lymph node dissection** is the treatment of choice. Stage I disease rarely has positive contralateral lymph nodes, and thus **ipsilateral lymphadenectomy** is sufficient. Most stage II disease can be treated with **modified radical vulvectomy** and separate inguinal incisions for resection of lymph nodes. Stage III and stage IV disease may require **radical vulvectomy**, bilateral inguinal-femoral lymph node dissection (Fig. 27-3), and **pelvic exenteration**. Most recently, preoperative radiation therapy and chemoradiation have been used to avoid the morbidity and mortality associated with pelvic exenteration.

If lymphadenectomy reveals metastatic disease, **pelvic radiation** is used as adjunct therapy. In patients for whom extensive surgery is contraindicated, the procedure may be confined to vulvectomy. In these patients, preoperative radiation therapy with and without chemotherapy has been used to reduce tumor burden. For recurrence, secondary excision or chemoradiation therapy can be used. Recurrences are usually near the primary site.

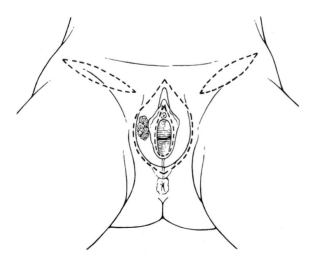

Figure 27-3 • Incision for radical vulvectomy with separate incisions for bilateral inguinofemoral lymph node dissection. (From Rock J, Jones H. *TeLinde's Operative Gynecology*, 10th ed. Philadelphia: Lippincott Williams & Wilkins, 2008.)

Melanoma of the vulva occurs predominantly in postmenopausal Caucasians. It can be treated similarly to SCC, except that **lymphadenectomy is rarely performed**. Depth of invasion is the key prognostic factor. **Once the melanoma has metastasized, the mortality rate is near 100%**. Basal cell carcinoma can be treated with wide local excision. These lesions rarely metastasize to the lymph nodes; thus, lymphadenectomy is not required.

Prognosis

The 5-year survival rate for all patients after surgical treatment of invasive squamous cell carcinoma is approximately 75%. The **most important prognostic factor is the number of positive inguinal lymph nodes**. In patients with metastases to local lymph nodes, 5-year survival rates are 90% to 95% for one positive lymph node, 50% to 80% for two positive lymph nodes, and less than 15% for three or more positive lymph nodes.

PREINVASIVE DISEASE OF THE VAGINA

Pathogenesis

Vaginal intraepithelial neoplasia (VAIN) is a **premalignant lesion** similar to those of the vulva and cervix. However, VAIN is much less common than either VIN or CIN. By definition, the squamous cell atypia seen in VAIN is limited to the epithelium. Lesions are designated as VAIN I, II, or III based upon the amount of epithelium with cellular changes. VAIN I and II encompass the lower one-third and two-thirds of the epithelium, respectively. **VAIN III** involved greater than two-thirds of the epithelium as well as full thickness abnormalities (**carcinoma in situ**). VAIN occurs most commonly as **multifocal lesions** in the **vaginal apex**. VAIN is associated with CIN, cervical cancer, condylomas, and history of **infection with HPV**.

Epidemiology

The peak incidence occurs in patients in their mid- to late 40s. At least 50% to 90% of patients with VAIN will have **coexistent or prior neoplasia** or cancer of the vulva or cervix.

Diagnosis

Patients with VAIN are **almost always asymptomatic**; however, some patients can present with vaginal discharge or postcoital spotting. Many patients are diagnosed due to an abnormality on **Pap smear**. In particular, suspicion of vaginal neoplasia should be raised in patients with **persistently abnormal Pap smears but no cervical neoplasia** on cervical biopsy. Patients who have undergone hysterectomy for a history of CIN or VAIN should continue to have annual Pap smears to screen for VAIN.

VAIN can be diagnosed with a thorough colposcopy of the cervix (if present) and upper vagina. Lesions are typically sharply demarcated areas of acetowhite epithelium with punctation. These lesions **should then be biopsied** to give a final pathologic diagnosis and rule out invasive disease.

Treatment

The primary treatment for VAIN is **local excision or laser ablation**. For focal lesions, local resection is both curative and the only way to rule out invasive disease. If lesions are found on the cervix and extend into the upper third of the vagina, they can be removed with hysterectomy. If invasive disease has been ruled out with extensive biopsies, the lesions can be treated with **laser vaporization** which heals well and has few side effects. Intravaginal **5-fluorouracil (5-FU)** is especially helpful in treating patients with multifocal lesions and immunosuppression. Many of these patients tend to have multifocal lesions of both the vulva and cervix and close follow-up with colposcopy on the entire lower genital tract is needed.

CANCER OF THE VAGINA

Pathogenesis

Vaginal cancer is extremely rare and comprises only 1% to 2% of malignant neoplasms of the female genital tract. The most common histologic type of vaginal cancer is **squamous cell carcinoma** (SCC [85%]); adenocarcinoma (6%), sarcomas, and melanomas are found in a much smaller percentage of patients. In the 1970s, **clear cell adenocarcinoma** was found to be associated with in utero exposure of **diethylstilbestrol** (DES).

SCC may appear ulcerated, nodular, or exophytic and usually involves the **posterior wall and upper one-third** of the vagina. Spread may occur via **lymphatic** drainage to the inguinal nodes and deep pelvic nodes or via **direct extension** to the bladder or rectum. Late in the disease process, **hematogenous spread** to liver, lungs, and bone is possible.

Epidemiology

Primary vaginal cancers make up only **1% to 2% of all gynecologic cancers**. In fact, secondary carcinoma of the vagina is more common than primary disease. The mean age for diagnoses of squamous cell cancer of the vagina is 60. The cause of squamous cell carcinoma of the vagina is **unknown**. Like vulvar and cervical cancer, vaginal cancers can be associated with HPV infection. However, because the vaginal mucosa is not undergoing constant metaplasia like cervical epithelium, the vagina is much less susceptible to the oncogenic effects of the virus.

Women who were exposed in utero to DES have a propensity to develop **clear cell adenocarcinoma** of the vagina. Even then, the incidence in DES-exposed women is only 0.1%. These cancers are typically found in DES exposed women under age 20. They present as polypoid masses on the anterior aspect of the vagina.

Diagnosis

Many patients (20%) with vaginal cancer are asymptomatic. The most common presenting symptoms are **pruritis, postmenopausal vaginal bleeding, postcoital bleeding, and/or watery, blood-tinged discharge**. In more advanced disease urinary (dysuria, hematuria, frequency) and gastrointestinal (constipation, melena) symptoms may be reported as well. As in VAIN, vaginal cancer may be diagnosed during Pap smear screening and follow-up colposcopy and biopsy. The differential diagnosis for vaginal cancer includes Gartner duct cyst, endometrial implant, and cancer of the urethra, bladder, or rectum.

Staging and Treatment

Invasive SCC of the vagina is often complicated by involvement with local structures such as the rectum or bladder (Table 27-3). Given this, patients diagnosed with vaginal cancer should undergo preoperative chest imaging, cystoscopy, proctosigmoidoscopy,

Stage	Clinical/Pathologic Findings
■ **TABLE 27-3** FIGO Staging for Carcinoma of the Vagina	
Stage 0	Carcinoma in situ, intraepithelial carcinoma
Stage I	The carcinoma is limited to the vaginal wall
Stage II	The carcinoma has involved the subvaginal tissue but has not extended to the pelvic wall
Stage III	The carcinoma has extended to the pelvic wall
Stage IV	The carcinoma has extended beyond the true pelvis or has clinically involved the mucosa of the bladder or rectum; bullous edema as such does not permit a case to be allotted to stage IV
Stage IVa	Spread of the growth to adjacent organs and/or direct extension beyond the true pelvis
Stage IVb	Spread to distant organs

and intravenous pyelogram (IVP) to assess for disease spread. At the time of presentation, 26% of vaginal cancer patients have stage I disease, 37% have stage II, 24% have stage III, and 13% have stage IV disease.

Small stage I lesions (<2 cm) in the upper third of the vagina are amenable to **surgical resection** (radical hysterectomy, upper vaginectomy, bilateral pelvic lymph node dissection). Lesions >2 cm, those in the lower two-thirds of the vagina, and stage III and IV lesions are treated with external and internal **radiation therapy** alone (Table 27-3). Comprehensive treatment should involve addressing the **psychosexual ramifications** of treatment.

Adenocarcinoma of the vagina is treated similarly to SCC. However, a clear-cut therapy for clear cell carcinoma has not been established. These lesions are often treated similarly with resection of earlier staged lesions and radiation for stage III and IV lesions and those involving the lower vagina.

Prognosis

The 5-year survival rate for SCC of the vagina is highly dependent on the clinical stage and tumor size at the time of diagnosis. The overall survival rate for primary vaginal cancer has improved over time and is now about 45% to 55%.

 KEY POINTS

- Vulvar intraepithelial neoplasia (VIN) is a premalignant disease confined to the vulvar epithelium. Histologic grades include VIN I, II, and III.

- VIN is often asymptomatic but can present with vulvar pruritus and vulvar irritation that are unresponsive to treatment with antifungals or steroids.

- Risk factors include HPV 16 and 18, cigarette smoking, and immunosuppression.

- The lesions are quite varied and vulvar biopsy is required for diagnosis and to rule out invasive disease.

- Treatments include wide local excision, simple or skinning vulvectomy, or laser vaporization of tissue with close colposcopic follow-up.

- Paget disease is another preinvasive intraepithelial neoplasia of the vulva; it is rare but it is associated with adenocarcinoma 20% of the time.

- These lesions are often velvety red in appearance and can eventually scar into white plaques. Diagnosis is made by biopsy.

- Treatment is with wide local excision; there is a high recurrence rate and close follow-up is important.

- Vulvar cancer makes up only 5% of gynecologic cancers. Risk factors include HPV, HIV, and history of cervical cancer.

- Patients with vulvar cancer often present with vulvar itching, pain, and bleeding, and diagnosis is made by vulvar biopsy.

- The most common histologic type of vulvar cancer is squamous cell carcinoma (90%).

Most treatment includes radical local excision (Stage I), or radical vulvectomy (Stage II, III, IV), and regional lymphadenectomy; pelvic exenteration or preoperative chemoradiation may also be used for advanced disease.

- Five-year survival rates are excellent for two or fewer positive nodes, but drops to 15% for three or more positive nodes.

- VAIN lesions are often asymptomatic but may present with vaginal discharge or postcoital spotting. They can also be picked up on cervical cytology.

- VAIN is much less common than CIN or VIN. Most lesions are multifocal and located in the vaginal apex. Diagnosis is made by colposcopically directed biopsy.

- Fifty-ninety percent of patients with VAIN have a coexistent intraepithelial lesion or invasive lesion of the cervix or vulva.

- Local excision, laser vaporization, and topical 5-FU are common therapies for VAIN.

- Patients require close follow-up with colposcopy to rule out recurrence.

- Vaginal cancer is often asymptomatic, with the most common presenting symptoms being vaginal pruritis, discharge, or bleeding.

- Diagnosis is made by colposcopic-assisted vaginal biopsy. Prior to treatment, patients should undergo chest imaging, cystoscopy, proctosigmoidoscopy, and intravenous pyelogram (IVP) to assess for disease spread.

- Small stage I lesions of the upper vagina can be treated with surgical excision; all other lesions are treated with internal and external radiation therapy for an overall 5-year survival rate between 45% and 55%.

Cervical Neoplasia and Cervical Cancer

Prior to the 20th century, cervical cancer was the most common cancer in women and the most common cause of cancer death in women in the United States. Since the advent of the **Papanicolaou (Pap) smear**, which gained widespread acceptance in the 1950s and 1960s, it has been easier to detect and treat premalignant changes before they develop into cancer (Fig. 28-1). As a result of public health initiatives involving population-based screening, detection, and treatment, cervical cancer has dropped to the 11th leading cause of death from cancer in women in the United States accounting for nearly 4,000 deaths per year.

Further advances in detection and screening have resulted from identification of the **human papillomavirus (HPV) as the causal agent** in the vast majority of cervical intraepithelial neoplasias and cervical cancers. By allowing us to pick up premalignant changes of the cervix, the combination of **Pap smear screening** and **HPV testing** reduces a woman's risk of dying of cervical cancer by 90%. Fortunately, vaccines have been developed that protect against HPV infection and reduce the risk of cervical cancer by 70%.

Because developing countries often lack available screening, vaccination, and treatment modalities, cervical cancer continues to be the second most common cancer in women worldwide and is the **number one cancer killer of women in the developing world.**

CERVICAL INTRAEPITHELIAL NEOPLASIA

PATHOGENESIS

Cervical intraepithelial neoplasia (CIN) (formerly cervical dysplasia) refers to **premalignant changes in the cervical epithelium** that have the potential to progress to cervical cancer. The histologic features most commonly associated with cervical dysplasia include cellular immaturity, cellular disorganization, nuclear abnormalities, and increased mitotic activity. The severity of CIN is determined by the **portion of epithelium showing disordered growth and development**. The changes start at the basal layer of the epithelium and can expand to encompass the entire epithelium (Fig. 28-2).

The nomenclature for cervical neoplasia divides the epithelial thickness into thirds to express the degree of abnormality (Table 28-1). In CIN I (formerly mild dysplasia), the changes are restricted to the lower one-third of the epithelium. In CIN II (formerly moderate dysplasia), two-thirds of the epithelium is involved. And, in CIN III (formerly severe dysplasia), more than two-thirds of the epithelium shows abnormal changes. The atypical cells in CIN III can expand the full thickness of the epithelium (formally CIS or carcinoma in situ).

During menarche, the production of estrogen stimulates metaplasia in the transformation zone (TZ) of the cervix. These metaplastic cells are more susceptible to oncogenic factors; therefore CIN **most commonly occurs during menarche and after pregnancy** when metaplasia is most active. CIN is thought to begin as a single focus in the TZ but develops into a **multifocal lesion**. It is twice as likely to be on the **anterior lip** as the posterior lip and rarely occurs in the lateral angles of the cervix.

HPV is now accepted as the **primary causative agent in CIN and cervical cancer**. DNA fragments of HPV have been found incorporated into the DNA of cells from 80% of all CIN lesions and 90% of all

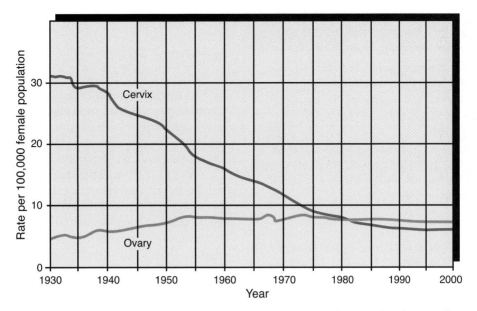

Figure 28-1 • Declining rates of cervical cancer in the United States since the introduction of the Pap smear. The Pap test was first used in the early 1930s and 1940s and became more commonly used in the 1950s.

(From Beckmann CRB, Ling FW, Laube DW, et al. *Obstetrics and Gynecology*, 4th ed. Baltimore: Lippincott Williams & Wilkins, 2002.)

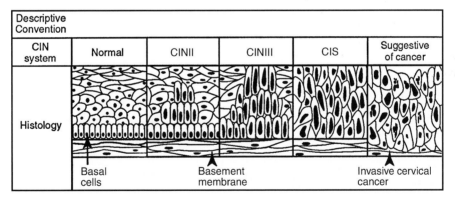

Figure 28-2 • Histologic classification of cervical intraepithelial neoplasia (CIN). The degree of CIN is determined by the portion of epithelium showing disordered growth and development. Changes are restricted to the lower one-third of the epithelium in CIN I. The lower two-thirds of the epithelium are involved in CIN II, and more than two-thirds of the epithelium shows abnormal changes in CIN III. If the entire epithelium is abnormal, this represents carcinoma in situ (CIS) but is still within the CIN III category. In invasive cervical cancer, the abnormalities invade through the basement membrane into the cervical stroma.

(From Beckmann CRB, Ling FW, Laube DW, et al. *Obstetrics and Gynecology*, 4th ed. Baltimore: Lippincott Williams & Wilkins, 2002.)

■ **TABLE 28-1** Classification of Cervical Intraepithelial Neoplasia (CIN)
CIN I: Cellular dysplasia confined to the basal third of the epithelium (formerly mild dysplasia)
CIN II: Cellular dysplasia confined to the basal two-thirds of the epithelium (formerly moderate dysplasia).
CIN III: Cellular dysplasia encompassing greater than two-thirds of the epithelial thickness (formerly severe dysplasia), including full-thickness lesions (formerly carcinoma in situ or CIS)

invasive cervical cancers. There are over 100 different serotypes of HPV. Serotypes 6 and 11 are among the **low-risk types** of HPV and are most commonly associated with **condylomas**. Serotypes such as 16, 18, 31, and 45 are considered **high-risk types** and are found in **cervical dysplasia and cancer**. We are now able to test for high-risk HPV types in Pap smear specimens. This testing allows providers to more accurately predict which precancerous lesions have the potential to progress to cancer if left untreated and which will regress spontaneously. Moreover, HPV vaccines are now available (e.g., Gardasil®) that prevent HPV infections and reduce the risk of cervical cancer by 70%.

EPIDEMIOLOGY

CIN is most commonly diagnosed in **women in their twenties**; carcinoma in situ is diagnosed most commonly in women 25 to 35 years of age; and invasive cancer is typically diagnosed after the age of 40.

Risk factors for cervical dysplasia include characteristics that predispose to multiple and early **exposure to HPV** (early intercourse, multiple sexual partners, early childbearing, "high-risk" partners, low socioeconomic status, sexually transmitted infections). Most of these behavioral and sexual risk factors are **proxies for HPV** infection rather than independent risk factors in and of themselves. At least **80% of sexually active women** will have acquired a genital HPV infection by age 50.

Other factors that influence CIN are **cigarette smoking**, exogenous or endogenous **immunodeficiency** (HIV infection, systemic lupus erythematosus, transplant recipients, chemotherapy, chronic steroid use), and multiparity. Approximately 10% of women with CIN have concomitant vulvar (VIN), vaginal (VAIN), or perianal (PAIN) intraepithelial lesions.

DIAGNOSIS

Pap Smear Screening

Because cervical dysplasia is otherwise **asymptomatic**, the Pap smear has revolutionized our ability to identify, monitor, and treat premalignant cervical changes before cancer arises. The Pap smear involves scraping cells from the external os of the cervix with a blunt spatula to gain cells from the **transformation zone** (Fig. 28-3A). Because the squamocolumnar junction may be in the endocervical canal, it is important to also sample the **endocervical canal** with a cytobrush. The sample is then placed directly on a glass slide (conventional Pap smear) or into a liquid-based medium that is then used to make a slide. The prepared slides are then examined by a cytopathologist (Fig. 28-3B).

Liquid-based Pap tests, such as ThinPrep® and SurePath™, have proven to be more sensitive than conventional glass slide Pap smears because the cells do not clump on top of each other in the liquid-based medium and there is **less debris** on the resulting slide. Additionally, fewer cells are required to make an adequate liquid-based specimen than with a conventional glass slide Pap smear. As a result, with liquid-based cytology tests, more **intraepithelial lesions are identified** and fewer Pap smears are considered nondiagnostic secondary to "insufficient material."

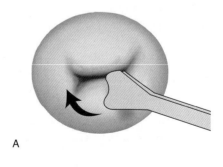

A

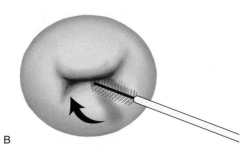

B

Figure 28-3 • Performing a Pap. **(A)** Spatula. **(B)** Endocervical brush.
(From Bickley LS, Szilagyi P. *Bates' Guide to Physical Examination and History Taking*, 8th ed. Philadelphia: Lippincott Williams & Wilkins, 2003.)

All women should begin cervical cancer screening **3 years after they begin having vaginal intercourse, but no later than age 21**. Screening should continue on an annual basis. Beginning at age 30, women who have had three normal Pap smears in a row may opt to be screened every 3 years. All women over age 30 should have high-risk HPV screening every 3 years.

The American Cancer Society guidelines for cervical cancer screening state that **women 70 years or older** who have had three or more normal Pap tests in a row and no abnormal Pap test results in the past 20 years may choose to stop having cervical cancer screening. Likewise, if a woman has had a **total hysterectomy** (uterine corpus and cervix) for a benign indication such as fibroids or dysfunctional bleeding and she does not have a history of abnormal Pap smears in the past 20 years, she does not need to continue Pap screening after the hysterectomy.

Importantly, women who have undergone a **supracervical hysterectomy** and have an intact cervix still need to continue regular Pap smear screening. And women with risk factors such as in utero DES exposure, HIV infection, or **immunosuppression** due to organ transplant, chemotherapy, or chronic steroid use should continue annual screening.

Abnormal Pap Smear Management

Pap smear reports may show findings consistent with normal cellular material, inflammatory changes, infection, dysplasia, or cancer. Nearly 3.5 million American women have abnormal Pap smear findings each year; this represents approximately 5% to 7% of Pap smears performed. Table 28-2 shows the major **classes of epithelial abnormalities** as they are reported using the 2001 Bethesda classification system.

Cytological abnormalities occur because actively replicating HPV produces characteristic cellular changes, such as nuclear enlargement, multinucleation, hyperchromasia, and perinuclear cytoplasmic clearing (halos), which are detected during the cytopathologic evaluation. These cytological features are used to classify the Pap smear as abnormal. Resolution of HPV infection is associated with regression of these abnormalities.

The cellular changes ascribed to the atypical squamous cells (ASC) category may represent benign inflammatory response to infection or trauma but may also herald a preinvasive neoplastic lesion. In fact, it is estimated that **10% to 15% of ASC Pap smears harbor severe dysplasia** histology that should be treated. To better delineate Pap smears with more benign appearing features from those which are more concerning, the atypical squamous cell category has been divided into two groups; **ASC-US** (atypical squamous cells of unknown significance) and **ASC-H** (atypical squamous cells—cannot rule out high-grade lesion). Patients in the ASC-H category should be evaluated with colposcopy. **Patients with ASC-US should undergo HPV testing to determine if colposcopy is indicated or not**.

Patients who receive an ASC-H, LSIL, or HSIL Pap smear result should **proceed directly to colposcopy** (Table 28-3). Because of the potential for both cervical and endometrial **adenocarcinoma**, patients with a Pap smear reading of **atypical glandular cells** (AGC) should undergo **colposcopy**, cervical biopsy, and endocervical sampling. Moreover, patients 35 and older and those younger than 35 with risk factors for endometrial hyperplasia or endometrial cancer should also have an **endometrial biopsy** (Table 28-3).

HPV Testing

With the advent of **HPV DNA testing**, it is now recommended that women with an ASC-US result be tested immediately for the presence of high-risk HPV subtypes. This process is known as **reflex HPV testing**. "Reflex" testing can be achieved either using the residual liquid from the liquid-based Pap test or using a separate sample collected at the time of the initial Pap for HPV testing. The HPV results are added to the initial Pap smear interpretation. This eliminates the need for the patient to return for repeat testing and it allows the clinician to predict a patient's risk for a high-grade lesion with more accuracy and to better direct the plan of care.

If the woman with an ASC-US Pap test is **positive for a high-risk HPV type, then she should be evaluated with colposcopy** (Table 28-3) where directed

■ **TABLE 28-2** Major Classes of Epithelial Cell Abnormalities Found on Pap Smears
ASC-US: Atypical squamous cells of undetermined significance
ASC-H: Atypical squamous cells cannot exclude high-grade squamous intraepithelial lesion
LSIL: Low-grade squamous intraepithelial lesion
HSIL: High-grade squamous intraepithelial lesion
SCC: Squamous cell carcinoma
AGC: Atypical glandular cells

■ **TABLE 28-3** Management of Abnormal Pap Smear Results in Adult Women*

ASC-US, High-risk HPV negative	→	Repeat Pap smear in 1 year
ASC-US, High-risk HPV positive	→	Colposcopy and cervical biopsies
ASC-H	→	Colposcopy and cervical biopsies
LSIL	→	Colposcopy and cervical biopsies
HSIL	→	Colposcopy and cervical biopsies
SCC	→	Colposcopy and cervical biopsies, potential cold-knife conization (CKC)
AGC	→	Colposcopy and cervical biopsies, endometrial biopsy**

*Adolescents (≤age 20) have slightly different management options.
**In women 35 or older and in women with risk factors for endometrial hyperplasia and endometrial cancer.

biopsies can be performed. However, if the patient **tests negative for a high-risk HPV type**, she can be followed by another Pap smear and high-risk HPV screen in 1 year. Not all providers are using HPV testing in their management of ASC-US Pap smears; some providers repeat the cytology in 6 months and then refer to colposcopy if the repeat Pap smear results are ASC or higher. Likewise, **no HPV testing is recommended for ASC-H, LSIL, and HSIL**, because nearly all of these lesions will be positive for high-risk HPV types.

Fortunately, many epithelial abnormalities found on Pap smears will **regress back to normal** over 1 to 2 years. Some of the abnormalities will **persist at their current level** and the remainder will **progress to** more serious lesions or cervical cancer (Table 28-4). ASC and LSIL lesions usually represent a transient infection with HPV so the majority will regress spontaneously on their own over time. However, HSIL lesions are more likely to be associated with persistent infection and progression to cancer. Therefore, patients who receive an ASC-H, LSIL, or HSIL Pap smear result should **proceed directly to colposcopy** (Table 28-3).

COLPOSCOPY AND CERVICAL BIOPSY

Once a *cytologic* diagnosis of epithelial abnormalities has been made on Pap smear, a *histologic* examination is needed to make the diagnosis of cervical dysplasia or cancer. This histologic evaluation can be achieved with **colposcopy and directed biopsies** to determine the severity of dysplasia and to identify any invasive carcinoma. The colposcope gives a magnified view of the cervix and, when stained with acetic acid, cervical lesions can be noted. Changes may include **acetowhite epithelium, mosaicism, punctations, and atypical vessels** (Fig. 28-4 and Color Plate 14). These lesions should be biopsied and the specimens sent to pathology where more definitive histologic diagnoses can be made.

Cervical dysplasia is classified as mild (CIN I), moderate (CIN II), or severe (CIN III) depending on the depth of involvement of the epithelium on cervical biopsy (Fig. 28-2). The treatment plan is then determined by the level of cervical dysplasia. In general, **CIN I** lesions can be followed with **repeat cytology** (every 6 months ×2) or **repeat HPV testing** (in 1 year). Because of their potential to progress to cervical cancer, **CIN II** and **CIN III** are typically treated with **surgical excision** (Table 28-5).

Treatment of Cervical Dysplasia

When the diagnosis of CIN is made on cervical biopsy, several treatments may ensue. **CIN I** is commonly followed with **repeat Pap smears** (every 6 months for

■ **TABLE 28-4** Natural History of Cervical Intraepithelial Lesions

CIN Level	Regress Spontaneously (%)	Persist at Same Level	Progression to CIN III	Progress to Invasive Cancer
CIN I	60	30	10	<1
CIN II	40	35	20	5
CIN III	30	50	N/A	12 to 22

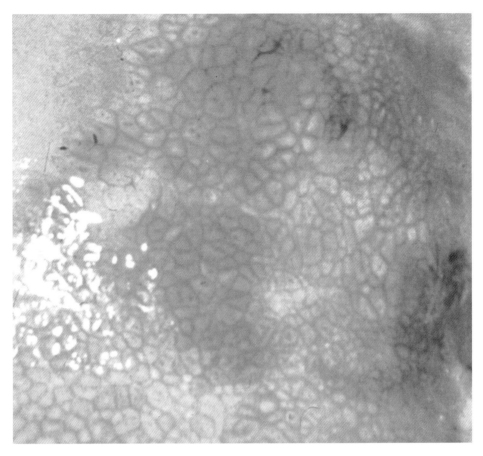

Figure 28-4 • Colposcopic view of the cervix. Abnormalities shown include acetowhite epithelium, punctuations, and mosaic patterns.
(From Rubin E, Farber JL. *Pathology*, 3rd ed. Philadelphia: Lippincott Williams & Wilkins, 1999.)

12 months) or **HPV testing** in 1 year. If either the repeat Pap smears are abnormal or if the testing for high-risk HPV is positive, the patient should have a **repeat colposcopy and biopsy**. If the repeat Pap smears are all within normal limits, then the patient can return to annual Pap smears.

Adult women who have CIN II or CIN III are treated with surgical excision. The same is true for -

■ TABLE 28-5 Management of Cervical Intraepithelial Neoplasia by Level

CIN I	→	Repeat Pap smear every 6 months ×1 year; or high-risk HPV screen in 1 year; if persistent ×2 yrs	→	LEEP procedure
CIN II	→	LEEP procedure		
CIN III	→	LEEP procedure		

patients with CIN I that persists for more than 2 years. Historically, a **cold-knife conization** (CKC) was performed, which removes a wedge-shaped portion of the cervical stroma and endocervical canal (Fig. 28-5). This is no longer the standard of care for CIN. The **loop electrosurgical excision procedure (LEEP) or large loop excision of the transformation zone** (Lletz) is now more commonly performed to treat CIN II and CIN III. LEEP, loop, and Lletz all refer to the same procedure that involves removing a cone-shaped piece of cervical portio (conization), typically with a cauterized fine-wire loop or with a laser (Fig. 28-6). The LEEP can be performed as an office procedure under local anesthesia and is quicker and has less blood loss than the CKC.

Table 28-6 describes the suggested means of surgical excision of CIN based on characteristics of the lesion or patient. For small lesions confined to the ectocervix, an **in-office LEEP** is the most common means of excision although cryotherapy or laser

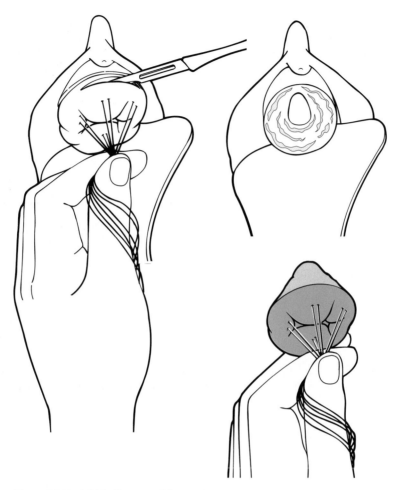

Figure 28-5 • Cold-knife cone of the cervix.

■ **TABLE 28-6** Various Surgical Excision Options Based on Characteristics of the Lesion or Patient

Characteristic		Suggested Procedure
Confined to ectocervix	→	LEEP*
Endocervix involved	→	2-stage LEEP or cold-knife conization (CKC)
Large lesion	→	Laser conization
Teenage patient	→	Laser conization
Upper vagina involved	→	Laser conization

*Cryotherapy is acceptable if lesion is small, limited to CIN I or CIN II, and there is no endocervical involvement.

therapy may be used. Lesions involving the endocervix are usually treated with **cold-knife conization or a two-stage LEEP** to allow more of the endocervix to be removed. In the two-stage LEEP procedure, the first LEEP is performed to remove the ectocervix and a second smaller, deeper LEEP is then done to remove a portion of the endocervical canal. This is also known as a "top hat" because the resulting defect in the cervix resembles the shape of a top hat. Lesions that are large or involve the vagina and those in teenagers are often treated with **laser conization** to allow for more precise removal of only abnormal tissue such that less normal cervix is removed.

In general, cervical excision procedures remove cervical tissue without causing extensive damage to the stroma of the cervix, although scarring of the en-

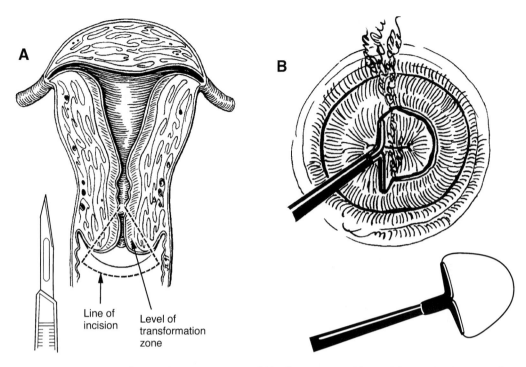

Figure 28-6 • Methods of cervical conization. **(A)** Cold-knife conization. **(B)** LEEP/Lletz conization procedure. (From Beckmann CRB, Ling FW, Laube DW, et al. *Obstetrics and Gynecology*, 4th ed. Baltimore: Lippincott Williams & Wilkins, 2002.)

docervical canal may still ensue. Infrequent complications include **cervical stenosis, cervical insufficiency, infection, or bleeding**. The persistence rate is about 4% for CIN II and III and the recurrence rate is 10% and 15%, respectively. Therefore, after surgical conization, patients should be followed every 6 months with a repeat Pap smear or repeat Pap smear and colposcopy for 1 year. If the results all remain normal, the patient can return to routine screening for at least 20 years. Alternatively, after a cervical conization, the patient can be followed with HPV testing 1 year after the procedure. If not high risk, the patient can return to routine screening for at least 20 years. In either scenario, any abnormal cytology or the presence of high-risk HPV should result in repeat colposcopic examination and cervical biopsies.

CERVICAL CANCER

PATHOPHYSIOLOGY

Squamous cell carcinoma (SCC) accounts for 80% of all cervical cancers. The route of metastasis is most often by direct extension (Fig. 28-7). **Adenocarcinoma** accounts for most of the remaining 20% of cervical cancers. One type of adenocarcinoma is clear cell carcinoma, which is correlated with in utero diethylstilbestrol **(DES) exposure**. Very rarely a sarcoma or lymphoma of the cervix is found.

EPIDEMIOLOGY

There are approximately 11,000 cases of invasive cervical cancer diagnosed annually in the United States, leading to an estimated 3,600 deaths. Annual Pap smear screening combined with HPV typing decreases a woman's risk of cervical cancer by 90%.

The median age of diagnosis of cervical cancer is 52 and the average is 45. Risk factors for cervical cancer and dysplasia include **high-risk HPV serotypes** (16, 18, 31, 45), cigarette smoking, high number of sexual partners, early age at onset of sexual activity, and **immunosuppression**. Additionally, patients with poorly controlled HIV (high viral loads and low CD4 counts) have an increased progression, persistence, and recurrence of disease. In fact, cervical cancer is now considered an **AIDS-defining illness**.

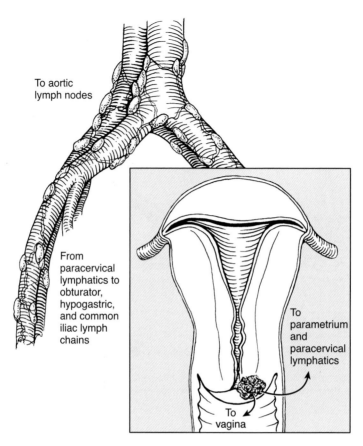

To aortic
lymph nodes

From
paracervical
lymphatics to
obturator,
hypogastric,
and common
iliac lymph
chains

To
parametrium
and
paracervical
lymphatics

To
vagina

Figure 28-7 • Spread patterns of cervical carcinoma.

CLINICAL MANIFESTATIONS

Even though the Pap smear has proved to be an excellent screening method for cervical dysplasia, some patients who still do not get routine Pap smears occasionally present with advanced stages of cervical cancer. Early disease is **usually asymptomatic**. When symptoms are present, the most common is **postcoital bleeding**. Other signs and symptoms that accompany cervical cancer include any abnormal vaginal bleeding, watery discharge, pelvic pain or pressure, and rectal or urinary tract symptoms. On speculum examination, a friable, bleeding cervical lesion or mass may be seen with possible invasion into the upper vagina. On bimanual examination, a mass within the cervix may be palpated as well as invasive lesions into the upper vagina, cul-de-sac, or adnexa.

DIAGNOSIS

Pap smears are not sufficient to diagnose cancer. Cervical cancer can only be diagnosed with a tissue biopsy. If an abnormal pap smear is found, a colposcopy and cervical biopsies should be obtained. If a visible lesion is found, it should also be **biopsied**. If the physical examination is abnormal, ultrasound (US) or computed tomography (CT) may be performed to confirm the findings and define the extent of disease.

CLINICAL STAGING

Cervical cancer is the only gynecologic cancer that is **still clinically staged** (Table 28-7) rather than surgically staged. This is due in large part to the fact that it is the leading cause of cancer death in women in developing nations where many diagnostic tools are not readily available. Clinical staging involves evaluating the patient for **invasion into adjacent structures** and metastatic involvement (Figs. 28-7 and 28-8). Acceptable diagnostic tools for staging of cervical cancer include exam under anesthesia, chest x-ray, cystoscopy, proctoscopy, intravenous pyelography (IVP), and barium enema. Magnetic

■ **TABLE 28-7**	FIGO Staging for Carcinoma of the Cervix Uteri
Stage	**Clinical/Pathologic Findings**
0	Carcinoma in situ, intraepithelial carcinoma
I	The carcinoma is strictly confined to the cervix (extension to the corpus should be disregarded)
Ia	Invasive cancer identified only microscopically. All gross lesions—even with superficial invasion—are stage Ib cancers. Invasion is limited to measured stromal invasion with maximum depth of 5.0 mm and no wider than 7.0 mm*
Ia-1	Measured invasion of stroma no greater than 3.0 mm in depth and no wider than 7.0 mm
Ia-2	Measured invasion of stroma greater than 3.0 mm and no greater than 5.0 mm and no wider than 7.0 mm
Ib	Clinical lesions confined to the cervix or preclinical lesions greater than stage Ia
Ib-1	Clinical lesions no greater than 4.0 cm in size
Ib-2	Clinical lesions greater than 4.0 cm in size
II	The carcinoma extends beyond the cervix but has not extended to the pelvic wall. The carcinoma involves the vagina but not as far as the lower third
IIa	No obvious parametrial involvement
IIb	Obvious parametrial involvement
III	The carcinoma has extended to the pelvic wall. On rectal examination, there is no cancer-free space between the tumor and the pelvic wall
	The tumor involves the lower third of the vagina
	All cases with hydronephrosis or nonfunctioning kidney are included unless they are known to be due to other causes
IIIa	No extension to the pelvic wall
IIIb	Extension to the pelvic wall and/or hydronephrosis or nonfunctioning kidney
IV	The carcinoma has extended beyond the true pelvis or has clinically involved the mucosa of the bladder or rectum. A bullous edema as such does not permit a case to be allotted to stage IV
IVa	Spread of the growth to adjacent organs
IVb	Spread to distant organs

*The depth of invasion should be no more than 5 mm taken from the base of the epithelium, either surface or glandular, from which it originates. Vascular space involvement, either venous or lymphatic, should not alter the staging.

resonance (MRI) imaging and CT may be used to define the extent of the disease but **cannot be used to determine the stage of the disease**. Likewise, once the stage has been assigned, it **does not change based on intraoperative findings** or progression of disease.

Stage I is confined to the cervix (Table 28-7 and Fig. 28-7). Stage II extends beyond the cervix but not to the pelvic sidewalls or the lower third of the vagina. Stage III extends to the pelvic sidewalls or lower third of the vagina. Stage IV is defined as extension beyond the pelvis, invasion into local structures including the bladder or rectum, or distant metastases.

TREATMENT

Preinvasive and Microinvasive Disease

In the case of preinvasive carcinoma (stage 0) and microinvasive carcinoma (stage Ia-1), the standard of care is **simple hysterectomy**. A **cold-knife cone** may be adequate therapy if the patient wants to maintain fertility (Table 28-8).

Early Disease

Early disease (stages Ia-2 to IIa) may be treated with either **radiation therapy or radical hysterectomy** (with

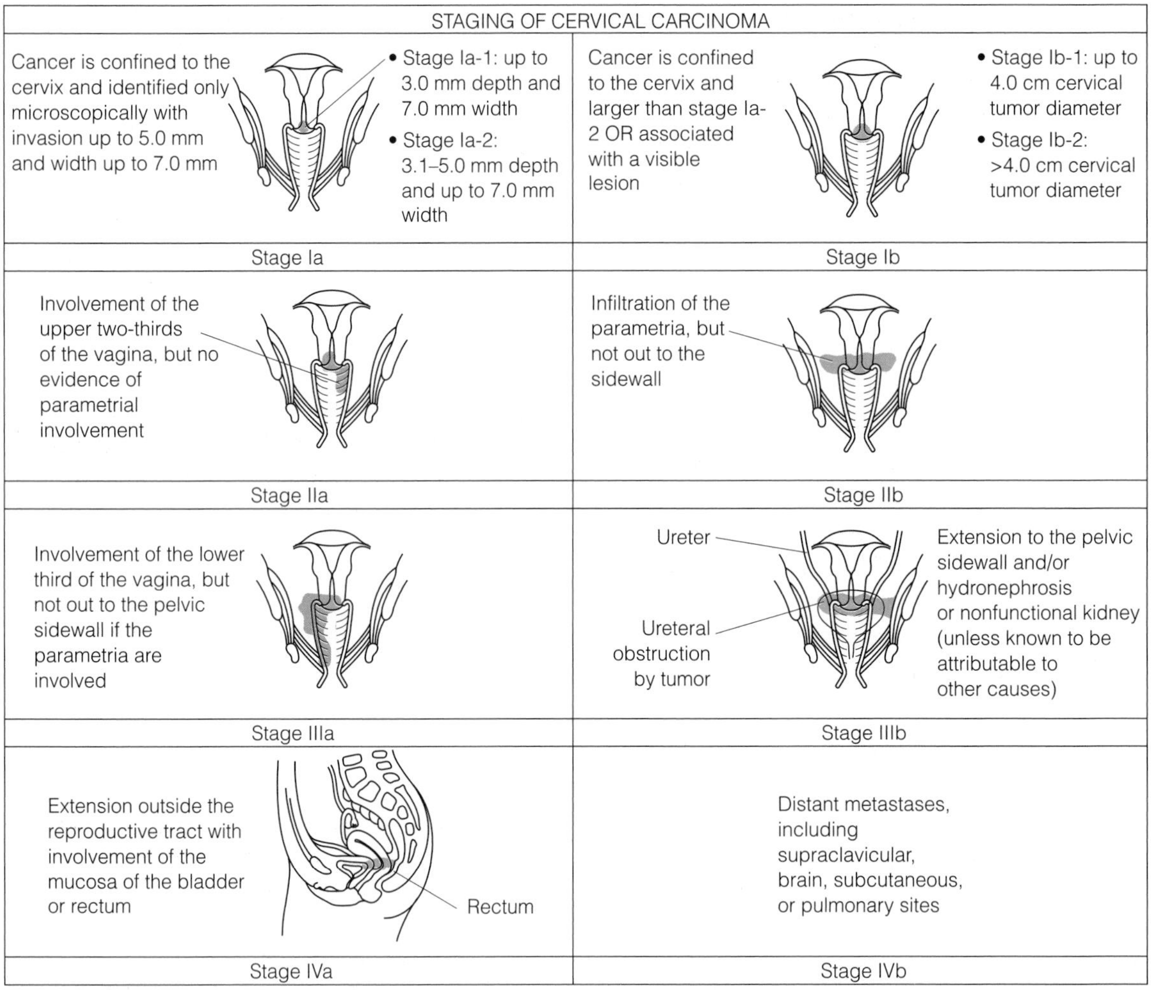

STAGING OF CERVICAL CARCINOMA

Cancer is confined to the cervix and identified only microscopically with invasion up to 5.0 mm and width up to 7.0 mm	• Stage Ia-1: up to 3.0 mm depth and 7.0 mm width • Stage Ia-2: 3.1–5.0 mm depth and up to 7.0 mm width
Stage Ia	
Cancer is confined to the cervix and larger than stage Ia-2 OR associated with a visible lesion	• Stage Ib-1: up to 4.0 cm cervical tumor diameter • Stage Ib-2: >4.0 cm cervical tumor diameter
Stage Ib	
Involvement of the upper two-thirds of the vagina, but no evidence of parametrial involvement	
Stage IIa	
Infiltration of the parametria, but not out to the sidewall	
Stage IIb	
Involvement of the lower third of the vagina, but not out to the pelvic sidewall if the parametria are involved	
Stage IIIa	
Ureter — Ureteral obstruction by tumor	Extension to the pelvic sidewall and/or hydronephrosis or nonfunctional kidney (unless known to be attributable to other causes)
Stage IIIb	
Extension outside the reproductive tract with involvement of the mucosa of the bladder or rectum — Rectum	Distant metastases, including supraclavicular, brain, subcutaneous, or pulmonary sites
Stage IVa	**Stage IVb**

Figure 28-8 • Staging of cervical carcinoma.

bilateral pelvic lymph node dissection) (Table 28-8). In addition to removing the uterus, a radical hysterectomy also removes the parametria, upper vaginal cuff, uterosacral/cardinal ligament complex, and local vascular and lymphatic supplies. For early disease, both radical hysterectomy and radiation therapy have **similar recurrence and survival rates**. The choice of treatment depends on the patient's age, ability to tolerate surgery, and proximity to radiation facilities. Young patients who are otherwise healthy are often treated with surgery to maintain ovarian function that would be diminished or terminated by radiation therapy.

Advanced Disease

For more advanced lesions (stages IIb to IV) that have spread to the pelvic sidewall or beyond (Fig. 28-8), the treatment is **chemoradiation therapy**.

■ **TABLE 28-8** Treatment of Cervical Cancer by Stage of Disease Invasion		
Level	**Stage**	**Treatment**
Preinvasive disease	0-Ia to 1	Cold-knife conization or simple hysterectomy
Early disease	Ia-2 to IIa	Radical hysterectomy or radiation
Advanced disease	IIb to IV	Chemoradiation*
*External beam radiation, cisplatin-based chemotherapy, and intracavitary radiation.		

Both external beam radiation and intracavitary radiation are used in combination with **cisplatin-based chemotherapy**. The goals of chemoradiation are to eradicate local disease and prevent metastatic disease. This combined treatment regimen has led to significantly prolonged disease-free survival when compared to radiation therapy alone.

Recurrent Disease

When cervical cancer recurs in a patient initially treated with surgery alone, radiation can be used to treat the recurrence. When the cancer recurs in a patient already treated with radiation, surgical treatment with **pelvic exenteration** can be used if the recurrence is centrally located. Exenteration involves removal of all of the pelvic organs including the uterus, tubes, ovaries, vagina, bladder, distal ureters, rectum, sigmoid colon, muscles of the pelvic floor, and the supporting ligaments. The 5-year survival rate after exenteration is about 50%.

■ **TABLE 28-9** Overall Five-Year Survival Rate for Cervical Cancer

Stage	5-Year Survival Rate (%)
I	85 to 90
II	60 to 75
III	35 to 45
IV	15 to 20

Palliative Care

Palliative **radiation** with external beam or intracavitary therapy may be used to control bleeding or for pain management. Cisplatin **chemotherapy** may also be used for palliative care.

PROGNOSIS

Overall survival rates for cervical cancer are shown in Table 28-9.

KEY POINTS

- Cervical cancer is the leading cause of cancer deaths in women in developing nations.
- Human papillomavirus (HPV) is the causative agent in cervical intraepithelial neoplasia CIN and cervical cancer. HPV types 16, 18, 31, and 45 are considered high-risk types.
- HPV testing can be used in the diagnosis and surveillance of CIN and cervical cancer. HPV vaccination can protect against some HPV infections thereby preventing 70% of cervical cancer.
- Regular Pap smear screening and HPV testing can reduce a woman's risk of cervical cancer by 90%.
- Regular Pap smear screening should begin 3 years after the first sexual activity or by age 21. Pap smears should then be repeated annually.
- Screening in women over 30 should include HPV typing every 3 years. Cytologic screenings may be spaced out by the provider in certain low-risk women.
- Pap smears are classified as positive for intraepithelial lesions and malignancy, atypical squamous cells (ASC-US and ASC-H), LSIL, HSIL, or SCC.
- ASC-H, LSIL, and HSIL Pap smears should be evaluated with colposcopy and directed biopsies as should ASC-US Pap smears which are positive for high-risk types of HPV.

- CIN I reflects abnormalities in the basal one-third of epithelial cells of the cervix. These changes can potentially lead to cancer but a high number will regress spontaneously.
- In general, patients with biopsies showing CIN I can be followed with repeat Pap smears every 6 months ×2 or HPV testing in 12 months.
- Adult women with CIN II and CIN III biopsies require treatment with surgical excision, typically with loop/LEEP/Lletz.
- Complications of cervical conization include bleeding and infection and much less likely cervical stenosis or cervical incompetence.
- Preinvasive (stage 0) and microinvasive disease (stage Ia-1) can be treated with cone biopsy or simple hysterectomy. Stage Ia-2 should be treated with radical hysterectomy.
- Early disease stages Ia-2 to IIa are equally responsive to radical hysterectomy or radiation therapy.
- More advanced lesions stage IIb or greater are treated with internal and external radiation, usually in combination with cisplatin chemotherapy.
- Radiation and/or chemotherapy may be used for palliative care.
- Five-year survival rates for cervical cancer vary from 85% to 90% for stage I disease, and 15% to 20% for stage IV disease.

Endometrial Cancer

Endometrial carcinoma is the **most common and most curable gynecologic cancer** in the United States. It is the fourth most common cancer in American women today, exceeded only by cancer of the breast, bowel, and lung. Over 39,000 women are diagnosed with this disease each year in the United States alone, accounting for 6% of all cancers in women. Fortunately, **early symptoms and easy and accurate diagnosis modalities** make endometrial cancer only the third most common cause of gynecologic cancer deaths (behind ovarian and cervical cancer) accounting for 7,400 deaths each year in the United States.

Factors such as **obesity, chronic anovulation, nulliparity, late menopause, exogenous estrogen use without progesterone, hypertension, and diabetes mellitus** lead to an increased risk of both endometrial hyperplasia (see Table 14-6) and endometrial cancer.

PATHOGENESIS

There are **two distinct pathogenic types** of endometrial cancer. The most common type, type I (80%), occurs in **younger perimenopausal women** with a history of chronic estrogen exposure unopposed by progestin. These are referred to as **estrogen-dependent neoplasms**. These tumors usually start as atypical endometrial hyperplasia and progress to carcinomas. The tumors tend to be well differentiated and usually have a more **favorable prognosis**.

Type II (20%) endometrial cancer is believed to be an **estrogen-independent** neoplasm that is unrelated to estrogen stimulation or endometrial hyperplasia. These tumors are not generally associated with endometrial hyperplasia and tend to occur in older, **postmenopausal, thin women**. These cancers

are less differentiated and occur more frequently in African American and Asian women.

Grossly, endometrial cancer itself may appear as a single mass within the endometrium or it may be spread diffusely throughout the endometrium. **Depth of myometrial invasion** is an important component in the staging and prognosis of endometrial cancer. The prognosis is dramatically worsened when the cancer has invaded greater than one-half of the thickness of the myometrium.

Endometrial carcinoma has four primary routes of spread. The most common route is **direct extension** of the tumor downward to the cervix or outward through the myometrium and serosa. When there is significant myometrial penetration, cells may spread through the **lymphatic system** to the pelvic and para-aortic lymph nodes. Exfoliated cells may also be shed **transtubally** through the fallopian tubes to the ovaries, parietal peritoneum, and omentum. **Hematogenous** spread occurs less frequently but can result in metastasis to the liver, lungs, and/or bone.

The most common type of endometrial cancer is **endometrioid adenocarcinoma** (75% to 80%). Other nonendometrioid tumor types include mucinous carcinomas (5%), clear cell carcinomas (5%), papillary serous carcinomas (4%), and squamous carcinomas (1%). These types are less common but also tend to be more aggressive. Invasive adenocarcinoma usually results from **proliferation of the glandular cells** of the endometrium in a back-to-back fashion without intervening stroma.

Histologic grade is the most important prognostic factor for endometrial carcinoma (Table 29-1). Poorly differentiated tumors have a higher grade and a higher percentage of solid (nonglandular) growth. High-grade tumors have a much poorer prognosis due

TABLE 29-1 Prognostic Factors for Endometrial Cancer: Histologic Grade—Degree of Differentiation

Grade	Percentage Solid Growth	Differentiation
Grade 1 (G1)	5% or less of the tumor shows a solid growth pattern	Highly differentiated
Grade 2 (G2)	6% to 50% of the tumor shows a solid growth pattern	Moderately differentiated
Grade 3 (G3)	More than 50% of the tumor shows a solid growth pattern	Poorly differentiated

to the likelihood of spread outside of the uterus. The **histologic type** of carcinoma also affects prognosis. Other prognostic factors are shown in Table 29-2.

EPIDEMIOLOGY

Endometrial cancer occurs in both premenopausal (25%) and postmenopausal (75%) women. 5% to 10% of those with premenopausal diagnoses are less than 40 years of age. The **average age of diagnosis is 61**; the largest affected group is between age 50 and 59. Most tumors are caught early when they are of low grade and low stage (Table 29-3); therefore, the overall prognosis for the disease is good and overall mortality rates are declining. Eighty percent of women have type I endometrial cancer while 20% have the more aggressive type II cancers.

RISK FACTORS

Several risk factors have been identified for type I endometrial cancer. These include a history of **unopposed estrogen exposure**, obesity, nulliparity, late menopause, chronic anovulation, and tamoxifen use

(Table 29-4). Other risk factors include diabetes mellitus; hypertension; cancer of the breast, ovary, or colon; and a family history of endometrial cancer.

Excess exogenous estrogen exposure can result from unopposed use of **estrogen replacement therapy (ERT)** in the absence of progesterone in a woman with a uterus. Studies show that 20% to 50% of women who are given ERT without progesterone will develop endometrial hyperplasia within 1 year. Similarly, **tamoxifen**, a selective serotonin reuptake inhibitor (SERM) can also act as a source of exogenous estrogen. It is typically used in women with estrogen-progesterone receptor positive breast cancer (see Chapter 32) to competitively inhibit estrogen at the estrogen receptor. Therefore, it works to block stimulation of breast tissue in women with estrogen-progesterone receptor positive breast cancer. However, in endometrial tissue, tamoxifen acts as a **partial agonist/weak estrogen** to stimulate endometrial proliferation.

Endometrial cancer can also be caused by prolonged exposure to **excess endogenous estrogen** without concomitant progesterone exposure. This mechanism of action is demonstrated in **obese women**. These women have higher endogenous estrogen levels due to **peripheral conversion of androgens to estrone and estradiol** in the adipocytes. These women also have lower SHBG levels. Many are also anovulatory as well.

Women with chronic anovulation and/or PCOS typically have more central obesity and therefore have more peripheral conversion of androgens to estrone

TABLE 29-2 Major Independent Prognostic Factors for Endometrial Cancer

Age
Depth of myometrial invasion
Histologic grade
Histologic type
Surgical stage
Peritoneal cytology
Tumor size
Lymphovascular invasion
Pelvic lymph node metastasis

TABLE 29-3 Stage at Which Endometrial Cancer Is Diagnosed

Stage I	70%
Stage II	12%
Stage III	13%
Stage IV	4%

■ **TABLE 29-4** Risk Factors for Endometrial Cancer

Risk Factor	Relative Risk
Nulliparity	2 to 4
Late menopause	2 to 4
Chronic anovulation (PCOS)	3
Diabetes mellitus	2 to 8
Tamoxifen use	2 to 3
Obesity	
21 to 50 lbs overweight	2 to 4
>50 lbs overweight	10
Unopposed estrogen therapy	2 to 10

and estradiol. These patients also have a **relative lack of progesterone** in luteal phase due to their **anovulatory cycles**. This mechanism of action may also explain the higher rates of endometrial cancer in **nulliparous women**. These women are thought to be at higher risk of infertility and subfertility secondary to **anovulatory cycles**. The increased risk of endometrial cancer in **early menarche** and **late menopause** are presumably due to prolonged endogenous estrogen stimulation without progesterone exposure.

Diabetes (type II > type I) and hypertension also impose a greater risk of endometrial cancer. This is due in part to the comorbid risk of **obesity and chronic anovulation** in diabetic and hypertensive patients. Even when these factors are controlled for, diabetes and hypertension still pose an independent increased risk of endometrial cancer. It is hypothesized that the presence of hyperinsulinemia, insulin resistance, and insulin-like growth factors may lead to **abnormal endometrial proliferation** in these patients.

There is an increased risk of endometrial cancer in women who have at least one **first-degree relative** (mother, sister) with uterine cancer. There has yet to be a specific gene implicated in these familial trends. Conversely, women with a known **family history of hereditary nonpolyposis colorectal cancer** (HNPCC) have an increased risk of endometrial cancer as well. HNPCC is also known as Lynch II syndrome and is associated with a genetic predisposition to breast, ovarian, colon, and endometrial cancers along with other noncolorectal cancers. Specific **germline gene mutations** are responsible for the cancers in the majority of these women with HNPCC. Patients with a **personal history of breast cancer** also have an increased risk of

endometrial cancer. This is attributed to the presence of similar risk factors (**obesity, nulliparity, high-fat diet**) in both cancers. It is unclear if the presence of *BRCA1* (the breast cancer susceptibility gene) plays a role in the development of endometrial cancer.

Endometrial hyperplasia is another risk factor for endometrial cancer. The degree of risk of malignant transformation of endometrial hyperplasia to endometrial cancer depends on the type of hyperplasia (see Table 14-5). Its mildest form, simple hyperplasia *without* atypia poses a 1% risk of endometrial cancer while its most severe form, complex hyperplasia *with atypia*, poses a 29% risk of developing endometrial cancer if left untreated.

Despite these known risk factors for type I endometrial cancer, there are **no effective screening mechanisms** for endometrial carcinoma. Neither annual Pap smears nor endometrial biopsies have been shown to offer cost-effective screening in asymptomatic patients.

Conversely, protective factors include those that **decrease lifetime estrogen exposure** including combination oral contraceptive pills (OCPs), progestin-containing contraceptives, and combination estrogen and progesterone hormone replacement (HRT). These patients have a lower rate of endometrial cancer compared to nonusers. The protection conferred to a woman who takes combination OCPs lasts for 10 years after the pills are stopped. Other **protective factors** include high parity, pregnancy, physical activity (decreased obesity, favorable immune function, and endogenous hormone levels), and smoking (causes increased hepatic metabolism of estrogen). Women can also lower their risk of endometrial cancer by **avoiding obesity, hypertension, and diabetes**, and by eating a **healthy diet and exercising**. Women who exercise regularly have one-half the risk of endometrial cancer as those who do not exercise.

Unfortunately, there are **no identifiable risk factors** for women who may be at risk for type II endometrial cancer.

CLINICAL MANIFESTATIONS

HISTORY

Ninety percent of women with endometrial cancer have either **postmenopausal bleeding** or some form of **abnormal vaginal bleeding** (menorrhagia, postcoital spotting, or intermenstrual bleeding). Ten percent of women may also present with a nonbloody vaginal discharge. As a result of these early symptoms, most endometrial cancers are diagnosed at an early stage (Table 29-3). **Pelvic pain**, **pelvic mass**, and **weight loss** are seen in women who present with more advanced disease.

PHYSICAL EXAMINATION

The physical examination may reveal obesity, acanthosis nigricans, hypertension, or stigmata of diabetes. The clinician should look for signs of metastatic disease including pleural effusion, ascites, hepatosplenomegaly, general lymphadenopathy, and abdominal masses.

Women with endometrial carcinoma typically have a **normal pelvic examination**. In more advanced stages of the disease, the cervical os may be patulous and the cervix may be firm and expanded. The uterus may be of normal size or enlarged. The adnexae should be carefully examined for evidence of extrauterine metastasis and/or coexistent ovarian carcinoma.

DIFFERENTIAL DIAGNOSIS

Most women with endometrial cancer present with a complaint of **abnormal uterine bleeding**. This may include menorrhagia, metrorrhagia, menometrorrhagia, or even oligomenorrhea. The differential diagnosis for premenopausal bleeding includes uterine fibroids, endometrial polyps, adenomyosis, endometrial hyperplasia, ovarian cysts, and thyroid dysfunction (see Fig. 22-1).

The differential diagnosis for **postmenopausal bleeding** is shown in Table 29-5. Note that endometrial cancer is responsible for only 10% to 15% of postmenopausal bleeding. However, the older the patient and higher the number of years since menopause, the higher the probability of malignancy.

■ TABLE 29-5 Differential Diagnosis of Postmenopausal Bleeding

Cause of Bleeding	Frequency (%)
Endometrial atrophy	60 to 80
Exogenous estrogens/HRT	15 to 25
Endometrial cancer	10 to 15
Endometrial or cervical polyps	2 to 12
Endometrial hyperplasia	5 to 10
Miscellaneous	10

The amount of bleeding does not correlate with risk of malignancy.

DIAGNOSTIC EVALUATION

Although dilation and curettage (D&C) was once the gold standard for evaluating irregular bleeding, modern office endometrial biopsy has an accuracy of 90% to 98% without the need for anesthesia and operative time. The **endometrial biopsy** (EMB) has therefore become the standard of care. If an adequate endometrial biopsy cannot be performed due to patient discomfort, cervical stenosis, or insufficient tissue sample, **D&C** ($\pm$ hysteroscopy) should be done to sample the endometrium. A D&C should also be done if there are suspicious findings (atypical hyperplasia or necrosis) on EMB or if the patient continues to have symptoms after a negative EMB.

In addition to endometrial sampling, the initial workup for a woman with abnormal vaginal bleeding should also include a **TSH**, a **prolactin level** (if oligomenorrheic), and possibly an **FSH** (to distinguish if the patient is truly menopausal). A complete blood count (**CBC**) should be obtained to rule out anemia preoperatively. Similarly, a **CA-125 level** is often drawn preoperatively. Very high CA-125 levels are suggestive of spread beyond the uterus. These levels can also be followed postoperatively to assess effectiveness of treatment.

An up-to-date **Pap smear** should also be obtained in women with abnormal bleeding although only 30% to 40% of patients with endometrial cancer will have an abnormal Pap smear. When the Pap smear cytology shows **endometrial cells** in a woman ≥40, an EMB should be performed to rule out endometrial cancer. These cytology reports are particularly concerning when **atypical endometrial cells** are found.

A **pelvic ultrasound** should also be performed to look for fibroids, adenomyosis, polyps, and endometrial hyperplasia. Due to estrogen deficiency, the endometrial stripe of a postmenopausal woman should be very thin (<4 to 5 mm). Postmenopausal women with an endometrial stripe <4 to 5 mm are unlikely to have endometrial hyperplasia or cancer. However, even if the endometrial stripe and the remainder of the pelvic ultrasound appear normal, the physician is **still obliged to obtain an endometrial sampling** via EMB or D&C if the bleeding is persistent. Likewise, even if another potential source for bleeding is identified, the endometrium must still be

■ TABLE 29-6 FIGO Surgical Staging of Endometrial Carcinoma (1988)

Stages	Grade*	Extent of Disease
Stage I		
Ia	G 1,2, or 3	Tumor limited to endometrium
Ib	G123	Invasion to less than half of the myometrium
Ic	G123	Invasion to greater than half of the myometrium
Stage II		
IIaa	G123	Endocervical glandular involvement only
IIb	G123	Cervical stromal invasion
Stage III		
IIIa	G123	Tumor invades serosa and/or positive peritoneal cytology
IIIb	G123	Vaginal metastases
IIIc	G123	Metastases to pelvic and/or para-aortic lymph nodes
Stage IV		
Iva	G123	Tumor invasion of bladder and/or bowel mucosa
IVb	G123	Distant metastases including intra-abdominal and/or inguinal lymph nodes

*Grade refers to the percentage of the tumor which is solid (see Table 29-1). The higher the grade, the higher the percent of solid growth, and the poorer the prognosis.

sampled. If bone pain is present, a chest radiograph, CT, or bone scan can be performed.

More than 50% of women at risk for hereditary nonpolyposis colorectal cancer (**HNPCC or Lynch II syndrome**) will develop endometrial and/or ovarian cancer before developing colon cancer. Given this, these women who carry HNPCC-associated mutations or who have a family member known to carry such a mutation should undergo yearly endometrial biopsy beginning at age 35.

TREATMENT

Although endometrial cancer was once clinically staged, in 1988 the International Federation of Gynecology and Obstetrics (FIGO) changed to a **surgical staging system** that more accurately identifies the true degree of disease progression. This system relies on **pathologic confirmation** of the extent of spread of the disease (Table 29-6).

■ TABLE 29-7 Treatment Recommendations for Endometrial Cancer by Stage

Stage I	TAHBSO; if high risk,* then pelvic and para-aortic LN sampling and radiation as well
Stage II	TAHBSO; if high risk, then pelvic and para-aortic LN sampling and radiation as well
Stage III	TAHBSO, pelvic and para-aortic LN sampling, radiation
Stage IV	TAHBSO, pelvic and para-aortic LN sampling, radiation
Recurrence, pelvic	High-dose progestins, +/− chemotherapy
Recurrence, vaginal	Vaginal radiation

*Grade 3 lesions, grade 2 lesion >2 cm, lower uterine segment involvement, cervical involvement, poor histologic differentiation, papillary serous or clear cell histology, > ⅓ myometrial penetration.

STAGE I AND STAGE II DISEASE

In general, treatment for endometrial carcinoma includes **total abdominal hysterectomy and bilateral salpingo-oophorectomy** (TAHBSO) for all stages of the disease (Table 29-7). The ovaries are removed to rule out metastasis and to eliminate them as a source of endogenous estrogen.

The uterus should be opened during surgery so that the depth of myometrial invasion can be determined. Patients with greater than 50% myometrial invasion have a poorer prognosis even if they have stage I or stage II disease confined to the uterus. These patients and those with other poor prognostic factors such as large tumor mass (>2 cm or filling the cavity), grade 3 tumor type (more than 50% of the tumor is solid), papillary serous or clear cell histologic types, or enlarged lymph nodes, will also require **pelvic and aortic lymph node dissection** and **radiation therapy** even if the disease is confined to the uterus.

STAGE III AND STAGE IV DISEASE

When the malignancy has spread to the uterine serosa or beyond it (stage III and IV disease), **pelvic and para-aortic lymph node sampling** should also be performed. These patients will also require **pelvic radiation** therapy in addition to their surgical treatment.

ADVANCED AND RECURRENT DISEASE

High-dose progestins are the first line of treatment for advanced and recurrent disease. **Chemotherapy** may also be used in advanced or recurrent disease but the best regimen and duration of use have yet to be determined.

PROGNOSIS

Because most endometrial cancers are stage I at diagnosis and endometrioid subtype, the **overall 5-year survival rate is quite good—65%**. Survival rates for the various stages of endometrial cancer are 87% for stage I, 76% for stage II, 59% for stage III, and 18%

TABLE 29-8 High-Risk Features for Endometrial Cancer

>50% Myometrial invasion
Papillary serous or clear cell tumors
Grade 3 tumors (>50% solid growth)
Large tumor (>2 cm or filling cavity)
Spread beyond the uterine fundus (Stage III and IV)
Lymphovascular involvement

for stage IV. The presence of certain high-risk features (Table 29-8) confers a higher risk of recurrence and lower survival rates.

FOLLOW-UP

After treatment for endometrial carcinoma, 75% of **recurrences are within the first 2 years** and 85% to 100% in the first 3 years after treatment. Recurrence is most common in women with high-risk features (Table 29-8). Most recurrences (60%) are distant recurrences to upper abdomen or lungs while 40% are local recurrences to the vagina or pelvis. Follow-up should include physical examination every 3 to 6 months for 2 years and then annually and vaginal cytology every 6 months for 2 years and then annually. The first line of treatment for recurrent disease is **chemotherapy** or **high-dose progestin therapy** (Table 29-7). These therapies, typically megestrol (Megace) or medroxyprogesterone (Provera), have been used with a 30% response rate and minimal side effects.

The use of **estrogen replacement therapy** (ERT) in patients treated for endometrial carcinoma has been controversial. A few preliminary studies suggest that ERT may not affect the rate of recurrence of endometrial cancer. However, at this time, ERT is usually reserved for those patients whose cancer was well differentiated and minimally invasive. Even then, ERT is initiated no sooner than 6 to 12 months after treatment. As with traditional use of hormone replacement, use of ERT should be initiated only for symptoms and then only continued for 6 to 12 months.

KEY POINTS

- Endometrial cancer is the most common gynecologic cancer but has the best survival rates because it is associated with early symptoms and easy and accurate diagnostic modalities. It is thus diagnosed and treated early.

- Endometrial cancers are classified as type I (80%) or type II (20%). Type I endometrial cancers can be caused by prolonged exposure to exogenous or endogenous estrogen in the absence of progesterone. Endometrial hyperplasia is the typical precursor to type I disease.

- Type II endometrial cancers are estrogen-independent neoplasms. They are not generally associated with endometrial hyperplasia and tend to occur in older, postmenopausal, thin, nonwhite women. They tend to be more aggressive and have a poorer prognosis than type I cancers.

- The most common type of endometrial cancer (80%) is endometrioid adenocarcinoma. Other types have poorer prognosis, including papillary serous and clear cell carcinomas.

- Endometrioid cancer is diagnosed at a median age of 61 with 25% of patients being diagnosed premenopausally and 75% postmenopausally.

- The major risk factors for type I endometrial cancer include unopposed estrogen exposure, endometrial hyperplasia, obesity, chronic anovulation, nulliparity, and late menopause. Hypertension and diabetes are also important risk factors.

- The most common presenting symptom is abnormal vaginal bleeding.

- Endometrial biopsy is the standard of care for diagnosing endometrial cancer.

- Currently, there are no cost-effective screening tools for endometrial cancer; however, because of abnormal bleeding most women are diagnosed early with 75% of lesions being at stage I at the time of diagnosis.

- Endometrial cancer is surgically staged. Treatment may involve TAHBSO for low-risk, low-stage disease (stages 1 and 2).

- In addition to TAHBSO, pelvic and para-aortic lymphadenectomy and pelvic radiation are used to treat women with stage 3 or 4 disease and those with high-risk features including papillary serous or clear cell types, grade 3 differentiation, large tumor size, lymphovascular invasion, or enlarged lymph nodes.

- Advanced or recurrent disease can be treated with chemotheraphy or high-dose progestin therapy.

- Overall 5-year survival rate is 65% with 85% to 100% of recurrences occurring in the first 3 years after treatment.

Chapter 30

Ovarian and Fallopian Tube Tumors

TUMORS OF THE OVARIES

There are many types of benign and malignant tumors of the ovaries (Table 30-1), each possessing its own characteristics. Fortunately, 80% of ovarian tumors are benign. While fallopian tube carcinoma is extremely rare, ovarian cancer is the **third most common cancer of the female genital tract**, second only to endometrial and cervical cancer (Fig. 30-1). Moreover, ovarian cancer is the fifth most common cause of cancer death in women in the United States and the most common cause of gynecologic cancer death.

Although ovarian carcinoma accounts for 25% of all gynecologic malignancies (21,700 new cases per year), it is **responsible for over 50% of deaths from cancer of the female genital tract** (15,500 deaths per year). This high mortality is due in part to the **lack of effective screening tools** for early diagnosis and in part to the spread by direct extension into the peritoneal cavity. Because the overall **5-year survival rate** for women with ovarian carcinoma is only **25% to 45%**, a high degree of suspicion and prompt diagnosis and intervention are critical.

PATHOGENESIS

Tumors of the ovaries are derived from one of the three distinct components of the ovary: the surface **epithelium**, the ovarian **germ cells,** or the ovarian **stroma** (Fig. 30-2). Over 65% of all ovarian tumors and **90% of all ovarian cancers originate from the epithelium** on the ovary capsule. About 5% to 10% of ovarian cancer is metastatic from other primary tumors in the body, usually from the gastrointestinal tract, breast, or endometrium, and are known as **Krukenberg tumors.**

Ovarian cancer is primarily spread by **direct exfoliation** of malignant cells from the ovaries. As a result, the sites of metastasis often follow the broad circulatory path of the peritoneal fluid. **Lymphatic spread** can also occur, most commonly to the retroperitoneal pelvic and para-aortic lymph nodes (Fig. 28-7). **Hematogenous spread** is responsible for more rare and distant metastases to the lung and brain. In advanced disease, intraperitoneal tumor spread leads to accumulation of ascites in the abdomen and encasement of the bowel with tumor. This results in intermittent bowel obstruction known as a **carcinomatous ileus**. In many cases, this progression results in malnutrition, slow starvation, cachexia, and death.

Although the cause of ovarian carcinoma is unclear, it is believed to result from **malignant transformation of ovarian tissue** after prolonged periods of **chronic uninterrupted ovulation**. Ovulation disrupts the epithelium of the ovary and activates the cellular repair mechanism. When ovulation occurs for long periods of time without interruption, this mechanism is believed to provide the opportunity for somatic **gene deletions** and **mutations** during the cellular repair process.

About 10% to 15% of women with ovarian cancer have a **familial cancer syndrome**. Patients with **Lynch II syndrome** (hereditary nonpolyposis colorectal cancer syndrome, or HNPCC) have a high rate of familial breast, ovarian, colon, and endometrial cancer. Patients with mutations in the **BRCA1** gene have an 85% chance of developing breast cancer and a 30% to 50% chance of developing ovarian cancer. A smaller proportion of patients with **BRCA2** gene mutations

■ TABLE 30-1 Benign and Malignant Ovarian Tumors

Epithelial tumors	Serous tumors	Germ cell tumors (cont.)	Monodermal or specialized (e.g., carcinoid, struma ovarii)
	Serous cystadenoma		Dysgerminoma
	Borderline serous tumor		Endodermal sinus tumor
	Serous cystadenocarcinoma		Choriocarcinoma
	Adenofibroma and cystadenofibroma		Embryonal carcinoma
	Mucinous tumors		Polyembryoma
	Mucinous cystadenoma		Mixed germ cell tumors
	Borderline mucinous tumor	Sex cord–stromal tumors	Granulosa–theca cell tumors
	Mucinous cystadenocarcinoma		Granulosa cell tumor
	Endometrioid carcinoma		Thecoma
	Clear cell adenocarcinoma		Fibroma
	Brenner tumor		Sertoli-Leydig cell tumor (androblastoma)
	Undifferentiated carcinoma		Gonadoblastoma
Germ cell tumors	Teratoma	Unclassified	Ex. lipoid-cell tumors and sarcomas
	Benign (mature, adult)	Metastatic tumors	Ex. from GI tract, female genital tract, or breast
	Cystic teratoma (dermoid cyst)		
	Solid teratoma		
	Malignant (immature)		

Reproduced with permission from Robbins S, Cotran R, Kumar V. *Robbins' Pathologic Basis of Disease*. Philadelphia: WB Saunders, 1991:1158.

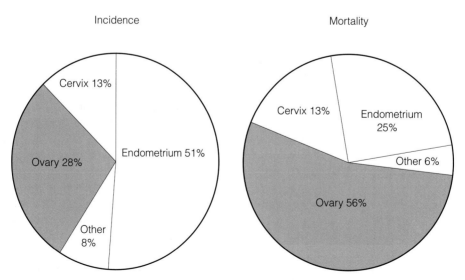

Figure 30-1 • Relationships of ovarian cancer to other gynecologic cancer for incidence and mortality; United States, 1996.
(Modified from Parker SL, Tong T, Bolden S, et al. Cancer statistics. *CA Cancer J Clin* 1996;46:5–27.)

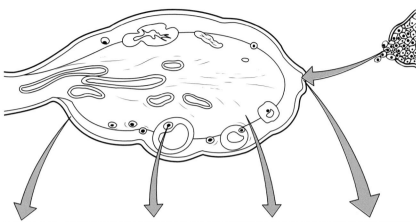

Origin	Surface epithelial cells (common epithelial tumors)	Germ cell	Sex cord–stroma	Metastasis to ovaries
Percent of all ovarian tumors	65–70%	15–20%	5–10%	5%
Age group affected	20+ years	0–25+ years	All ages	Variable
Types	• Serous tumor • Mucinous tumor • Endometrioid tumor • Clear cell tumor • Brenner tumor • Undifferentiated	• Teratoma • Dysgerminoma • Endodermal sinus tumor • Choriocarcinoma • Embryonal carcinoma	• Granulosa–theca cell tumor • Sertoli-Leydig cell tumor • Fibroma	

Figure 30-2 • Classification of various ovarian neoplasms (benign, borderline, and malignant).

(25%) also have an increased risk of ovarian cancer. High dietary fat and agents such as talc and asbestos have also been proposed as possible etiologic agents in the pathogenesis of ovarian carcinoma.

EPIDEMIOLOGY

The average woman has a **1 in 70 chance of developing ovarian carcinoma** over her lifetime and a 1 in 95 chance of dying from invasive ovarian cancer. The median age of diagnosis is 61 years with two-thirds of women with ovarian cancer being over the age of 55 at the time of diagnosis. Hereditary ovarian cancers typically occur in women who are, on average, 10 years younger than those with nonhereditary ovarian cancer, whereas non epithelial ovarian cancers are more common in girls and young women. There is a slight increased frequency in Caucasian women compared to the incidence in Hispanic, Asian, and African American women.

RISK FACTORS

Table 30-2 highlights the major risk factors and protective factors for ovarian cancer. Women with a **familial ovarian cancer syndrome** (BRCA1, BRCA2, or Lynch II syndrome/HNPCC) have the highest risk of ovarian cancer (30% to 50%). Women with a **family history** of ovarian cancer have the next highest risk (5% to 15%). Women with a mother, sister, or daughter with ovarian cancer are at increased risk of developing the disease. The younger the relative is at the time of diagnosis, the higher the risk to first-degree relatives. Similarly, women with a personal history of **breast cancer** have a twofold increase in the incidence of ovarian cancer.

Because the mechanism of ovarian cancer is thought to be linked to mutations occurring during ovulation, women with a history of long periods of **uninterrupted ovulation** (early menarche, infertility, nulliparity, delayed childbearing, late-onset menopause) are at

TABLE 30-2 Risk Factors and Protective Factors for Ovarian Cancer

Risk factors
Familial Ovarian Cancer Syndrome
Family history of breast and/or ovarian cancer
Personal history of breast cancer
Increasing Age
Early menarche (<12 yo)
Infertility
Nulliparity
Late-onset menopause (>50 yo)
Obesity (BMI >30)
Protective factors
Use of oral contraceptives (5+ years)
Multiparity
Breastfeeding
Tubal Ligation
Hysterectomy

increased risk of ovarian cancer. For the same reason, **increasing age** is another major risk factor for ovarian cancer. Fifty percent of all women diagnosed with ovarian cancer are 63 years of age or older.

Other proposed risk factors include the use of talcum powder on the perineum and obesity (BMI >30). It has been suggested that women who undergo ovulation induction with clomiphene citrate (Clomid) for longer than 1 year may be at increased risk of developing ovarian carcinoma. These findings may be confounded by OCP use, infertility, and/or nulliparity.

PROTECTIVE FACTORS

Many of the factors found to be protective from ovarian cancer (Table 30-2) are also linked to the **incessant ovulation** hypotheses. This speculates that ovulation suppression results in less disruption of the ovarian epithelium and less need for activation of the cellular repair mechanism. Thus, there are fewer opportunities for gene deletions and mutations. **Oral contraceptives** (OCPs) have been found to have a protective effect against ovarian cancer by suppressing ovulation. Use of OCPs for greater than 5 years can reduce the risk of ovarian cancer by 50%. Similarly, **breastfeeding**, **multiparity**, and **chronic anovulation**

have also been found to be protective agents that act by interrupting or suppressing ovulation. **Tubal ligation** and **hysterectomy** have been associated with a 67% and 30% reduction in ovarian cancer, respectively; even in patients with a familial cancer syndrome. This may be due to impairment of ovarian blood supply by these procedures and/or decreased migration of carcinogens from the lower genital tract up to the ovaries.

CLINICAL MANIFESTATIONS

History

Patients with ovarian cancer are most often **asymptomatic** or have **vague**, **nonspecific complaints** until the disease has progressed to the advanced stages. Some patients may present with **vague lower abdominal pain**, abdominal distension, bloating, and **early satiety** (Table 30-3). As the tumors progress, other symptoms may develop, including gastrointestinal complaints (nausea, anorexia, indigestion), urinary frequency, dysuria, and pelvic pressure. Ascites may develop in later stages and cause shortness of breath secondary to pleural effusion. Ventral hernia may also be seen due to increased intra-abdominal pressure.

Physical Examination

There is no evidence to suggest that routine pelvic examination improves the early diagnosis of ovarian

TABLE 30-3 Symptoms of Ovarian Cancer

Initial symptoms
Bloating
Early satiety
Dyspepsia
Abdominal pain
Pelvic pain
Later Symptoms
Back pain
Urinary frequency/urgency
Constipation
Fatigue
Dyspareunia
Menstrual changes

TABLE 30-4 Evaluation of Pelvic and Abdominal Masses Found on Physical Exam

	Benign	Malignant
Mobility	Mobile	Fixed
Consistency	Cystic	Solid
Tumor surface	Smooth	Irregular
Bilateral or unilateral	Unilateral	Bilateral

cancer. As the disease progresses, the primary findings on examination are a **solid, fixed, irregular pelvic mass** (Table 30-4) that may extend into the upper abdomen and **ascites** (Color Plate 15). Ovarian cancer metastasis to the umbilicus is known as **Sister Mary Joseph nodule**. When a mass is located on exam, there is an increased likelihood of cancer in postmenopausal women (30% to 60%) compared with premenopausal women (5% to 15%).

DIAGNOSTIC EVALUATION

Pelvic ultrasound is the primary diagnostic tool for investigating an adnexal mass. These sonographic traits help to distinguish between benign and malignant tumors (Table 30-5). Other studies, including **computed tomography** (CT) and **magnetic resonance imaging** (MRI) of the pelvis and abdomen, can assist in diagnosis and in delineation of the spread of disease. Because malignant cells can spread via direct exfoliation, paracentesis and cyst aspiration should be avoided. Once the diagnosis is made, studies are undertaken to look for **metastatic disease** and to distinguish between primary and secondary ovarian cancer. **Barium enema and intravenous pyelography** (IVP) are helpful in looking for GI and GU sources of disease.

Depending on the type of tumor, ovarian malignancies can be monitored using the **serum tumor markers** CA-125, α-fetoprotein (AFP), lactate dehydrogenase (LDH), and human chorionic gonadotropins (hCG).

SURGICAL STAGING

Ovarian carcinoma is **surgically staged** (Table 30-6). Primary staging includes total abdominal hysterectomy, bilateral salpingo-oophorectomy (**TAHBSO**), **omentectomy, peritoneal washings,** Pap smear of the diaphragm, and **sampling the pelvic and paraaortic lymph nodes.** Because there are no reliable screening tools for ovarian cancer and few early symptoms, nearly 75% of patients present with stage III or IV. Subsequently, the 5-year survival is low overall (25% to 45%) and decreases with increasing age. The different types of ovarian cancers are discussed below.

EPITHELIAL TUMORS

PATHOGENESIS

Epithelial cell tumors of the ovaries are derived from malignant transformation of the **epithelium cells** of the surface of the ovary. These cells come from the primitive mesoderm and are capable of undergoing metaplasia. The six primary types of epithelial tumors are serous, mucinous, endometrioid, clear cell, Brenner, and undifferentiated (Fig. 30-2). The neoplasms in this group range in malignant potential from benign to borderline (tumors of **low malignant potential**) to frankly malignant. **Serous cystadenocarcinomas** are the most common malignant epithelial cell tumors.

TABLE 30-5 Ultrasound Findings in Patients with a Pelvic Mass

	Benign	Malignant
Size	<8 cm	>8 cm
Consistency	Cystic	Solid or cystic and solid
Solid components	Not present	Nodular, papillary
Septations	Not present or singular	Multilocular, thick (>2 mm)
Doppler flow	Not present	Present in solid component
Bilateral or unilateral	Unilateral	Bilateral
Associated features	Calcification, esp. teeth	Ascites, peritoneal masses, lymphadenopathy

■ **TABLE 30-6** Staging of Ovarian Carcinoma
Stage I: Growth limited to the ovaries
Ia — one ovary involved
Ib — both ovaries involved
Ic — Ia or Ib and ovarian surface tumor, ruptured capsule, malignant ascites, or peritoneal cytology positive for malignant cells
Stage II: Disease extension from the ovary to the pelvis
IIa — extension to the uterus or fallopian tube
IIb — extension to other pelvic tissues
IIc — IIa or IIb and ovarian surface tumor, ruptured capsule, malignant ascites, or peritoneal cytology positive for malignant cells
Stage III: Disease extension to the abdominal cavity
IIIa — abdominal peritoneal surfaces with microscopic metastases
IIIb — tumor metastases >2 cm in size
IIIc — tumor metastases >2 cm in size or metastatic disease in the pelvic, para-aortic, or inguinal lymph nodes
Stage IV: Distant metastatic disease
Malignant pleural effusion
Pulmonary parenchymal metastases
Liver or splenic parenchymal metastases (not surface implants)
Metastases to the supraclavicular lymph nodes or skin

Malignant epithelial tumors extend through the capsule of the ovary to seed the peritoneal cavity. They rarely invade the underlying ovary. These are **slow-growing tumors** that often remain undiagnosed until they are very large and at an advanced stage. In over 75% of patients, tumors have spread beyond the ovary at the time of diagnosis; thus the prognosis is very poor.

EPIDEMIOLOGY

Epithelial tumors tend to occur in patients who are in their 50s with a peak incidence from 56 to 60 years of age. **Epithelial cell cancers account for 65% of all ovarian tumors** and more than **90% of ovarian cancers. Serous tumors** (serous cystadenocarcinomas) are the most common type of epithelial ovarian cancer. These tumors are large, cystic, and bilateral 65% of the time.

CLINICAL MANIFESTATIONS

The serum tumor marker **CA-125** is elevated in 80% of epithelial cell cancers. Because CA-125 levels correlate with the progression and regression of these

tumors, it has been useful in **tracking the effect of treatment and recurrence** of epithelial ovarian carcinoma. Its value as a screening tool for the detection of ovarian cancer has not yet been established. One reason for this is the high number of benign and malignant gynecologic and nongynecologic conditions associated with an elevated CA-125 level (Table 30-7).

TREATMENT

Surgery is the mainstay of treatment for epithelial cell tumors, including TAHBSO, omentectomy, cytoreduction or "debulking," and bilateral pelvic and paraaortic lymph node sampling. The goal of debulking is to leave behind no tumor mass greater than 1 cm. When this is achieved, the patient is said to have undergone optimal debulking. When optimal debulking is not achieved, there is a greater chance of recurrent or persistent disease.

After surgery, epithelial ovarian cancer is treated with combination chemotherapy, most commonly **carboplatin and paclitaxel** (Taxol) or docetaxel (Taxotere). Patients who have had optimal debulking may be offered **intraperitoneal chemotherapy** which

■ TABLE 30-7 Gynecologic and Nongynecologic Conditions Associated with Elevated CA-125 Levels

Gynecologic cancers
Epithelial ovarian cancer
Fallopian tube cancer
Endometrial cancer
Endocervical cancer
Nongynecologic cancers
Pancreatic cancer
Lung cancer
Breast cancer
Colon cancer
Benign gynecologic conditions
Normal and ectopic pregnancy
Endometriosis
Fibroids
Pelvic inflammatory disease
Benign nongynecologic conditions
Pancreatitis
Cirrhosis
Peritonitis
Recent laparotomy

can be more effective but also has more complications than traditional intravenous chemotherapy.

In the past, after completion of chemotherapy, a second-look laparoscopy or laparotomy was performed to evaluate the patient's response to treatment. This is no longer the standard of care and is generally reserved for the research setting. The tumor marker **CA-125** and **CAT scan imaging** are most commonly used to evaluate the success of treatment and to diagnose recurrent disease. Unfortunately, the tumors **frequently recur** despite aggressive treatment. Recurrent or persistent cancer is treated with combination chemotherapy. Recurrent ascites is treated with paracentesis.

The overall **5-year survival rate is 20%** for patients with epithelial cell ovarian cancer (80% to 95% for stage I, 40% to 70% for stage II, 30% for stage III, and less than 10% for stage IV disease).

GERM CELL TUMORS

PATHOGENESIS

Germ cell ovarian tumors arise from primordial germ cells of the ovary and may be benign (95%) or malignant (5%). These undifferentiated, totipotent germ cells are capable of differentiating into any of the three germ cell layers: yolk sac, placenta, and fetus. This accounts for the various subtypes of germ cell tumors (Fig. 30-3).

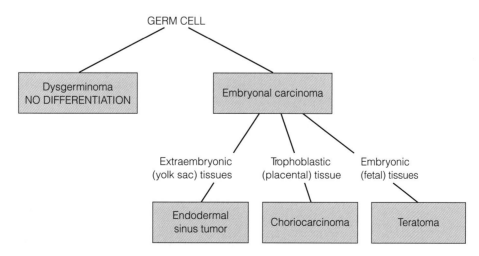

Figure 30-3 • Histogenesis of tumors of germ cell origin. Because they are totipotent, germ cells may remain undifferentiated or they may develop into any of the three germ layers: yolk sac or placental or fetal tissue.

The most common type of germ cell tumor is the **benign cystic mature teratoma**, also known as **dermoid cysts**. Dermoids are cystic masses containing mature adult tissue such as skin, hair, and teeth mixed in sebaceous material giving them a very characteristic appearance (Color Plate 16). Cystectomy is recommended for definitive diagnosis and to rule out malignancy.

The most common malignant germ cell tumors are **dysgerminomas (50%)**, **immature teratomas (20%)**, and endodermal sinus (yolk sac) tumors (20%). Embryonal carcinoma (composed of undifferentiated cells), nongestational choriocarcinoma (composed of placental tissue), and mixed germ cell tumors are much less common.

Many of these tumors produce **serum tumor markers** that can be useful in the diagnosis of a pelvic mass and in assessing a patient's response to therapy (Table 30-8). Although there is wide variation in the type of serum tumor markers produced by ovarian tumors, in general, dysgerminomas produce LDH, endodermal sinus (yolk sac) tumors produce AFP, and choriocarcinomas produce hCG. The undifferentiated embryonal carcinomas that give rise to the more differentiated germ cell tumors produce both AFP and hCG.

In contrast to epithelial tumors, most germ cell tumors **grow rapidly**, are **limited to one ovary**, and are at **stage I** at the time of diagnosis. The prognosis for germ cell tumors is therefore far better than that for epithelial tumors. In most cases, **these tumors are considered curable.**

EPIDEMIOLOGY

Germ cell tumors account for 20% to 25% of all ovarian tumors but make up less than 5% of ovarian cancers. Although **95% are benign**, the remaining 5% of germ cell tumors are malignant and found primarily in children and young women. This makes germ cell tumors the **most common ovarian malignancy in women less than 20 years of age**. Malignant germ cell tumors are three times more common in **black and Asian women** compared to Caucasian women.

CLINICAL MANIFESTATIONS

Unlike the slow-growing epithelial ovarian cancers, germ cell tumors **grow rapidly** and thus cause symptoms leading to earlier diagnosis. Most commonly, distension of the ovarian capsule from rapid growth, **hemorrhage**, **and necrosis** results in acute **pelvic pain**. Patients may also complain of **pressure symptoms** on the bladder or rectum or pain from **torsion or rupture** of the tumor. Eighty-five percent of women will have abdominal pain and a pelvic mass at the time of presentation.

TREATMENT

Women with benign germ cell tumors such as mature teratomas (dermoid cysts) are diagnosed and cured by removing the part of the ovary containing the tumor (ovarian cystectomy) or by removing the entire ovary (oophorectomy).

Because most germ cell cancers are diagnosed in the early stage and are **rarely bilateral**, surgery is typically limited to **unilateral salpingo-oophorectomy** if fertility is desired. However, complete surgical staging should still be performed. If childbearing is complete or if the cancer is bilateral, total abdominal hysterectomy and bilateral salpingo-oophorectomy **(TAH/BSO)** is required along with surgical staging.

With the exception of stage IA dysgerminomas and immature teratomas, all germ cell malignancies require **multiagent chemotherapy** after surgery. The most common regimen is BEP: bleomycin, etoposide, and cisplatin (Platinol). In patients who have elevated **serum tumor markers** prior to treatment, these markers can be used to judge the effectiveness of therapy between chemotherapy cycles.

In the past, **radiation therapy** was used as the primary treatment for **dysgerminomas**, which are exquisitely sensitive to radiation. However, current combination chemotherapy regimens have proven to be as good as or better than radiation therapy. Chemotherapy is also more protective of future fertility when only one ovary is removed.

■ **TABLE 30-8** Primary Serum Tumor Marker for Germ Cell Cancers	
Tumor Type	**Primary Tumor Marker**
Dysgerminoma	LDH
Immature teratoma	N/A
Endodermal sinus (yolk sac) tumor	AFP
Embryonal carcinoma	AFP and hCG
Choriocarcinoma	hCG

Fortunately, most cases of germ cell cancer are **considered curable** with surgery and chemotherapy. The overall 5-year survival rate is 85% for dysgerminomas, 70% to 80% for immature teratomas, and 60% to 70% for endodermal sinus tumors.

SEX CORD-STROMAL TUMORS

PATHOGENESIS

Ovarian stromal cell tumors originate from either the cells surrounding the oocyte (before the differentiation into male or female) or from the ovarian stroma (Fig. 30-2). In general, these tumors are **low-grade malignancies,** which can **occur at any age.** They are **usually unilateral** and **do not often recur.** Granulosa-theca cells are low-grade malignancies and the most common (70%) type of tumor in this group. Sertoli-Leydig tumors are very rare.

Both granulosa-theca cell tumors and Sertoli-Leydig cell tumors are known as **functional tumors** because they are characterized by **hormone production.** Ovarian stroma can develop into an ovary or a testis. As a result, ovarian **granulosa-theca cell tumors** resemble fetal ovaries and produce large amounts of estrogens. Microscopically, the granulosa cells have grooved "coffee-bean" nuclei and the cells are arranged in small clusters around a central cavity. These histologic configurations are known as **Call-Exner bodies** which are pathognomonic for granulosa cell tumors. Conversely, ovarian **Sertoli-Leydig cell tumors** resemble fetal testes and produce testosterone and other androgens.

The third type of germ cell tumor, the **ovarian fibroma,** is derived from mature fibroblasts and, unlike the other sex cord-stromal tumors, is not a functioning tumor. Occasionally, fibromas are associated with ascites. The presence of ovarian **tumor, ascites, and right hydrothorax** is known as **Meigs syndrome.**

EPIDEMIOLOGY

Sex cord-stromal ovarian tumors can affect women of any age but occur most commonly in women between ages **40 and 70.** The mean age at diagnosis is 50. Due to estrogen stimulation, 25% to 50% of women with granulosa cell tumors will have **endometrial hyperplasia** and 5% will have concurrent **endometrial cancer.** Most Sertoli-Leydig tumors occur in women under 40.

CLINICAL MANIFESTATIONS

Granulosa-theca cell tumors often produce **estradiol and inhibin A/B.** The estrogen stimulation can cause feminization, precocious puberty, menstrual irregularities, secondary amenorrhea, or postmenopausal bleeding. This estrogen stimulation can lead to endometrial hyperplasia and/or endometrial cancer; therefore **endometrial sampling** is very important in this setting. Sertoli-Leydig cell tumors produce **androgens** (testosterone, androstenedione) that can cause **virilizing effects** in 75% of patients including breast atrophy, hirsutism, deepened voice, acne, clitoromegaly, and receding hairline. Patients may also have oligomenorrhea or amenorrhea.

TREATMENT

Because most sex cord-stromal tumors are low-grade lesions, unilateral, and do not often recur, the usual treatment is **unilateral salpingo-oophorectomy.** In women who have completed their childbearing, hysterectomy and bilateral salpingo-oophorectomy (TAH/BSO) should be performed. Chemotherapy and radiation have no regular role in treating sex cord-stromal cell cancers.

The 5-year survival rate for patients with sex cord-stromal carcinomas is 70% to 90%. However, granulosa cell tumors are slow growing and late recurrences can be detected 15 to 20 years after removal of the primary lesion.

CANCER OF THE FALLOPIAN TUBES

PATHOGENESIS

Fallopian tube carcinoma is **extremely rare,** comprising only 0.5% of all cancers of the female genital tract. The etiology of the cancer is unknown. Most fallopian tube cancers are **adenocarcinomas** arising from the mucosa of the tube. Sarcomas and mixed tumors are less common. The tube is often hugely dilated and the lumen is filled with papillary growth of solid tumor. The fimbriated end is closed in 50% of cases. The disease progression of these tumors is **similar to that of ovarian cancer,** including wide **peritoneal spread** and **ascites** accumulation. The cancer is bilateral in 10% of cases and is **often the result of metastasis** from other primary tumors.

EPIDEMIOLOGY

Primary fallopian tube carcinoma is very rare. These tumors can occur at any age (18 to 80), but the mean age at diagnosis is 55 to 60. Like epithelial ovarian cancers, fallopian tube cancers occur **more frequently in Caucasian women** as compared with African American women. Risk factors include **familial cancer syndromes** (BRCA1 and BRCA2), **nulliparity**, and **infertility**.

CLINICAL MANIFESTATIONS

Fallopian tube cancer is typically **asymptomatic** and is usually diagnosed during pelvic surgery for other indications. The classic triad of **profuse watery discharge, pelvic pain,** and **pelvic mass** is known as Latzko's triad. Although the triad is seen in only 15% of cases, it is considered pathognomonic for fallopian tube carcinoma. The same is true for **hydrops tubae profluens** (intermittent hydrosalpinx), the phenomenon of spontaneous or pressure-induced discharge of watery or blood-tinged vaginal discharge resulting in shrinkage of the adnexal mass. Patients may also report low back pain.

DIAGNOSIS

The diagnosis of fallopian tube cancer is almost never made preoperatively. **Ultrasound** may reveal a complex adnexal mass or ascites. The **CA-125** is often elevated in these patients and **cervical cytology** may rarely show malignant cells with subsequent negative cervical and endometrial biopsy.

TREATMENT

Fallopian tube cancers are **surgically staged**. One-third of patients are stage I at the time of diagnosis, one-third are stage II, and one-third are stage III or IV. The treatment of fallopian tube cancer is the same as that of epithelial ovarian cancer including TAHBSO, omentectomy, cytoreduction, peritoneal cytologic studies, and retroperitoneal lymph node sampling. After surgery, adjunctive chemotherapy is given including **carboplatin and paclitaxel (Taxol)**. CA-125 levels can be used to monitor the effectiveness of treatment.

The prognosis for fallopian tube cancer is slightly better than that of epithelial ovarian cancer. The overall 5-year survival rate is 45% (71% for stage I, 48% for stage II, 25% for stage III, and 17% for stage IV disease).

 KEY POINTS

- Epithelial tumors of the ovary are derived from the ovarian epithelium and account for 90% of ovarian cancers.

- Epithelial tumors of the ovary are slow-growing so most patients are asymptomatic or may have non-specific vague complaints. Therefore, over 75% of patients are diagnosed at stage III or higher.

- When symptoms are present, they might include low abdominal pain, bloating, early satiety, pelvic mass, and ascites. Pelvic ultrasound and abdominal-pelvic CT often reveal a fixed, solid, nodular mass.

- Epithelial ovarian cancers are staged surgically and treated with surgery (TAHBSO, omentectomy, pelvic and paraaortic lymph node sampling, and cytoreduction) followed by Taxol and carboplatin chemotherapy.

- The tumor marker CA-125 can be used to evaluate the success of treatment and look for recurrence of disease but is not appropriate to use as a screening tool for ovarian cancer.

- The 5-year survival rate for epithelial ovarian cancer is less than 20%.

- Germ cell tumors arise from totipotential germ cells capable of differentiating into yolk sac, placental or fetal tissues; 95% are benign and 5% are malignant.

- The most common germ cell tumor is the benign mature cystic teratoma (dermoid cyst). The most common malignant germ cell tumors are dysgerminomas (50%) and immature teratomas (20%).

- Germ cell tumors occur primarily in women under age 20, grow rapidly, are usually unilateral, and are diagnosed at early stages. They often produce serum tumor markers (LDH, AFP, and/or hCG) that can be used in the diagnosis of a pelvic mass and to assess response to therapy.

- Most germ cell tumors are treated by removal of the affected ovary, staging, and combination chemotherapy with bleomycin, etoposide, and cisplatin (BEP) with good 5-year survival rates (60% to 85%) depending on the type of tumor.

- Sex cord-stromal germ cell tumors are derived from the cells surrounding the oocyte that produce steroid hormones or from the ovarian stroma.

- Sex cord-stromal tumors are slow-growing tumors with low malignant potential and are often found only incidentally, usually in women between 40 and 70 years old. Sertoli-Leydig cell tumors are rare and occur most often in women under 40.

- Granulosa cell tumors are the most common type (70%) of sex cord-stromal tumor. They secrete inhibin and estradiol, resulting in feminization and potentially endometrial hyperplasia and/or cancer. Microscopic Call-Exner bodies are pathognomonic for granulosa cell tumors.

- Sertoli-Leydig cell tumors are rare. They secrete androgens causing virilization in patients.

- Ovarian fibromas are derived from mature fibroblasts. These are nonfunctioning tumors. Meigs syndrome consists of the triad of ovarian tumor, ascites, and right hydrothorax.

- The sex cord-stromal tumors are treated surgically, usually with unilateral salpingo-oophorectomy in younger women or TAHBSO in women who have completed their childbearing.

- Sertoli-Leydig cell tumors do not frequently recur, but granulosa cell tumors often have late recurrences 15 to 20 years later.

- Fallopian tube cancers are rare malignancies that can occur at any age. They behave very similar to epithelial ovarian cancers.

- These are usually adenocarcinomas arising from the mucosa or metastases from other primary tumors. Fallopian tube cancers are usually asymptomatic and are rarely diagnosed preoperatively.

- The classic triad of pain, profuse watery discharge (hydrops tubae profluens), and pelvic mass is considered pathognomonic for fallopian tube carcinoma but only occurs in 15% of patients.

- Fallopian tube cancers are treated similar to epithelial ovarian cancers with TAHBSO, omentectomy, cytoreduction, and pelvic lymph node sampling followed by combination chemotherapy with carboplatin and Taxol.

- The overall 5-year survival rate is 45%.

31 Gestational Trophoblastic Disease

Gestational trophoblastic disease (GTD) is a diverse group of interrelated diseases resulting in the **abnormal proliferation of trophoblastic (placental) tissue**. GTD can be grouped into four major classifications (Table 31-1): molar pregnancies (80%), persistent/invasive moles (10% to 15%), choriocarcinoma (2% to 5%), and very rare placental site trophoblastic tumors (PSTTs). These tumors are unique in that the maternal tumor results from **abnormal fetal tissue** rather than maternal tissue. These neoplasms also share the ability to **produce human chorionic gonadotropin (hCG)**, which serves both as a tumor marker for diagnosing the disease and as a tool for measuring the effects of treatment. GTD is also **extremely sensitive to chemotherapy** and is therefore the most curable gynecologic malignancy and one of the few that may allow for the **preservation of fertility**.

BENIGN GESTATIONAL TROPHOBLASTIC DISEASE

Benign GTD consists of molar pregnancies, also known as **hydatidiform moles**. Complete and partial moles account for 80% of all GTD. Ninety percent of molar pregnancies are classified as **classic** or **complete moles** and are the result of molar degeneration but have no associated fetus. Ten percent of molar pregnancies are classified as **partial or incomplete moles** and are the result of molar degeneration in association with an abnormal fetus. The characteristics of complete and partial molar pregnancies are compared in Table 31-2.

EPIDEMIOLOGY

The incidence of molar pregnancy is about **1 in 1,000 pregnancies** among white women in the United States. There is a decreased rate of GTD in black women in the United States. The worldwide incidence of molar pregnancy **varies from region to region**. Low and intermediate rates are seen in North America and Europe while Latin America and Asia have moderate to high rates. The global rate is **highest among Asian women**, particularly in Japan, where molar pregnancies occur in 1 in 500 pregnancies.

RISK FACTORS

Extremes in age and **prior history of GTD** are two of the major risk factors for molar pregnancy. There is a slight increase in women under 20 and a significant increase in women over 35 years old. Women over 35 also have an increased risk of malignant disease. Similarly, women with a **history of GTD** are at increased risk to have subsequent pregnancies affected by gestational trophoblastic disease. The baseline risk of GTD in a woman with no previous history of the disease is 0.1%. That risk increased to 1% in women with one prior molar pregnancy and can be as high as 16% to 28% in a woman with two prior molar pregnancies.

Over 70% of women with GTD have never given birth, making **nulliparity** another important risk factor. Conversely, the rate of GTD seems to decrease with increasing parity. Higher incidences have also been found in geographic areas where the **diet is low in beta-carotene, folic acid, and animal fat**. Other possible associated factors include **smoking, infertility**, and a history of **OCP use**.

COMPLETE MOLAR PREGNANCIES

PATHOGENESIS

Although the cause of molar pregnancy is unknown, it is believed that most **complete moles** result from the fertilization of an enucleate ovum or **empty egg**, one whose nucleus is missing or nonfunctional, by **one normal sperm** which then replicates itself (Fig. 31-1). All of the resultant chromosomes are therefore **paternally derived**. The most common chromosomal pattern for complete moles is 46,XX. Rarely, a complete mole may be formed by the fertilization of an empty egg by two normal sperm. In this case as well, all chromosomes are parentally derived.

■ **TABLE 31-1** Classification of GTD
Benign GTD (80%)
Complete mole (classic mole)
Partial mole (incomplete mole)
Malignant GTD (20%)
Persistent/invasive mole
Choriocarcinoma
Placental site trophoblastic tumors

The placental abnormality in a complete mole is characterized by noninvasive **trophoblastic proliferation** associated with diffuse swelling of the chorionic villi. This **hydropic degeneration** gives the complete mole the appearance of grape-like vesicles filling the uterus in the **absence of a fetus** villi (Fig. 31-2).

■ **TABLE 31-2** Comparison of Characteristics of Complete and Partial Molar Pregnancies		
Features	**Complete (Classic) Mole (90%)**	**Partial (Incomplete) Mole (10%)**
Genetics		
Most common karyotype	46,XX	69,XXY
Chromosomal origin	All paternally derived	Extra paternal set
Pathology		
Coexistent fetus	Absent	Present
Fetal red blood cells	Absent	Present
Chorionic villi	Hydropic (swollen)	Few hydropic
Trophoblasts	Severe hyperplasia	Minimal/no hyperplasia
Clinical presentation		
Associated embryo	None	Present
Symptoms/signs	Abnormal vaginal bleeding	Missed abortion
Classic symptoms*	Common	Rare
Uterine size	50% large for dates	Size equals dates
Theca lutein cysts	present in 25%	Rare
hCG levels	High (>100,000)	Slightly elevated
Malignant potential		
Nonmetastatic disease	15% to 25%	2% to 4%
Metastatic disease	4%	0%
Follow up		
Weeks to normal hCG	14 weeks	8 weeks
* Hyperemesis gravidarum, early preeclampsia, hyperthyroidism, anemia, excessive uterine enlargement.		

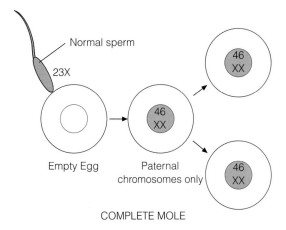

Figure 31-1 • A complete mole arises from the fertilization of an empty enucleate egg by a normal sperm. The sperm duplicates its own chromosomes, resulting in a 46,XX diploid karyotype; all of the chromosomes are, therefore, of paternal origin. (From Beckmann C & Ling F. *Obstetrics & Gynecology*, 5th ed. Philadelphia: Lippincott Williams & Wilkins, 2006.)

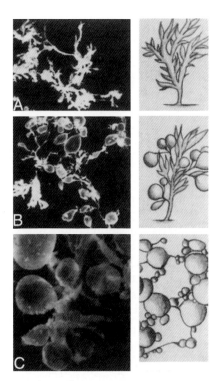

Figure 31-2 • Gross morphology of villi. **(A)** Normal chorionic villi. **(B)** Partial mole with normal villi admixed with swollen ones (case of triploidy, 69,XXY). **(C)** Complete mole with swollen, vesicular villi.

In complete molar pregnancy there is abnormal proliferation of the syncytiotrophoblasts which produce hCG. This is responsible for the extremely **high hCG levels** (>100,000 mIU/mL) that can be associated with complete moles. These high hCG levels explain many of the signs and symptoms associated with complete moles. Recall that hCG has both an alpha and a beta subunit. While the beta subunit is unique to hCG, the **alpha subunit is also found in LH, FSH, and TSH**. Therefore, high hCG levels associated with complete moles can act as a homolog to LH and FSH resulting in stimulation of **large theca lutein cysts** (>6 cm). hCG can similarly act as a homolog to TSH resulting in **hyperthyroidism** in patients with complete moles. The high hCG levels can also cause **hyperemesis gravidarum** and early **preeclampsia** in these patients as well.

Although most molar pregnancies are benign, complete moles have a **higher malignant potential** than do partial moles (Table 31-2).

CLINICAL PRESENTATION

History

The most common presenting symptom of molar pregnancy is **irregular or heavy vaginal bleeding** during early pregnancy (97%). The bleeding is due to separation of the tumor from the underlying decidua resulting in disruption of the maternal vessels. Table 31-3 lists other conditions associated with complete molar pregnancy, in descending order of frequency. Many of these symptoms can be attributed to the **high hCG levels** including severe nausea and vomiting (from **hyperemesis gravidarum**); irritability, dizziness, and photophobia (from **preeclampsia**); or nervousness,

■ **TABLE 31-3** Symptoms Associated with Molar Pregnancy	
Symptoms	**Percent**
Vaginal bleeding	90 to 97
Passage of molar vesicles	80
Anemia	50
Uterine size greater than dates	30 to 50
Bilateral theca lutein cysts	25
Hyperemesis gravidarum	10 to 25
Pre-eclampsia before 20 weeks' gestation	10 to 15
Hyperthyroidism	10
Trophoblastic pulmonary embolic	2

anorexia, and tremors (from **hyperthyroidism** although subclinical hyperthyroidism is more common than overt hyperthyroidism). In fact, in the absence of chronic hypertension, preeclampsia occurring prior to 20 weeks' gestation is pathognomonic for molar pregnancy. Fortunately, due to earlier diagnosis and treatment of molar pregnancy, these conditions are seen less often than they were historically.

Physical Examination

In complete molar pregnancy, the physical examination may show sequelae of **preeclampsia** (hypertension) or **hyperthyroidism** (tachycardia, tachypnea). The abdominal examination in molar pregnancy may be remarkable for the **absence of fetal heart sounds** since there is no associated fetus in complete molar pregnancy. The **uterine size is greater** than the anticipated "gestational age" due to the presence of tumor, hemorrhage, and clot in the uterus. The pelvic examination may reveal the expulsion of **grape-like molar clusters** into the vagina or blood in the cervical os. Occasionally, the provider may palpate large bilateral **theca lutein cysts** (Fig. 31-3).

DIAGNOSTIC EVALUATION

In the presence of a molar pregnancy, quantitative serum **hCG levels can be extremely high** (>100,000 mIU/mL), relative to values for normal pregnancy. The hCG level reflects the amount of tumor volume and can be used for diagnosis and risk stratification and assessment of treatment effectiveness. Confirmation of GTD is usually made using **pelvic ultrasound**. In the case of a complete mole, no fetus or amniotic fluid is present. Instead, the intrauterine tissue appears as a **"snowstorm" pattern** due to swelling of chorionic villi (Fig. 31-3). The scan may also reveal **bilateral theca lutein cysts**, which appear as large (>6 cm) multilocular cysts on both ovaries. The definitive diagnosis of molar pregnancy is made on **pathologic examination of the intrauterine tissue** once the uterus is evacuated.

DIFFERENTIAL DIAGNOSIS

The differential diagnosis for gestational trophoblastic disease includes conditions that can result in abnormally high hCG levels, vaginal bleeding in pregnancy, and/or enlarged placentas such as multiple gestation pregnancy, erythroblastosis fetalis, intrauterine infec-

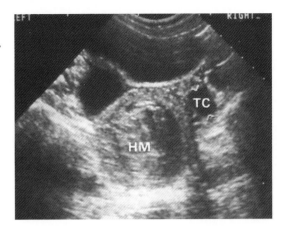

Figure 31-3 • Ultrasound scan of a complete molar pregnancy demonstrating the classic "snow storm" appearance. Large theca lutein cysts can sometime be seen on the ovary (not pictured here).

tion, uterine fibroids, threatened abortion, ectopic pregnancy, or normal intrauterine pregnancy.

TREATMENT

The treatment for molar pregnancy, regardless of the duration of pregnancy, is **immediate removal of the uterine contents** with suction curettage (D&C). Prior to evacuation of the uterus, laboratory examination should include a baseline hCG level, a complete blood count (CBC), coagulation studies, along with renal, thyroid, and liver function tests. Maternal blood type and antibody screen should also be obtained to determine **Rh(D) status** and to prepare for the possibility of heavy vaginal bleeding during the procedure. A chest x-ray (CXR) is not longer routinely necessary. If a patient is demonstrating signs of preeclampsia, **antihypertensives** may be used to decrease risk of maternal stroke. Similarly, patients with sequelae of hCG-induced hyperthyroidism benefit from the use of **beta blockers** such as propranolol to avoid precipitation of **thyroid storm** by the anesthesia and the surgical procedure.

Prior to the procedure, **cross-matched blood** should be made available in case of heavy bleeding and **intravenous (IV) access** should be maximized. **General anesthesia** is typically used given the risk of hemorrhage and complications such as thyroid storm and **trophoblastic embolization**. Dilation and suction curettage (D&C) is the definitive treatment for most patients with complete molar pregnancy. After the uterine contents have been removed, **intravenous oxytocin** can be administered to stimulate uterine contraction and minimize blood loss. Even though no fetal tissue is present, Rh immunoglobulin (**RhoGAM**) should be given to all Rh-negative women. Patients with **theca lutein cysts** can be managed expectantly. In general, the cysts will slowly resolve as the hCG levels decrease following the procedure.

If the patient with a molar pregnancy has completed childbearing, **hysterectomy** is an alternate therapy. While this will eliminate the risk of local invasion, hysterectomy does not prevent metastasis of the disease.

FOLLOW-UP

The prognosis for molar pregnancy is excellent, with **95% to 100% cure rates** after suction curettage. Persistent disease will develop in 15% to 25% of patients with complete moles and in 4% of patients with partial moles. For this reason, close follow-up is essential even after hysterectomy.

After evacuation of a molar pregnancy, **serial hCG titers** should be monitored to ensure complete resolution of the disease. For this monitoring, a radioimmunoassay specific for GTD should be used and the same lab should be used for each measurement. Levels should be measured within 48 hours of uterine evacuation and then **weekly until negative for 3 consecutive weeks**. The levels should then be followed monthly for 6 months. Figure 31-4 demonstrates the normal regression of hCG titers after molar evacuation. The average time to normalization of levels is **14 weeks** for a complete mole compared to 2 to 4 weeks following a normal pregnancy, miscarriage, or termination. A **plateau or rise** in hCG levels during monitoring or the presence of **hCG greater than 6 months after the D&C** is indicative of persistent/invasive disease.

To ensure resolution of the disease, hCG monitoring is critical. Therefore, it is essential to **prevent pregnancy** during the follow-up period. Oral contraceptive pills are typically used given their low failure rate and low risk of irregular bleeding.

Patients who are cured of the disease can have normal pregnancies after treatment with no increase in the rate of spontaneous abortion, complications, or congenital malformations. However, all subsequent pregnancies should be closely monitored with **early ultrasound** and **hCG levels** to exclude recurrent disease. Following delivery, an **hCG level** should be checked at the 6-week postpartum visit. It is no longer necessary to send the placenta for pathologic examination but any tissue obtained from a miscarriage or

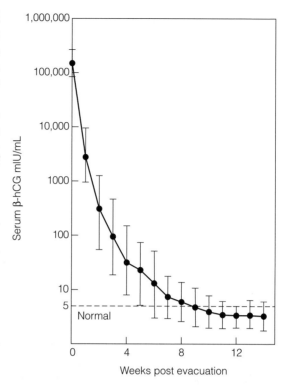

Figure 31-4 • Normal regression of β-hCG levels after molar evacuation of the uterus. The average time to normalization of levels is 8 to 14 weeks.

termination should be evaluated for molar tissue. The risk of developing **recurrent GTD** is approximately **1% to 2% after one molar pregnancy** (compared to 0.1% in the general population) but as high as 16% to 28% after two molar pregnancies. This holds true even after hysterectomy.

PARTIAL MOLAR PREGNANCY

PATHOGENESIS

A **partial or incomplete mole** is formed when a normal ovum is fertilized by two sperm simultaneously (Fig. 31-5). This results in a **triploid karyotype** with 69 chromosomes, of which two sets are paternally derived. The most common karyotype is **69,XXY** (80%). The placental abnormality in a partial mole is characterized by focal hydropic villi and trophoblastic hyperplasia primarily of the cytotrophoblast. Since cytotrophoblasts do not produce hCG, hCG levels in partial molar pregnancies are **normal or only slightly elevated** compared with the extreme elevations seen in complete moles.

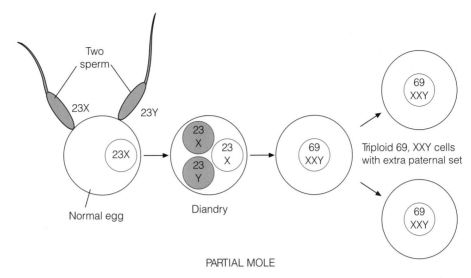

PARTIAL MOLE

Figure 31-5 • An incomplete mole arises from the simultaneous fertilization of a normal ovum by two sperm (diandry). The resulting triploid karyotype is most commonly 69,XXY.

Partial moles are the only histologic type of GTD associated with the **presence of a fetus**. In fact, amniotic fluid and a fetal heart rate may also be present. The karyotype of the fetus may be normal diploid or triploid. These fetuses often have **multiple anomalies** such as syndactyly or hydrocephalus and are often **growth restricted**. Most fetuses associated with partial moles survive only several weeks **in utero** before being spontaneously aborted in the late first or early second trimester. As a result, partial moles are often misdiagnosed as spontaneous or missed abortions. Partial moles are almost always benign and have a much **lower malignancy potential** than complete moles.

CLINICAL PRESENTATION

History

Partial molar pregnancy often presents with **delayed menses** and **a pregnancy diagnosis**. The hCG levels are **normal or only slightly elevated**. As a result, patients with partial moles may have similar but **much less severe symptoms** than those with complete molar pregnancy. Ninety percent of patients with partial moles present with **vaginal bleeding** from miscarriage or incomplete abortion in late first trimester or early second trimester. Consequently, partial moles may be **diagnosed somewhat later** than complete molar pregnancies. Diagnosis is often made on pathologic examination of the products of conception.

PHYSICAL EXAMINATION

In partial molar pregnancy, the physical examination is typically normal. Given the relatively normal hCG levels, hyperemesis, hyperthyroidism, and preeclampsia are rarely seen in women with partial moles. Fetal heart sounds may be present since there is a coexistent fetus. These pregnancies are often complicated by intrauterine growth restriction (IUGR) so the abdominal exam may be notable for size less than dates.

DIAGNOSTIC EVALUATION

Unlike complete molar pregnancy, quantitative serum **hCG levels** are likely to be relatively normal in partial molar pregnancies. **Pelvic ultrasound** may reveal a fetus with cardiac activity, congenital malformations, and/or intrauterine growth restriction. Amniotic fluid is usually present but reduced and these patients generally do not have theca lutein cysts seen in complete molar pregnancy. The intrauterine tissue may contain anechoic spaces juxtaposed against chorionic villi giving the tissue a **Swiss-cheese appearance**. The definitive diagnosis of molar pregnancy is made on **pathologic examination of the intrauterine tissue** once the uterus is evacuated.

TREATMENT

Treatment is immediate removal of the uterine contents via **suction curettage (D&C)** as described in the complete molar pregnancy treatment section. Less than 4% of patients with partial moles will develop persistent malignant disease (Table 31-2).

FOLLOW-UP

Meticulous follow-up with **serial hCG levels**, as described in the previous section on complete molar pregnancy, is critical to treatment of this disease. The average time to normalization of levels is **8 weeks** for a partial mole compared to 2 to 4 weeks following a normal pregnancy, miscarriage, or termination and 14 weeks for a complete mole. **Reliable contraception** is also important to prevent pregnancy and allow accurate hCG measurement.

MALIGNANT GESTATIONAL TROPHOBLASTIC DISEASE (GTD)

OVERVIEW

Molar pregnancies (complete and partial) are typically benign and make up 80% of all gestational trophoblas-tic disease; however, 20% of patients with GTD are diagnosed with a malignant form of the disease so named because of their potential **for local invasion and metastasis**. Malignant GTD is divided into three histologic types (Table 31-1): **persistent/invasive moles (75%)**, **choriocarcinoma (25%)**, and **PSTT (extremely rare)**. In 50% of cases, malignant GTD occurs **months to years after a molar pregnancy**. Another 25% occur after an antecedent normal pregnancy and 25% occur after a miscarriage, ectopic pregnancy, or abortion. Malignant GTD that occurs after a molar pregnancy is most commonly persistent/invasive GTD and malignant GTD that occurs after a nonmolar pregnancy is most commonly choriocarcinoma.

For the purpose of treatment and prognosis, malignant GTD (persistent/invasive moles, choriocarcinoma, PSTT) can be classified as **nonmetastatic** if the disease is confined to the uterus or **metastatic** if the disease has progressed beyond the uterus (Fig. 31-6). Metastatic disease can further be classified as **good prognosis or poor prognosis** depending on factors such as length of time since antecedent pregnancy, hCG level, presence of brain or liver metastases, type of antecedent pregnancy, and the result of prior chemotherapy trials (Fig. 31-6).

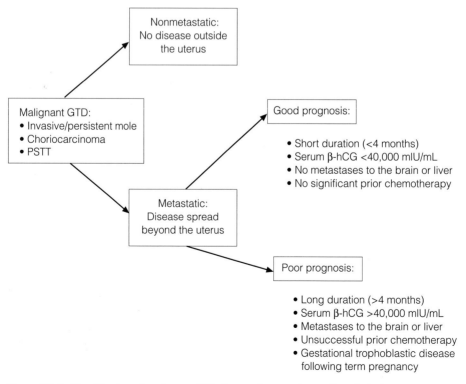

Figure 31-6 • Classification of malignant GTD. Anatomic spread as well as clinical presentation impact the prognosis of malignant disease.

TABLE 31-4 Staging of Gestational Trophoblastic Tumors

Stage	Extent of Disease*
I	Confined to the uterus
II	Metastases to the pelvis or vagina
III	Metastases to the lung
IV	Distant metastases

*Metastasis sites in order of frequency are lung, vagina, pelvis, brain, and liver.

TABLE 31-6 Risk Factors for Persistant/Invasive Moles

hCG >100,000 mIU/mL
Uterine size > 14 to 16 weeks
Large theca lutein cysts
Coexistent viable fetus

The staging for gestational trophoblastic disease is shown in Table 31-4. This system has not been found to be clinically useful because it does not account for important prognostic factors such as degree of metastasis, type of antecedent pregnancy, or duration of disease. In the United States, the World Health Organization (WHO) and National Institutes of Health (NIH) have devised systems that incorporate these prognostic factors to better reflect disease outcome. Table 31-5 shows the WHO system.

One distinguishing feature of malignant GTD is its **extreme sensitivity to chemotherapy. Surgery does not generally play a role** in the treatment of malignant GTD except for high-risk patients and those with PSTT. As with benign forms of GTD, **serum hCG levels** are monitored after treatment of malignant GTD. Newer assays which measure hyperglycosylated hCG are being investigated as possible markers for GTD.

PERSISTENT/INVASIVE MOLES

PATHOGENESIS

Persistent/invasive moles almost always occur after the evacuation of a molar pregnancy. Following D&C, about 15% of patients will have persistent local disease (mostly invasive/persistent GTD) and 4% will have metastatic disease (mostly choriocarcinoma). Characteristics which are most frequently associated with persistent/invasive disease are shown in Table 31-6.

Invasive moles are characterized by the penetration of large, swollen **(hydropic) villi and trophoblasts** into the myometrium. This proliferation can sometimes reach through the myometrium to the peritoneal cavity to invade the uterine vasculature. In rare cases persistent/invasive GTD can cause uterine rupture, hemoperitoneum, and severe anemia. Despite this, invasive moles **rarely metastasize** and are capable of **spontaneous regression**.

TABLE 31-5 WHO Scoring System Based on Prognostic Factor for GTD*

Risk Factor	0	1	Score 2	4
Age (y)	≤39	≥40		
Antecedent pregnancy	Mole	Abortion	Term	
Pregnancy event to treatment interval (mo)	<4	4 to 6	7 to 12	>12
Pretreatment hCG level (IU/mL)	$<10^3$	10^3 to 10^4	10^4 to 10^5	$>10^5$
No. of metastases		1 to 4	4 to 8	>8
Site metastases	Lung	Spleen, kidney	Bowel, liver	Brain
Largest tumor mass, including uterine (cm)			3 to 5	>5
Prior no. of failed chemotherapy drugs			Single drug	Two +

*The total score for a patient is obtained by adding the individual scores for each prognostic factor. Total score: <4 = low risk; 5–7 = middle risk; ≥8 = high risk.

EPIDEMIOLOGY

Invasive moles have an overall incidence of 1 in 15,000 pregnancies.

CLINICAL PRESENTATION

History

Most patients with persistent/invasive moles are identified as a result of **plateauing or rising hCG** after treatment for a molar pregnancy and are usually asymptomatic at the time of diagnosis. The most common symptom is **abnormal uterine bleeding**.

Physical Examination

The physical examination in patients with invasive moles is similar to that for molar pregnancy. Women with persistent/invasive GTD are more likely to have hCG levels above 100,000 mIU/mL, excessive uterine size for dates, and prominent theca lutein cysts.

DIAGNOSTIC EVALUATION

As with benign forms of GTD, **hCG levels and pelvic ultrasound are the cornerstones of diagnosis**. Pelvic ultrasound may reveal one or more **intrauterine masses** with possible invasion of the myometrium. Doppler examination typically shows **high vascular flow**.

TREATMENT

Persistent/invasive moles are typically **nonmetastatic** and respond well to **single-agent chemotherapy** with methotrexate or actinomycin-D. When metastases are present, low-risk patients are treated with **single-agent chemotherapy** and high-risk patients are treated with **multiagent chemotherapy** (EMA/CO).

FOLLOW-UP

As with other forms of GTD, careful follow-up with **serial hCG levels** as described is critical to demonstrating resolution of disease (Fig. 31-4). Likewise, **reliable contraception** is critical in order to maintain accurate measurement of hCG levels.

CHORIOCARCINOMA

PATHOGENESIS

Choriocarcinoma is a **malignant necrotizing tumor** that can arise weeks to years after any type of pregnancy. Although 50% of patients who develop choriocarcinoma have had a **preceding complete molar pregnancy**, 25% develop the disease after a normal-term pregnancy and 25% after miscarriage, abortion, or ectopic pregnancy.

Choriocarcinoma is a **pure epithelial tumor**. The characteristic histologic pattern of choriocarcinoma includes **sheets of anaplastic cytotrophoblasts and syncytiotrophoblasts in the absence of chorionic villi**. Choriocarcinoma invades the uterine wall and uterine vasculature, causing destruction of uterine tissue, necrosis, and potentially severe hemorrhage. These tumors are often metastatic and usually **spread hematogenously** to the lungs, vagina, pelvis, brain, liver, intestines, and kidneys. These lesions tend to be very vascular and bleed easily.

EPIDEMIOLOGY

Choriocarcinoma is very rare in the United States, where its incidence is only 1 in 20,000 to 40,000 pregnancies, but in Africa it is one of the leading causes of cancer in women.

CLINICAL PRESENTATION

History

Patients with choriocarcinoma often present with **late postpartum bleeding** (beyond 6 to 8 weeks postpartum) but can also present with **irregular uterine bleeding** years after an antecedent pregnancy. Unlike patients with persistent/invasive moles, patients with choriocarcinoma often present with symptoms of **metastatic disease**. Metastases to the **lungs** may cause cough, dyspnea, respiratory distress, or hemoptysis. Central nervous system (**CNS**) **lesions** may cause headaches, dizziness, blackouts, or other symptoms common to space-occupying lesions. Hepatic, urologic, and gastrointestinal symptoms are often signs of metastatic disease. Vaginal metastases may cause **vaginal bleeding**.

PHYSICAL EXAMINATION

Patients with choriocarcinoma often have **signs of metastatic disease**, including uterine enlargement, vaginal mass, bilateral theca lutein cysts, and neurologic signs from CNS involvement.

DIAGNOSTIC EVALUATION

The primary workup for choriocarcinoma includes measurement of quantitative **hCG levels** and assessment for metastasis to the lungs, liver, kidneys, spleen, and brain. This entails **laboratory tests** including a complete blood count (CBC), coagulation studies, along with renal and hepatic function tests. **Pelvic ultrasound** may reveal a uterine mass with hemorrhage and necrosis. These tumors are typically **highly vascular** as demonstrated by Doppler analysis. Other imaging studies should include **a chest x-ray or chest CT** to look for lung metastases as well as an **abdominal/pelvic CT or MRI** to look for metastatic disease. If vaginal or lung metastases are present, **a CT or MRI of the brain** should also be obtained.

DIFFERENTIAL DIAGNOSIS

Choriocarcinoma has been found to metastasize to virtually every tissue in the body. It is known as **"the great imitator"** because its signs and symptoms are similar to those of many disease entities. Also, given that choriocarcinoma can occur from weeks to years after any type of gestation and is relatively rare, the **diagnosis is often delayed** when the disease occurs outside the context of a prior molar pregnancy.

TREATMENT

Classification and treatment of choriocarcinoma mirror those of persistent/invasive GTD (Fig. 31-6). Nonmetastatic and good-prognosis metastatic disease are treated with **single-agent chemotherapy**. Poorprognosis metastatic choriocarcinoma is treated with **multiagent chemotherapy**. The cure rate for good prognosis disease is 95% to 100%, and the cure rate for poor prognosis disease is 50% to 70%.

FOLLOW-UP

As with all other forms of GTD, choriocarcinoma requires close monitoring of **hCG levels** in conjunction with **reliable contraception**.

PLACENTAL SITE TROPHOBLASTIC TUMORS

PATHOGENESIS

Placental site trophoblastic tumors (PSTTs) are extremely rare tumors that arise from the **placental implantation site**. In this form of malignant GTD, intermediate cytotrophoblasts from placental site infiltrate the myometrium and then invade the blood vessels. Histologically, these tumors are characterized by the **absence of villi** and the proliferation of intermediate trophoblasts (as opposed to proliferation of syncytiotrophoblasts and cytotrophoblasts seen in other forms of GTD).

CLINICAL PRESENTATION

Persistent **irregular vaginal bleeding** is the most common symptom of PSTT and may occur weeks to years after an antecedent pregnancy. Physical exam may reveal an **enlarged uterus**.

DIAGNOSTIC EVALUATION

Unlike other forms of GTD, these tumors produce **chronic low levels of hCG** because these tumors lack proliferation of syncytiotrophoblasts (the placental layer responsible for hCG production). The **pelvic ultrasound** may show a uterine mass but there is typically less hemorrhage than seen in choriocarcinomas. Both cystic and solid components may be present. Like other forms of malignant GTD, the tumor can invade the uterine wall and surrounding tissues.

TREATMENT

PSTTs are also generally **not sensitive to chemotherapy** but, fortunately, they rarely metastasize beyond the uterus. Therefore, **hysterectomy is the treatment of choice** for PSTT. Multiagent chemotherapy (EMA/CO) is given one week after surgery to prevent recurrent disease.

KEY POINTS

- GTD is a group of related diseases resulting from abnormal proliferation of trophoblastic (placental) tissue.

- Eighty percent of GTD is benign disease (complete and partial moles) and 20% is malignant disease (persistent/invasive moles, choriocarcinoma, and placental site trophoblastic tumors/PSTT).

- Of benign GTD, 90% are complete moles. Complete moles result from the fertilization of an empty ovum by one sperm. The most common karyotype is 46,XX—all chromosomes are parentally derived.

- There is no associated fetus in complete molar pregnancy and patients usually present with irregular vaginal bleeding, an enlarged uterus, or passage of vesicles.

- Complete molar pregnancy can have very high hCG levels (>100,000 mIU/mL) resulting in classic symptoms of hyperemesis gravidarum, preeclampsia before 20 weeks' gestation, hyperthyroidism, and/or theca lutein cysts.

- Complete molar pregnancy is diagnosed by hCG levels and pelvic ultrasound showing a "snowstorm" pattern and is treated with immediate suction D&C to empty the uterus. Oxytocin is often given to encourage hemostasis.

- Complete molar pregnancy requires close follow-up with weekly, then monthly, hCG levels for 6 months. Concurrent reliable contraception is imperative during this time.

- Complete molar pregnancy results in persistent malignant disease in 15% of cases and has a risk of recurrence of 1% after one molar pregnancy and 16% to 28% after two molar pregnancies.

- Partial moles account for 10% of molar pregnancies and result from the simultaneous fertilization of a normal ovum by two sperm. The most common karyotype is 69,XXY.

- Partial moles have a coexistent abnormal fetus and usually present with vaginal bleeding from spontaneous or incomplete abortion.

- Partial moles are diagnosed by hCG levels and pelvic ultrasound and treated with D&C. Persistent malignant disease develops in only 4% of cases. Follow-up is similar to complete moles with serial hCG levels and reliable contraception.

- Persistent/invasive moles make up 75% of malignant GTD. They are usually diagnosed by detecting plateauing or rising hCG levels after molar evacuation.

- These moles have an overall incidence of 1 in 15,000 normal pregnancies. They are generally confined to the uterus and respond well to single-agent chemotherapy (95% to 100% cure rate).

- Choriocarcinoma is a rare form of GTD with an overall incidence of 1 in 20,000 to 40,000 pregnancies in the U.S. It is a malignant, necrotizing tumor that can occur weeks to years after any type of gestation.

- Patients present with signs and symptoms of metastases to the lungs, vagina, liver, brain, or kidneys. Choriocarcinoma is diagnosed by pelvic ultrasound, hCG levels, and a thorough work-up for metastatic disease.

- Choriocarcinoma is treated with single- or multi-agent chemotherapy depending on the presence of disease outside the uterus and on the disease prognosis category.

- PSTTs are extremely rare tumors that arise from the placental implantation site. They are characterized by the absence of villi and the proliferation of cytotrophoblasts. This results in chronic low levels of hCG (<100 mIU/mL).

- PSTTs spread by invasion into the myometrium and blood vessels. Patients most commonly present with vaginal bleeding and persistently low levels of hCG (<100 mIU/mL).

- PSTTs are treated by hysterectomy followed by multiagent chemotherapy to prevent recurrences.

Disease and Breast Cancer

Breast cancer is the most common malignancy in women in the United States, representing approximately 30% of female cancers and 210,000 **new diagnoses** each year. It is also the second most common cause of **cancer deaths** in women (after lung cancer deaths), accounting for some 41,000 deaths per year. A woman has a **1 in 8 chance of having breast cancer** in her lifetime (birth to death). Yet, despite its incidence, the cause of breast cancer remains unknown.

In addition to breast cancer, as many as 50% of women will have benign breast lesions over their lifetime. Therefore, understanding the range of benign and malignant breast lesions and their symptoms is enormously important. Obstetrician-gynecologists, primary care providers, and surgeons perform the evaluation of breast pain, nipple discharge, and breast masses and also screen for breast cancer. The anatomy and physiology of the breast as well as how to diagnose and treat these lesions should be understood by all physicians involved in the care of women.

ANATOMY

Breast parenchyma is divided into segments containing **mammary glands** that consist of 20 to 40 lobules drained by **lactiferous ducts** that open individually into the nipple (Fig. 32-1). Fibrous bands spanning between two fascia layers—called **Cooper suspensory ligament**s—support the breast. The breast is divided into four quadrants for ease of description: upper outer quadrant (UOQ), lower outer quadrant (LOQ), upper inner quadrant (UIQ), and lower inner quadrant (LIQ).

The **major blood supply** to the breast is from the **internal mammary** and **lateral thoracic arteries** (Fig. 32-2). The medial and central aspects are supplied by the anterior perforators of the internal mammary artery and the UOQ is supplied by the lateral thoracic.

The **axillary lymph nodes** drain up to 97% of the ipsilateral breast, and secondarily drain the supraclavicular and jugular nodes. These nodes are subdivided into three levels for the purposes of specifying disease progression. The **internal mammary nodes** are responsible for 3% of drainage, mainly of the UIQ and LIQ. The interpectoral nodes (Rotter nodes) lie between the pectoralis major and pectoralis minor muscles.

The **innervation** of the breast requires careful attention during surgical dissection. Nerves at risk of injury include the **intercostobrachial nerve** that transverses the axilla to supply sensation to the upper medial arm; the **long thoracic nerve** (of Bell) of C5, C6, and C7 that innervates the serratus anterior muscle, injury of which can lead to the "winged" scapula; the **thoracodorsal nerve** that innervates the latissimus dorsi muscle; and the lateral pectoral nerve that innervates the pectoralis major and minor muscles.

PHYSIOLOGY

Breast development is classified into **Tanner stages 1 to 5** (see Chapter 20 and Fig. 20-3). The breast responds to cyclic hormones, as well as to changes

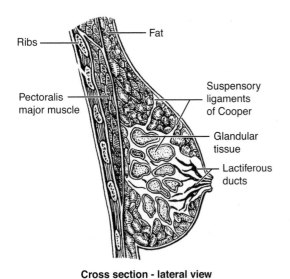

Cross section - lateral view

Figure 32-1 • Clinical anatomy of the female breast and chest wall.
(From Beckmann C, Ling F. *Obstetrics & Gynecology*, 5th ed. Philadelphia: Lippincott Williams & Wilkins, 2006.)

during pregnancy and menopause. **Estrogen** promotes ductal development and fat deposition. **Progesterones** promote the lobular-alveolar (stromal) development that makes lactation possible. **Prolactin** is involved in milk production, whereas **oxytocin** from the posterior pituitary causes milk letdown. In **postmenopausal women**, the decreased estrogenic state is associated with **tissue atrophy**, loss of stroma, and replacement of atrophied lobules with fatty tissue.

EVALUATION OF THE BREAST

ROUTINE EVALUATION

Routine **monthly self-examination** and **yearly clinician evaluation** are recommended for all women over age 20. Self-examination should be performed approximately 5 days after menses when the breast is least engorged and tender. Physical examination involves careful inspection of the skin for contour or

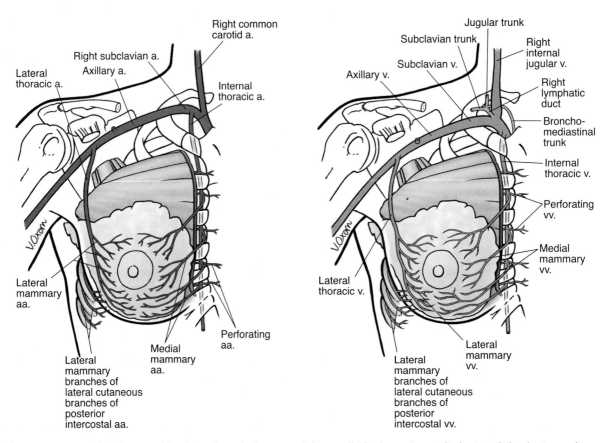

Figure 32-2 • Arterial and venous blood supply to the breast and chest wall. The breast is supplied primarily by the internal thoracic arteries and the lateral thoracic arteries.
(From Moore KL, Agur A. *Essential Clinical Anatomy*, 2nd ed. Philadelphia: Lippincott Williams & Wilkins, 2002.)

color changes with the patient in upright and supine positions. This is followed by palpation for lymphadenopathy, masses, nipple discharge, or pain. The breast self-exam should be reviewed at each annual gynecology visit. Patients are often motivated by the fact that the many breast masses are found by patients or their partners.

In addition to clinician and breast self-exams, the third part of routine breast care is **screening mammography** (Fig. 32-3). Current mammography screening guidelines by the American Cancer Society include a mammogram every year starting at age 40 and continuing for as long as a woman is in good health. There is **no upper age limit** at which mammogram screening is no longer indicated. Women with a strong family history of breast cancer (mother, sister) should begin mammogram screening 5 years earlier than the age at which the youngest family member was when diagnosed with breast cancer; 10 years earlier if the breast cancer was premenopausal.

Digital mammography has been found to be better imaging of changes than conventional film mammography. It may have particular benefit in women with dense breasts, women under 50 years of age, and perimenopausal women. The role of **breast MRI** in breast screening is currently limited to differentiating between scar tissue and cancer in patients with previous surgery or radiation, assessing the integrity of silicone breast implants, and looking for breast cancer in patients with axillary node metastases in the setting of negative mammographic imaging. At this time, other appropriate and cost-effective uses of breast MRI are under investigation.

EVALUATION OF BREAST PAIN

Breast pain (mastalgia, mastodynia) is a **common complaint** (65%) in women but is not always reported to a healthcare provider. The pain is **typically mild** and may be **cyclic** (67%) or **noncyclic** (33%) in nature. Breast pain can be a normal physiologic response to hormonal fluctuations or it can be a pathologic response to trauma or malignancy. Mastalgia may be a component of premenstrual syndrome (PMS), associated with hormone replacement therapy (HRT), or caused by menstrual irregularities or fibrocystic change. Only 1% to 6% of women with breast pain will have underlying malignancy.

The patient's **medical history**, including benign or malignant diseases of the breast, is relevant. Clinicians need to establish if the pain is cyclic or noncyclic, bilateral or unilateral, diffuse or focal. They must also ask about **associated symptoms** (back/neck pain, erythema, fever) and use of medications such as OCPs and HRT. Also relevant are any history of trauma, radiation or surgery to the breast, family history of breast disease, and constitutional symptoms such as weight loss or gain, chest wall pain, or amenorrhea.

The history and physical exam are typically enough to provide **reassurance** to a patient. Focal lesions or areas of trauma can be evaluated with an **ultrasound** in women. Women at high risk of cancer should be evaluated with **mammography**. The vast majority of breast pain is benign and can be treated with **NSAIDs**, a **supportive bra or sports bra**, and the use of warm and cool **compresses**. Management of breast pain associated with specific benign and malignant processes is further discussed below.

EVALUATION OF NIPPLE DISCHARGE

As many as 50% to 80% of women will have nipple discharge at some point during their reproductive years. The vast majority of nipple discharge is due to normal physiology or benign processes and only 5% is associated with underlying malignancy (Table 32-1). The **most concerning discharge is** spontaneous, **bloody** or serosanguineous, **unilateral**, **persistent**, from a **single duct** and **associated with a mass**. Bilateral, nonbloody, multiductal secretion is usually benign regardless of color.

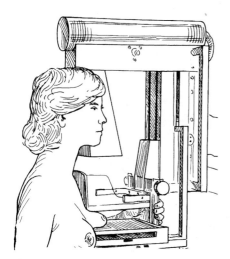

Figure 32-3 • Mammogram.

■ TABLE 32-1 Causes of Nipple Discharge

Etiology class	Conditions
Benign breast disease	Ductal papilloma, ductal hyperplasia, duct ectasia, fibrocystic breast changes
Premalignant and malignant breast disease	Intraductal carcinoma (in situ or invasive), diffuse papillomatosis
Systemic disease	Hyperprolactinemia, hypothyroidism, pituitary adenomas, sarcoidosis, chronic renal failure, liver cirrhosis
Medications	Oral contraceptives, phenothiazines, methyldopa, reserpine, imipramine, amphetamines, metoclopramide
Chest wall lesions	Thoracotomy, chest wall trauma and burns, herpes zoster
Skin changes mistaken for nipple discharge	Paget disease, insect bites, local infection, eczema
Chronic breast stimulation	Poorly fitted bra, stimulation by partner, self-stimulation

Bloody discharge is associated with intraductal papilloma or invasive papillary cancer. **Galactorrhea** is associated with pregnancy, pituitary adenomas, hypothyroidism, stress, and medications such as oral contraceptive pills (OCPs), antihypertensives, and psychotropic drugs. **Serous discharge** is associated with normal menses, OCPs, fibrocystic change, or early pregnancy. **Yellow-tinged discharge** is associated with fibrocystic change or galactocele. **Green, sticky discharge** is associated with duct ectasia. **Purulent discharge** indicates superficial or central breast abscess.

When a patient presents with nipple discharge, it is important to find out the nature of any nipple discharge: its **color**, whether it is **bilateral**, the number of **duct openings** involved, and if it occurs **spontaneously** or with manual expression. The physical exam should look for **skin changes**, associated **masses** or lymphadenopathy. An attempt should be made to elicit secretion by applying pressure to the base of the areola. Bloody or serosanguineous discharge should be tested on a **guaiac card** and sent for **cytologic evaluation**. Routine culture is not indicated. Women with associated amenorrhea, menstrual irregularities, headaches, or visual disturbances should have **prolactin and thyroid levels** drawn. Women with associated masses should have **ultrasound and/or mammography** evaluation depending on their age.

Most nipple discharge is benign and does not require treatment. When indicated, treatment should be individualized to the specific cause of the discharge.

EVALUATION OF BREAST MASSES

If a patient is found to have a **breast mass** on the physician's exam or her own self-exam, a thorough history and exam are crucial. Importantly, up to **20% of new breast cancers are not seen or detected via mammography**; therefore, a suspicious mass should never be dismissed just because the mammogram is negative.

■ TABLE 32-2 Breast Imaging Reporting and Database System (BI-RADS) for Characterization of Mammogram Findings

Cat	Assessment Category	Recommended Action	Risk of Malignancy
0	Incomplete	Additional imaging needed	N/A
1	Negative	Routine follow-up	0%
2	Benign finding(s)	Routine follow-up	0%
3	Probably benign	Short-interval (6 mo) follow-up	≤2%
4	Suspicious of malignancy	Core-needle biopsy ASAP	2% to 95%
5	Highly suspicious of malignancy	Core-needle biopsy ASAP	≥95%
6	Known, biopsy-proven malignancy	Definitive treatment ongoing	100%

When evaluating a breast mass, it's important to ascertain the manner in which it was discovered, associated tenderness or trauma, and the relationship of changes to the menstrual cycle. Likewise, its location, size, shape, consistency, and mobility should be noted, as well as any overlying skin changes. Worrisome lumps are dominant, discrete, and dense. **Malignant masses are usually firm, nontender, poorly circumscribed, and immobile**. Lymph nodes are worrisome if larger than 1 cm, fixed, irregular, firm, or multiple.

Abnormal breast masses should also be **evaluated radiographically**. For **women under age 30, ultrasound** is the preferred method of imaging and is also useful in assessing whether a mass that is greater than 0.5 cm is **solid or cystic** in women of any age. For **women 30 or older, mammography** is used to further evaluate suspicious masses. To standardize mammogram reporting, a collaborative scoring system was devised and published by the American College of Radiology. It is known as the **Breast Imaging Reporting and Database System** (BI-RADS). This system (Table 32-2) categorizes mammographic findings to translate the radiologist's opinion of the absence or likelihood of breast cancer. Findings which are most suggestive of malignancy include a spiculated mass; architectural distortion with retraction; asymmetric localized fibrosis; microcalcifications with linear, branched patterns; increased vascularity; or altered subareolar duct pattern (Fig. 32-4).

Any concerning palpable mass or abnormality seen on radiologic imaging should be biopsied to obtain a **pathologic diagnosis** (Table 32-3). The goal of tissue biopsy is to obtain an adequate sample for diagnosis using the least invasive sampling possible. If a palpable cystic mass is found on examination and confirmed on ultrasound, it can be drained and sampled for diagnosis using **needle aspiration** (Fig. 32-5). This

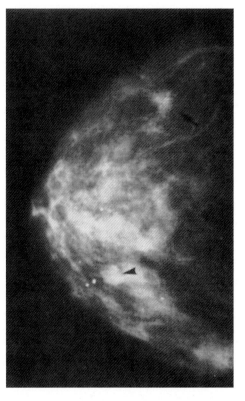

Figure 32-4 • A cephalocaudal mammogram film contrasting a small speculated mass carcinoma (*arrow*) versus a well-marginated fibroadenoma (*arrowhead*).
(From Beckmann C, Ling F. *Obstetrics & Gynecology*, 5th ed. Philadelphia: Lippincott Williams & Wilkins; 2006.)

treats the cyst and also provides fluid for cytology if indicated by turbid or bloody aspirate. The **cyst should be excised** if the fluid is bloody, a mass persists after fluid is removed, the cyst is persistent after two aspirations, or the fluid reaccumulates within 2 weeks.

■ TABLE 32-3 Evaluation of Abnormal Breast Masses and Abnormal Mammogram Findings

Abnormal Finding		Appropriate Evaluation
Palpable cystic lesion	→	Needle drainage
Recurrent cyst, bloody fluid	→	Excision
Solid, palpable mass (<30 yo)	→	Fine-needle aspiration (FNA)
Nondiagnostic FNA of solid mass	→	Excisional biopsy
Solid, palpable mass (≥30 yo)	→	Core-needle biopsy
Nondiagnostic core-needle biopsy	→	Excisional biopsy
Nonpalpable abnormal mammogram finding	→	Wire-guided excision

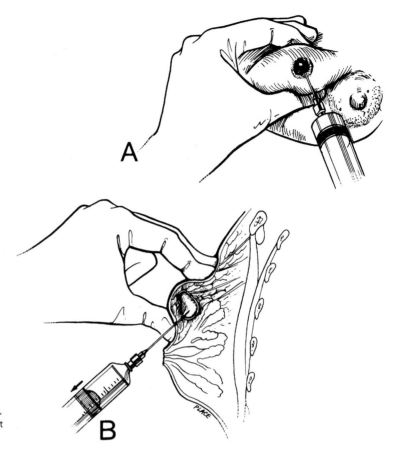

Figure 32-5 • Needle aspiration of a breast cyst.

When a palpable solid mass is found on exam and confirmed with ultrasound or mammography, a tissue sample should be obtained for diagnosis. In women <30 years old, **fine-needle aspiration** (FNA) can be used to sample solid masses (Fig. 32-6). This technique involves making multiple passes through the mass from different angles while aspirating the syringe on a 20- to 22-gauge needle. Diagnostic accuracy approaches 80% to 90%. An **excisional biopsy** is performed if the FNA does not obtain fluid or tissue. Excisional biopsy is also performed if cytology or histology is nondiagnostic. In women 30 years of age or older with a palpable solid mass, a core-needle biopsy is recommended.

When a **nonpalpable lesion** is found by mammography, excisional biopsy can also be performed under **needle or wire guidance**. The goal should be to excise the abnormal tissue along with a 1-cm rim of normal tissue to qualify for lumpectomy, thus avoiding the need for repeat surgery if the mass is malignant.

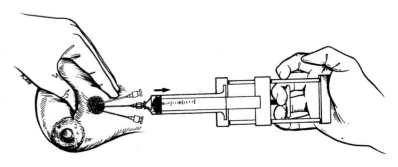

Figure 32-6 • Fine-needle aspiration of a solid breast mass.

BENIGN BREAST DISEASE

Benign breast symptoms and findings are common and occur in approximately 50% of women, with a higher incidence in younger women. The decision to biopsy any abnormal breast findings for definitive diagnosis is influenced by the patient's risk factors for malignant disease. Two-thirds of tumors in reproductive-age women are benign, whereas half of palpable masses in perimenopausal women and the majority of lesions in postmenopausal women are malignant.

FIBROCYSTIC BREAST CHANGE

Pathophysiology

Fibrocystic change of the breast includes a spectrum of clinical findings due to **exaggerated stromal response** to hormones and growth factors. It typically presents as **painful breast masses** that are **often multiple and usually bilateral**. There can be rapid fluctuation in the size of the masses. The associated breast changes can include cystic change, nodularity, stromal proliferation, and epithelial hyperplasia. In the absence of atypical hyperplasia, **fibrocystic change is not associated with increased cancer risk**.

Epidemiology

Peak incidence is between ages 30 and 40, but changes can persist throughout a woman's entire life. The changes are rare in postmenopausal women.

Diagnosis

Patients with fibrocystic changes present with breast swelling, pain, and tenderness. Fibrocystic disease may have more focal symptomatic areas, involve both breasts, and vary throughout the menstrual cycle. The pain is commonly worse as the mass size increases during the **premenstrual part of the cycle**. Evaluation with mammogram, ultrasound, and/or biopsy should be performed for suspicious lesions (dominant mass that does not fluctuate in size).

Treatment

The pain of fibrocystic breast changes can be ameliorated with **reduction of caffeine, tea, and chocolate** although the role of caffeine reduction is controversial.

Avoiding trauma and wearing a support bra may also help decrease the pain associated with fibrocystic change. Although the data have been inconsistent, other recognized treatments include **evening primrose oil, vitamins E and B6, danazol, progestins, bromocriptine, and tamoxifen** (not approved for this indication).

FIBROADENOMA

Pathogenesis

Breast fibroadenomas are benign tumors with glandular and stromal components. Most masses are 1 to 5 cm in diameter at the time of detection. Lesions larger than 5 cm are termed *giant fibroadenomas* and need to be ruled out as **cystosarcoma phyllodes**. Fibroadenomas are **usually solitary** but can be multiple, and occur bilaterally up to 25% of the time (Fig. 32-4). The etiology is unknown but is likely related to the hormonal milieu.

Epidemiology

Fibroadenomas are the most common benign tumors of the breast. They usually occur in women ages 20 to 35. The can also be found in teenagers and are more common than breast cysts in women under 25. They very rarely occur after menopause.

Diagnosis

Fibroadenomas are often palpated on physical examination as round, well-circumscribed, mobile firm lesions that are **rubbery and nontender**. The patient may report changes in the lesion during the menstrual cycle, pregnancy, and with OCP use. Classic fibroadenoma in a woman <30 years old may be the only solid breast mass that does not require tissue diagnosis.

Treatment

A young patient (<30 years old) with classic presentation of a fibroadenoma and no family history of breast cancer can be **followed clinically if stable**. Otherwise, FNA for cytology is highly sensitive for detecting cancer or phyllodes tumors. If the fibroadenoma is large or worrisome, excisional biopsy is recommended to remove the tumor and establish pathologic diagnosis.

CYSTOSARCOMA PHYLLODES

Pathogenesis

Phyllodes tumors are a **rare variant of fibroadenoma** and involve epithelial and stromal proliferation.

Epidemiology

It is diagnosed most commonly in premenopausal women, although it can occur at any age.

Diagnosis

This lesion appears as a **large, bulky, mobile mass**. The overlying skin is warm, erythematous, shiny, and engorged. The mass is **large** (4 to 5 cm), smooth, and well circumscribed and is characterized by **rapid growth**. Most lesions are benign; however, some physicians consider cystosarcoma phyllodes a **low-grade malignancy** and a few tumors do develop true sarcomatous potential. These tumors are worrisome for aggressive malignancies; pathologic diagnosis must therefore be made.

Treatment

The clinical course of these tumors is unpredictable as most appear benign, but **10% do contain malignant cells**. There is also a high rate of local recurrence after simple excision. Recommended therapy is therefore **wide local excision** with a 1-cm margin for small tumors and simple mastectomy for large lesions.

INTRADUCTAL PAPILLOMA

Pathogenesis

Intraductal papilloma is a benign solitary lesion that involves the **epithelial lining of lactiferous ducts**. It is the most common cause of **bloody nipple discharge** in the absence of a concurrent mass.

Diagnosis

Intraductal papilloma usually appears with bloody nipple discharge in premenopausal women. The serosanguineous discharge is **sent for cytology** to rule out invasive papillary carcinoma, which has similar symptoms 25% of the time. To identify the papilloma, the physician can open the involved duct to visualize the tumor.

Treatment

Definitive diagnosis and treatment is by **excision of the involved ducts** after localization by physical examination. Intraductal papillomas rarely undergo malignant transformation.

MAMMARY DUCT ECTASIA (PLASMA CELL MASTITIS)

Pathogenesis

This subacute inflammation of the ductal system causes dilated mammary ducts. There are infiltration of plasma cells and significant periductal inflammation.

Epidemiology

This lesion most commonly occurs **at or after menopause**.

Diagnosis

Patients present with **nipple discharge**, noncyclic **breast pain**, **nipple retraction**, or subareolar masses. The discharge is multicolored, sticky, originating from multiple ducts, and **often bilateral**. The patient should have a mammogram and excisional biopsy is indicated to rule out carcinoma.

Treatment

Definitive treatment is **local excision** of the inflamed area, occasionally requiring extensive subareolar duct excision.

MALIGNANT BREAST DISEASE

Epidemiology

Breast cancer is the most common nonskin malignancy affecting women in the United States. One in every eight American women will develop this disease during her lifetime and will have a 3.5% chance of dying from it. It accounts for 30% of all cancers in women and 20% of women's cancer deaths. Although black women in the United States have a lower incidence of breast cancer, they have a higher mortality rate compared to white women in the United States. This difference in mortality rates is not completely understood.

The risk of getting breast cancer increases with age. Four out of every five women with breast cancer and are over age 50. While the incidence of diagnosis is increasing, the death rate is decreasing, likely due to earlier detection and improved therapies. Currently, breast cancer is the leading cause of death in U.S. women age 40 to 55. The average age of diagnosis is 60 to 61.

Risk Factors

Numerous risk factors are associated with breast cancer (Table 32-4). One major risk factor is **increasing age**. For example, an American woman's annual risk of invasive breast increases from 1 in 2,000 by age 30,

to "1 in 8" by age 80. Similarly, **a personal history of breast cancer** increases the risk of developing invasive cancer in the contralateral breast. For women with invasive breast cancer, the risk of developing cancer in the contralateral breast is 1% per year for premenopausal women and 0.5% per year for postmenopausal women.

A **family history** of gynecologic malignancies also significantly increases a patient's risk of breast cancer. Having a first-degree relative with breast cancer increases a woman's risk greatly depending on the number of affected relatives, their age at diagnosis, and the bilaterality of their disease. Having one affected first-degree family member increases the patient's risk by nearly two times and having two first-degree families increases a patient's risk by nearly three times. These risks are even further amplified if the family member was premenopausal at the time of diagnosis.

A strong family history is suspicious for a **genetic predisposition**. Although **10% of women with breast cancer have a family history** of the disease, inherited genetic mutations are still rare. Six familial syndromes have been identified with an increased risk of breast cancer. The best known of these are the BRCA1 and BRCA2 genes associated with **bilateral premenopausal breast cancer** and breast cancer associated with ovarian cancer.

Exposure to **ionizing radiation** of the chest at a young age (such as used in the treatment of Hodgkin lymphoma) and alcohol abuse can significantly increase the risk of breast cancer. Diagnosis of atypical **ductal or lobular hyperplasia** on biopsy increases risk by a factor of 5. The presence of ductal or lobular carcinoma in situ or noninvasive carcinomas also increases cancer risk.

Between 0.5% and 4.0% of breast cancer is diagnosed surrounding **pregnancy or lactation**. Compared to nonpregnant women with breast cancer at similar stage and age, **survival rates seem equivalent** for pregnant or lactating women with breast cancer. Younger age at menarche, nulliparity, later date of first live birth, and later age at menopause have all been linked with increased risk of breast cancer. This is thought to be due to cumulative lifetime estrogen exposure.

The question of whether or not **postmenopausal HRT** changes the risk of breast cancer has been hotly debated. It is now generally believed that patients who use combination HRT for more than 5 years are at a slightly **increased risk** of developing invasive breast cancer. **Past and current oral contraceptive (OCP)** use has not been shown to **increase risk** of

■ **TABLE 32-4** Breast Cancer Risk Factors	
Risk Factors	**Relative Risk**
Sex	99% in women
Age	85% over age 40
Proliferative fibrocystic change	2 to 5:1
Previous breast cancer, 1 breast	5:1
Nulliparous versus parous	3:1
First birth after age 34	4:1
Menarche before age 12	1.3:1
Menopause after age 50	1.5:1
Affluent versus poor	2:1
Jewish versus non-Jewish	2:1
Western hemisphere	1.5:1
Cold climate versus warm climate	2:1
Chronic psychologic stress	2:1
Obesity	2:1
Obesity, hypertension, diabetes	3:1
High dietary fat	3:1
White versus Asian	5:1
Second-degree relative	1.5:1
First-degree relative	
Unilateral premenopausal	1.8:1
Bilateral premenopausal	8.8:1
Unilateral postmenopausal	1.2:1
Bilateral postmenopausal	4:1

Adapted from DiSaia PJ, Creasman WT. *Clinical Gynecologic Oncology*, 5th ed. St. Louis: Mosby-Yearbook, 1997:403.

breast cancer. Nor has the use of caffeine, breast implants, electric blankets, hair dyes.

Prevention

Early pregnancy, prolonged lactation, chemical or surgical sterilization, exercise, abstinence from alcohol, and a low-fat diet may help prevent breast cancer. The studies linking phytoestrogens to a reduction of breast cancer risk have been inconclusive. These are naturally occurring plant substances similar to estradiol and are composed mainly of isoflavones such as those found in soybeans—a major component of tofu. Similarly, no protective effect has been proven with the use of aspirin and other NSAIDs.

Increasing evidence suggests that tamoxifen may be effective in suppressing the development of breast cancer. By binding to the estrogen receptor, **tamoxifen competitively inhibits estrogen binding** and maintains inhibition of breast cancer cells. Tamoxifen is currently used widely in patients with early-stage, surgically treated breast cancer and has been shown to decrease contralateral breast cancer by 40%.

Diagnosis

The trifecta of routine breast care is the monthly **breast self-exam**, the annual **clinician breast exam**, and annual **mammography** for women age 40 and over or those who are at high risk for breast cancer. Thirty percent to 50% of breast cancers are diagnosed as a result of an abnormality detected via mammography.

Patients may present clinically with **breast masses**, **skin change**, **nipple discharge**, or symptoms of metastatic disease. **Skin dimpling** can occur due to tethering of Cooper ligaments from the mass underneath. The skin can appear erythematous and warm, with nipple retraction or inversion. Tissue edema or a peau d'orange appearance may occur due to dermal lymphatic invasion and blockage. The superficial epidermis of the nipple may appear eczematous or ulcerated, as in Paget disease.

Bloody discharge needs to be evaluated to rule out invasive papillary carcinoma. Palpable masses are often detected by the patient or partner on self-exam and are usually nontender, irregular, firm, and immobile. **Fifty percent of tumors occur in the UOQ** (Fig. 32-7). These tumors can be multifocal, multicentric, or bilateral. Mammography is the best tool to detect early lesions, reducing mortality by 32% to 50%. Recent studies have shown that mammography is less effective in women with dense breast tissue—for

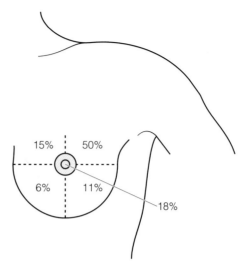

Figure 32-7 • Most common locations of malignant lesions.

example, in African American women. Furthermore, up to **20% of new breast cancers are not detectable on mammography** so any suspicious lesion should be biopsied if clinically indicated, even if the mammogram is negative.

A nonpalpable suspicious lesion found on mammogram requires **localized needle biopsy** or **stereotactic FNA** for pathologic diagnosis.

The evaluation for metastatic disease with a thorough history, physical, and imaging is also an important part of breast disease management. Breast cancer tends to metastasize to the **bone, liver, lung, pleura, brain,** and **lymph nodes**. Patients may present with constitutional symptoms of weight loss, anorexia, night sweats, and fatigue. They may have symptoms of dyspnea, cough, or bone pain.

NONINVASIVE DISEASE

Lobular Carcinoma in Situ (LCIS)

Pathogenesis

Lobular carcinoma in situ (LCIS) is the proliferation of **neoplastic epithelial cells** contained within breast lobules with no invasion of the stroma (Fig. 32-8). It is usually multicentric and is bilateral 50% to 90% of the time. LCIS is considered by some to be a premalignant lesion that is, itself, not a true cancer. Most agree, however, that the importance of LCIS is as **an indicator for subsequent risk of invasive breast cancer** (25% to 30% within 15 years) in the ipsilateral or contralateral breast or in both breasts.

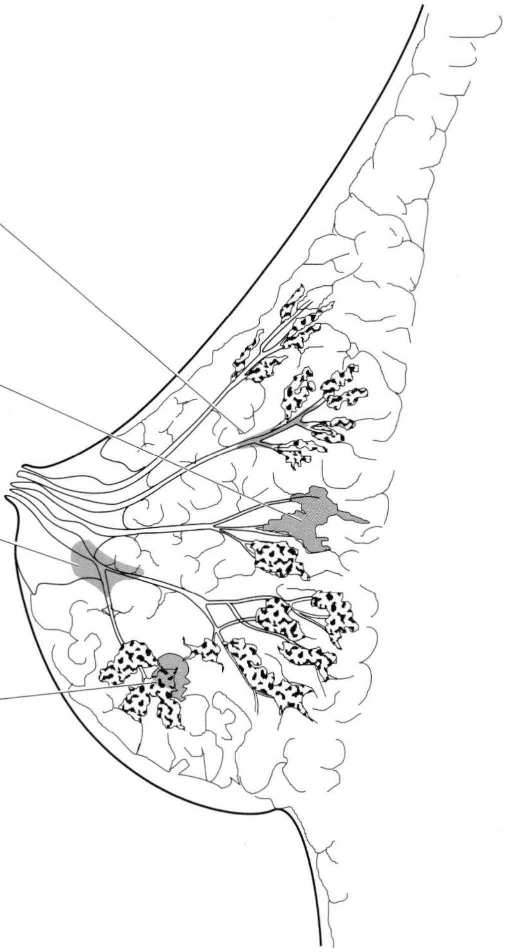

Ductal carcinoma
in situ (DCIS) (15%)

Lobular carcinoma
in situ (LCIS) (4%)

Infiltrating (Invasive)
ductal carcinoma (70%)

Infiltrating (Invasive)
lobular carcinoma (10%)

Figure 32-8 • Subtypes of breast cancer. DCIS is believed to be a precursor to invasive ductal carcinoma; LCIS is, in contrast, more akin to atypical hyperplasia and carries a risk of future ductal or invasive lobular carcinoma anywhere in the breast. Invasive ductal carcinoma is the most common type of breast cancer in women.

Epidemiology

The average age at diagnosis is the mid-40s. Patients are typically premenopausal.

Diagnosis

LCIS is usually diagnosed incidentally on biopsy for another finding as it **is not palpable** and **not seen on mammograms**.

Treatment

Observation without further therapy is needed after biopsy confirms LCIS; however, selective estrogen receptor modulators (**SERMs**) such as tamoxifen or raloxifene may reduce the risk of subsequent invasive cancer by 50% and should be considered. Subsequent cancers may be intraductal, invasive ductal, or lobular carcinoma and may be in the ipsilateral or contralateral breast.

Ductal Carcinoma in Situ

Pathogenesis

Ductal carcinoma in situ (DCIS)—also called intraductal carcinoma—involves proliferation of **malignant epithelial cells** in mammary ducts without spread to the breast stroma (Fig. 32-8). It is more common than lobular carcinoma in situ, and, if left untreated, has a **higher potential to progress to invasive carcinoma** than does LCIS.

Epidemiology

Average age at diagnosis is mid-50s.

Diagnosis

Ninety percent of DCIS is detected by **screening mammography** revealing **clustered microcalcifications**. Ten percent present with a palpable mass.

Diagnosis can be established by needle localization biopsy or excisional biopsy of a palpable lesion. Thirty-five percent of lesions are multicentric; bilateral disease is rare.

Treatment

Current treatment involves conservative surgical **excision of all microcalcifications with wide margins**. Simple **mastectomy** is occasionally necessary for extensive lesions, but is considered overly aggressive for treatment of all women with DCIS. If resection margins are inadequate (<10 mm), **radiation therapy** may be used to reduce the risk of local recurrence but has no impact on survival. The risk of subsequent invasive ductal carcinoma or local recurrence of intraductal carcinoma is approximately 5% per year. Of recurrent disease, 50% will be DCIS; the other 50% will be invasive carcinoma.

INVASIVE BREAST CANCERS

Infiltrating Ductal Carcinoma

This is the **most common breast malignancy**, accounting **for 70% of all breast cancers**. The tumor arises from the ductal epithelium and infiltrates the supporting stroma (Fig. 32-8). Less common but more favorable subtypes include medullary carcinoma, colloid carcinoma, tubular carcinoma, and papillary carcinoma.

Invasive Lobular Carcinoma

Lobular carcinoma arises from the lobular epithelium and infiltrates the breast stroma (Fig. 32-8). It accounts for 8% to 10% of all breast cancers and tends to be bilateral.

Paget Disease of the Nipple

Paget disease accounts for 1% to 3% of all breast malignancies. It is often concomitant with DCIS or invasive carcinoma in the subareolar area. The malignant cells enter the **epidermis of the nipple**, causing the classic eczematous changes of the nipple. Examination reveals crusting, scaling, erosion, discharge, and possibly a breast mass.

Inflammatory Breast Carcinoma

This is an **extremely aggressive** malignancy, accounting for 1% to 4% of all breast cancers. It is a poorly differentiated tumor characterized by **dermal lymphatic invasion**. Symptoms include edema, erythema, warmth, and diffuse induration of the skin described as **peau d'orange**. It is usually accompanied by axillary lymphadenopathy, and has distant metastases on presentation 17% to 36% of the time.

Strategies for the Treatment of Invasive Breast Cancer

Primary Surgical Treatment

Surgical resection is required in all patients with invasive breast cancer. In the past, radical mastectomy was the standard of care; however, most patients today are able to undergo breast-conserving therapy, modified radical mastectomy with reconstruction at the time of surgery, or modified radical mastectomy with or without reconstruction later.

Breast-conserving therapy (BCT) with **lumpectomy and radiation therapy results in identical survival as modified radical mastectomy** in appropriately selected patients. The type of primary treatment depends largely upon **the size and histology of the cancer** and on the **presence of palpable lymph nodes** preoperatively. Large tumors and those that have spread to the lymph nodes tend to recur more often, so BCT is not recommended. Patients with large tumors (>5 cm) benefit from mastectomy coupled with postoperative radiation therapy. Despite these limitations, **60% to 75% of women will be candidates for BCT** with lumpectomy and radiation.

Breast Reconstruction

Breast reconstruction carries significant **psychosocial benefits** for women with breast cancer. Reconstruction can be achieved with **implants or with autogenous tissue** (Fig. 32-9). The need for reconstruction is determined by the type of primary surgery. BCT doesn't typically require reconstruction unless a large mass is removed from a small breast. Also, reconstruction can be performed **at the time of initial surgery or deferred** until later without any adverse oncologic impact. In either case, the reconstructive surgeon should be consulted before the initial surgery.

Axillary Lymph Node Evaluation

Since **axillary node status** is one of the **most important outcome predictors** of breast cancer, evaluation of the axillary nodes must always take place. In the past, this has been accomplished using full **axillary lymph node dissection** (ALND). ALND has been

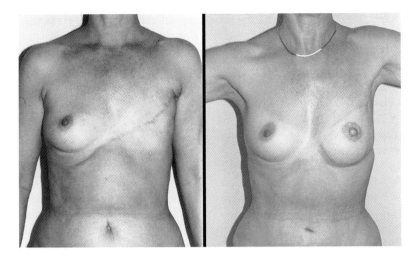

Figure 32-9 • Postmastectomy breast reconstruction.
(From Georgiade NG, Reifkohl R, Levine LS. *Georgiade Plastic, Maxillofacial and Reconstructive Surgery*, 3rd ed. Baltimore: Lippincott Williams & Wilkins; 1997.)

proven to increase survival, decrease recurrence, and provide valuable prognostic information. However, this can result in arm morbidity including arm edema, seroma formation, loss of sensation, and shoulder dysfunction. As a result, many centers are now looking at **sentinel lymph node biopsy** (SLNB) as an alternative to ALND. This less morbid procedure involves intradermal injection of dye or radioactive colloid prior to surgery around the primary tumor to identify the sentinel lymph nodes which are either sampled prior to the surgical resection of the cancer or sent for frozen section at the time of surgery. If these nodes are negative for cancer, there is a very low likelihood that the remaining nodes are positive and the patient can be spared ALND. If these nodes return positive, ALND must be performed.

Radiation Therapy

Radiation therapy is necessary for **all patients who undergo conservative therapy** because of the risk of recurrence. Radiation therapy has also been indicated for patients who undergo modified radical mastectomy if they are at a high risk for recurrence. Factors which indicate a **high risk of recurrence** include ≥4 positive nodes, a large primary tumor, positive resection margins, and grossly evident extracapsular nodal resection. Some authorities advocate the use of radiation therapy for all patients regardless of node.

Tumor Receptor Status

The **hormone receptor status** has significant implications for **prognosis and treatment** options. To ascertain the status, special assays are run to look for estrogen receptors (ER) and progesterone receptors (PR), S-phase analysis (measure of cell growth), and Her2/neu status in the excised tumor. In general, **estrogen and progesterone receptor** positive (ER+, PR+) tumors are well differentiated and exhibit a less aggressive clinical behavior, including lower recurrence rate and lower capacity to proliferate. Estrogen and progesterone-positive status therefore carries a **more favorable prognosis** than negative hormone receptor status. In addition to estrogen and progesterone receptor status, **HER2/neu status** has become an important assessment for treatment options. Overexpression of HER2/neu indicates more **aggressive tumors**.

Systemic Adjuvant Chemotherapy

Systemic adjuvent therapy with hormonal therapy, chemotherapy, or both may also be indicated based on lymph node status, tumor size, tumor grade, menopausal status, and tumor receptor status (ER, PR, Her2). Adjuvant chemotherapy results in significantly **decreased risk of recurrence** and **decreased morbidity**.

Women with **positive lymph node status** are twice as likely to metastasize to other parts of the body and chemotherapy is indicated. Women with **negative lymph node status but at higher risk** (tumor size >1 cm, high tumor grade) should also undergo chemotherapy with the goal of controlling micrometastases. Various chemotherapy regimens are currently in use. A typical regimen might include a combination of cyclophosphamide (C), methotrexate (M), and 5-fluorouracil (F).

Systemic Adjuvant Hormone Therapy

Systemic hormonal therapy with or without chemotherapy is also utilized for patients with receptor positive cancers (ER+, PR+) regardless of the patient's age or menopausal status. **Tamoxifen** is available for women with positive estrogen and/or progesterone receptor status. This antiestrogen works by competitively binding estrogen receptors, thus inhibiting the effect of estrogen on breast tissue. Tamoxifen stops estrogen from stimulating growth of the cancer cells. It is generally used for 5 years after the primary surgical treatment.

Aromatase inhibitors such as letrozole, anstrozole, and exemstane are now available for postmenopausal women with receptor-positive cancers. These newer agents have **antiestrogenic properties** and have been shown to have a longer disease-free survival when compared to tamoxifen.

HER2/neu status is another prognostic factor for more aggressive tumors. Monoclonal antibodies such as Trastuzumab are used for adjuvent treatment. Trastuzumab works by binding to the HER2/neu receptor and preventing proliferation.

Treatment of Metastatic or Recurrent Disease

Estrogen receptor negative patients with metastatic or recurrent disease are best treated with combination chemotherapy that may include doxorubicin (Adriamycin [A]) and vincristine (V), in addition to CMF. There is a 75% response to chemotherapy but this is only temporary (6 to 8 months) with the average additional survival being 1.5 to 2 years from the time of recurrence.

Estrogen receptor positive patients with metastatic or recurrent disease benefit most from hormonal therapy rather than chemotherapy. Premenopausal women may be treated with oophorectomy or gonadotropin-releasing hormone (GnRH) antagonists, whereas postmenopausal women are treated with tamoxifen or aromatase inhibitors.

Prognosis

The most reliable predictor for survival is the **stage of breast cancer** at the time of diagnosis (Table 32-5). Other prognostic indicators include lymph node status, hormone receptor status, tumor size, nuclear grade, histologic type, proliferative rate, and oncogene expression. The current overall 5-year survival rate for breast cancer has increased to 94%. The 5-year disease-free survival rate is 80% for stage I, 60% for stage II, 20% for stage III, and minimal for stage IV disease. **Positive estrogen and progesterone receptor status carries a more favorable prognosis as does negative lymph node status**.

Follow-Up

Follow-up after breast cancer treatment should include **a physical exam** every 3 to 6 months for 3 years, every 6 to 12 months for years 4 and 5, and annually thereafter. In women who receive breast-conserving surgery, the first **follow-up mammogram** is usually performed 6 months after completion of radiation treatment. Unless otherwise indicated, breast cancer patients should have **annual mammograms**.

Routine CBC, blood chemistries, tumor markers, chest x-ray, CT, and bone scans are not recommended for routine breast cancer follow-up or for asymptomatic patients. These tests have been replaced with **clinical monitoring for metastatic disease** (dry cough, exertional dyspnea, bone and body pains, pleuritic chest pain, etc.). Women taking **tamoxifen** should be followed for irregular bleeding given the possibility of increased endometrial cancer with tamoxifen use. Endometrial biopsy should be performed where indicated.

Hormone Use after Breast Cancer Treatment

Some premenopausal patients may wish to become pregnant after breast cancer treatment. Traditionally, this has been discouraged for fear that pregnancy-related estrogens may stimulate dormant cancer cells. Studies now suggest that **there is no difference in survival rates in women who become pregnant after breast cancer treatment**. For women who wish to avoid fertility after cancer treatment, there has been **no adverse effect shown with the use of oral contraceptives** containing estrogen.

The use of postmenopausal HRT in breast cancer survivors has been widely debated. Several well-constructed, long-term studies such as the Women's Health Initiative have identified an increased risk of breast cancer in women utilizing combination hormone therapy (HRT). For this reason, **HRT should not be used in women with a personal history of breast cancer**.

■ **TABLE 32-5** TNM Staging of Breast Cancer

Cancer Stage	Primary Tumor Size	Lymph Node Involvement	Distant Metastases
0	T_{is}	N_0	M_0
I	T_1	N_0	M_0
IIa	T_0	N_1	M_0
	T_1	N_1	M_0
	T_2	N_0	M_0
IIb	T_2	N_1	M_0
	T_3	N_0	M_0
IIIa	T_0	N_2	M_0
	T_1	N_2	M_0
	T_2	N_2	M_0
	T_3	N_1	M_0
	T_3	N_2	M_0
IIIb	T_4	Any N	M_0
	Any T	N_3	M_0
IV	Any T	Any N	M_1

Key: TNM Classification	
T:	Primary Tumor
T_x	Primary tumor unassessable
T_0	No evidence of primary tumor
T_{is}	Carcinoma in situ; intraductal carcinoma, lobular carcinoma in situ, or Paget disease of the nipple with no tumor
T_1	Tumor <2 cm in largest dimension
T_{1a}	Tumor <0.5 cm
T_{1b}	Tumor <1 cm but >0.5 cm
T_{1c}	Tumor <2 cm but >1 cm
T_2	Tumor <5 cm but >2 cm
T_3	Tumor >5 cm
T_4	Tumor any size extending to chest wall or skin
T_{4a}	Extension to chest wall
T_{4b}	Edema or ulceration of skin of breast or satellite skin nodules on ipsilateral breast
T_{4c}	Both T4a and T4b
N	Regional lymph nodes
N_x	Regional lymph nodes cannot be assessed
N_0	No regional lymph node metastases
N_1	Metastasis to mobile ipsilateral axillary lymph node
N_2	Metastasis to the ipsilateral axillary lymph node, fixed
N_3	Metastasis to ipsilateral internal mammary lymph node

continues

■ **TABLE 32-5** TNM Staging of Breast Cancer *(continued)*	
Key: TNM Classification	
M	Distant metastasis
M_x	Presence of distant metastasis cannot be assessed
M_0	No evidence of distant metastasis
M_1	Distant metastasis, including metastasis to ipsilateral supraclavicular lymph nodes

Adapted from American Joint Committee on Cancer. *Manual for Staging of Cancer*, 4th ed. Philadelphia: J.B. Lippincott; 1992:147.

KEY POINTS

- Breast cancer is the most common neoplasm in women, with a lifetime risk of 1 in 8 women in the United States.

- Routine monthly self-examination and annual physician evaluation are recommended for all women over age 20.

- Current routine mammogram recommendations include a mammogram every 1 to 2 years from age 40 to 50, and yearly after age 50.

- Women with a strong family history of breast cancer should begin screening mammograms 5 years earlier than the age of diagnosis of the youngest family member with breast cancer; 10 years earlier in the case of premenopausal breast cancer.

- Evaluation of breast masses includes careful physical exam, evaluation with mammography and ultrasound of any abnormal findings, and biopsy of suspicious findings to rule out malignancy.

- Benign breast symptoms and findings are common and occur in approximately 50% of women, with a higher incidence in younger women.

- Two-thirds of tumors in reproductive-age women are benign, whereas half of palpable masses in perimenopausal women and the majority of lesions in postmenopausal women are malignant.

- The most common benign breast illness are fibrocystic changes and fibroadenomas.

- Patients with fibrocystic change often have cyclic breast pain and masses due to an exaggerated stromal response to hormones and growth factors. Reduction in caffeine, tea, and chocolate, and treatment with vitamin E, progestins, danazol, and tamoxifen, have been found to help symptoms.

- Fibroadenomas are benign rubbery breast tumors that are usually solitary. They can be followed with expectant management. When large, they should be biopsied to rule out cystosarcoma phyllodes.

- Intraductal papilloma is the most common cause of bloody nipple discharge.

- Numerous risk factors have been identified for breast cancer (increasing age, family history, high-fat diet, ionizing radiation, late childbearing, atypical hyperplasia; prolonged HRT use); however, most patients have no known risk factors.

- Only 5% to 10% of breast cancer is related to genetic predisposition.

- DCIS (15%) is a preinvasive disease and is treated with lumpectomy and radiation therapy. LCIS (4%) is treated with observation and possible use of tamoxifen to prevent subsequent invasive breast cancer.

- Invasive breast disease—including infiltrating ductal carcinoma (70%) and infiltrating lobular carcinoma (10%)—is treated with lumpectomy and radiation or with modified mastectomy with equal risk of recurrence and survival in properly selected patients.

- Breast reconstruction can be an important part of recovering from breast cancer. It can be done during the primary surgery or delayed until later.

- All women with invasive breast disease should have ipsilateral lymph node evaluation with ALND or SLN dissection. The resected tumors should also be checked for hormone receptor status.

- The standard adjuvant treatment for women with positive lymph nodes is combination chemotherapy.

- All hormone receptor positive patients should receive hormone therapy aimed at suppressing estrogen and thereby suppressing stimulation of cancer cells. This is most commonly achieved with tamoxifen (an estrogen agonist/antagonist) or aromatase inhibitors (e.g., letrozole, anastrazole) which have antiestrogen activity.

- Follow-up for patients with invasive breast cancer includes annual mammography and frequent physical exam to evaluate for recurrent metastatic disease. Other routine blood and imaging studies are not indicated in the asymptomatic patient.

- The use of HRT should be avoided in breast cancer survivors.

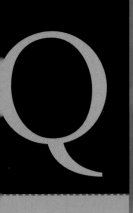

Questions

1. A couple comes in to see you because they have been un-successfully trying to conceive for the past 14 months. After a thorough history, you learn that the woman has never been pregnant and that the man has fathered no children to his knowledge. You also learn that the timing of their intercourse has been appropriate for conception. As an initial workup, what do you do next?
   a. Semen analysis for the husband and menstrual tracking, ovulation tracking, and thyroid-stimulating hormone, follicle-stimulating hormone, and prolactin levels for the wife
   b. Semen analysis and testicular biopsy for the husband and ovulation tracking, hysterosalpingogram, and lap-aroscopy for the wife
   c. Offer the couple clomiphene citrate (Clomid) because it has few side effects and the best success rate in couples with unexplained infertility
   d. Refer the couple to an infertility specialist capable of performing in vitro fertilization
   e. Do nothing because this couple is not "technically" infertile until they have been trying to conceive for 18 months

2. A 41-year-old G3 P2 Caucasian woman presents with heavy, prolonged vaginal bleeding. She has no other complaints. Up until 8 months ago she had regular monthly menses which lasted 4 to 5 days. Over the past 8 months, her periods have become progressively heavy and a bit longer. The current bleeding episode began 13 days ago. She has no other significant medical history. On physical exam she weighs 122 pounds and her blood pressure is 117/68. On pelvic exam she has a small amount of blood in the vaginal vault. Her uterus is normal size, nontender, and mobile. Her ovaries are not palpable. The patient had a normal Pap smear 3 months ago and no history of abnormal Pap smears. On pelvic ultrasound, she has an 8-cm uterus with a normal myometrium and nor-mal endometrial–myometrial junction. The endometrium

is 14 mm and there is a 2 cm × 1.2 cm lesion in the uter-ine cavity. Her β-hCG, TSH, and endometrial biopsy are all normal. Which of the following is the most likely cause of this patient's bleeding?
   a. Endometrial polyp
   b. Endometrial hyperplasia
   c. Fibroid uterus
   d. Adenomyosis
   e. Dysfunctional uterine bleeding

3. A 47-year-old G3 P3 black female comes in to see you for a second opinion. She has had fibroids all of her life and has always had regularly timed menses but they were very heavy. She has never bled after intercourse or between her periods. She has become accustomed to these symptoms but is concerned because her last period lasted 10 days and she was changing her menstrual pad nearly every 2 to 3 hours. Her TSH and endometrial biopsy were within nor-mal limits. Her hematocrit at the visit is 31%. A repeat pelvic U/S shows a multifibroid uterus that is 18 cm in overall size. Three years ago her uterus was 15 cm in size and 4 years before that it was 13 cm in size. Her primary gynecologist has suggested that she may need a hysterec-tomy and she wants your opinion. In this situation, the patient's symptoms would best be treated with:
   a. oral contraceptive pills.
   b. total abdominal hysterectomy.
   c. depo-lupron.
   d. hysteroscopic myomectomy.
   e. abdominal myomectomy.

4. A 29-year-old G3 P1 presents complaining of no menses for 4 months after stopping her birth control pills. She is con-cerned that the use of the oral birth control pills (OCPs) has left her with amenorrhea. The patient has had no recent changes in weight, exercises two to three times a week, and notes no particular changes in either her work or home

355

life. Her obstetric history includes a therapeutic abortion at age 21, a normal spontaneous delivery at age 25, and a miscarriage at age 27. After the dilation and curettage at the time of the miscarriage, the patient was hospitalized with an infection of her uterus. Since that time she has taken OCPs. Given this history, which of the following is the most likely etiology of this patient's amenorrhea?

a. Vaginal agenesis
b. Asherman's syndrome
c. Mayer-Rokitansky-Küster-Hauser syndrome
d. Testicular feminization
e. Hypogonadotropic hypogonadism

5. You are assisting in a gynecologic oncology clinic when you see a 57-year-old G3 P3 female patient who is a former nurse. She presents with 6 months of pelvic discomfort, increasing abdominal girth, and early satiety. Physical exam reveals a large abdominopelvic mass. A pelvic ultrasound and CT scan show a 10-cm right ovarian mass, ascites, and studding of the peritoneum. In your discussion with the patient you predict that this most likely represents a malignant ovarian neoplasm. She asks about the primary method of treatment for ovarian carcinoma. You explain that the mainstay of treatment for epithelial ovarian cancer is:

a. radiation therapy alone.
b. surgery alone.
c. surgery followed by chemotherapy.
d. surgery followed by radiation therapy.
e. chemoradiation alone.

6. You are seeing a 23-year-old G0 P0 who is interested in obtaining more information on available contraceptive methods. She is a nonsmoker who has had chlamydia once in the past. She has had four male sexual partners in the past and uses condoms intermittently. Her family history is notable for postmenopausal breast cancer in her mother, who was recently diagnosed and is doing well. She denies any family history of endometrial, colon, or ovarian cancer. The patient wants to know if she is a candidate for oral contraceptive pills. You tell her that the absolute contraindications for the use of estrogen-containing oral contraceptives include:

a. a history of migraine headaches.
b. a history of pulmonary embolism.
c. current smoking.
d. symptomatic fibroid uterus.
e. current hypertension.

7. A 28-year-old G2 P1 woman with a history of a prior cesarean delivery presents at 36 weeks' gestation with a complaint of vaginal bleeding. She notes no contractions, but awoke this morning with vaginal bleeding equivalent to heavy menstrual flow. You obtain an ultrasound as part of her workup for third trimester bleeding. Ultrasound is the primary diagnostic tool for which cause of third trimester bleeding?

a. Uterine rupture
b. Placental abruption
c. Placenta previa
d. Cervical neoplasm
e. Vaginal laceration

8. A 22-year-old G2 P0 at 33 weeks' gestation is found to have a BP of 166/114 mm Hg on a routine office visit. Her BP at her first prenatal visit at 7 weeks was 124/72. Her urine dip at this most recent visit shows 3+ protein although it previously had 0 to trace protein. The patient is also complaining of a persistent headache although she has no history of migraines. Her ALT and AST are elevated at 92 and 105, respectively. After starting an antihypertensive agent, magnesium sulfate, and betamethasone, what do you do next?

a. Order bed rest for the remainder of the pregnancy
b. Order bed rest until week 37, then amniocentesis for fetal lung maturity, then deliver
c. Immediate induction of labor for anticipated vaginal delivery
d. Immediate delivery via cesarean section
e. Continue expectant management

9. The patient described above has a last menstrual period of May 4, 2006. What is estimated date of confinement using the Nägele rule?

a. January 11, 2007
b. January 12, 2007
c. February 4, 2007
d. February 11, 2007
e. February 12, 2007

10. A 19-year-old G3 P1 at 31 weeks' gestation presents with contractions every 3 to 4 minutes. On examination, her cervix is found to be dilated 2 cm and 50% effaced. The patient's history is remarkable for a delivery at 33 weeks' gestation in her last pregnancy of a 5 lb 3 oz infant 3 years ago, and a miscarriage 2 years ago. She has a history of a half pack per day smoking for 6 years. Which of the following is the most predictive risk factor for recurrent preterm labor?

a. History of spontaneous abortion
b. Prior preterm delivery
c. Large fetus
d. Cigarette smoking
e. Teenage pregnancy

11. A 19-year-old primigravid patient presents for an initial prenatal visit at 7 weeks' gestation. She is concerned because she used both cocaine and heroin in the month before

she discovered she was pregnant. In a long discussion with her about the risks of substance abuse during pregnancy, you tell her that use of which of the following has the highest correlation with congenital abnormalities?

a. Alcohol
b. Caffeine
c. Cocaine
d. Opiates
e. Smoking tobacco

12. Your next patient is returning to see you to get her pelvic ultrasound results. She is 32-year-old G2 P1011 who presents with menorrhagia for the past year. She denies any intermenstrual bleeding or postcoital spotting. However, when her menses come, she needs to wear an overnight pad and a super tampon at the same time. For the first 3 days, she has to change her pad and tampon about every 2 hours. She's already ruined several pairs of pants and has had to leave work twice for heavy bleeding. Her pelvic ultrasound is notable for an 8-cm uterus with two intramural fibroids about 2 cm each. She has a third fibroid that is 3.1 cm. About one-half of that fibroid is reported as being submucosal. Her ovaries are both normal. Her TSH from last visit was normal, her hematocrit is 33%, and her endometrial biopsy showed proliferative endometrium. She wants your advice for what to do next. How would this patient be best managed?

a. Intravenous estrogen
b. Oral contraceptive pills
c. Hysteroscopic myomectomy
d. Abdominal myomectomy
e. Abdominal hysterectomy

13. A 19-year-old G3 P1 patient with a history of a miscarriage in her last pregnancy presents to the emergency department with some vaginal spotting. She reports that her last menstrual period occurred 6 weeks earlier. She has had no vaginal discharge other than the spotting, no cramping, and no abdominal pain. Her physical examination reveals a slightly enlarged uterus, no tenderness, and a closed cervical os. A serum β-hCG level is sent off and returns 346. A pelvic ultrasound shows no intrauterine pregnancy, a 2-cm left ovarian cyst, and no free fluid. Your diagnosis of this patient is which of the following?

a. Threatened abortion/rule out ectopic pregnancy
b. Ectopic pregnancy
c. Inevitable abortion
d. Missed abortion
e. Normal pregnancy

14. In the patient described above, when should a repeat β-hCG be drawn?

a. 24 hours
b. 48 hours

c. 72 hours
d. 1 week
e. It does not need to be drawn again

15. A 29-year-old G0 woman presents for a routine examination. Her physical examination is entirely normal; however, her Pap smear shows a high-grade squamous intraepithelial lesion (HSIL). She is otherwise healthy and is a moderate smoker. You perform an immediate colposcopy and the biopsies read as squamous cell carcinoma in situ (CIS). The patient would like to preserve her fertility if possible. How would you manage this patient?

a. Simple hysterectomy
b. Cryotherapy
c. Loop electrosurgical excision procedure
d. Radical hysterectomy
e. Cold-knife cone biopsy

16. A 27-year-old nonpregnant woman comes to the emergency department complaining of a vaginal discharge. On speculum exam, you observe that she has a mucousy yellow discharge and that her cervix appears erythematous. On bimanual exam, the patient has cervical motion tenderness, no uterine tenderness, and no adnexal tenderness. Her temperature is 36.7°C, white blood cell count is 8.4, and the rest of the vital signs and laboratory results are within normal limits. The treatment of choice for this patient is:

a. azithromycin 1 g PO for 7 days.
b. doxycycline 100 mg PO BID for 7 days.
c. ceftriaxone 250 mg IM times 1 and doxycycline 100 mg PO BID for 7 days as an outpatient.
d. cefoxitin 2 g IV Q6h and doxycycline PO as an inpatient.
e. ampicillin, gentamicin, and clindamycin IV as an inpatient.

17. A 32-year-old G2 P2 patient is 7 days' postpartum after repeat cesarean section. She presents to labor and delivery complaining of fever and chills. She is breastfeeding and her breasts are sore and tender. In your differential diagnosis of fever in this patient, which of the following is unlikely because of the timing of the presentation?

a. Endomyometritis
b. Wound infection
c. Mastitis
d. Pyelonephritis
e. Onset of lactation, or milk letdown

18. A 32-year-old woman presents for her first prenatal visit. She has a history of two singleton births, at 39 and 40 weeks; a twin birth at 28 weeks; and two miscarriages. All four of her children are alive and well. Which of the following is her designation of gravidity (G) and parity (P)?

a. G5 P3024
b. G5 P2224

c. G6 P3024
d. G6 P2124
e. G6 P2224

19. A 19-year-old G1 P0 at 38 weeks' gestation presents to labor and delivery. On arrival, she is having contractions every 2 to 3 minutes and claims that her water broke 2 days earlier but that she didn't come in because she hadn't reached her due date. She has a temperature of 101.2°F, heart rate of 110, blood pressure of 116/72 mm Hg, and uterine tenderness on palpation. The fetal heart rate is in the 170s with small accelerations and no decelerations. Which of the following is your diagnosis of this patient?
a. Labor
b. Preterm labor
c. Chorioamnionitis
d. Maternal fever
e. Preterm rupture of membranes

20. During your pediatric gynecology rotation, you see a 13-year-old girl who is brought in by her mother. The daughter has been very healthy and is a great student and an avid gymnast. The mother is concerned that her daughter has not yet begun to menstruate. The mother had her own menarche at age 11 and she is concerned that something is wrong with her daughter. After a thorough history you perform a physical examination that reveals age-appropriate pubic and axillary hair and breast buds, which the mother says developed 1 year ago. What assessment about this patient's pubertal development is likely to be most accurate?
a. She was right to be concerned since something is most likely wrong with her daughter's development.
b. Her daughter will most likely begin to menstruate around age 14.
c. Her daughter is ahead of the expected pubertal development and should be evaluated for precocious puberty.
d. Her daughter most likely has a congenital abnormality which is responsible for the lack of menses.
e. The daughter very likely has an eating disorder which is responsible for the lack of menses.

21. A healthy 28-year-old G0 comes in to see you for increasingly painful periods. She and her husband have been trying to conceive for the past year. The patient reports regular menses each month, which are normal in length and amount of blood. However, a couple days before her menses are due to begin she gets severe abdominal pain and cramping. The pain usually subsides within a day or two of her menses beginning. More recently, her pain is lasting through her entire period and she misses at least a day or two of work each month. She is also beginning to have pain with intercourse as well. She takes ibuprofen with minimal pain relief for at least 7 days each month. Her only other

medication is the Ortho-Evra birth control patch, which she stopped using 1 year ago. On exam, her uterus is retroverted and not easily mobile. There is nodularity noted on the uterosacral ligaments. A pelvic ultrasound reveals a normal uterus and normal bilateral adnexa. What is the most appropriate initial management for this patient?
a. Diagnostic laparoscopy
b. Oral contraceptive pills and NSAIDs
c. Depot Lupron with estrogen add-back
d. Danazol
e. Expectant management

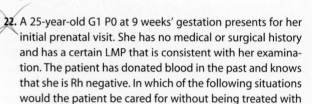

22. A 25-year-old G1 P0 at 9 weeks' gestation presents for her initial prenatal visit. She has no medical or surgical history and has a certain LMP that is consistent with her examination. The patient has donated blood in the past and knows that she is Rh negative. In which of the following situations would the patient be cared for without being treated with RhoGAM?
a. First trimester bleeding
b. Second trimester bleeding
c. Routinely at the beginning of the third trimester
d. Contractions at 34 weeks' gestation
e. At the time of an amniocentesis

23. A 52-year-old woman presents with no menses for 10 months, hot flashes, vaginal dryness, and mood swings. Her medical history is otherwise without complications. Her physical examination is within normal limits and her thyroid and pituitary function are normal. Her FSH is elevated and her endometrial biopsy shows inactive endometrium with no evidence of hyperplasia or cancer. She has no liver or renal dysfunction and has never been diagnosed with cancer or abnormal vaginal bleeding. How would you counsel this patient regarding the use of combination hormone replacement therapy?
a. She still has her uterus so she should use progestin therapy alone.
b. She still has her uterus so she should use estrogen and progestin therapy.
c. HRT will increase her risk of osteoporosis.
d. HRT will decrease her risk of breast cancer.
e. HRT will decrease her risk of uterine cancer.

24. A 23-year-old G1 P0 at week 38 is being managed with magnesium sulfate while she undergoes induction of labor for severe preeclampsia. She received a 4-g bolus followed by a constant infusion of 1.0 g/hr. However, the nurse found the patient to have absent patellar reflexes and a respiratory rate of 6 breaths/minute. The patient can be aroused but is very drowsy. In addition to discontinuing the magnesium, what should your next management step be?
a. Administer terbutaline
b. Intubate immediately

c. Administer calcium gluconate

d. Give betamethasone

e. Do nothing further

25. A 28-year-old class A2 diabetic at 34 weeks of gestation presents for a prenatal appointment. In addition to managing her insulin regimen and performing routine counseling, you also discuss plans for delivery. In general, in the well-controlled, insulin-requiring gestational diabetic woman, which mode and timing of delivery is usually employed?

a. Expectant management; await the natural onset of labor

b. Offer cesarean section in labor

c. Offer expectant management until week 42, and vaginal delivery in labor

d. Offer induction of labor between weeks 39 and 40 of gestation

e. Offer cesarean section if expected fetal weight is >4,000 g

26. A 37-year-old G7 P6 with a dichorionic/diamnionic, vertex/vertex twin gestation at 38 weeks presents to labor and delivery for induction of labor. She is started on oxytocin and begins having contractions after several hours. The patient progresses slowly over the next 16 hours until she is 5 cm dilated and, at this point, develops a fever and fetal tachycardia. The woman is diagnosed with chorioamnionitis and antibiotic therapy is started. She delivers the babies vaginally 6 hours later. Right after delivery of the second infant, there is a large, continuous hemorrhage from the vagina. The most likely cause of this is:

a. vaginal laceration.

b. cervical laceration.

c. uterine atony.

d. uterine rupture.

e. placenta accreta.

27. A 27-year-old G1 P0 African American woman presents at 16 weeks' gestation for a prenatal visit. She has had one prior prenatal visit and no known medical complications of pregnancy. Which of the following genetic tests would only be offered if one of the other tests was positive?

a. Screening for thalassemia

b. Screening for sickle-cell anemia

c. Amniocentesis

d. Expanded maternal serum α-fetoprotein

e. Screen for cystic fibrosis

28. A 69-year-old woman presents for her annual examination. Her last menstrual period was 20 years ago. She has had no vaginal bleeding since then. During the process of performing her pelvic examination, you notice a thinning

and whitening of the vulva and perianal area. When questioned, the patient reports that she has never noticed the changes before. On further examination the patient has an atrophic vulva with fusion of the labia majora and minora. What would you do next?

a. Treat with topical testosterone

b. Treat with topical ketoconazole

c. Treat with topical corticosteroid

d. Treat with vaginal estrogen

e. Biopsy representative areas of the lesion

29. Your next patient in clinic is a young woman who recently underwent a dilation and evacuation of the uterus for a complete molar pregnancy. She is now being followed with weekly β-hCG levels to monitor for recurrent disease. Initially, her β-hCG levels declined. Unfortunately, the levels then plateaued and, 8 weeks after evacuation, began to rise. They have continued to rise over the past 2 weeks. The patient has not been sexually active since the evacuation and has been reliably taking oral contraceptive pills. You inform her of the rising levels and your suspicion of a persistent/invasive molar pregnancy. The evaluation for metastatic disease is negative. Together you make a plan for her follow-up care. How do you manage her disease at this stage?

a. Continue expectant management

b. Repeat D&C

c. Total abdominal hysterectomy

d. Single-agent chemotherapy

e. Multiagent chemotherapy

30. A 25 yo G1 with a singleton pregnancy at 27 weeks' gestation presents to labor and delivery with contractions and vaginal spotting. External tocometry demonstrates regular contractions every 3 to 4 minutes, and her cervical exam is 3 cm dilated. Fetal heart rate monitoring is reassuring. She is initiated on tocolysis in order to achieve steroid benefit. Which of the following is a tocolytic whose mechanism of action is to directly block the influx of calcium into smooth muscle cells?

a. Indomethacin

b. Nifedipine

c. Magnesium sulfate

d. Betamethasone

e. Terbutaline

31. A 34-year-old G3 P1102 presents for routine prenatal visit at 32 weeks' gestational age. Fetal heart tones are measured at 140 by Doppler. Fundal height is 28 centimeters, slightly increased from 27 centimeters at her last visit 3 weeks ago. The patient undergoes an ultrasound evaluation which demonstrates an estimated fetal weight of 2,120 g, the 44th percentile for age, and an obvious scarcity of amniotic fluid with an amniotic fluid index (AFI)

of 3. Which of the following conditions could be responsible for oligohydramnios in this pregnancy?

a. Poorly controlled maternal diabetes
b. Fetal renal agenesis
c. Fetal duodenal atresia
d. Maternal-fetal Rh incompatibility
e. Fetal tracheo-esophageal fistula

32. A 32-year-old G1 with a history of systemic lupus erythematosus (SLE) presents for a routine prenatal visit at 33 weeks' gestation. She complains of headaches and an overall feeling of malaise starting 2 days ago. Upon further evaluation, the patient is found to have an elevated blood pressure of 156/98 mm Hg. Which of the following pieces of data will best help you to determine whether her findings are secondary to a lupus flare or preeclampsia?

a. Catheterized urinalysis
b. Platelet count
c. Serial blood pressure measurements
d. Complement levels (C3, C4)
e. Transamonitis

33. A 21-year-old G0 presents for her first gynecologic exam. She states that she is not sexually active and is a virgin. She is a college senior who plays volleyball on the club team and has no significant medical history. She has regular menses with some mild dysmenorrhea. On speculum exam, you observe a small raised lesion 0.5 cm in diameter on the face of the cervix. It is smooth and blue in color with the appearance of a bubble underneath the cervical surface. What is your diagnosis?

a. Bartholin cyst
b. Nabothian cyst
c. Skene's gland cyst
d. Cervical dysplasia
e. Cervical cancer

34. A 25-year-old nulliparous female presents to her gynecologist with chief complaint of infertility. She states that she and her husband have been trying to get pregnant for the past year. She has regular periods that she considers somewhat heavy associated with cramping pain during the first 2 to 3 days of her menses. She undergoes a hysterosalpingogram which confirmed tubal patency but demonstrated an irregular uterine cavity surface consistent with submucosal leiomyomata (fibroids). Considering this patient's desire for a pregnancy, what is the most appropriate treatment for her fibroids?

a. Uterine artery embolization
b. Combined oral contraceptives
c. Depot medroxyprogesterone
d. Hysteroscopic myomectomy
e. Total hysterectomy

35. An otherwise healthy 32-year-old G5 P3013 presents for her first prenatal visit at 8 weeks' gestation. She had a spontaneous miscarriage 9 years ago before having two term vaginal deliveries 7 years ago and 5 years ago before undergoing a cesarean section 2 years ago. You request the operative note from that procedure. Which of the following would be an absolute contraindication for a trial of labor after cesarean and attempt at vaginal birth after cesarean (VBAC)?

a. A classical cesarean section for transverse presentation
b. An emergent low-transverse cesarean section for nonreassuring fetal status
c. A low-vertical cesarean section for cephalopelvic disproportion
d. A scheduled low-transverse cesarean section for active herpes simplex lesions
e. A low-transverse cesarean section for breech presentation

36. A 21-year-old G1 P0 at 42 weeks' gestation presents with mild contractions every 4 to 5 minutes and a cervical examination of 1 cm dilation, 50% effaced at −2 station. The fetal heart rate tracing reveals a baseline in the 140s with repetitive variable decelerations. The patient has had routine prenatal care and a normal fetal survey at 18 weeks' gestation. Which of the following is the most likely cause of these decelerations?

a. Uteroplacental insufficiency
b. Maternal hypotension
c. Oligohydramnios
d. Fetal acidemia
e. Fetal head compression

37. A 23-year-old G0 P0 woman presents to the emergency room complaining of a sudden onset of LLQ pain which began a few hours ago. The pain is now dull and achy but persistent. She has regular menses and is not sexually active. Her last period was 4.5 weeks ago. She says that she is a few days overdue for her menses. This is not typical for her. She denies any nausea, vomiting, or diarrhea. She is afebrile, normotensive, and her abdominal exam is notable for moderate LLQ tenderness with palpation. She has no rebound, her abdomen is not rigid, and she has no involuntary guarding. Her labs show a hematocrit of 38% and a β-hCG that is negative. A pelvic ultrasound reveals a 4-cm complex left ovarian cyst and a small amount of complex free fluid in the cul-de-sac. After a few hours' observation, you reexamine the patient and her exam has improved a bit and a repeat hematocrit is 37%. How would you proceed with this patient?

a. Take her to the OR for a left ovarian cystectomy
b. Start her on an oral contraceptive pill to suppress cyst formation and reevaluate her at her next annual visit

c. Reassure her and have her follow up in 2 weeks; if stable then, repeat the pelvic ultrasound in 60 to 90 days

d. Reassure her that all is well and prescribe a nonsteroidal anti-inflammatory drug (NSAID) for her discomfort

e. Take her to the OR for a left oophorectomy

38. A 37-year-old G2 P0 at 42 weeks' gestation with diet-controlled Class A1 gestational diabetes presents in labor. The fetal heart rate tracing is reassuring, and the patient is contracting well every 2 to 3 minutes. She progresses slowly over the course of the day until she is fully dilated. She begins the second stage of labor and pushes for 1.5 hours. Finally the head delivers, but once it does there is a shoulder dystocia. Which of the following actions is likely to worsen the shoulder dystocia?

a. Suprapubic pressure

b. Fundal pressure

c. Increased flexion of the hips

d. Delivery of the posterior arm

e. Episiotomy

39. A 42-year-old G3 P3 comes in to see you for a second opinion. She has had fibroids all of her life but her periods have always been regular and she has never had postcoital spotting or intermenstrual bleeding until recently. Over the past year or so her periods have become very heavy with more cramping and she also had some prolonged menses lasting 7 to 10 days (normal for her is 4 days). She is sexually active with her husband but had a tubal ligation after their last child was born. Her TSH was normal and her β-hCG was negative. Her FSH level showed her to be pre-menopausal. Her pelvic ultrasound showed an 8-cm uterus with two 2-cm intramural fibroids. There was thickening of the junction between the endometrium and myometrium up to 15 mm in some locations. The junction was indiscernible in other places. Her ovaries were both normal. This was confirmed on pelvic MRI. Her primary gynecologist has suggested that she may need a hysterectomy and she wants your opinion. In this situation, the patient's symptoms would best be treated with:

a. total abdominal hysterectomy and bilateral salpin-gooophorectomy.

b. hysteroscopic myomectomy.

c. abdominal myomectomy.

d. total abdominal hysterectomy.

e. vaginal hysterectomy.

40. Your next patient is a 24-year-old graduate student who comes in 36 hours after she and her partner experienced a condom break while having intercourse. She is using no other form of contraception and her last menstrual period started 2 weeks ago. She is in the middle of her graduate

studies and does not wish to be pregnant at this time. What do you tell this patient?

a. You have nothing to offer her because there is no way to prevent pregnancy once a contraceptive accident has occurred.

b. You have nothing to offer her because, although there is a "morning after" pill, it must be given within the first 24 hours after unprotected intercourse.

c. Take 2 35-g birth control pills now, and 2 more 24 hours from now.

d. Take 1 0.75-mg levonorgestrel now, and another 12 hours from now.

e. It is very unlikely that she will get pregnant and she should come back if she doesn't get a period within 6 weeks.

41. A 36-year-old G1 with a singleton pregnancy at 27 weeks' gestation presents for routine prenatal care and undergoes a diabetes screening with a 50-g oral glucose load. Her serum glucose 1 hour after glucose administration is 147. What is the next appropriate action for this patient?

a. Have patient return for diabetic teaching and nutritional counseling

b. Have patient record fasting and postprandial glucose readings via glucometer

c. Have patient return for 3-hour 100-g glucose tolerance test

d. Have patient return for fasting serum glucose

e. Have patient return for hemoglobin A1c

42. An otherwise healthy 26-year-old G1 with a pregnancy at 34 weeks' gestation presents for routine prenatal care complaining of dyspnea. The patient reports that she is increasingly short of breath as her pregnancy progresses, and she is unable to walk up a flight of stairs without becoming winded. Which of the following is a normal maternal physiologic change of pregnancy that contributes to dyspnea of pregnancy?

a. Decreased tidal volume

b. Decreased $PaCO_2$

c. Increased total lung capacity

d. Increased expiratory reserve volume

e. Decrease in minute ventilation

43. A 17-year-old G1 presents in term labor and progresses to complete dilation and +3 station. She pushes for 2 hours and progresses to +4 station but cannot deliver the fetal head. Which of the following is a theoretical benefit to performing a mediolateral episiotomy compared to a median (or midline) episiotomy?

a. Less painful for patient

b. Decreased risk of infection

c. Ease of repair
d. Decreased risk of fourth-degree laceration
e. Improved healing

44. A 29-year-old G2 P1001 with a singleton pregnancy at 35 weeks' gestation presents for routine prenatal visit. As part of her visit, her physician performs Leopolds maneuvers and suspects her fetus is in the breech position. An ultrasound confirms breech positioning, and the patient is counseled on her options for delivery. She has a history of previous vaginal delivery at term, delivering an 8 lb 3 oz baby. She would prefer a vaginal delivery. What would you recommend for this patient?
   a. Recheck fetal position at 37 weeks and if still breech, attempt external version
   b. Recheck fetal position at 39 weeks and if still breech, repeat cesarean section
   c. Admit to L&D at 35 weeks, administer an epidural, and attempt external version as version is more successful earlier in gestation
   d. Plan for repeat cesarean section at 39 weeks as fetus is unlikely to spontaneously convert to vertex position
   e. Wait for spontaneous labor and if still breech, repeat cesarean section

45. A 23-year-old woman presents with multiple lesions on her labia and perineum. These tender ulcers have been causing discomfort for 36 hours. The patient also complains of dysuria and fatigue. On physical exam, she also has bilateral inguinal adenopathy. A Tzanck prep of one of the lesions reveals multinucleated giant cells. The woman is concerned that this was transmitted sexually and would like to be tested for other sexually transmitted diseases.
   Which of the following tests should be ordered?
   a. Rapid plasma reagin (RPR)
   b. HIV
   c. Chlamydiazyme DNA probe
   d. Gonorrhea culture or DNA probe
   e. All of the above

46. Which of the following regimens can be used to cure the patient described in Question 45?
   a. Acyclovir 400 mg PO TID
   b. Ceftriaxone 250 mg IM × 1
   c. Azithromycin 1 g PO × 1
   d. Metronidazole 500 mg PO BID
   e. None of the above

47. A colleague asks for your opinion with a patient she is currently examining. The patient is a 37-year-old G2 P2 who is presenting with postcoital spotting. Her menstrual periods are regular in amount and timing. She has never had this symptom before and has had the same sexual partner, her husband, for 8 years. On exam she has normal external female genitalia and a normal vagina. Her cervix shows no discharge or cervical motion tenderness. The cervical os is noted to contain a 3-mm fleshy pedunculated mass. Her uterus is normal in size, mobile, and nontender. Her last Pap smear was 6 months ago and was negative for malignancy. How would this patient be best managed?
   a. Observation and menstrual calendar
   b. Repeat Pap smear
   c. Pelvic ultrasound
   d. Remove the mass in the office at that time
   e. Abdominal hysterectomy

48. A 17-year-old gymnast presents in generally good health except for the absence of menses. She states that she developed breasts later than her friends and never began menstruation. On physical examination, she has Tanner stage V development of breasts and pubic hair. On speculum exam, her cervix appears normal and she has a normal bimanual exam. The most likely etiology of this patient's primary amenorrhea is:
   a. anorexia nervosa.
   b. gonadal agenesis.
   c. transverse vaginal septum.
   d. testicular feminization.
   e. hypogonadotropic hypogonadism.

49. A 46-year-old woman was diagnosed with metastatic breast cancer. She underwent mastectomy and axillary node dissection, which showed positive lymph node involvement. She underwent breast reconstruction at the same time as her primary surgery. The tissue was sent for estrogen and progesterone receptor evaluation and both were positive. What would be your next step in treatment?
   a. No further therapy is needed
   b. Chemotherapy and hormone therapy
   c. Chemotherapy alone
   d. Hormone therapy alone
   e. Radiation therapy alone

50. A 27-year-old woman presents complaining of foul-smelling vaginal discharge. On exam she has a gray-green discharge and the cervix has punctate epithelial papillae, giving it a "strawberry" appearance. On wet prep a unicellular organism with flagella can be seen. This organism is most likely:
   a. Candida albicans.
   b. Trichomonas vaginalis.
   c. Gardnerella vaginalis.
   d. Bacteroides fragilis.
   e. Haemophilus ducreyi.

51. A 27-year-old G1 P0 at 40 weeks' gestation presents to labor and delivery in active labor. Over the course of

several hours, she progresses from 3 cm to 8 cm dilation. At this point, she is in:

a. stage I of labor, latent phase.
b. stage I of labor, active phase.
c. stage II of labor, latent phase.
d. stage II of labor, active phase.
e. stage III of labor.

52. A 27-year-old woman presents to the emergency department complaining of vaginal discharge and abdominal pain. On physical examination she has a temperature of 38.1°C and on abdominal exam has tenderness in the right upper quadrant and lower abdomen with minimal peritoneal signs. On speculum exam, the patient has a mucousy yellow discharge. On bimanual exam, she has cervical motion tenderness and bilateral adnexal tenderness. Her white blood cell count is 14.3 and a pelvic ultrasound shows a normal uterus and normal ovaries bilaterally. The most likely diagnosis for this patient is which of the following?

a. Cervicitis
b. Endomyometritis
c. Pelvic inflammatory disease
d. Tubo-ovarian abscess
e. Appendicitis

53. A 68-year-old woman presents with vulvar pruritis for the prior year that has been increasing over the past few months. She has tried antifungal medications, which seem to help but the symptoms always return and have persisted for several months. She went through menopause at age 49 and has not been sexually active for 10 years. She does not use douching products and is not on any antibiotics. On physical examination, you note thin white epithelium of the labia, perineum, and perianal area which is consistent with lichen sclerosis. How do you proceed?

a. Wide local excision of the lesion
b. Perform a punch biopsy of the vulvar lesion
c. Use cryotherapy to eradicate the lesion
d. Culture the vagina and treat with a long course of antifungals
e. Treat with moderate-potency topical steroids

54. A 29-year-old G3 P2 at 38 weeks' gestation presents to labor and delivery complaining of the sudden onset of abdominal pain and bright-red vaginal bleeding. On examination, her uterus is firm and tender to palpation and the tocodynamometer reveals regular contractions every 1 to 2 minutes. The fetal heart monitor shows no evidence of fetal distress. The patient had a normal ultrasound at week 34 that showed the infant in the vertex presentation. Which of the following is the most likely diagnosis in this patient?

a. Labor
b. Premature rupture of membranes

c. Placenta accreta
d. Placenta previa
e. Placental abruption

55. A 45-year-old G4 P4 Caucasian female comes in to see you for an annual exam. During this time she mentions that she has had some pelvic pressure and an uncomfortable sensation in her vagina, which has worsened over the past year or so. She describes a pressure sensation in her vagina, which feels as if she is "sitting on a small ball." She also complains of urinary frequency but denies any leaking of urine or irregular bleeding. Her past obstetric/gynecologic history is notable for four term spontaneous vaginal deliveries and two of the children were over 10 pounds at birth. She has regular menses and denies any symptoms of menopause. She has no major medical problems. She has worked for a national package delivery business for the past 15 years. As such, she loads and unloads heavy boxes much of the day. Her pelvic exam is notable for a large bulging anterior vaginal wall. In this situation, how would the patient's symptoms best be treated?

a. Bladder suspension/sling procedure
b. Vaginal pessary
c. Anterior colporrhaphy
d. Anticholinergics drugs
e. Kegel exercises

56. A 23-year-old woman presents with a single papule on her right labia. It is nontender and approximately 1 cm in diameter. The rest of her physical exam is negative except for palpable inguinal adenopathy. She has never had a lesion like this before. She last had intercourse 2.5 weeks ago and wants to be tested for sexually transmitted diseases. Which of the following would likely not be ordered in a routine STI screen?

a. Gonorrhea culture or DNA probe
b. Chlamydiazyme DNA probe
c. Rapid plasma reagin
d. HIV
e. HSV Ab titers

57. Dark-field microscopy is performed on the above patient, revealing motile spirochetes. You treat the patient with which of the following?

a. 1 g azithromycin PO
b. Acyclovir 400 mg PO TID
c. Acyclovir 400 mg IV TID
d. Benzathine penicillin G 2.4 M units × 1
e. Penicillin G 2.4 M units IV Q4h

58. Your next patient is a 43-year-old G2 P1 Caucasian female who comes in to see you for involuntary loss of urine. Her history is notable for a radical hysterectomy and bilateral

salpingo-oophorectomy for cervical cancer. Unfortunately, she had a recurrence of her cancer but it was controlled with pelvic radiation. She is feeling well but is concerned about constantly leaking urine. The leaking is painless but continuous. When methylene blue is instilled into the bladder in a retrograde fashion, there is no blue leakage onto the vaginal tampon. However, when indigo-carmine is intravenously administered, the dye leaks onto the tampon. What is the most likely source of this patient's incontinence?

a. Urethrovaginal fistula
b. Vesicovaginal fistula
c. Ureterovaginal fistula
d. Overflow incontinence
e. Genuine stress urinary incontinence

59. A 27-year-old G1 P0 at 40 weeks' gestation presents to labor and delivery with contractions every 6 to 8 minutes. Of the following findings, which is the most worrisome on the fetal heart tracing?

a. Repetitive early decelerations, minimal variability
b. No heart rate decelerations, minimal variability
c. Repetitive late decelerations, absent variability
d. No heart rate decelerations, moderate variability
e. Repetitive variable decelerations, moderate variability

60. You are seeing a patient in follow-up after your partner started her on hormone replacement therapy (HRT) 3 months ago. She had severe menopausal symptoms including hot flashes, vaginal atrophy, and mood swings. She has no history of liver disease, cancer of any kind, DVT, or pulmonary embolism. She has never been diagnosed with abnormal vaginal bleeding. She is very happy with the symptom relief she has received but wonders how long she should continue using HRT. What do you recommend for her?

a. Continuous therapy for the next 5 years and then stop to see if symptoms return.
b. You inform her that there's no risk in continuing HRT indefinitely.
c. You suggest she continue HRT until her symptoms are completely gone.
d. You recommend a 6- to 12-month course and then changing to other options to address any remaining symptoms.
e. You apologize for your colleague and explain that she should have never been started on HRT and should try other remedies for her symptoms.

61. A 23-year-old G1 P0 at 35 weeks' gestation presents with a vaginal gush of fluid. On sterile speculum examination, the patient has a pool of clear fluid in the vagina that is nitrazine and fern positive. She is contracting every 3 to 4 minutes, and her cervix on visualization appears to be dilated 2 to 3 cm. Which of the following is the best course of action?

a. Tocolysis with magnesium or terbutaline
b. Betamethasone and tocolysis
c. Betamethasone and no tocolysis
d. Expectant management
e. Amnio/dye test

62. A 19-year-old woman presents with complaints of no periods for the past 7 months. During this time she started college and feels her stress level has increased. The patient has also changed her eating habits, which has led to a weight decrease from 120 to 105 pounds. She has noted no other changes in her health. Which of the following tests should be ordered initially?

a. Thyroid-stimulating hormone (TSH), prolactin
b. β-hCG, prolactin, TSH
c. Follicle-stimulating hormone, β-hCG
d. Prolactin, β-hCG, DHEAS
e. Testosterone, β-hCG

63. The labs ordered for the patient discussed above were all normal. Which of the following would be the best way to assess this patient's estrogenization?

a. Progesterone challenge test
b. ACTH stim test
c. LH/FSH ratio
d. Estradiol levels
e. Endometrial biopsy

64. A 29-year-old G0 has been a type 1 diabetic for 17 years and now presents for pregestational counseling. In addition to the standard pregestational advice such as checking a rubella titer and to take folic acid, you counsel her regarding tight blood sugar control prior to becoming pregnant. Assuming that the patient lowers her HgbA1c prior to pregnancy, the risk of which of the following complications will be unchanged?

a. Caudal regression syndrome
b. Cardiac anomalies
c. Fetal macrosomia
d. Neural tube defects
e. All of the above

65. A 43-year-old patient presents with 2-cm breast mass in the right upper outer quadrant of her left breast. On examination in your office there is no skin change, nipple discharge, enlarged lymph nodes, or tenderness. She has no known family history of breast cancer. She reports the mass has not changed after her menstrual cycle and the mass is still present. An ultrasound shows that the mass is not a cyst. You obtain a mammogram, which is

negative. What is the next management step for this patient?

a. No further follow-up is needed
b. Follow with clinical exams
c. Reexamine at her annual exam in 4 months
d. Excisional biopsy
e. Fine-needle aspiration or core biopsy

66. A 19-year-old woman presents with a complaint of 6 months of amenorrhea. She notes that she has not had a period since starting college last fall. The patient notes no weight loss during that time and has, in fact, gone from 173 to 181 pounds over the past few months but believes the weight gain is secondary to change in diet during college. She denies nipple discharge, frequent headaches, and vaginal discharge. She notes no other symptoms. Which of the following tests is most likely to be abnormal, indicating her diagnosis?

a. Thyroid-stimulating hormone
b. Follicle-stimulating hormone
c. Prolactin
d. Luteinizing hormone
e. β-hCG

67. A 38-year-old G0 P0 woman comes in to see you at the urging of her friend. She is concerned because she has not had a period in 8 months. She regrets not coming in sooner but she is 275 pounds and felt embarrassed about her weight. She says that she has skipped menstrual periods all of her life and has never has a regular monthly period. She denies headaches, visual changes, or nipple discharge. She denies any hot flashes, mood swings, and vaginal dryness. She and her husband have tried to conceive for years but have been unable to become pregnant. They still desire a child. Her past medical history is notable for morbid obesity, hypertension, and infertility. Her TSH and PRL are both normal and her FSH is at a premenopausal level. You perform an endometrial biopsy, which shows complex endometrial hyperplasia without atypia. What would be the most important next step in her management?

a. Progestin therapy and repeat an endometrial biopsy in 3 to 6 months
b. OCPs for menstrual regulation
c. Progesterone for menstrual regulation
d. Abdominal hysterectomy
e. Recommend weight loss

68. A 52-year-old menopausal patient comes in for a complaint of involuntarily leaking urine. These episodes occur without warning and may happen any time during the day or night. The leaking occasionally occurs with coughing or laughing but there is no clear association between her leaking and any specific activity. Occasionally, if she even sees a bathroom, she feels the urge to void. This has become more and more of a problem for her since she has an active work life and social life. You perform some simple tests in your office and send her for further urodynamic testing. Her physical exam is largely unremarkable. Her urinalysis and cultures are negative. Urodynamic evaluation shows the presence of spontaneous bladder contractions even after filling the bladder with small amounts of fluid. What treatment would you offer this patient?

a. Bladder suspension/sling procedure
b. Vaginal pessary
c. Kegel exercises
d. Anticholinergics
e. Anterior colporrhaphy

69. A 17-year-old G1 P0 presents for a first prenatal visit. She has had minimal symptoms, but she has gained 10 pounds over the past 2 to 3 months. She does not know when her last menstrual period (LMP) was. Which of the following would be the most useful to determine her estimated date of delivery?

a. Physical examination
b. Maternal perception of fetal movement
c. Abdominal ultrasound at 16 weeks' gestation
d. Transvaginal ultrasound at 8 weeks' gestation
e. Her best guess at LMP

70. A 19-year-old woman presents complaining of 7 months of amenorrhea. She notes that she has not had a period since 2 to 3 months after starting college. She notes weight loss during that time from 131 to 114 pounds over the past few months but believes the weight loss is secondary to a change in diet during college. She also has insomnia, heat intolerance, and occasionally hot flashes. Which of the following tests would most likely indicate her diagnosis?

a. Thyroid-stimulating hormone
b. Luteinizing hormone
c. Prolactin
d. β-hCG
e. ACTH stim test

71. A 21-year-old G1 P1001 is now 36 hours status post a primary low transverse cesarean section for failure to progress after a prolonged attempt at a vaginal delivery. She is complaining of abdominal pain that is worsening. Her temperature is 38.5°C, BP is 115/70 mm Hg, P 106, O_2 saturation of 97%, and respirations are 16. Her uterine fundus is exquisitely tender to palpation. Lungs are clear to auscultation, no signs or erythema or tenderness of the breasts, and she has no swelling or pain in her lower extremities. There is no incisional erythema or induration. Labs reveal a WBC of 22

and hematocrit of 34. What is the most appropriate next step to evaluate and treat this patient?

a. CT of the abdomen and transfuse 2 units of packed RBCs.
b. Do nothing as these are all normal findings after a cesarean delivery.
c. Culture for *Gonorrhea* and *Chlamydia* and treat with azithromycin.
d. Perform a bimanual exam and start IV clindamycin and gentamycin.
e. Dopplers of the lower extremities and start heparin or lovenox.

72. A 68-year-old postmenopausal G4 P4004 is seen in your clinic for her annual exam. She complains of occasional urinary incontinence with sneezing or coughing, and also reports heaviness in the lower abdomen and mild bulging from the vagina that is more prominent at the end of the day. She has no fecal incontinence and no vaginal dryness. Her PMH is significant for obesity, COPD, CHF, and poorly controlled diabetes. She has smoked 1/2 PPD for the last 40 years. Three of her children weighed more than 9 lbs at birth. On pelvic exam you note second-degree pelvic relaxation. What treatment would you recommend for this patient?

a. Placement of a mesh transobturator sling for urethral support.
b. Vaginal hysterectomy and McCall culdoplasty
c. Anterior colporrhaphy
d. Posterior colporrhaphy
e. Placement of a pessary and encourage Kegal exercises

73. Mrs. M brings her 13-year-old daughter to see you because she is concerned that her daughter has not yet started menstruation. The young girl is well nourished, but not overweight. Her mother was 11 years old at menarche. She states that her daughter first started developing breast tissue 6 months ago, which is when she started wearing a training bra. Shortly thereafter she started to develop a small amount of pubic and axillary hair. On examination you find that the patient has a small amount of hair covering the labia majora only and does not extend onto the mons pubis. She has development of breast buds and papilla and areolar enlargement, but there is no separation in contour between the breast and areola. What Tanner stage would you assign this patient?

a. Tanner stage I
b. Tanner stage II
c. Tanner stage III
d. Tanner stage B
e. Tanner stage C

74. A 16-year-old female presents to your clinic with primary amenorrhea. She is not sexually active and to confirm you check a pregnancy test which is negative. She had normal breast development that began at age 12 and is now

at a Tanner stage V. Pelvic exam reveals a blind pouch that represents a very shortened vagina. Abdominal ultrasound reveals bilateral normal appearing ovaries and a pelvic mass consistent with a uterus. Chromosome analysis reveals that she is 46, XX. Which is the most likely diagnosis?

a. Testicular feminization
b. Gonadal agenesis
c. Mayer-Rokitansky-Kuster-Hauser syndrome
d. Swyer's syndrome
e. Turner's syndrome

75. A young married couple returns to your clinic with 2 years of infertility. She has regular menses and per the ovulation predictor kits and basal body temperature charting, she ovulates regularly on day 13 or 14. They have been practicing timed intercourse with no success. Hysterosalpingogram shows that both of her fallopian tubes are patent. Semen analysis collected at the last visit shows that the he has a low sperm count, but normal motility and morphology. He is otherwise healthy and takes no medications except for an over-the-counter multivitamin and does not smoke. What is the best recommendation for this couple to achieve conception?

a. With a low sperm count it will be nearly impossible for this couple to conceive. Their best options would be to pursue adoption or donor sperm.
b. This couple may be able to achieve pregnancy with intrauterine insemination in which washed sperm is inserted into the uterus at the time of ovulation.
c. This couple should be referred to a reproductive endocrinologist so that intracytoplasmic sperm injection can be performed.
d. The husband should begin to routinely take warm baths to encourage a better sperm count for the next month.
e. The next best step for this couple would be for the woman to start clomiphene citrate and practice timed intercourse accordingly.

76. A 27-year-old G2 P2 returns to your clinic after her Pap smear returned as high-grade squamous intraepithelial lesion (HSIL). On colposcopic exam you note an area on the anterior cervix at the squamocolumnar junction that turns opaque white with administration of acetic acid. A mosaic pattern surrounds this area with small red punctate lesions within the mosaicism. You biopsy this area and send it to pathology. An endocervical curettage is also performed. She tolerated the procedure without any difficulties. The lesion appears to be confined to the ectocervix. The pathology on the cervical biopsy returns as CIN II. The endocervical curettings were within normal limits (negative for dysplasia). What treatment recommendations would you make for this patient?

a. Repeat Pap and colposcopy in 6 months
b. LEEP to be performed in the office.

c. Cold-knife conization in the operating room.
d. Two-stage or "top-hat" LEEP procedure
e. Hysterectomy

77. At the end of her visit for a blood pressure check, a 48-year-old G3 P3 mentions that she has been having an embarrassing problem with leaking a small amount of urine when she cough, laughs, or sneezes. She denies any dysuria, hematuria, or nocturia and denies the urge to void when hearing running water or passing a ladies room. Mostly, she finds her symptoms to be inconvenient and embarrassing. She's otherwise healthy and has regular monthly menses and has had three vaginal deliveries. What initial therapy would best address her symptoms?
a. Bladder suspension/sling procedure
b. Vaginal pessary
c. Anterior colporrhaphy
d. Anticholinergics
e. Kegel exercises

78. A 35-year-old G3 P2 comes to you for help in selecting a new birth control method. She is 2 months' postpartum and no longer breastfeeding. She used combination OCPs in the past but they exacerbated her migraines and she had trouble remembering the pill, given her busy life with her husband and two young children. Her past history is notable for mild depression and obesity. She had mildly heavy but regular periods with moderate uterine cramping that is somewhat controlled with NSAIDs. Her current weight is 214 lbs. She denies any history of STDs, ectopic pregnancy, or fibroids. She and her husband are considering having more children but not for a few more years. She is using the hope of a future pregnancy as an inspiration to quit smoking. She is down to one pack per day of cigarettes. What contraceptive method would best meet this patient's needs?
a. Depo-Provera
b. Nuvaring
c. Mirena IUD (levonorgestrel IUD)
d. ParaGard IUD (copper T IUD)
e. Ortho-Evra patch

79. Of the following, which classic triad characterizes preeclampsia?
a. Visual changes, proteinuria, pitting pedal edema
b. Headache, visual changes, right upper quadrant pain
c. Hypertension, visual changes, right upper quadrant pain
d. Hypertension, proteinuria, and nondependent edema
e. Hypertension, proteinuria, and pitting pedal edema

80. Your next patient is a 39-year-old G2 P1 at 19 weeks' gestation. You sent her for an anatomic fetal survey that showed multiple fetal anomalies incompatible with life.

The patient and her husband are devastated. They have received genetic counseling and decided to terminate the pregnancy at this time. Her gestational dating is very accurate and was confirmed with a first trimester ultrasound. They would like to know everything possible about what caused the anomalies and how to prevent a future problem. They ask for your advice regarding methods of termination in their situation. Which method of termination of pregnancy would be most suitable for this couple's needs?
a. A single dose of RU-486 (mifepristone) followed by vaginal prostaglandin administration
b. A single dose of methotrexate followed by vaginal prostaglandin administration
c. Suction curettage
d. Dilation of the cervix with laminaria, followed by evacuation of the uterus using forceps and suction curettage
e. Cervical ripening followed by induction of labor with high-dose oxytocin

81. You are seeing a 57-year-old woman who presents with vulvar pruritis for 1 year. Her husband died 4 years ago and she has a new male sexual partner. You perform a wet prep that is negative for yeast, clue cells, and trichomonads. Cervical cultures for gonorrhea and chlamydia are both negative. She had an abnormal Pap smear last year that showed atypical squamous cells, but cervical biopsies and two follow-up Pap smears were negative for dysplasia. Vulvar biopsies reveal a single focus of moderate vulvar intraepithelial neoplasia (VIN). How would you treat this patient?
a. Antifungal agents
b. High-potency topical steroids
c. Wide local excision
d. Skinning vulvectomy
e. Laser ablation

82. A 26-year-old G2 P2 woman presents for a routine examination. Her physical examination is entirely normal; however, her Pap smear shows atypical squamous cells of undetermined significance (ASC-US). Her high-risk HPV screen is positive. You explain the results to the patient and recommend that she have a colposcopy. Subsequent colposcopy reveals a lesion on the anterior aspect of the cervix. The transformation zone is entirely visualized. The lesion turns white after treatment with acetic acid and both punctations and mosaicism are noted. The cervical biopsy is read as moderate dysplasia (CIN II). Which of the following is the standard of care for management of this patient?
a. Imiquimod (Aldara) treatment
b. Cryotherapy
c. Cold-knife cone biopsy
d. Loop electrosurgical excision procedure (LEEP)
e. Simple hysterectomy

83. A 15-year-old G0 woman presents with a history of no menarche. Both she and her mother are concerned about this, and want to discuss the possible causes. Of the following, which can cause both primary and secondary amenorrhea?
    a. Asherman's syndrome
    b. Gonadal agenesis
    c. Anorexia nervosa
    d. Sheehan's syndrome
    e. Kallmann's syndrome

84. A 63-year-old G0 P0 woman comes to you with 6 weeks of postmenopausal bleeding. Review of her history reveals menarche at age 10 and menopause at age 54. She has never been on hormone replacement therapy. She reports being overweight most of her life and currently weighs 237 pounds and is 5 feet 4 inches tall. She is basically healthy except for borderline hypertension and adult-onset diabetes mellitus, for which she takes oral hyperglycemic agents. A TSH and prolactin are normal. The endometrial biopsy shows grade 1 adenocarcinoma of the endometrium. Which is the patient's most concerning risk factor for endometrial cancer?
    a. Nulliparity
    b. Obesity
    c. Early menarche
    d. Late menopause
    e. Diabetes mellitus (NIDDM)

85. A 49-year-old woman presents complaining of vulvar pain that increases with ambulation and intercourse. She also notes a lump on her right labia that has increased in size over the past 48 hours and is quite painful. The patient has had these same symptoms in the past. On examination she has a 5-cm tender cyst on the medial aspect of her right labia, with a surrounding erythema of the labia that extends 1 to 2 cm away. What would be your first step in management of this patient?
    a. Sitz baths
    b. Insertion of Word catheter
    c. Antibiotics
    d. Biopsy of the cyst and insertion of Word catheter
    e. Marsupialization of the cyst

86. You are seeing a 64-year-old G3 P1 patient for an annual exam. When you ask her about the date of her last menstrual period, you are surprised when she responds that her last period was 2 months ago. When you probe further, you find that she has been having vaginal bleeding every 2 to 3 years for the past 10 years. You begin an evaluation, which shows a normal TSH and prolactin and an elevated FSH level consistent menopause. Her Pap smear was done 4 months ago at her primary care physician's office and was within normal limits. A pelvic ultrasound shows a 7-mm

endometrial stripe and a normal myometrium. The adnexa also appear normal. You attempt an endometrial biopsy but the patient has cervical stenosis and you are unable to sample the cavity. You are reassured by your findings thus far. How do you proceed?
    a. Take her to the OR for a cervical dilation and curettage of the uterus
    b. Take her to the OR for an endometrial ablation
    c. Take her to the OR for a total abdominal hysterectomy
    d. Recommend oral estrogen for the likely diagnosis of endometrial atrophy
    e. Reassure her that a thin endometrial stripe likely excludes cancer so you can follow expectantly

87. A 29-year-old G2 P1 comes for prenatal care. She has a history of delivery of a 4,250-g baby. She herself had been a big baby at birth. The patient is concerned because her prepregnancy weight was 162 pounds and she gained 70 pounds during this pregnancy. At 26 weeks' gestation the patient had a glucose-loading test of 50 g glucose. When her blood glucose level was measured 1 hour later, it was 164. As her obstetrician, what would you do next?
    a. Check a hemoglobin A1c
    b. Start her on an appropriate insulin regimen
    c. Check a 3-hour glucose tolerance test
    d. Start her on an oral hyperglycemia agent
    e. Start her on a diabetic diet

88. A 44-year-old woman comes in with a complaint of unilateral bloody nipple discharge. On examination in your office there is no skin change, nipple discharge, enlarged lymph nodes, or tenderness. There is no mass on clinical breast exam and she has no known family history of breast cancer. A mammogram and ultrasound are both negative. The most likely diagnosis is:
    a. intraductal papilloma.
    b. mammary duct ectasia.
    c. Paget disease of the breast.
    d. carcinoma in situ.
    e. invasive breast cancer.

89. A 67-year-old woman presents with light vaginal bleeding. She has no other complaints. The bleeding began 10 months ago and she has bled three or four times since then. An endometrial biopsy at that time was negative for hyperplasia and cancer. She has no other medical history. On physical exam she is a thin woman in no apparent distress. Her vagina and introitus are atrophic with no lesions and she has no obvious hemorrhoids. Her uterus is small and her ovaries are not palpable. Her FSH is elevated to the menopausal level, her TSH is normal, and her prolactin level is normal. The patient had a normal Pap smear 8 months ago and no history of abnormal Pap smears. Her

pelvic ultrasound shows a 6-cm uterus with a 3-mm endometrial stripe. You attempt a repeat endometrial biopsy in the office but her os is stenotic and you are unable to obtain an adequate tissue specimen for evaluation. How do you proceed?

a. Start combination hormone replacement therapy
b. Start estrogen replacement therapy
c. Take her to the operating room for a D&C
d. Take her to the operating room for a hysterectomy
e. Expectant management

90. A 28-year-old G2 P1 woman with a history of a prior cesarean delivery presents at 36 weeks of gestation with a complaint of vaginal bleeding, passing several golf ball-sized clots. She notes frequent contractions that begin as menstrual cramps, but have increased over the past hour. As you begin your work-up you consider that risk factors for placental abruption include all of the following except:

a. hypertension.
b. advanced maternal age.
c. cocaine use.
d. preterm premature rupture of membranes.
e. heroin abuse.

91. A 33-year-old G3 P0 S3 comes to you for a history of recurrent miscarriage. Each of her miscarriages occurred during the first trimester and presented with heavy but self-limited bleeding. She had a thrombophilia evaluation, which was normal. Evaluation of the uterine cavity with hysterosalpingogram and sonohysterogram both suggest a uterine septum. An MRI was obtained that also showed a uterine septum and no evidence of bicornuate uterus. The remainder of the pelvic and urologic structures appeared to be within normal limits. The patient and her husband would like to conceive again but are very afraid of another miscarriage. How would you advise them to proceed?

a. Surgical resection of the uterine septum prior to attempting conception again.
b. Inform them that the uterine septum is not related to their history of recurrent miscarriage and they can start attempting pregnancy again.
c. Proceed to infertility evaluation and in vitro fertilization.
d. Plan for a gestational carrier.
e. Attempt to adopt.

92. A 53-year-old G0 presents to your clinic as a new patient with the complaints of vaginal bleeding. She is aggravated because over the last 3 years she has continued to have occasional vaginal bleeding occurring every 6 months even though she thought she had gone through menopause at the age of 51. Since going through menopause she has been taking an estrogen supplement to relieve the hot flashes. She has never had surgery and is essentially healthy. She does not smoke or drink alcohol. She has no

pain with intercourse and denies any vaginal dryness. Her last Pap smear was just over 3 years ago and she has never had an abnormal Pap or a sexually transmitted infection. Her BMI is 35. On exam you note well-estrogenized vaginal mucosa without signs of atrophy or laceration or abrasion and a normal appearing cervix. How would you proceed in evaluating this patient?

a. Perform a Pap smear and order an FSH and estradiol level
b. Dilation and curettage and endometrial ablation
c. Order a CT of the pelvis and perform a Pap smear
d. No further evaluation is needed. Schedule a total hysterectomy
e. Endometrial biopsy, transvaginal ultrasound, TSH, prolactin, FSH, Pap

93. A 58-year-old G0 presented for her annual exam last week with complaints of abdominal bloating and heaviness over the last month. She denies vaginal bleeding, unusual or excessive hair growth, or weight loss. Her mother and sister both had breast cancer in their 50s. She has had up-to-date and normal mammograms. Her Pap smear was negative and her bimanual exam at that time was notable for mild adnexal fullness on her right side. Her ultrasound reveals a 7-cm right adnexal mass with cystic and solid components with multiple septations. There is a similar 3-cm mass on the left adnexa. Endometrial stripe is 3 mm. There is moderate free fluid noted within the pelvis. She also has an elevated CA-125 and a normal CEA-1 antigen and hCG. What is this patient's most likely diagnosis?

a. Serous cystadenocarcinoma
b. Endodermal sinus tumor
c. Sertoli-Leydig cell tumor
d. Choriocarcinoma
e. Brenner tumor

94. An 18-year-old G0 presents to your clinic with primary amenorrhea. She has normal breast development, but has limited development of pubic or axillary hair. On pelvic exam you note that she has a foreshortened vagina. Transvaginal and transabdominal ultrasound is unable to identify a uterus. Chromosomal analysis shows that the patient is 46, XY. What is this patient's diagnosis?

a. Testicular feminization
b. Gonadal agenesis
c. Mayer-Rokitansky-Kuster-Hauser syndrome
d. Swyer syndrome
e. Turner syndrome

95. A 32-year-old G4 P2022 presents to the infertility clinic and reports 18 months of infertility with her new husband of 3 years. She had no difficulties conceiving her two living children. She had two elective abortions after her children were born and also had a D&C following delivery of her

second child for retained placenta. Her husband has never fathered any children. His semen analysis shows normal count, motility, and morphology. She has light but regular menses and per the ovulation predictor kits, usually ovulates on day 14. Her endocrine evaluation was normal. How would you best evaluate this couple's infertility?

a. Repeat semen analysis, perform an endocrine evaluation on the male partner, and perform a testicular biopsy
b. Recommend use of clomiphene citrate to induce ovulation along with timed intercourse. No further evaluation is needed
c. Until this patient has been infertile for at least 24 months, there is no need for further evaluation
d. Perform a pelvic exam, a hysterosalpingogram, and a sonohysterogram to look for intrauterine abnormalities
e. Perform a transvaginal ultrasound to look for fibroids or polyps that could be the cause of the infertility

96. A 31-year-old G3 P2002 presents to labor and delivery with vaginal bleeding at 33 weeks' gestation. She woke up in the middle of the night with blood-stained sheets, and proceeded immediately to the hospital. She has a history of a repeat cesarean section 2 years ago after a primary cesarean section for breech presentation 5 years ago. She reports her baby is moving well, and she is comfortable with stable vital signs. The baby's fetal heart rate tracing is reassuring and the bleeding has slowed substantially. You review her records and notice a second trimester ultrasound report which identifies the placenta as "low-lying." What is the next immediate step in management?

a. Perform a contraction stress test to evaluate for fetal well-being
b. Perform a cervical examination to evaluate patient for preterm labor
c. Obtain a fetal cell stain to evaluate patient for abruption
d. Perform a bedside ultrasound to evaluate placental location
e. Obtain coagulation studies to evaluate patient for coagulopathy

97. A 23-year-old G3 P1102 presents to labor and delivery at 28 weeks' gestation with painful uterine contractions and vaginal bleeding. On tocometry, the patient is found to have frequent low-amplitude contractions occurring every 1 to 2 minutes. FHR tracing demonstrates baseline in the 150s with minimal variability. Upon further questioning, the patient admits to using a substance in the past 12 hours. Which of the following substances could be directly responsible for the events taking place?

a. Cocaine
b. Tobacco
c. Alcohol

d. Marijuana
e. Caffeine

98. A 19-year-old G0 presented to the emergency room 3 days ago with gastrointestinal symptoms and abdominal pain. She has had a regular menstrual history and denies any excessive hair growth or loss. Her pregnancy test was negative. A CT was performed and an incidental finding of a 4-cm right adnexal mass was made. Ultrasound revealed a heterogeneous mass with multiple septations and solid components in the right adnexa and a normal appearing left adnexa. There is flow to the mass and good flow to both ovaries. You were consulted and requested that tumor markers be drawn and to have her follow up in the oncology clinic. The results of the tumor markers are as follows: elevated AFP, normal CA-125, normal LDH, and serum β-hCG <5. What is the patient's most likely diagnosis?

a. Serous cystadenocarcinoma
b. Endodermal sinus tumor
c. Sertoli-Leydig cell tumor
d. Choriocarcinoma
e. Brenner tumor

99. A 61-year-old postmenopausal female presents for her annual exam without complaints. You notice a white patchy area between the posterior forchette of the vagina and the anus. When questioned about this area, the patient denies any pruritis or irritation. You obtain a biopsy of this area, and the pathology report diagnoses lichen sclerosis. What is the first line treatment for this lesion?

a. Wide local excision
b. Clobetasol cream
c. Laser vaporization
d. Topical antifungals
e. Topical estrogen cream

100. A 65-year-old G2P2002 presents to the urogynecology clinic with complaints of urinary incontinence. She leaks urine occasionally when she coughs, but also leaks urine without any provocation. She often has difficulty making it to the restroom in time. She has even leaked urine shortly after having normal emptying of her bladder. She normally gets up at least 2 to 3 times per night to urinate. Urinalysis and urine culture performed last week at her PCP's office are both negative. What is the most likely diagnosis and appropriate treatment for this type of incontinence?

a. Stress urinary incontinence, Ditropan (oxybutynin chloride)
b. Detrusor overactivity, Detrol (tolterodine)
c. Overflow incontinence, cholinergic agent
d. Detrusor overactivity, suburethral sling
e. Stress urinary incontinence, suburethral sling

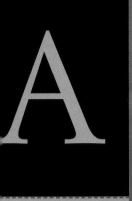

Answers

1. a (Chapter 26)

Infertility is the inability to conceive after 12 months of unprotected intercourse. At this point, it is reasonable to begin an initial diagnostic evaluation. Care should be taken to evaluate both the female and the male partner, since 40% of infertility is due to female factors and 40% is due to male factors. For the female partner, the initial investigation should include a thorough history and physical, demonstration of ovulation (tracking the menstrual cycle, measuring the basal body temperature using ovulation prediction kits, measuring the midluteal progesterone, and documenting any premenstrual or ovulatory symptoms), and some baseline lab values (TSH, FSH, and prolactin). For the male partner, the initial investigation should include a thorough history and physical and a semen analysis to evaluate the sperm volume, motility, and morphology. This basic workup can be done easily and without the assistance of a reproductive endocrinologist.

2. a (Chapter 22)

The lesion in this woman's uterus is most likely an endometrial polyp given the endometrial mass. Endometrial polyps are typically benign masses that most commonly present in women over age 40. They can cause heavy and/or prolonged bleeding similar to fibroids and adenomyosis. The pelvic ultrasound showing a normal myometrium and normal endometrial–myometrial junction make fibroids and adenomyosis much less likely. Endometrial hyperplasia and endometrial cancer can also present with abnormal bleeding and endometrial mass. However, this patient has none of the risk factors for endometrial cancer such as obesity, hypertension, or diabetes. Dysfunctional uterine bleeding is a diagnosis of exclusion describing bleeding with no identifiable etiology. In this case, there is an identifiable cause of the patient's symptoms. The most likely next step would be a sonohysterogram to better characterize the endometrial mass hysteroscopy to remove it.

3. b (Chapter 14)

Most women with fibroids are asymptomatic. However, when fibroids cause symptoms such as pelvic pain, heavy bleeding, or infertility, treatment can be considered. Oral contraceptive pills are a relative contraindication in patients with fibroids because they result in increased estrogen levels, which can stimulate fibroid growth (similar to growth from increased estrogen levels during pregnancy). Medical treatment of fibroids can range from use of NSAIDs, Provera (medroxyprogesterone), Danazol (danocrine), and Depo-Lupron (leuprolide acetate). All of these work to decrease circulating estrogen levels and thereby shrink fibroids. Unfortunately, leiomyoma often recurs after discontinuation of these medicines and a patient with a uterus of this size is unlikely to have her bleeding controlled long-term with medical management alone. Similarly, IUDs are contraindicated in the fibroid uterus when the cavity is affected. Surgical treatment will vary depending on the location of the fibroids and desire for future fertility. Submucosal fibroids, which can cause bleeding and result in fertility difficulties, can be resected via hysteroscopy. This patient's symptoms—heavy bleeding and mild anemia—are most likely due to the presence of multiple fibroids, which have grossly enlarged the uterus. Intramural and subserosal fibroids, which are often the cause of pelvic pressure, pain, and urinary symptoms, can be removed via laparoscopic or abdominal myomectomy if future fertility is desired. However, for a patient with multiple symptomatic fibroids and a very large uterus, abdominal hysterectomy is the best choice. Given the size of her uterus, vaginal hysterectomy would not be an option. Given that she is over 45 years old, you could also offer her a bilateral salpingo-oophorectomy as well.

4. b (Chapter 21)

When considering the differential diagnosis of amenorrhea, it should be classified as primary or secondary. Primary amenorrhea is the absence of menses at age 16. Anatomic etiologies include vaginal agenesis, transverse vaginal septum, Mayer-Rokitansky-Küster-Hauser syndrome, and other müllerian anomalies that lead to no development of either the vagina or the uterus. Secondary amenorrhea is the absence of menses for three menstrual cycles or a minimum of 3 months. Hormonal etiologies are related to the lack of either release or response to GnRH, FSH, or LH. Noninherited etiologies of hypogonadotropic hypogonadism include anorexia, stress, and athletics. Asherman's syndrome, which is intrauterine scarring, is usually secondary to infection or instrumentation.

5. c (Chapter 30)

The mainstay of treatment for ovarian cancer is surgery with complete surgical staging, including total abdominal hysterectomy, bilateral salpingo-oophorectomy (TAHBSO), omentectomy, and cytoreduction of any visible tumor. The patient then undergoes chemotherapy, typically with cisplatin and taxol.

6. b (Chapter 24)

Absolute contraindications for oral contraceptives (OCPs) include deep venous thrombosis (DVT), pulmonary embolism, cardiovascular disease, stroke, breast or endometrial cancers, melanoma, hepatic tumor, or abnormal liver function (impacts clearance of hormones). Smoking over age 35 is a relative contraindication given the increased risk of DVT, stroke, heart disease, pulmonary embolism, and so on if patients take OCPs. Other relative contraindications include migraines, diabetes mellitus, sickle-cell disease, hypertension, depression, and hyperlipidemia. Smokers over age 35 and lactating women are strongly encouraged to use progesterone-only contraception such as the progesterone only pill, or the Mirena (IUD) Depo-Provera. Lactation itself is only a relative contraindication to combined OCP use.

7. c (Chapter 4)

Ultrasound can be very useful in diagnosing potential causes of third trimester bleeding. Placenta previa can be diagnosed with 90% accuracy on ultrasound. Most placental abruptions, however, are not seen on ultrasound. Diagnosis of placental abruption is made based on a detailed history of risk factors and the clinical picture of bleeding associated with abdominal pain. About 30% of abruptions are small and asymptomatic and are diagnosed after delivery. The presentation of uterine rupture can also be quite variable and requires a detailed history and physical. Uterine rupture can cause sudden abdominal pain, vaginal bleeding, fetal distress, abnormal abdominal contouring, cessation of uterine contractions, and regression of the presenting part. Cervical neoplasm is usually best diagnosed with Pap smear, colposcopy, biopsy, and CT. Vaginal laceration diagnosis requires a careful speculum exam.

8. c (Chapter 8)

Severe preeclampsia is defined as having any of the following: blood pressure higher than 160/110 mm Hg; >5,000 mg (5 g) of proteinuria in 24 hours; symptoms such as severe headache, epigastric or RUQ pain, or visual symptoms; findings of oliguria or pulmonary edema; or any of the elements of hemolysis, elevated liver enzymes, or low platelets (HELLP) syndrome. This woman meets several of these criteria. The ultimate treatment for severe preeclampsia is delivery of the fetus. Steps should be taken to stabilize the mother with antihypertensives to maintain BP between 120/70 and 160/110 and magnesium sulfate for seizure prophylaxis. Prior to 32 weeks' gestation, it is common to use expectant management in order to gain fetal maturity and administer betamethasone. However, delivery should not be delayed in the setting of a headache or liver function test elevations. Immediate induction of labor for an anticipated vaginal delivery is therefore the management plan of choice. As part of this treatment, cervical ripening with prostaglandins, amniotomy, and oxytocin may be used. This induction of labor is likely to take 20 to 30 hours, and thus the fetus will gain some benefit from the treatment with betamethasone prior to 34 weeks' gestation.

9. d (Chapter 1)

The Nägele rule of dating a pregnancy stems from the fact that the estimated date of delivery (EDD) is 280 days from the last menstrual period (LMP). On average, that will be 9 months and 1 week from the LMP. Thus, the Nägele rule is to subtract 3 months and add 7 days (and 1 year).

10. b (Chapter 6)

Preterm labor is described as contractions leading to cervical change before 37 weeks' gestation. Risk factors include prior preterm delivery, prior preterm labor, PPROM, uterine abnormalities, polyhydramnios, bacterial vaginosis, placental abruption, preeclampsia, chorioamnionitis, and pregestational weight less than 50 kg. Multiple (3 or more) prior dilations of the cervix in a therapeutic or spontaneous abortion—particularly in the second trimester—have been associated with cervical incompetence; this would be unlikely in this patient, who has reached 31 weeks' gestation. A large fetus can be correlated with polyhydramnios, which is correlated with preterm labor, but this association is weaker than prior preterm delivery. Teenage pregnancy is correlated with lower socioeconomic status, which is correlated with many complications of pregnancy, including preterm delivery, but again this is weaker than prior preterm delivery. Smoking is correlated more with lower birth weight than with preterm delivery.

11. a (Chapter 11)

Although none of the substances is recommended in pregnancy, only alcohol, which is associated with fetal alcohol syndrome and with cardiac defects in particular, is associated with congenital anomalies. Cocaine use during pregnancy has been correlated with central nervous system effects and developmental delay in the exposed child. Tobacco use has been correlated with small-for-gestational-age fetuses and increased respiratory disease in childhood. Caffeine and opiates do not have particularly noted fetal effects, although fetuses exposed to opiates throughout pregnancy will need to be weaned off the drug postpartum.

12. c (Chapter 14)

This patient's heavy bleeding is most likely due to the presence of a submucosal fibroid. Fibroids that impinge on the endometrial cavity are more likely to cause heavy bleeding than those in an intramural or subserosal location. Because this patient has become anemic, expectant management would not be an acceptable long-term option. Oral contraceptive pills are useful in regulating menstrual bleeding but this is most applicable when the etiology of bleeding is hormonal. Also, the estrogen from OCPs can stimulate fibroid growth in some patients. The etiology of this patient's bleeding is structural; therefore, a structural solution is typically needed; in this case, a myomectomy. Because the fibroid of concern is submucosal it can be surgically removed from a hysteroscopic approach with less morbidity and mortality than an abdominal approach. A hysterectomy would not be needed in this case since her other fibroids are very small and likely asymptomatic. Depo-Lupron is often used to stop bleeding temporarily to help raise a patient's hematocrit before a planned myomectomy. The patient's hematocrit in this case is high enough that iron supplementation would likely be adequate to raise the blood count prior to surgery.

13. a (Chapter 2)

This patient has the diagnosis of a threatened abortion. If the physical exam shows a closed cervical os in the setting of vaginal bleeding and either a viable intrauterine pregnancy (IUP) or a pelvic ultrasound and β-hCG that are too early to show a viable IUP, the diagnosis is threatened abortion. If the IUP cannot be seen, but there is not enough evidence to confirm an ectopic pregnancy, the patient is also considered to have a diagnosis of rule-out ectopic pregnancy. A patient in early pregnancy who presents with abdominal or pelvic pain and vaginal bleeding is at risk for ectopic pregnancy. The diagnostic workup includes a history, physical examination, β-hCG, CBC, type and screen (T&S), and pelvic ultrasound. The definitions of ectopic pregnancy and the different types of abortions are described in Chapter 2.

14. b (Chapter 2)

In patients who have the diagnosis of rule-out ectopic pregnancy because their β-hCG is still too low for an intrauterine pregnancy (IUP) to be seen on ultrasound, the β-hCG should be checked every 48 hours. In a normally developing IUP, the β-hCG should double every 48 hours or at least increase by a minimum of 67%. In a failed pregnancy the β-hCG will decrease. In an ectopic pregnancy, the β-hCG will rise but commonly at a rate less than 67–100% every 48 hours.

15. e (Chapter 28)

This patient has biopsy confirmed squamous cell carcinoma in situ (CIS) of the cervix. By definition, this cancer is limited to the cervical epithelium. The standard of care for patients with early preinvasive cancer or microscopic cervical cancer is simple hysterectomy. However, the option for a cold-knife cone biopsy does exist for women who wish to retain their fertility. These patients should be counseled strongly regarding follow-up care and the risk of recurrence with CKC. She should also be strongly counseled for smoking cessation since women who smoke have a higher rate of cervical dysplasia and cancer. Because the patient wishes to preserve her fertility, simple hysterectomy and radical hysterectomy would not be appropriate options. Radical hysterectomy is the treatment of choice for early invasive cervical cancer and chemoradiation is used to treat advanced cervical cancer. Cryotherapy can be used to treat small foci of cervical dysplasia when LEEP/LOOP is not available. It is not appropriate in this setting.

16. c (Chapter 16)

Cervical motion tenderness with no other findings on exam is most consistent with cervicitis. The two most common organisms that cause cervicitis are *N. gonorrhoeae* and *C. trachomatis*. The treatment for cervicitis should cover both *Gonococcus* and *Chlamydia*. The most common way to treat this is with a single IM dose of ceftriaxone and a week of PO doxycycline. Because of concern for patient compliance, a single dose of azithromycin is often used to treat chlamydia rather than the week course of doxycycline. Choices d and e reflect treatment options for severe PID and tubo-ovarian abscess, respectively.

17. e (Chapter 12)

Although the onset of lactation can commonly cause a fever in the first 24 to 72 hours postpartum, it is unlikely to do so 7 days postpartum. However, mastitis, a wound infection, or endomyometritis are all quite likely to result in fever. Patients who deliver by cesarean section, as well as many patients who deliver vaginally, may have had an indwelling catheter for 24 hours, which can predispose them to urinary infections. Thus, while pyelonephritis is not the most likely diagnosis, it should be in the differential diagnosis and ruled out with urinalysis and culture and physical examination.

18. d (Chapter 1)

The gravidity and parity designation is as follows: gravidity is the number of pregnancies that a patient has had, and parity is the number of deliveries that a patient has had, in which a twin delivery counts as one delivery. Parity is further broken down into the four-digit designation of term, preterm, aborted, and living (TPAL). A term pregnancy is any gestation at or past 37 weeks. A preterm pregnancy is any gestation that is longer than 20 weeks but less than 37 weeks or results in a fetus that weighs more than 500 g. Aborted pregnancies include both spontaneous abortions and elective terminations of pregnancy. Living refers to the total number of living children. This patient has had 5 previous pregnancies and is currently pregnant, so her gravidity is 6. She has had 2 term deliveries, 1 preterm pregnancy (remember, a twin delivery is one delivery), 2 miscarriages, and 4 living children. Thus, her parity would be 2-1-2-4.

19. c (Chapter 6)

Chorioamnionitis is an infection of the fluid around the fetus that usually involves the uterus and the fetus as well. The five diagnostic signs include elevated maternal white blood count and temperature, fetal tachycardia, uterine tenderness, and vaginal discharge. If diagnosis is uncertain, amniocentesis can be performed and tested for Gram's stain, glucose, white blood count, and culture. Neither the sensitivity nor the specificity of the first three tests is over 80%, and although culture is the gold standard, it can take several days to obtain results. Recently, it has been suggested that IL-6 in the amniotic fluid is more sensitive. This patient is likely in labor, but this cannot be confirmed without a cervical exam. She does not have either preterm labor or preterm rupture of membranes because she is not preterm (<37 weeks). The patient does have a fever, but that is not a diagnosis.

20. b (Chapter 20)

The four stages of puberty include gonadarche—the initiation of luteinizing hormone and follicle-stimulating hormone release; thelarche—the onset of breast development; pubarche—the development of pubic and axillary hair; and menarche—the onset of menstruation. The mean ages of the stages of puberty are as follows: gonadarche at age 8, thelarche at around age 10, pubarche at age 11, menarche at age 12. Your patient and her mother will be relieved to find that her pubertal development is within normal limits and that menstruation usually begins about 2 years after the development of breast buds. Therefore, your patient will likely experience menarche in the coming year. Menarche can be delayed in gymnasts, long-distance runners, and ballet dancers. This is thought to be related to decreased body fat. There is no reason to assume that this patient has an eating disorder at this point in the evaluation. If menstruation has not occurred by age 16, then a complete evaluation can be done to look for etiologies of primary amenorrhea such as congenital malformations, chromosomal abnormalities, and hypothalamic-pituitary disorders.

21. a (Chapter 15)

This patient's symptoms are most consistent with endometriosis. Endometriosis is the presence of endometrial cells outside the uterine cavity. The treatment options vary widely. For a patient in whom endometriosis is suspected but symptoms do not severely affect quality of life, symptoms can be managed with NSAIDs, oral contraceptive pills, or Depo-Provera, which induce a state of pseudopregnancy by suppressing ovulation and menstruation. Danazol, an androgen derivative, and Lupron, a GnRH agonist, can be used to induce a reversible state of pseudomenopause by suppressing FSH and LH and consequently decreasing the level of estrogen. These are all temporizing measures and do not increase the likelihood of conceiving. In this patient who is trying to conceive and whose symptoms are worsening and not controlled by conservative medical management, a diagnostic laparoscopy is indicated. Ablation of endometrial implants has been found to increase the rate of fertility depending on the stage of the disease. If this patient was not attempting to get pregnant, the laparoscopic ablation of endometriosis should be followed with medical management to suppress recurrence of the endometriosis and its symptoms.

22. d (Chapter 7)

Management of Rh-negative patients with RhoGAM has led to a marked reduction in women who have been sensitized to the Rh antigen. The recommendations for treatment with RhoGAM include use anytime in the first two trimesters with vaginal bleeding or amniocentesis, at the beginning of the third trimester at approximately 28 weeks' gestation, during the third trimester if there are signs of a fetal-maternal hemorrhage that is greater than can be negated by the 28-week dose of RhoGAM, and postpartum if the infant is Rh positive. RhoGAM is not routinely given during preterm labor unless the patient has not yet received a dose in the pregnancy.

23. b (Chapter 20)

It is generally accepted that the indications for hormone replacement therapy (HRT) include short-term symptomatic relief of postmenopausal symptoms. Estrogen replacement in a postmenopausal patient has been shown to decrease the risk of osteoporosis, urogenital atrophy, and hot flashes. However, because unopposed estrogen can increase the risk of endometrial cancer, estrogen is given in conjunction with either continuous or cyclic progesterone (combination therapy) to protect the uterus from hyperplasia and cancer. HRT also carries an increased risk of breast cancer, endometrial cancer, thromboembolic disease, and gallbladder disease. Therefore, it is now generally accepted that HRT therapy should be used only for relief of menopausal symptoms and the duration of use should be short, generally 6 to 12 months. Contraindications to HRT use include hepatic dysfunction, undiagnosed abnormal vaginal bleeding, history of acute venous thrombosis (DVT, PE) and history of an estrogen-sensitive cancer (e.g., breast, endometrial).

24. c (Chapter 8)

Magnesium sulfate is often used in obstetrics for tocolysis in the management of preterm labor and for seizure prophylaxis in the management of preeclampsia. The therapeutic range is between 4 and 8 mEq/mL. Patellar reflexes are generally lost at 10 and respiratory depression occurs at 12. Levels of 20 or greater are associated with respiratory and cardiac arrest. This patient is at risk for respiratory and cardiac arrest. She should be given calcium gluconate to reverse the effects of magnesium sulfate. Because the patient is breathing on her own, intubation is not necessary at this point, although constant assessment is necessary in case the patient's condition should deteriorate. The MagPIE trial demonstrated that a 1 g/hr infusion was efficacious in reducing seizures in preeclamptic women, and this lower infusion rate is likely to lead to less magnesium toxicity. However, in severe preeclamptics who have decreased renal function, even this infusion can eventually lead to toxicity. Because of the progression of findings with rising magnesium levels, the best way to identify such toxicity is to have hourly reflex checks. If the reflexes become absent, at that time, a magnesium level can be checked. Terbutaline is a tocolytic used to treat preterm labor and betamethasone is a steroid used antenatally to encourage fetal lung development when preterm delivery is anticipated between 28 and 34 weeks' gestation.

25. d (Chapter 9)

Offer induction of labor at 39 to 40 weeks' gestation. This is done given the increased risk of intrauterine fetal demise (IUFD) after 40 weeks in diabetic pregnancies. Alternatively, in patients who are poorly controlled or are interested in earlier induction, induction is offered from 37 to 39 weeks' gestation. However, before electively inducing labor prior to 39 weeks in these patients, fetal lung maturity should be verified. Cesarean section is commonly offered if the estimated fetal weight is greater than 4,500 g to avoid the increased incidence of shoulder dystocia and Erb palsy.

26. c (Chapter 12)

Postpartum hemorrhage is defined as blood loss greater than 500 mL after vaginal delivery or greater than 1,000 mL after cesarean delivery. It can be caused by any of the answers mentioned here, including abnormal placentation; uterine atony; maternal trauma of the perineum, vagina, cervix, or uterus; and coagulation defects. Of all the etiologies mentioned, this patient's hemorrhage is most consistent with uterine atony. This patient has multiple risk factors for uterine atony, including a multiple gestation, chorioamnionitis, prolonged labor, exposure to oxytocin, and multiparity.

27. c (Chapter 3)

How patients are managed with genetic screens depends on their risk factors. African Americans are at an increased risk of carrying the sickle-cell disease and thalassemias. They are not at increased risk for cystic fibrosis (CF); however, CF testing is now offered to all women during their prenatal care. The expanded maternal serum α-fetoprotein (MSAFP) that is used to screen for neural tube defects and Down syndrome is also offered to all women. Invasive prenatal diagnosis with amniocentesis or chorionic villus sampling (CVS) is offered only to those women of advanced maternal age or who are known to be at high risk for chromosomal or other genetic anomalies (e.g., balanced translocations). If the patient and her partner are known to be carriers of thalassemia, sickle-cell anemia, or cystic fibrosis, an amniocentesis should be performed to diagnose the fetus. Further, if the MSAFP was positive for a risk of either chromosomal abnormality or neural tube defect, an amniocentesis can be performed to confirm or rule out these diagnoses.

28. e (Chapter 13)

Postmenopausal women presenting with vulvar pruritus or vulvodynia should usually always have a biopsy to rule out vulvar dysplasia or cancer if the symptoms are long-standing or persistent. If vulvar candidiasis seems to be the etiology of the symptoms, topical antifungals such as ketoconazole may be used first. In this case, the findings are most consistent with a diagnosis of lichen sclerosis but a biopsy should still be performed to rule out underlying malignancy. The treatment for lichen sclerosis is a medium- to high-potency topical steroid. A topical 2% testosterone cream can also be used for lichen sclerosis only if there is evidence of atrophy secondarily. Surgical treatment of the effects of lichen sclerosis is rarely indicated. If the etiology of a vulvar biopsy is vulvar eczema, a topical hydrocortisone should be used. If it is secondary to atrophy, topical estrogen is the treatment of choice. Further, in a patient with vulvar atrophy who is not on hormone replacement therapy, oral supplementation should be offered as well.

29. d (Chapter 31)

This patient most likely has an invasive molar pregnancy that may be the result of persistent molar disease. Most patients with invasive moles are diagnosed as a result of plateauing or rising β-hCG levels following molar evacuation. Invasive moles typically penetrate locally into the myometrium and into the peritoneal cavity. Despite this, invasive moles rarely metastasize, but it is still important that the patient be evaluated for possible metastatic disease. The mainstay of treatment for invasive molar pregnancies is chemotherapy; single-agent chemotherapy (typically methotrexate or adrianycin) for nonmetastatic disease as this patient has, or multiagent chemotherapy for metastatic disease. Radiation therapy is indicated only for treatment of brain and liver metastases. As with all forms of gestational trophoblastic disease, close follow-up with serial β-hCG levels and reliable birth control during the surveillance period is imperative to successful treatment. There is no contraindication to contraceptives containing estrogen or progesterone.

30. b (Chapter 6)

Nifedipine is a calcium channel blocker which decreases the influx of calcium into smooth muscle cells. Indomethacin is a cyclooxygenase inhibitor that decreases levels of prostaglandins, therefore decreasing intracellular levels of calcium in smooth muscle cells. Magnesium is a calcium antagonist. Terbutaline is a beta-mimetic that converts ATP to cAMP which decreases intracellular levels of calcium in smooth muscle cells. Betamethasone is not a tocolytic but rather a glucocorticoid administered to enhance fetal lung maturity from 24 to 34 weeks' gestation.

31. b (Chapter 7)

Of the answers listed, only fetal renal agenesis would result in oligohydramnios with the remaining answers associated with polydramnios. Fetal renal agenesis and other fetal genitourinary tract malformations causing decreased fetal urine output will consequently decrease the amniotic fluid volume resulting in oligohydramnios. Poorly controlled maternal diabetes results in high circulating levels of glucose for mother and fetus which acts as an osmotic diuretic, causing increased fetal urine output and polyhydramnios. Fetal duodenal atresia or tracheo-esophageal fistula will decrease fetal swallowing of amniotic fluid and result in polyhydramnios. Maternal-fetal Rh incompatibility would lead to hydrops which is associated with polyhydramnios as well.

32. d (Chapter 11)

In order to distinguish a lupus flare from preeclampsia, complement levels (C3, C4) should be obtained. Decreased C3 and C4 will signal a lupus flare. Thrombocytopenia and transamonitis are common both to a lupus flare and preeclampsia with HELLP syndrome. Catheterized urinalysis will demonstrate proteinuria in either case, and serial blood pressures will likewise not help to distinguish between the two disease processes.

33. b (Chapter 13)

The lesion described is a nabothian cyst, a normal variant among menstruating women. They appear as a bubble under the surface of the cervix and are often bluish in color. Cervical dysplasia or cancer would not have this appearance. Bartholin cysts are found in the labia majora when the duct leading to the gland becomes occluded. Skene's glands are located near the urethral meatus.

34. d (Chapter 14)

This patient has been diagnosed with submucosal fibroids which may or may not be impacting her fertility. Treatment in this scenario should be tailored to preserve fertility and should take place after a full infertility evaluation of both the patient and her husband. Hysteroscopic myomectomy could treat her fibroids at least temporarily and possibly improve fertility. Uterine artery embolization, while less invasive, is only recommended for those who have completed their childbearing. Oral contraceptives and depot medroxyprogesterone can improve symptoms from fibroids, but they will prevent pregnancy in this patient. A total hysterectomy is the definitive treatment for fibroids but would clearly prohibit a future pregnancy for this patient.

35. a (Chapter 4)

Although nonrecurring indications (transverse or breech presentation, active HSV lesions, and nonreassuring fetal status) usually predict a more successful vaginal delivery after cesarean (VBAC), a classical hysterectomy is a strict contraindication for VBAC with its higher risk of uterine rupture. Low-transverse and low-vertical incisions are considered candidates for VBAC. A history of previous cesarean section for cephalopelvic disproportion does decrease likelihood of a successful VBAC, but it is not a strict contraindication.

36. c (Chapter 7)

Repetitive decelerations are never reassuring and indicate that close attention needs to be paid to the fetal heart tracing until their resolution. The most worrisome repetitive decelerations are late ones that can be a result of uteroplacental insufficiency or maternal hypotension. Repetitive early decelerations can result from descent of the fetal head that leads to head compression with contractions. Variable decelerations result from cord compression. In the postdate patient, spontaneous or repetitive variable decelerations most likely result from oligohydramnios, which leads to more frequent cord compression. Fetal acidemia usually leads to decreased fetal heart rate variability rather than decelerations.

37. c (Chapter 14)

This patient's clinical course is characteristic of a patient with a ruptured hemorrhagic cyst. Management of ovarian cysts varies with the age of the patient and the size and characteristics of the cyst. Cysts of any size in a premenarchal or postmenopausal female should be evaluated via laparoscopy or laparotomy. In reproductive age women, cysts larger than 6 cm generally require surgical exploration and management given the risk of torsion and neoplasm. Cysts smaller than 6 cm are typically physiologic cysts and will generally resolve on their own. This patient's cyst is small and hemostatic and her abdomen is nonacute, so no surgical management is indicated. Her discomfort can be managed with NSAIDs and future cyst formation can be suppressed with oral contraceptive pills, which suppress follicle formation and ovulation (Chapter 22). It is critical, however, that she be followed to ensure that bleeding from the cyst has stopped and that a repeat pelvic ultrasound be performed to assure regression of the complex cyst.

38. b (Chapter 6)

The management of shoulder dystocia, as with any emergency situation, should be discussed and considered frequently so that clinicians can react quickly and efficiently to its occurrence. A common algorithm would be to begin with suprapubic pressure to dislodge the anterior shoulder and the McRobert's maneuver increases hip flexion to increase the pelvic diameter. An episiotomy is commonly performed if these maneuvers fail. This is usually followed with the Wood screw maneuver, delivery of the posterior arm, or the Rubin maneuver. If none of these maneuvers works after several attempts, more aggressive interventions include fracturing the fetal clavicle. A final maneuver that has been described, the Zavanelli maneuver, is to place the fetal head back into the maternal pelvis and perform a cesarean delivery. Fundal pressure, which would further impact the anterior fetal shoulder behind the maternal pubic symphysis, is not recommended.

39. e (Chapter 15)

This patient's symptom and studies are most consistent with the presence of adenomyosis. Adenomyosis is the presence of endometrial tissue that breaks through the basalis layer of the endometrium to invade the myometrium. This is demonstrated by the widened and indistinct junction between the endometrium and myometrium in this patient. Although the patient does have two small fibroids, they are in an intramural location and are not likely to be the source of the patient's heavy bleeding. Patients with adenomyosis, however, tend to have heavy prolonged bleeding and a slightly enlarged boggy-feeling uterus. In adenomyosis, the ectopic endometrial tissue is not generally responsive to hormonal therapy, so OCPs are less likely to work. Depo-Lupron is often used to treat endometriosis and to shrink fibroids prior to surgical resection. It is not a good solution for this patient since it carries the risk of bone demineralization with long-term use. The only definitive means of diagnosing and treating adenomyosis is with a hysterectomy. This patient has a normal-sized uterus and has completed her childbearing so she would be a candidate for vaginal hysterectomy. Since she is less than 45 years old and her ovaries appear normal, you would not likely plan to perform a bilateral salpingo-oophorectomy.

40. d (Chapter 24)

Emergency contraception can be offered to a patient if unprotected intercourse or contraceptive failure has occurred no more than 72 hours prior to treatment. It would be highly recommended for this patient since her contraceptive failure occurred 36 hours ago and was around her expected time of ovulation. There are three current regimens available: high-dose progesterone-only pills (POPs), high-dose combination OCPs, and copper IUD insertion (ParaGard). None of the current methods is an abortifacient and none disrupts an implanted pregnancy. The medical hormone methods (POPs and OCPs) both involve taking a high dose of hormone and then taking a second dose 12 hours later. POPs come prepackaged as "Plan B." Each tablet contains 0.75 mg of levonorgestrel. This is the preferred method of emergency contraception if available because it is more effective and has fewer side effects. The combination OCP method is a two-dose regimen of 100 mcg of ethinyl estradiol combined with levonorgestrel or norgestrel, given 12 hours apart. The dose recommended in the question is too low and the length of time between dose is 12 hours, not 24. The Copper IUD (ParaGard) can be used for emergency contraception if placed within 5 days of unprotected intercourse. Mifepristone (RU-486) is as effective as Plan B in preventing pregnancy but it is not currently available as an emergency contraceptive in the United States.

41. c (Chapter 1)

The patient in this scenario has an abnormal screening test for gestational diabetes (GDM) but will need a 3-hour glucose tolerance test (GTT) to confirm this diagnosis. Should she have two or more elevated values on her 3-hour GTT, she should undergo diabetic teaching and nutritional counseling as well as record fasting and postprandial glucose readings at home. Fasting serum glucose and hemoglobin A1c are not typically used for diagnosis of GDM.

42. b (Chapter 1)

During pregnancy, there is a physiologic decrease in $PaCO_2$ with a corresponding mild respiratory alkylosis. Tidal volume increases during pregnancy with a resultant increase in minute ventilation. Total lung capacity and expiratory reserve volume are both decreased during pregnancy.

43. d (Chapter 4)

A mediolateral episiotomy likely leads to fewer third- and fourth-degree extensions than a median episiotomy because the apex of the incision is angled away from the rectum.

However, mediolateral episiotomy is thought to be more painful for the patient with a higher rate of infection and slower healing. The difficulty of repair for a mediolateral or median episiotomy should be equivalent.

44. a (Chapter 6)

If the patient desires a vaginal delivery, an attempt at external version should be performed. The ideal time for an attempt at external version is 37 weeks when the pregnancy reaches term status, understanding that as the fetus continues to grow, a successful version becomes less likely. It is important to recheck position at 37 weeks because some fetuses will spontaneously convert to vertex. If a version is unsuccessful, the physician's comfort level and experience should dictate whether an attempt at vaginal breech delivery is appropriate considering the fetal size and maternal obstetric history.

45. e (Chapter 16)

This patient's history is most consistent with a primary outbreak of genital herpes. Patients will commonly present with systemic symptoms of fever, malaise, and fatigue. Locally, the pain secondary to the lesions can require hospital admission for pain control and the dysuria can require a Foley catheter placement. Whether this is primary or secondary can be confirmed by sending HSV 1&2 IgG and IGM titers. If the IgG is elevated, it is a secondary outbreak. These tests are expensive and generally are not sent unless there is some question regarding management. In addition, other sexually transmitted diseases should be screened for including gonorrhea, chlamydia, syphilis, hepatitis B, hepatitis C, and HIV.

46. e (Chapter 16)

This is a bit of a trick question, as there is no cure for a herpes simplex virus infection. Therefore, patients with oral and genital herpes may experience recurrent lesions. Acyclovir and several other antiviral medications (most commonly valacyclovir or Valtrex) can be used to decrease symptom outbreak by several days. Common dosing regimes of acyclovir for primary HSV are 400 mg TID or 200 mg 5× per day. In patients who get recurrent lesions, these medications can be used prophylactically to prevent outbreaks; often 400 mg BID will suffice, but some patients will need TID to prevent outbreaks. Ceftriaxone is used to treat *Gonococcus,* azithromycin to treat *Chlamydia,* and metronidazole to treat bacterial vaginosis.

47. d (Chapter 13)

This patient's symptoms are consistent with a cervical polyp. Most polyps are fleshy and soft and easily removed in the office at the time that they are diagnosed. Although cervical polyps are almost always benign, the tissue should still be sent for pathologic evaluation. Likewise, the patient should still undergo a complete evaluation for metrorrhagia including TSH, pelvic ultrasound, and endometrial biopsy to rule out other sources of abnormal uterine bleeding including fibroids, adenomyosis, endometrial polyps, hyperplasia, and cancer. As long as the polyp is benign there is no need to repeat the Pap smear at this time.

48. e (Chapter 21)

This patient likely has primary amenorrhea due to a lack of GnRH pulsatility, which is secondary to the exercise and stress from her competitive athletics. Anorexia nervosa should also be considered in all women with primary and secondary amenorrhea, but there is no other evidence in this patient to support that diagnosis. The anatomic causes were each ruled out on physical exam. A transverse vaginal septum was ruled out by visualization of the cervix. In testicular feminization, the patient would have breast development, but no uterus— a normal bimanual exam of the pelvic organs and a visualized cervix rules this out. Patients with gonadal agenesis with either 46,XY or 46,XX karyotypes will not have breast development, although those with 46,XX will have a uterus.

49. b (Chapter 32)

Both lymph node status and hormone receptor status are major prognostic factors for recurrence and morbidity with invasive breast cancer. For instance, once the cancer has spread to the lymph nodes, it is twice as likely to metastasize to other parts of the body and to recur. Contrastingly, hormone receptor positive tumors are well differentiated, less aggressive clinically, and have a lower recurrence rate. Thus, estrogen and progesterone positive status carries a more favorable prognosis than negative hormone receptor status. It is therefore generally accepted that all women, whether treated with lumpectomy and radiation or with mastectomy, should be evaluated for lymph node spread and hormone receptor status. Women with positive lymph nodes should receive adjuvant chemotherapy regardless of hormone receptor status. Most typically, a combination of cyclophosphamide (C), methotrexate (M), and 5-fluorouracil (F) is used. Patients with hormone receptor positive tumors should receive adjuvant hormone therapy with tamoxifen or anastrozole, regardless of the patient's age or menopause status. Patients with hormone receptor negative tumors do not benefit from hormone therapy. This patient should receive both chemotherapy and hormone therapy.

50. b (Chapter 16)

This history and exam are most consistent with *Trichomonas vaginalis* infection. The finding of a "strawberry cervix" is considered pathognomonic for *Trichomonas,* but is only present about 10% of the time. Diagnosis is most often confirmed by visualizing the motile organism on wet prep. Overgrowth with *Gardnerella vaginalis* can lead to bacterial vaginosis. Diagnosis is made by a positive "whiff" test and identification of clue cells on the wet prep. This patient's history is not consistent with candidiasis, which is diagnosed by symptoms and identification of yeast on potassium hydroxide prep.

51. b (Chapter 4)

Labor is described as having three stages. Stage I is from the onset of labor until complete dilation of the cervix, stage II is from the end of stage I until delivery of the infant, and stage III is from the end of stage II until delivery of the placenta. Stage I of labor is divided into the latent and active phases. The latent phase is from the onset of labor until the rate of change of cervical dilation reaches its maximum; this usually occurs between 3 and 5 cm. The active phase is from the point of maximum rate of change until almost full dilation, where some patients will go through a transition or deceleration phase as they dilate the remaining 0.5 to 1.0 cm.

52. c (Chapter 17)

This patient's constellation of findings is most consistent with pelvic inflammatory disease (PID), likely complicated by Fitzhugh-Curtis syndrome with a perihepatitis leading to the right upper quadrant tenderness. Tubo-ovarian abscess should be on the differential diagnosis, but is unlikely with a normal pelvic ultrasound. Appendicitis should also be considered and, if the appendix is not visualized on ultrasound, a CT would more definitively rule this out.

53. b (Chapter 27)

Vulvar pruritus is a common symptom of many benign and malignant diseases of the vulva. When a postmenopausal patient presents with vulvodynia or vulvar pruritus that is refractory to treatment, a punch biopsy should always be performed to identify the lesion and guide the choice of treatment. If there are no obvious lesions, colposcopy can be performed with acetic acid and any acetowhite lesions can be biopsied. Even in this patient, where lichen sclerosis is the most likely diagnosis, biopsy should still be performed to confirm the diagnosis and rule out any underlying malignancy prior to starting therapy. Surgical treatment is not indicated at this point in the evaluation since lichen sclerosis can easily be treated with 6 to 12 weeks of topical steroids such as clobetasol or halobetasol. Destruction of the lesion with cryotherapy should never be performed without a pathologic tissue diagnosis.

54. e (Chapter 5)

The classic signs of placental abruption include the sudden onset of painful contraction and vaginal bleeding. The uterus is typically firm and tender, and the irritation from the placental separation will often initiate regular contractions. Placental abruption can be more common in the setting of hypertension, abdominal trauma, and the use of cocaine or methamphetamines. Thus, a good history of domestic violence and drug use is important, and a urine toxin screen should be sent. The diagnosis can be made with evidence of a fetal-maternal bleed by sending a Kleihauer-Betke test. Rarely, the retroplacental bleed can be seen on ultrasound, but generally placental abruption is a clinical diagnosis. Even though the patient is having regular contractions, no cervical change is described; therefore, a diagnosis of labor cannot be made. Given the normal ultrasound, a placenta previa is unlikely. While placenta accreta can occur outside of the setting of a placenta previa, bleeding associated with this form of abnormal placentation occurs after delivery when the placenta does not separate entirely from the uterine wall. The most common presentation of rupture of membranes is a gush of clear fluid rather than blood.

55. c (Chapter 18)

This patient's symptoms and exam are consistent with a large cystocele. Her risk factors for pelvic relaxation include four vaginal deliveries, particularly with large babies. Her pelvic relaxation is likely worsened by years of heavy lifting resulting in pressure on the anatomic pelvic support mechanisms. The cystocele can be repaired surgically with an anterior colporrhaphy to plicate the endopelvic fascial support of the bladder and remove any redundant attenuated vaginal mucosa. This patient has no urinary incontinence at this time so a bladder suspension would not be necessary. Vaginal pessaries are generally reserved for very elderly patients or for patients who are poor candidates for surgery. Anticholinergic medications can be used to treat incontinence due to detrusor instability. Mild pelvic relaxation and urinary incontinence can often be improved with Kegel exercises and HRT (in postmenopausal patients). This patient is not menopausal nor does she have incontinence.

56. e (Chapter 16)

This patient's history is most consistent with syphilis, and is least consistent with genital herpes. Because of concern for other sexually transmitted diseases (STDs) with the transmission of syphilis, the battery of tests sent would include those for gonorrhea, chlamydia, HIV, hepatitis B, and hepatitis C. Syphilis would be screened for with an RPR or VDRL and confirmed with an FTA-ABS or MHA-TP. There would be no reason to send for antibody titers of HSV because even if the patient were exposed, it would not change the management of the situation. If the patient did develop lesions more consistent with HSV, it would be reasonable to send IgG and IgM titers if there is any question about whether this is a primary or secondary outbreak. These antibody titers are not sent routinely in patients requesting STD screens.

57. d (Chapter 16)

The history is now confirmed with the identification of the causative organism of syphilis, *Treponema pallidum,* which is seen as a motile spirochete on dark-field microscopic inspection of a slide made from the contents of the chancre. Of note, the most common way that syphilis is diagnosed is with one of the two confirmatory tests, FTA-ABS or MHA-TP. Because this patient clearly has primary syphilis of only several weeks' duration, she can be treated with a single dose of IM benzathine penicillin G. A positive screen for syphilis without any symptoms would be considered of unknown duration and the patient would be treated with 3 weekly dosages of benzathine penicillin G. Tertiary syphilis and neurosyphilis both require treatment with IV penicillin. Because of the efficacy of penicillin, in patients who are allergic, they should go through the trouble of desensitization and still receive penicillin.

58. c (Chapter 19)

This patient most likely has total urinary incontinence, also known as bypass incontinence. This form of involuntary urinary leakage is due to fistulas between the urethra and the vagina (urethrovaginal fistula), the bladder and the vagina (vesicovaginal fistula), or the ureter and the vagina (ureterovaginal fistula). Total incontinence typically presents as painless continuous incontinence and is most commonly associated with pelvic surgery or pelvic radiation in developed countries and with obstetric trauma in developing nations. The fact that there was no leakage onto the vaginal tampon when the bladder was back-filled with dye means that the fistula is not in the urethra or the bladder. The presence of dye on the tampon after IV indigo-carmine is a sign that the fistula is higher up in the ureter and leakage is occurring after the dye is passed through the kidney and traveling via the ureter to the bladder. Overflow incontinence usually presents with involuntary dribbling of urine from an overdistended hypotonic bladder. Stress urinary incontinence usually presents with leaking with increased intra-abdominal pressure such as with coughing, laughing, or sneezing.

59. c (Chapter 4)

Fetal heart rates are evaluated, paying attention to baseline rate, variability, accelerations, and decelerations. The baseline rate should be between 110 and 160 bpm. Minimal and absent variability are worrisome for hypoxia and acidemia of the fetus, with absent variability being worse than minimal. Three types of decelerations have been described—early, variable, and late. Early decelerations begin and end with contractions and are thought to be a result of fetal head compression. Variable decelerations are sharp drops in the fetal heart rate with quick return to baseline and can be either isolated or correlated with contractions; these are believed to result from compression of the umbilical cord. Late decelerations begin after the contraction has begun and end after it has ended. These are usually shallow and can be quite subtle and difficult to detect. Late decelerations are correlated with decreased placental perfusion that can be secondary to inadequate

blood flow to the uterus or increased vascular resistance of the placenta (aka uteroplacental insufficiency).

60. d (Chapter 20)

Hormone replacement therapy (HRT) can be very useful and effective in treating the symptoms of menopause and in preventing bone loss in postmenopausal women. However, HRT also carries an increased risk of breast cancer, endometrial cancer, thromboembolic disease, and gallbladder disease. Therefore, it is now generally accepted that HRT therapy should be used only for relief of menopausal symptoms and the duration of use should be short, generally 6 to 12 months. Contraindications to HRT use include hepatic dysfunction, undiagnosed abnormal vaginal bleeding, history of acute venous thrombosis (DVT, PE), and history of an estrogen-sensitive cancer (e.g., breast, endometrial). If a patient completes a short course of HRT or declines HRT, the symptoms of menopause (hot flashes, night sweats, vaginal dryness, bone loss) can be treated using alternative therapies.

61. d (Chapter 6)

The management of PPROM is widely debated. Before 32 to 34 weeks' gestation, most institutions use betamethasone to help induce fetal lung maturity; however, it is rarely used beyond 34 weeks' gestation. The use of tocolysis varies greatly, ranging from no use whatsoever to tocolysis at less than 26 to 28 weeks' gestation to tocolysis until 34 weeks, as in preterm labor. Many patients with PPROM go into labor within 48 to 72 hours; for those who do not, the risks of prolonged ROM include chorioamnionitis, abruption, and cord prolapse. With these risks weighed against the risks of prematurity, induction of labor has been considered between 32 and 36 weeks' gestation. Some institutions send the amniotic fluid for fetal lung maturity testing and induce labor if it is mature. Tocolysis at 35 weeks' gestation would not be used in this patient; thus the most appropriate plan presented would be expectant management. If the patient stopped contracting, many practitioners would induce or augment labor at that point.

62. b (Chapter 21)

This patient has secondary amenorrhea. Although it is possible that her weight loss and stress have led to the secondary amenorrhea, it is still important to rule out other causes. The most common cause of secondary amenorrhea is pregnancy; thus a β-hCG test should be ordered. Thyroid dysfunction and elevated prolactin levels can both lead to amenorrhea and should be ordered. An elevated follicle-stimulating hormone level would be seen in someone with early menopause; however, this 19-year-old patient with no other complaints is unlikely to have premature ovarian failure. Secondary amenorrhea can also be seen in patients with polycystic ovarian syndrome and, if these patients are showing signs of masculinization, a testosterone or dehydroepiandrosterone sulfate (DHEAS) level is reasonable; however, in this patient, without any particular symptoms, it is unnecessary as the initial screen. Because of her 15-lb weight loss, the patient should also be carefully screened for an eating disorder such as anorexia or bulimia. A careful exercise history should be taken as well, as the stress from hours of daily exercise can lead to secondary amenorrhea.

63. a (Chapter 21)

The progesterone challenge test involves giving 7 to 10 days of progesterone, usually 10 mg of medroxyprogesterone acetate (Provera). Within a few days after the last dose of progesterone, the patient should undergo a withdrawal bleed that may be lighter than usual, indicating that the uterus is receiving some estrogen stimulation. Estradiol levels are a poor way to measure estrogenization, particularly when the day of the cycle is unknown. An endometrial biopsy can show that the endometrial lining has had estrogen stimulation and can be done in the luteal phase. However, in this patient, it is unclear where in the cycle she is, so this test is not useful in this setting. The adrenocorticotropic hormone stim test for Addison and CAH disease and the LH:FSH ratio once used in polycystic ovarian disease have little bearing on this clinical situation.

64. c (Chapter 9)

The fetal complications of diabetes vary widely, including abnormalities in growth ranging from intrauterine growth-restricted and small-for-dates infants to fetal macrosomia with delayed organ maturity. Congenital anomalies are increased two- to threefold over pregnancies without diabetes. These range from cardiovascular abnormalities to neural tube defects and the rare caudal regression syndrome. These infants are also at increased risk for sudden intrauterine fetal demise (IUFD). Prepregnancy HgbA1c is predictive of the risk of congenital anomalies, but is not well associated with fetal macrosomia which is more dependent on blood glucose control during pregnancy, particularly the latter half.

65. e (Chapter 32)

A mammogram is used to assess breast masses in women and for annual screening for breast cancer. However, 20% of all breast cancers will not be visible or detected via mammogram. Since this mass is not characteristic of a breast cyst, fibrocystic change, or a fibroadenoma, it should not be dismissed just because the mammogram is negative. Any dominant palpable mass or suspicious nonpalpable mammogram finding requires a biopsy and tissue diagnosis. This can be accomplished with a fine-needle aspiration (FNA) or core biopsy using a large cutting needle. If this is nondiagnostic, an excisional biopsy should be performed for histologic diagnosis. If the cytology from the FNA or core biopsy is negative and the mass is still concerning, an excisional biopsy should be performed.

66. e (Chapter 21)

The most common cause of secondary amenorrhea is pregnancy, which is the most likely diagnosis that can be made from the tests being ordered. You would expect her to have an elevated hCG level confirming a pregnancy diagnosis. She does not have symptoms of either hypo- or hyperthyroidism or of elevated prolactin, but these tests are usually ordered as well. LH and FSH would not be ordered and would offer no helpful information in making a diagnosis. Many women who become pregnant may not realize they are until quite late into the pregnancy, particularly if they are obese and/or have a history of oligomenorrhea.

67. a (Chapter 14)

Endometrial hyperplasia is the abnormal proliferation of glandular and stromal elements of the endometrium. It is a premalignant condition, not a preinvasive cancer. Like endometrial cancer, risk factors include conditions that predispose the patient to prolonged exposure to unopposed endogenous or exogenous estrogen such as obesity, early menarche, late menopause, chronic anovulation, and unopposed exogenous estrogen administration. Both hypertension and diabetes also increase the risk of endometrial hyperplasia and endometrial cancer. Endometrial hyperplasia, if left untreated, could develop into endometrial cancer, depending on the degree of cytologic atypia. The risk of progression to endometrial cancer is 1% with simple hyperplasia, 3% with complex hyperplasia, 8% with atypical simple hyperplasia, and 29% with atypical complex hyperplasia. This patient can be treated with continuous progestin therapy but absolutely needs a repeat endometrial biopsy to confirm regression of the hyperplasia. This goal in her management is treatment of the hyperplasia and then menstrual regulation to prevent recurrence of the hyperplasia.

Menstrual regulation should be done with progestins in this case since the use of estrogen is contraindicated in patients with hypertension. A weight loss of 10% of her body weight will also help achieve menstrual regulation. A hysterectomy is not indicated in this patient since the endometrial hyperplasia and chronic anovulation can both be managed without removing the uterus.

68. d (Chapter 19)

This patient's history is consistent with incontinence due to detrusor overactivity, also known as urge incontinence. This form of incontinence is due to a defect in the filling stage of bladder function. As a result, involuntary bladder contractions can occur at anytime and result in urine leakage. Most detrusor overactivity is idiopathic but UTIs, bladder cancer, bladder diverticula, bladder stones, and many neurologic illnesses can cause detrusor overactivity. Medical management for detrusor overactivity is designed to relax the bladder, prevent bladder contractions, and improve bladder storage capacity. This can be achieved with smooth muscle relaxants (oxybutynin, flavoxate, tolterodine), anticholinergics (oxybutynin, tolterodine, propantheline), and tricyclic antidepressants (imipramine). Vaginal pessaries, Kegel exercises, and bladder suspension/sling procedures are used to treat pelvic relaxation and stress urinary incontinence. An anterior colporrhaphy is a surgical repair for a cystocele due to pelvic relaxation.

69. d (Chapter 1)

Dating of a pregnancy is important to establish as soon as possible. Usually, 280 days from the LMP is used as the EDD, which is then confirmed by physical examination and eventually a second trimester ultrasound. However, physical examination is not a particularly accurate way to date a pregnancy, and ultrasound becomes less accurate as a pregnancy continues. Ultrasound is considered to have a 7% to 10% range of accuracy, and a rule of thumb is that it can be off by up to 1 week in the first trimester, 2 weeks during the second trimester, and 3 weeks during the third trimester. Thus, in a patient who had no clear LMP to date the pregnancy, a transvaginal ultrasound performed as early as possible would be the best way to date this pregnancy.

70. a (Chapter 21)

This patient has signs and symptoms of hyperthyroidism with the weight loss, insomnia, and heat intolerance. These could also be put together as a constellation of stress or even anorexia; however, there is no specific test to diagnose either of these. If your suspicion for hyperthyroidism, and particularly Graves disease, is high with other physical findings such as a goiter and exophthalmos, other initial tests might include a free T4 and TSI (thyroid-stimulating immunoglobulin). If the patient has hyperthyroidism, most commonly PTU (propyl thiouracil) is begun, though methimazole is another medical treatment. Some patients will opt for thyroid ablatement with I-131 and then will need replacement with synthroid thereafter. If you are particularly concerned about thyroid storm with hypertensive crisis, you might even initiate treatment immediately without waiting for the lab results.

71. d (Chapter 17)

This patient has severe endometritis which is a clinical diagnosis based upon extreme tenderness on bimanual exam, elevated WBC, and fever. She is at a higher risk for such an infection due to her prolonged labor course and cesarean section. Treatment should be with IV clindamycin and gentamycin. Answer A suggests concern for a hematoma, which is not likely given her normal postsurgical hematocrit of 34. A CT would reveal if there was an abscess, but this should be reserved unless there is no improvement with treatment using IV antibiotics. There is some leukocytosis to be expected in the postpartum period, but this should not exceed a WBC of 20 and fever is not

a normal consequence of a cesarean delivery. Gonorrhea and chlamydia are common pathogens in PID, but not in endometritis and treatment with azithromycin would not provide sufficient broad spectrum coverage. While fever can be associated with a DVT or PE, this patient does not complain of leg pain or swelling and has appropriate O_2 saturation.

72. e (Chapter 18)

Nonoperative methods should be attempted first, as this patient is not a good surgical candidate given her medical history and current smoking history. Placing a mesh in someone with poor glucose control and tobacco abuse puts the patient at a much higher risk of erosion of the mesh and poor wound healing. Vaginal pessaries often provide adequate mechanical support to relieve many of the symptoms associated with pelvic organ prolapse and are most appropriate for elderly patients or poor surgical candidates. This patient should also be counseled regarding weight loss and smoking cessation.

73. b (Chapter 20)

This patient would be assigned Tanner stage II. The description is consistent with presexual pubic hair and breast development at the breast bud stage. This patient will likely start menstruation within the next 1 to 1.5 years since the onset of menses is usually within 2 years of breast bud development.

74. c (Chapters 21 and 14)

This patient has MRKH syndrome which can often be repaired with creation of a neovagina that will allow connection to the upper genital tract. Testicular feminization will have 46,XY chromosomes and often have undescended testes. With gonadal agenesis there is no development of internal female organs. Patients with Swyer syndrome will develop female genitalia externally and internally; however, they will not develop breasts. Turner syndrome is 45,XO and often has minimal breast development as a result of low estradiol levels.

75. b (Chapter 26)

A low sperm count can be overcome by washing the sperm and placing it into the uterine cavity through intrauterine insemination (IUI). Intracytoplasmic injection of sperm (ICSI) is an in vitro technique used for patients with notable low sperm density or motility and is a more invasive procedure that should be reserved if IUI is not successful. This couple's infertility is likely due to male factor infertility, since she appears to be ovulating at regular intervals and he has a low sperm count. Therefore, adding Clomid (clomiphene), which is an ovulation induction agent, would not benefit this couple. Men should avoid hot baths, saunas, tight fitting underwear, radiation exposure, excessive heat, marijuana or alcohol intake if trying to increase the sperm count. The male should also have a complete physical examination and endocrine evaluation.

76. b (Chapter 28)

CIN II that is confined to the ectocervix can be treated with a LEEP procedure. This can be performed as an office procedure with prudent patient selection. Patients who do not tolerate the biopsy very well will likely not tolerate an in-office LEEP and may need this procedure performed in the operating room. Cold-knife cones are reserved for lesions thought to involve the endocervix; however, many of these lesions can be adequately treated with a two-step or "top-hat" LEEP. The advantage to LEEP over cold-knife cone is less blood loss, healing, and the need for only local anesthesia. Hysterectomy is not an appropriate next step in the management of CIN II.

77. e (Chapter 19)

This patient's history is consistent with mild stress urinary incontinence. SUI incontinence can be treated in a variety of ways. Prior to moving to surgical repair with a bladder suspension/sling procedure more conservative treatments should be attempted. Kegel exercises can strengthen the underlying pelvic support muscles and can sometimes reverse SUI. Vaginal pessaries and incontinence pessaries are generally reserved for very elderly patients or for patients who are poor candidates for surgery. This patient does not fit those criteria. Anticholinergic medications can be used to treat incontinence due to detrusor over activity. Mild pelvic organ prolapse and urinary incontinence can often be improved with HRT in postmenopausal patients by increasing mucosal coaptation and urethral sphincter pressure. However, this patient is not menopausal. Anterior colporrhaphy is surgical procedure used to repair a cystocele by plicating the endopelvic fascia and removing excess vaginal mucosa to re-elevate the bladder.

78. c (Chapter 24)

The best contraceptive method for this patient would be the Mirena IUD. The failure rate of an intrauterine device (IUD) is extremely low and she would have reliable birth control for 5 years. The Mirena would also offer her the added benefit of decreased bleeding and cramping. Conversely, since the ParaGard IUD can cause increased bleeding and cramping, this method would not be appropriate for this patient. Her smoking history, age, weight over 200 pounds, and history of migraines make estrogen-containing methods (such as OCPs, Nuvaring, and Ortho-Evra patch) inappropriate for this patient. Likewise, her depression and obesity could be potentially worsened by Depo-Provera and return to fertility may be delayed.

79. d (Chapter 8)

The classic triad of preeclampsia includes hypertension, proteinuria, and nondependent edema in the face and hand. Because edema can be nonspecific, clinicians decreasingly use it as a part of diagnosis. The generalized vasoconstriction seen in preeclampsia can result in visual changes, headaches, strokes, seizures, pulmonary edema, oliguria, renal failure, or liver capsule pain or rupture. These symptoms, along with worsening blood pressure, or changes in liver function tests, platelets, and creatinine level are used to monitor the severity of the disease.

80. e (Chapter 25)

The method of termination of pregnancy should be based on the gestational age of the pregnancy and on the particular needs of the patient. Where available, safe and effective elective termination can be provided for pregnancies up to 24 weeks' gestation. Suction curettage is the most common method of termination (90% of all terminations) but is safe for use only in the first trimester. RU-486 and methotrexate (where available) are both highly effective means of medical abortion but are only indicated for use in the first 49 days (7 weeks) of pregnancy. This couple has a second trimester pregnancy so options for termination include dilation and suction evacuation (D&E) and induction of labor. In this case, the couple would likely benefit most from induction of labor since it would allow for the delivery of an intact fetus, which could undergo pathologic evaluation. Prior to termination of pregnancy, the patient should have her Rh status checked and should be given RhoGAM (Rh IgG) if indicated.

81. c (Chapter 27)

When a postmenopausal patient presents with vulvodynia or vulvar pruritus that is refractory to treatment, cancer must always be ruled out by performing an office biopsy of any visualized lesions. If there are no obvious lesions, colposcopy can be performed with acetic acid and any acetowhite lesions can be biopsied. This patient is at particular risk for a premalignant or malignant disease since her symptoms have persisted for some time, she has a new sexual partner, and she has evidence of exposure to the human papillomavirus (and 60% of women with VIN have cervical intraepithelial [CIN] lesions as well). Since her biopsy shows vulvar intraepithelial neoplasia (VIN), the treatment of choice is wide local excision. As long as a 5-mm negative margin could be obtained, skinning vulvectomy or laser ablation would not be needed. These techniques are generally reserved for large or multifocal lesions. Destruction of the lesion with laser ablation should never be performed without first having a pathologic tissue diagnosis. Antifungal agents and steroids that failed to ameliorate her symptoms in the past would be ineffective in treating this neoplastic lesion caused by human papillomavirus.

82. d (Chapter 28)

This patient has moderate cervical dysplasia (CIN II). The standard of care for patients with CIN II or CIN III (and persistent CIN I) is to perform a cervical conization also known as a LEEP, LLETZ, or loop using electrocautery. Cryotherapy can be used when the lesion is small and fully visualized and LEEP/LLETZ/

loop is not available. A cold-knife cone biopsy could also be performed, but is more invasive, more costly, and must be done in the OR. CKC biopsies are generally reserved for patients with endocervical disease or microscopic preinvasive disease (CIS). Simple hysterectomy is usually reserved for patients with early or preinvasive cervical cancer and for those who have completed childbaring. Although cervical dysplasia and condyloma are both associated with exposure to the human papillomavirus, imiquimod (Aldara) is a topical therapy for vulvar condyloma and is not indicated in the direct treatment of cervical dysplasia.

83. c (Chapter 21)

Anorexia nervosa, exercise, weight loss, and stress can all lead to primary or secondary amenorrhea depending on their timing in a woman's life. Kallmann's syndrome, which is the congenital absence of GnRH and gonadal agenesis, causes only primary amenorrhea. Sheehan's syndrome, which is pituitary infarction, usually postpartum, and Asherman's syndrome are primarily associated with secondary amenorrhea.

84. b (Chapter 29)

Endometrial cancer is an estrogen-dependent neoplasm. Therefore, conditions that increase a woman's lifetime exposure to unopposed endogenous or exogenous estrogen will put her at an increased risk for both endometrial hyperplasia and endometrial cancer. Although the mode of action is unclear, both HTN and diabetes mellitus also increase the risk of endometrial hyperplasia and cancer. The relative risk conferred by nulliparity is 2 to 3, late menopause is 2 to 4, and diabetes mellitus is 2 to 8. Other risk factors include tamoxifen use (2 to 3), unopposed estrogen therapy (4 to 8), and atypical endometrial hyperplasia (8% to 29% risk). Obesity is a major risk factor for endometrial cancer. The risk varies by the degree of obesity; being 21 to 50 pounds overweight increases a woman's risk of endometrial cancer by a factor of 3, and being greater than 50 pounds overweight, as is the case for this patient, increases the risk 10-fold.

85. d (Chapter 13)

This patient has a Bartholin abscess. The normal course of treatment for a Bartholin abscess should be an I&D with placement of a Word catheter. However, in this setting, because this patient had been over age 40 when she first developed her Bartholin cyst, the cyst wall should first be biopsied to rule out the rare possibility of Bartholin cyst malignancy. If malignancy was present, total excision would be indicated. In addition to biopsy and I&D with Word catheter placement, the patient should do sitz baths three to four times a day as well. If there is surrounding cellulitis as in this case, antibiotics to cover skin flora are used as well. If the patient merely had an enlarged Bartholin cyst, sitz baths alone could be considered. With an abscess or cyst of this size, needle drainage would not be used because the cavity of the cyst would continue to be or become infected. If the Word catheter failed to treat the Bartholin cyst, marsupialization could then be attempted.

86. a (Chapter 29)

The most common cause of postmenopausal bleeding is endometrial atrophy. However, endometrial hyperplasia and cancer must always be ruled out as part of the evaluation. The diagnostic evaluation of postmenopausal bleeding with an endometrial stripe >3–4mm requires an endometrial tissue sample. This can usually be obtained in the office setting with an endometrial biopsy. Modern endometrial biopsy is 95% to 98% as accurate as a D&C, which was formally the gold standard in evaluation of postmenopausal bleeding. D&C, however, only becomes necessary if an office endometrial biopsy cannot be obtained (e.g., cervical stenosis, patient intolerance of the procedure). Once a pathologic diagnosis is confirmed, this can direct your treatment appropriately. While other diagnostic tools such as a pelvic ultrasound are helpful in evaluation of postmenopausal bleeding, sampling of the endometrium is required. A hysterectomy is not indicated without a pathologic diagnosis and an endometrial ablation should never be done in the case of undiagnosed bleeding.

87. c (Chapter 8)

Check a glucose tolerance test by administering 100 mg of oral glucose and measuring a fasting blood glucose level immediately before the dose, then measuring levels at 1, 2, and 3 hours after the dose. This is the test used to confirm diabetes in pregnancy. Once the diagnosis is made, you can proceed to the next stage in management by diet, exercise, and/or insulin administration. Recently oral hyperglycemic agents have begun to be used in pregnancy both alone and to decrease amounts of insulin required. They are still not used postpartum in breastfeeding women. Hemoglobin A1c levels measure the concentration of glycosylated hemoglobin and are best used in patients with overt previously existing diabetes mellitus to correlate with glucose control over 6 to 8 weeks, not for the initial diagnosis of diabetes mellitus. Hemoglobin A1c levels below 6.5% at conception are associated with a 3% incidence of congenital anomalies, whereas levels above 8.5% at conception are associated with a 22% incidence of congenital anomalies.

88. a (Chapter 32)

Intraductal papilloma is the most common cause of bloody nipple discharge in the absence of a concurrent mass. It is a benign solitary lesion that involves the epithelial lining of lactiferous ducts. Intraductal papilloma usually presents with bloody nipple discharge in premenopausal women. The discharge should be sent for cytology to rule out invasive papillary carcinoma, which has similar symptoms 25% of the time. Definitive diagnosis and treatment are achieved by opening of the duct and excision of the involved areas. Mammary duct ectasia is a subacute inflammation of the duct system. The discharge is usually green or multicolored, bilateral, and sticky. Paget disease is a rare form of breast cancer that can also present with bloody nipple discharge. It only makes up 1% to 3% of breast cancers and is often associated with a characteristic nipple lesion caused by erosion of the nipple and areola from the underlying breast lesion.

89. c (Chapter 22)

This patient has postmenopausal bleeding (PMB). The most common cause of PMB is endometrial atrophy. In fact, endometrial cancer is only responsible for 10% to 15% of PMB. However, as with other forms of abnormal vaginal bleeding, it is imperative to sample the endometrium to rule out endometrial hyperplasia and endometrial cancer. An ultrasound showing a thin endometrial stripe is not sufficient to rule out cancer when the patient continues to bleed. This patient should be taken to the OR where a D&C (with or without hysteroscopy) can be performed to evaluate the endometrium. Hormone replacement therapy is contraindicated in undiagnosed vaginal bleeding and estrogen replacement therapy is contraindicated in a woman who still has her uterus in situ. A hysterectomy is not indicated without a tissue diagnosis and expectant management would be inappropriate.

90. e (Chapter 5)

The primary cause of placental abruption is unknown but there are many associated precipitating and predisposing factors for abruption. Maternal hypertension is the most common risk factor for placental abruption, accounting for 50% of cases, half of which are due to chronic hypertension and half of which are due to pregnancy-induced hypertension. Other risk factors for abruption include prior history of abruption, advanced maternal age, multiparity, cocaine abuse, and vascular disease. Some precipitating factors include trauma (external fetal version, motor vehicle accidents, abdominal trauma), sudden uterine volume loss (delivery of first twin, rupture of membranes with polyhydramnios), preterm premature rupture of membranes, and short umbilical cord. While abuse of most illicit drugs are associated with fetal complications, heroin abuse is not associated with placental abruption.

91. a (Chapter 14)

This couple's recurrent miscarriages are most likely due to the presence of the uterine septum. Although septums are often asymptomatic, they can result in an increased rate of early miscarriage when the implantation occurs on the largely avascular septum. Given that the couple has had three fetal losses, the septum should be hysteroscopically resected and pregnancy can again be attempted. The cou-

ple has been able to conceive, so a full infertility evaluation and advanced reproductive technologies are not yet indicated, especially given the maternal age less than 35. Similarly, a gestational carrier and adoption are not necessary at this point.

92. e (Chapter 29)

This patient has multiple risk factors for endometrial cancer including nulliparity, obesity, unopposed estrogen use. Proper evaluation includes a transvaginal ultrasound to evaluate the endometrial stripe as well as an endometrial biopsy. Pap smear should also be performed. An endocrine evaluation is also warranted which should include a TSH, FSH, and prolactin. Ultrasound is a better technique for evaluating the uterine cavity than CT because it can detect endometrial polyps, fibroids, and reliably predict the thickness of the endometrial layer. D&C is no longer the first diagnostic measure of choice because endometrial biopsies have accuracies of 95% to 98% without exposing the patient to unnecessary anesthesia. A hysterectomy should not be performed until a definitive diagnosis is made.

93. a (Chapter 30)

Epithelial cell cancers account for 65% of all ovarian tumors and 90% of all ovarian cancers. The most common of these are the serous tumors which include serous cystadenoma, borderline serous, serous cystadenocarcinoma, and cystadenofibroma. Brenner tumors are very rare epithelial tumors. Endodermal sinus tumors usually have an elevated AFP and normal CA-125 and affect a younger subset of patients that are usually younger than 20 years old. Sertoli-Leydig cell tumor is a sexcord–stromal tumor that produces androgens and often causes vaginal bleeding from endometrial hyperplasia and virilization. Choriocarcinoma is a germ cell carcinoma associated with trophoblastic tissue and elevated hCG levels.

94. a (Chapters 21 and 14)

This patient has testicular feminization syndrome. These patients often have undescended testes that will need to be removed due to the risk of developing testicular cancer. They are not able to reproduce. Patients with MRKH syndrome have a uterus and 46,XX karyotype. With gonadal agenesis there is no development of internal female organs and no development of breasts. Patients with Swyer syndrome will develop female genitalia externally and internally; however, they will not develop breasts. The Turner syndrome karyotype is 45,XO and these women often have minimal breast development as a result of low estradiol levels.

95. d (Chapter 26)

This patient likely has uterine cavity scarring called Asherman syndrome as a result of the three separate D&Cs

that were performed. Transvaginal ultrasound is helpful in evaluating the uterine cavity; however, it is most effective with instillation of saline into the cavity to look for synechiae that are best visualized with distension of the cavity. As a result of the Asherman syndrome she may also have scarring of the tubal ostia, preventing sperm from getting to the fallopian tubes and ovum. Tubal patency can be evaluated with a hysterosalpingogram, which forces contrast into the tubes if they are patent. Infertility is the inability to conceive after 1 year of unprotected intercourse. The normal semen anaylsis suggests that this couple's infertility is not related to male factor infertility.

96. d (Chapter 5)

The patient in this scenario presents with painless vaginal bleeding at 33 weeks and a previous ultrasound indicating a low-lying placenta. Since the patient is stable and fetal reassurance is obtained, the next appropriate step would be to evaluate for placenta previa with a bedside ultrasound. In this situation, a digital exam should not be performed until confirmation of placental location away from the os is obtained. If no placenta previa is identified, other causes of bleeding should be evaluated such as placental abruption, preterm labor, or nonobstetrical causes.

97. a (Chapter 11)

The patient in this scenario appears to be having a placental abruption given her frequent painful contractions, vaginal bleeding, and nonreassuring fetal status. Of the substances listed, only cocaine can be directly responsible for a placental abruption secondary to its vasoconstrictive and hypertensive effects. While smoking overall increases the risk of abruption, it is not a direct causative factor. Caffeine, alcohol, and marijuana use do not cause abruption.

98. b (Chapter 30)

This patient most likely has an endodermal sinus tumor. These tumors often grow rapidly and are more common in younger patients. They are often unilateral and respond well to unilateral salpingo-ophorectomy and BEP chemotherapy. Epithelial tumors are more common in older patients and are often bilateral. Brenner tumors are a very rare type of epithelial tumor. Sertoli-Leydig cell tumor is a sexcord–stromal tumor that produces androgens and often causes vaginal bleeding from endometrial hyperplasia and virilization. Choriocarcinoma is a germ cell carcinoma associated with trophoblastic tissue that will have an elevated serum β-hCG.

99. b (Chapter 13)

Lichen sclerosis is a benign vulvar lesion common among postmenopausal women and often asymptomatic. The first-line treatment of lichen sclerosis is a high-potency topical steroid such as clobetasol. It is important to remember that this lesion is associated with vulvar cancer and close surveillance should be maintained.

100. b (Chapter 19)

This patent has symptoms consistent with detrusor overactivity, also known as urge incontinence. There are several medications on the market targeted at decreasing bladder contractions such as Ditropan (oxybutynin chloride), Detrol (tolterodine), Uripas (flavoxate hydrochloride), and Pro-Banthine (propantheline bromide). There are no surgical options currently available to treat detrusor instability. Cholinergic agents, such as bethanecol, increase bladder contractility and are used in overflow incontinence. Stress urinary incontinence presents with loss of urine while coughing, laughing, and/or sneezing. It can be treated with Kegel exercises, pessary use (if elderly or a poor surgical candidate), or urethral sling procedures.

Index

Page numbers followed by *t* refer to tables; page numbers followed by *f* refer to figures.